# POCKET MEDICAL TERMINOLOGY

£10.32

*For Churchill Livingstone:*

*Commissioning Editor:* Sarena Wolfaard
*Development Editor:* Kim Benson
*Production Manager:* Yolanta Motylinska
*Design:* Steven Gardiner Ltd, Cambridge

# POCKET
# MEDICAL
# TERMINOLOGY

# Andrew R. Hutton

Lecturer in Life Sciences
Edinburgh, UK

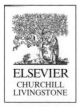

ELSEVIER
CHURCHILL
LIVINGSTONE

# ELSEVIER
## CHURCHILL
## LIVINGSTONE

POCKET MEDICAL TERMINOLOGY                    ISBN 0 443 07456 9

---

### Note

Knowledge and best practice in this field are constantly changing. As new
research and experience broaden our knowledge, changes in practice,
treatment and drug therapy may become necessary or appropriate. Readers
are advised to check the most current information provided (i) on
procedures featured or (ii) by the manufacturer of each product to be
administered, to verify the recommended dose or formula, the method and
duration of administration, and contraindications. It is the responsibility of
the practitioner, relying on their own experience and knowledge of the
patient, to make diagnosis, to determine dosages and the best treatment for
each individual patient, and to take all appropriate safety precautions. To
the fullest extent of the law, neither the publisher nor the author assumes
any liability for any injury and/or damage.

---

First published 2004

**British Library Cataloguing in Publication Data**
A catalogue record for this book is available from the British Library.

**Library of Congress Cataloging in Publication Data**
A catalog record for this book is available from the Library of Congress.

The
publisher's
policy is to use
**paper manufactured
from sustainable forests**

Printed in China

A051924

# Contents

W15

# Preface

Rapid changes to the management and practice of health care have brought an increased demand for professional training. This pocket book provides a valuable resource for those wishing to expand their use and understanding of medical terms.

Unlike a conventional medical dictionary, words in this pocket book have been listed according to the root words associated with a particular body system or speciality. This arrangement enables the reader to view numerous medical terms associated with the same medical root without looking up separate entries.

The book includes twenty-nine informative diagrams associating anatomical parts with combining forms of medical roots. These also act as guides to the meaning of medical terms. The appendices contain units of measurement, normal values of body fluids, chemical symbols, and formulae adopted from other Elsevier publications. They have been revised to ensure continuous relevance and usefulness to medical students and registered nurses.

I hope this pocket book will enhance the knowledge of all readers and help those delivering high-quality health care fulfil their training needs.

Andrew R. Hutton
Lecturer in Life Sciences
Edinburgh 2004

# About this book

Many medical and health care courses begin the study of the human body with system-based programmes. This handy pocket book lists medical terms associated with specific body systems and medical specialities and can be used to find the meanings of medical roots, prefixes and suffixes as you study a particular system. This arrangement will enable you to find the meaning of medical terms quickly and complement your medical studies.

The introduction Components of Medical Words explains how medical terms are constructed, how to split them into their components and how to understand their meaning. Using knowledge gained in this section and the glossary on page 344 you will be able to elucidate the meaning of hundreds of medical terms.

Sections 1–22 list medical terms associated with body systems and medical specialities. Quick reference guides at the beginning of each section contain combining forms of roots and common names that direct you to pages containing relevant medical terms and their definitions. The sections on body systems also contain labelled diagrams that associate the combining forms of word roots with anatomical parts to direct you to appropriate medical words.

Combining forms of medical roots are listed in alphabetical order within each section. Each root word is listed with its common prefixes, suffixes, definitions, and etymology. The simplest literal meaning of each term is given based on the meaning of its components.

Readers should be aware that many medical terms have more complex meanings than they imply. For example, the components of the medical term *schizophrenia* simply denote a condition of a split mind, but to a psychiatrist, it is a type of severe mental illness in which the personality is fragmented, with loss of emotional stability, judgment and reality, and is accompanied by hallucinations and delusions. Where the meaning of a medical term from its components is obscure, additional information is included with the definition.

The abbreviation Syn., meaning synonym, appears with some definitions. It indicates the word entry has the same meaning as another; for example, oophoritis is synonymous with ovaritis.

The medical terms listed in each section have been split into their components for ease of understanding, for example . . .

gastr/o-enter-itis
**gastr/o**   is the combining form of the medical root *gastr*, meaning stomach
-enter-   is the medical root, meaning intestine(s)
-itis   is a suffix, meaning inflammation of.

This medical term is listed in all other common medical words containing the root **gastr** as:

**gastr/o**-enter-itis, inflammation of the intestines and stomach

Where possible the meaning of a word is given reading its components from right to left, as in this example.

**gastr/o**[3]-enter[2]-itis[1]   1 inflammation of
                                  2 intestines (and)
                                  3 stomach

We read the word in the order of its components 1, 2 and 3 to give the full meaning as *inflammation of the intestines and stomach*.

This book also includes:

| | |
|---|---|
| Abbreviations | a list of common medical acronyms |
| Glossary | a list of word components and their meaning |
| Appendix 1 | units of measurement |
| Appendix 2 | normal values of blood, CSF, urine, and faeces |
| Appendix 3 | chemical symbols and formulae |

# Acknowledgements

Common medical terms included in this book were selected with reference to the following Elsevier publications:

*Dictionary of Nursing,* published by Churchill Livingstone
*Dorland's Pocket Medical Dictionary,* published by W.B. Saunders Company
*Pocket Medical Dictionary,* published by Churchill Livingstone in association with
   The Royal Society of Medicine
*Nurse's Pocket Dictionary,* published by Mosby.

   Appendix 1 and Appendix 2 were adapted from *Dictionary of Nursing* (eighteenth edition), with permission from Churchill Livingstone and Appendix 3 from *Nurse's Pocket Dictionary* with permission from Mosby.
   Fig. 8a and Tables 3 and 4 were adapted from *Anatomy and Physiology in Health and Illness* by Ross and Wilson (ninth edition), with permission from Churchill Livingstone.
   I would like to thank the staff at Elsevier for their enthusiasm and support for this venture.

# Introduction
## The components of medical words

## Objectives

**Once the introduction is complete you should be able to:**

- name and identify components of medical words
- split medical words into their components
- read medical words from their components.

Students beginning any kind of medical or paramedical course are faced with a bewildering number of complex medical terms. Surprisingly it is possible to understand many medical terms by learning relatively few words that can be combined in a variety of ways. Even the longest medical terms are easy to understand if you know the meaning of each component of the word.

In this section you will learn how to split medical terms into their components and deduce their meanings. Skills developed here will enable you to derive the meanings of unfamiliar medical words and improve your ability to understand medical literature.

Let us begin by using a medical word associated with an organ with which you are familiar, the stomach:

*Example 1  GASTROTOMY*

First we can split the word and examine its individual components:

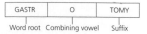

| GASTR | O | TOMY |
|-------|---|------|
| Word root | Combining vowel | Suffix |

## The word root

Roots are the basic medical words. Most are derived from Greek and Roman (Latin) words. Others have their origins in Arabic, Anglo-Saxon and German. Some early Greek words have been retained in their original form while others have been latinized. In their migrations throughout Europe and America many words have changed their spelling, meaning and pronunciation. In our first example we have used the root **gastr**, which always means stomach.

## The combining vowel

Combining vowels are added to word roots to aid pronunciation and to connect the root to the suffix. In our first example the combining vowel **o** has been added to join the root and suffix. All the combining vowels a, e, i, o and u are used but the most commonly used is o. In our first example we have added the combining vowel **o** to the root **gastr**.

## The suffix

The suffix follows the word root and is found at the end of the word. It also adds to or modifies the meaning of the word root. In our first example we have used the suffix **-tomy**, which always means to form an incision.

We can now fully understand our first medical word, gastrotomy means – *to form an incision into the stomach*. Gastrotomy is a name used by surgeons for an operation in which a cut is made into the wall of the stomach.

## The combining form

In our first example the root **gastr** is combined with the vowel **o** to make **gastro**. This word component is called a **combining form** of a word root, i.e.

$$\frac{\text{Word}}{\text{root}} + \frac{\text{combining}}{\text{vowel}} = \frac{\text{combining}}{\text{form}}$$

gastr + o = gastro

Most combining forms end in **o** and many are listed in the sections that follow.

Now we have learnt the meaning of our first root we can use it again with a new word component:

*Example 2 EPIGASTRIC*

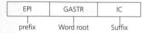

| EPI | GASTR | IC |
|-----|-------|-----|
| prefix | Word root | Suffix |

Here we have split the word into its components and we can see it begins with a prefix that appears before the root **gastr**.

## The prefix

The prefix precedes the word root and changes its meaning. The prefix **epi-** means upon and so it modifies the word to mean upon or above the stomach. Prefixes, like roots and suffixes are also derived from Greek and Latin words.

The suffix **-ic** meaning pertaining to was also used in our second example so we can now write the full meaning of epigastric:

The full meaning of epigastric is *pertaining to above or upon the stomach.*

### Key Point

The components of medical words are:

- prefixes
- roots
- suffixes
- combining vowels
- combining forms.

## Identifying word components

In Sections 1–22 medical terms are divided into prefixes, combining forms or roots and suffixes. You can identify these components in any word if you understand the way it has been constructed. When medical terms are built, the following simple rules are applied:

### Rule 1: Joining a combining form to a suffix

The suffixes **-logy**, meaning *study of* and **-ic**, meaning *pertaining to* can be added to the combining form gastr/o to make two words:

gastr/o + -logy =
gastrology (study of the stomach)

gastr/o + -ic =
gastric (pertaining to the stomach)

Notice in gastrology the combining vowel o is left in place while in gastric it is dropped. The o is dropped in gastric because -ic begins with i, a vowel. Gastroic is not used because it would be more difficult to pronounce.

### Key Point

When a combining form of a root is joined to a suffix, the combining vowel is left in place if the suffix begins with a letter other than a vowel.

Here are some more examples where the vowel is left in place because the suffix begins with a letter other than a vowel:

gastr/o + -tomy =
gastrotomy (incision into the stomach)

gastr/o + -scope =
gastroscope (instrument to view the stomach)

Here are some examples where the vowel is dropped:

gastr/o + -itis =
gastritis (inflammation of the stomach)

gastr/o + -ectomy = gastrectomy (removal of the stomach)

## Rule 2: Joining the combining forms of two word roots

Some medical words contain two or more combining forms of roots, as in Example 3 :

### Example 3 GASTROENTEROLOGY

| GASTR O | ENTER O | LOGY |
|---------|---------|------|
| Combining form meaning stomach | Combining form meaning intestines | Suffix meaning study of |

The full meaning of gastroenterology is the study of the intestines and stomach. Notice that the vowel **o** between the two roots **gastr** and **enter** is left in place.

### Key Point

When the combining forms of two roots are joined, the combining vowel of the first root is kept in place.

Here are some more examples:

pylor/o + gastr/o + ectomy = pylorogastrectomy

duoden/o + enter/o + stomy = duodenoenterostomy

Note: There are a few exceptions to this rule, in which the 'o' is retained and hyphenated, *e.g.* pharyngo-oral.

## Rule 3: Joining a prefix to a root

When a prefix that ends in a vowel is added to a root that begins with a vowel or 'h', the *vowel of the prefix is dropped*. If we look again at our second example, **epigastric**, here the vowel 'i' of **epi-** was retained because the root **gastr** begins with 'g', which is not a vowel.

Consider another example, which may be familiar to you – antacid, a drug used to neutralize stomach acid. This word is made from:

| anti | + acid | = antacid |
|------|--------|-----------|
| Prefix meaning against | Root meaning acid | (a drug that acts against or neutralizes acid) |

The 'i' is dropped because acid begins with the vowel 'a'.

Here are some more examples:
Here the vowel of the prefix is retained:

hemi + col/o + ectomy = hemicolectomy

Here the vowel of the prefix is dropped:

endo + arter/i + ectomy = endarterectomy

anti + helminth + ic = anthelminthic

Note. This is not a strict rule and there are many exceptions to it, e.g. periosteitis.

### Key Point

When a prefix that ends in a vowel is joined to a root, the vowel of the prefix is dropped if the root begins with a vowel or 'h'.

## Reading and understanding medical words

Now you have learnt the basic principles of building medical words, you should be able to deduce the meaning of an unfamiliar word from the meaning of its components. To illustrate this we will use two examples :

### Example 1 Gastroenteropathy

**First**

Split the word into its components gastro/entero/pathy

**Then**

Think of or look up the meaning of these components.

**Finally**

Read the meaning of the word *beginning with the suffix and reading backwards*:

For example: gastr/o[3], enter/o[2], -pathy[1]

1 disease of
2 the intestines and
3 stomach

We read the full meaning of gastro-enteropathy as *disease of the intestines and stomach*.

### Example 2  Pararectal

Here the prefix *para-* has modified the meaning of the root *rect-* to mean *beside the rectum*:

**First**

Split the word into its components

para/rect/al

**Then**

Think of or look up the meaning of these components.

**Finally**

Read the meaning of the word *beginning with the suffix followed by the meaning of the modified root*:

For example: pararect[2], al[1]

1 pertaining to
2 beside the rectum

We read the full meaning of pararectal as *pertaining to beside the rectum*.

---

### Key Point

When deducing the meanings of compound medical words, begin with the meaning of the suffix followed by those of the root(s) and prefix (from right to left).

---

Once you can split words in the ways described here and have learnt the meanings of common word components, you will be able to deduce the literal meaning of many familiar and unfamiliar medical terms

In Sections 1–22 the medical terms have been split into prefixes, word roots or combining forms and suffixes for ease of understanding. These word lists and their definitions will complement your studies of anatomy, physiology and health care.

# Section 1
# Cells, tissues, organs and systems

The human body consists of basic units of life known as **cells**. Groups of cells similar in appearance, function and origin join to form **tissues**. Different tissues then interact with each other to form **organs**. Finally, groups of organs interact to form body **systems**. Each system performs specific actions that contribute to the maintenance of homeostasis.

The four levels of organization in the human body are:

- cells
- tissues
- organs
- systems.

Figures 1–4 show combining forms of roots associated with levels of organization.

**A cell**
cellul/o
cyt/o

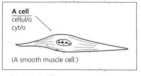

(A smooth muscle cell.)

Figure 1  A cell

**A tissue**
hist/o
cyt/o

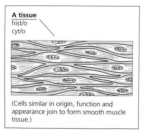

(Cells similar in origin, function and appearance join to form smooth muscle tissue.)

Figure 2  A tissue

**An organ**
organ/o

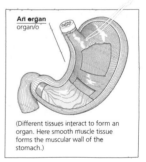

(Different tissues interact to form an organ. Here smooth muscle tissue forms the muscular wall of the stomach.)

Figure 3  An organ

### Quick Reference

Combining forms of roots relating to cells, tissues and levels of organization:

|  |  | Page |
|---|---|---|
| **Blast/o** | embryonic cell, immature cell | 6 |
| **Cellul-** | cell | 7 |
| **Clon/o** | clone of cells | 7 |
| **Collagen/o** | collagen | 8 |
| **Cyt/o, -cyte** | cell | 8 |
| **Elast/o** | elastic, elastic tissue, elastin | 12 |
| **Endotheli/o** | endothelium | 12 |
| **Epitheli/o** | epithelium | 12 |
| **Fibr/o** | fibre, fibrous tissue | 13 |
| **Hist/o** | tissue | 13 |
| **Kary/o** | nucleus of a cell | 14 |
| **Micro-** | small | 15 |
| **Nucle/o** | nucleus of a cell | 17 |
| **Organ/o** | organ | 17 |
| **-ploidy** | a set of chromosomes | 18 |
| **Somat/o** | the body | 18 |
| **System-** | system | 19 |

### Quick Reference

Common words and combining forms relating to cells, tissues and levels of organization:

|  |  | Page |
|---|---|---|
| Body | **somat/o** | 18 |
| Cell | **cellul-, cyt/o** | 7/8 |
| Chromosome set | **-ploidy** | 18 |
| Clone of cells | **clon/o** | 7 |
| Collagen | **collagen/o** | 8 |
| Elastic | **elast/o** | 12 |
| Elastic tissue | **elast/o** | 12 |
| Elastin | **elast/o** | 12 |
| Embryonic cell | **blast/o** | 6 |
| Endothelium | **endotheli/o** | 12 |
| Epithelium | **epitheli/o** | 12 |
| Fibre | **fibr/o** | 13 |
| Fibrous tissue | **fibr/o** | 13 |
| Immature cell | **blast/o** | 6 |
| Nucleus of a cell | **kary/o, nucle/o** | 14/17 |
| Organ | **organ/o** | 17 |
| Small | **micro-** | 15 |
| System | **system-** | 19 |
| Tissue | **hist/o** | 13 |

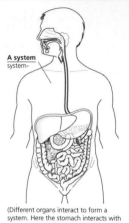

(Different organs interact to form a system. Here the stomach interacts with other organs to form the digestive system that breaks down food and absorbs nutrients.)

Figure 4  A system

### Roots and combining forms, meanings

**Blast/o**, a cell that forms . . . , embryonic cell, immature cell

From a Greek word **blastos**, meaning bud or germ. Here blast/o means an immature stage in cell development, an undifferentiated cell, embryonic cell or stem cell that is forming something.

angi/o-**blast**, a (blood) vessel-forming cell

**blast/o**-coele, a fluid-filled central cavity of a blastula

**blast/o**-cyst, 1. bladder of immature cells 2. early embryonic stage consisting of trophoblast cells around a fluid filled cavity and an inner cell mass

**blast/o**-cyte, an immature or undifferentiated embryonic cell

**blast/o**-derm, a skin of immature cells (a layer of cells forming the blastocyst that gives rise to the germ layers)

**blast/o**-disc, a disc-like convex structure formed by blastomeres (immature or undifferentiated cells) at the animal pole of an ovum

**blast**-oma, a tumour of immature cells (embryonic cells)

**blast/o**-mere, an immature cell produced by cleavage of a fertilized ovum

**blast**-ula, 1. a little bud or germ 2. a blastocyst (a bladder of immature cells, an early embryonic stage consisting of trophoblast cells around a fluid-filled cavity and an inner cell mass)

collagen/o-**blast**, an immature cell that forms a collagen-producing cell when mature

cyt/o-**blast**, 1. an immature or embryonic cell 2. a cell that has not begun to differentiate or specialize

derm/o-**blast**, a layer of embryonic cells (the mesoderm) that develops into skin

diplo-**blast**-ic, pertaining to two germ layers (of cells)

fibr/o-**blast**, 1. an immature cell that forms (collagen) fibres or fibrous connective tissue 2. an immature cell that forms precursor cells that produce connective tissue

haem/o-cyt/o-**blast**, 1. a cell that forms blood cells 2. an immature blood cell

hetero-**blast**-ic, pertaining to forming from different types of tissue

hist/o-**blast**, an immature cell or embryonic cell that forms tissues

leuco-**blast**, an immature granular leucocyte

leuco-erythro-**blast**-osis, abnormal condition of immature red cells and white cells (granulocytes) in the circulation

macro-**blast**, a large immature red blood cell with a nucleus

megalo-**blast**, a large immature cell that forms abnormal erythrocytes

megalo-**blast**-ic, pertaining to megaloblasts

micro-**blast**, a small immature cell (an erythroblast < 5 microns in diameter)

mono-**blast**, an immature cell that forms the monocyte series of cells

neur/o-**blast**, an immature cell or embryonic cell that forms nervous tissue

pro-megalo-**blast**, before the megaloblast, it refers to an immature abnormal erythrocyte that develops into a megaloblast

spermat/o-**blast**, an immature spermatozoon or spermatid

spongi/o-**blast**, an immature cell that forms spongiocytes

oste/o-**blast**, 1. a bone forming cell 2. an immature bone cell

---

### Cellul-, cell

From a Latin word *cella*, meaning compartment and *-ula*, meaning little. Here cellula- means the cell, the basic unit of life. Each cell has a cell membrane enclosing cytoplasm, a mix of chemicals and organelles that perform its metabolic activities. Within the cytoplasm is a nucleus that controls the metabolism, growth and development of the cell. The human body is composed of many different types of cell specialized for particular functions.

See the combining form cyt/o also meaning cell.

a-**cellul**-ar, pertaining to without cells or cellular structure, non-cellular

hetero-**cellul**-ar, pertaining to composed of different types of cell

iso-**cellul**-ar, pertaining to having the same or identical cells

multi-**cellul**-ar, 1. pertaining to many cells 2. made of many cells

uni-**cellul**-ar, 1. pertaining to one cell 2. made of a single cell

---

### Clon/o, clone

From a Greek word *klon* meaning a cutting used for propagation. Here clon/o means a clone of cells. Cells that form a clone are similar genetically and are derived by cell division from a single cell.

**clon**-al, pertaining to a clone

**clon**-al-ity, state or ability to form a clone

mono-**clon**-al, pertaining to a clone from a single cell

poly-**clon**-al, pertaining to many clones (derived from different cells)

**clon/o**-gen-ic, pertaining to forming a clone of cells

---

**Collagen/o**, collagen

From a Greek word **kolla** meaning glue and **genein** meaning to produce. Here, collagen/o means collagen, the protein found in the white fibres of connective tissues.

**collagen**-ase, an enzyme that breaks down collagen

**collagen**-ation, act or process of forming collagen (in cartilage)

**collagen**-ic, 1. pertaining to or of the nature of collagen 2. producing collagen

**collagen**-itis, inflammation of collagenous fibres in connective tissues

**collagen/o**-blast, an immature cell that forms a collagen-producing cell when mature

**collagen/o**-cyte, a collagen-producing cell

**collagen/o**-gen-ic, pertaining to forming collagen or collagen fibres

**collagen/o**-lysis, breakdown or disintegration of collagen

**collagen/o**-lyt-ic, pertaining to breakdown or disintegration of collagen

**collagen**-osis, abnormal condition or disease of collagen

**collagen**-ous, pertaining to or of the nature of collagen

pro-**collagen**, before collagen, it refers to a precursor of collagen formed by fibroblasts

---

**Cyt/o**, -cyte, cell

From a Greek word *kytos*, meaning cell. Here cyt/o means the cell, the basic unit of life. Each cell has a cell membrane enclosing cytoplasm, a mix of chemicals and organelles that perform its metabolic activities. Within the cytoplasm is a nucleus that controls the metabolism, growth and development of the cell. The human body is composed of many different types of cell specialized for particular functions.

The study of cells is known as cytology, a topic of great importance in medicine as many diseases and disorders can be diagnosed by studying cells. See the combining form cellula-also meaning cell.

**a-granul/o-cyte**, a cell without granules, for example a lymphocyte

**a-granul/o-cyt**-osis, abnormal condition of being without granulocytes, it refers to a decrease in polymorphonuclear leucocytes

**astr/o-cyte**, a star-shaped cell, it refers to a neuroglial cell of the CNS

**astr/o-cyt**-oma, a malignant tumour of astrocytes (neuroglial cells of the CNS)

**aux/o-cyte**, a cell necessary to increase growth or reproduction (an early oocyte or spermatocyte)

**chondr/o-cyte**, a cartilage cell

**collagen/o-cyte**, a collagen-producing cell

**cyt/o-architecture**, the arrangement of cells in a tissue or organ

**cyt/o-bio-logy**, the study of biology in relation to cells

**cyt/o-blast**, 1. an immature or embryonic cell 2. a cell that has not begun to differentiate or specialize

**cyt/o-chemistry**, the chemistry of cells or branch of biological science concerned with the chemical activities of cells

**cyt/o-chromes**, cell colours, it refers to cell proteins containing iron or copper whose main function is electron transport in reduction–oxidation reactions within mitochondria of cells. From a Greek word *chroma*-meaning colour

**cyt/o-cide**, an agent that kills cells

**cyt/o-cid-al**, 1. pertaining to killing cells 2. pertaining to an agent that kills cells

**cyt/o-clasis**, 1. the breaking or fragmentation of cells 2. cell necrosis

**cyt/o**-clast-ic, pertaining to the breaking or fragmentation of cells

**cyt/o**-clesis, influence on cells by other cells. From a Greek word *klesis* meaning calling for

**cyt/o**-desma, an intercellular substance that holds or bands cells together. From a Greek word *desmos* meaning a band

**cyt/o**-diagnosis, diagnosis based on the study or examination of cells

**cyt/o**-differentiation, 1. cell specialization 2. the development of special structures within embryonic cells

**cyt/o**-dist-al, pertaining to further away from a cell 'body' of a nerve cell

**cyt/o**-genet-ic, 1. pertaining to the genetic material (genes or chromosomes) in cells 2. pertaining to cytogenetics

**cyt/o**-genet-ical, 1. pertaining to or dealing with the genetic material (genes and chromosomes) in cells 2. pertaining to cytogenetics

**cyt/o**-genet-ics, a branch of science concerning the genetic material (genes and chromosomes) in cells

**cyt/o**-gen-ous, pertaining to forming cells

**cyt/o**-glyc/o-pen-ia, condition of reduced or deficient glucose in (blood) cells

**cyt/o**-hist/o-genesis, formation of cells and their structure

**cyt**-oid, resembling a cell

**cyt/o**-kines, signalling chemicals secreted by cells of the immune system *e.g.* interleukin

**cyt/o**-kin-esis, condition of movement of cells, it refers to the movement or changes that take place in a cell during cell division

**cyt/o**-log-ical, pertaining to or dealing with cells

**cyt/o**-log-ist, a specialist who studies cells

**cyt/o**-logy, the study of cells

**cyt/o**-lys-in, a chemical or antibody that lyses or breaks up cells

**cyt/o**-lysis, breakdown or disintegration of cells

**cyt/o**-lyt-ic, pertaining to the breakdown or disintegration of cells

**cyt/o**-meta-plas-ia, condition of change in growth, form or function of cells

**cyt/o**-meter, a device for measuring cells (number and/or size)

**cyt/o**-metry, technique of measuring cells (number and/or size) often of blood cells

**cyt/o**-morph/o-logy, the study of the form and structure (morphology) of cells

**cyt/o**-morph-osis, condition of change (to form and structure) in a cell during its life

**cyt/o**-myc-osis, abnormal condition of fungi affecting cells

**cyt/o**-path-ic, 1. pertaining to disease of cells 2. pertaining to capable of injuring or causing pathological change in a cell

**cyt/o**-path/o-genesis, 1. formation of pathogenic changes in cells 2. formation of disease of cells

**cyt/o**-path/o-gen-ic, 1. pertaining to formation of disease of cells 2. pertaining to cytopathogenesis

**cyt/o**-path/o-log-ist, a specialist who studies disease (pathological changes) in cells

**cyt/o**-path/o-logy, the study of disease of cells

**cyt/o**-pathy, disease of cells

**cyt/o**-pen-ia, condition of deficiency of cells (of blood)

**cyt/o**-phagy, the eating or ingestion of cells by phagocytes

**cyt/o**-pheresis, separation or removal of cellular components (from blood) and transfusion of the plasma and remaining cells into the donor

**cyt/o**-phil-ic, pertaining to having an affinity for cells

**cyt/o**-phylaxis, 1. protection of cells (against infection or cytolysis) 2. increase in cellular activity for defence against infection

**cyt/o**-plasm, the contents of a cell invested by the cell membrane excluding the nucleus

**cyt/o**-plasm-ic, pertaining to cytoplasm

**cyt/o**-proxim-al, pertaining to nearer to a cell 'body' of a nerve cell

**cyt**-osis, abnormal condition in which there are more than the norma number of cells (often prefixed by a combining form, for example reticulocytosis)

**cyt/o**-skeleton, internal reinforcing parts of a cell (micro filaments)

**cyt/o**-smear, a smear (thin film) of cells (for cytological examination)

**cyt/o**-sol, liquid medium of the cytoplasm minus organelles and insoluble inclusions

**cyt/o**-some, the body of a cell excluding the nucleus

**cyt/o**-stasis, slowing or stopping of the movement of cells (of blood)

**cyt/o**-stat-ic, 1. pertaining to stopping cells (growth and multiplication) 2. an agent that stops cells (growth and multiplication)

**cyt/o**-stome, a cell mouth (it refers to the aperture through which food enters protozoan cells)

**cyt/o**-tax-ia, condition of ordered movement of cells (attraction or repulsion of cells for one another)

**cyt/o**-taxis, movement and arrangement of cells in response to a stimulus

**cyt/o**-thesis, restoration of an injured cell to a condition of health. From a Greek word *thesis*- meaning a placing

**cyt/o**-tox-ic, pertaining to poisonous to cells

**cyt/o**-tox-in, an agent or antibody having a toxic (poisonous) action upon cells

**cyt/o**-tropho-blast, cellular layer of the trophoblast (cell layer covering the blastocyst stage of the developing ovum)

**cyt/o**-trop-ism, 1. process of cell movement in response to a stimulus 2. process of attraction of certain cells to particular micro-organisms or drugs

**cyt/o**-zo-ic, pertaining to an animal of a cell (a parasite of a cell)

**cyt/o**-zoon, an animal living within a cell, it refers to a parasite such as a protozoon

**cyt**-ur-ia, condition of cells in the urine

endo-**cyt**-osis, condition of cells in which large molecules move into them by formation of a vesicle at the cell membrane (the opposite of exocytosis)

epi-**cyte**, 1. upon a cell, it refers to a cell's plasma membrane 2. an epithelial cell

erythr/o-**cyte**, a red (blood) cell

erythr/o-**cyt/o**-pen-ia, condition of deficiency (in number) of red blood cells

erythr/o-**cyt**-osis, abnormal condition of (too many) red blood cells

exo-**cyt**-osis, condition of cells in which large molecules leave by moving to the outside through the cell membrane (the opposite of endocytosis)

fibr/o-**cyte**, a fibre cell

gangli/o-**cyte**, a ganglion cell

granul/o-**cyte**, a granular cell (a cell that contains granules)

hepat/o-**cyte**, a liver cell

histi/o-**cyte**, a macrophage (a phagocytic cell)

histi/o-**cyt**-osis, abnormal condition of histiocytes or macrophages (an increase in number in the blood)

homo-**cyt/o**-trop-ic, pertaining to having an affinity for cells of the same species

hypo-**cyt**-haem-ia, condition of below normal number of cells (erythrocytes) in the blood

keratin/o-**cyte**, an epidermal cell that synthesizes keratin

lept/o-**cyte**, a thin cell, it refers to a thin erythrocyte containing a clear area within its haemoglobin

leuco-**cyte**, a white (blood) cell

leuco-**cyt/o**-lysis, disintegration or breakdown of leucocytes

leuco-**cyt**-osis, abnormal condition of (too many) leucocytes in the blood

lymph/o-**cyte**, a lymph cell

lymph/o-**cyt/o**-lysis, disintegration or breakdown of lymph cells (lymphocytes)

lymph/o-**cyt/o**-pen-ia, condition of deficiency (in number) of lymphocytes in the blood

macro-**cyte**, a large cell, it refers to an abnormally large erythrocyte

macro-**cyt**-haem-ia, condition of macrocytes in the blood

macro-**cyt**-ic, pertaining to macrocytes

macro-**cyt**-osis, condition of macrocytes in the blood Syn. macrocythaemia

mega-kary/o-**cyte**, a large nucleated cell (of bone marrow from which platelets form)

melan/o-**cyte**, 1. a pigment cell 2. a cell that produces melanin found in the epidermis

mening/e-**cyte**, a cell of the meninges (a histiocyte)

micro-**cyte**, an (abnormally) small cell (red blood cell)

micro-erythr/o-**cyte**, a small red cell or small erythrocyte Syn. microcyte

micro-pino-**cyt**-osis, condition of forming small pinocytic vesicles (vesicles formed by cell membranes invaginating fluid). From a Greek word *pinein* meaning to drink

micro-spher/o-**cyte**, a small, spherical cell, it refers to an abnormal erythrocyte called a spherocyte

mono-**cyte**, a large cell (leucocyte) with a single nucleus found in normal blood

mono-**cyt**-ic, pertaining to or of the nature of monocytes

mono-**cyt**-osis, abnormal condition of (too many) monocytes in blood

myel/o-**cyte**, a marrow cell, it refers to an early differentiated leucocyte normally seen in bone marrow

neur/o-**cyte**, a nerve cell (of any type)

neur/o-gli/a-**cyte**, a nerve glue cell, it refers to a type of supporting cell of nervous tissue

neur/o-gli/o-**cyte**, a nerve glue cell, it refers to a type of supporting cell of nervous tissue

norm/o-**cyte**, a normal cell, it refers to a red blood cell normal in size and shape

oligo-dendr/o-**cyte**, a small tree-like cell. From a Greek word *dendron* meaning tree, it refers to a non-neural cell forming the neuroglia (supporting cells) of the central nervous system

oo-**cyte**, an egg cell

oste/o-**cyte**, a bone cell

pan-**cyt**/o-pen-ia, condition of deficiency (in number) of all types of blood cell

peri-**cyte**, a (contractile) cell that is found around arterioles

phag/o-**cyte**, an eating cell, it refers to a cell capable of engulfing other cells and debris in tissues

pino-**cyte**, a cell that 'drinks' or performs pinocytosis. From a Greek word *pinein* meaning to drink

pino-**cyt**-osis, condition of cells 'drinking', it refers to the process of forming pinocytic vesicles (fluid-filled vesicles formed by cell membranes). From a Greek word *pinein* meaning to drink

pitui-**cyte**, a cell of the pituitary gland (found in the neurohypophysis)

ple/o-**cyt**-osis, condition of more (than normal number) of cells in the CSF

pneum/o-**cyte**, a lung cell (Type 1 cells that line the alveoli, Type 2 cells that secrete surfactant)

pneumon/o-**cyte**, a lung cell (the term includes Type 1 cells that line the alveoli, Type 2 cells that secrete surfactant and alveolar macrophages)

pod/o-**cyte**, a foot-like cell, it refers to the foot-like epithelial cells covering the capillaries of the renal glomeruli

poly-**cyt**-haem-ia, condition of too many blood cells (usually an increase in number of red cells)

pre-mono-**cyte**, a cell before the monocyte, it refers to a cell that forms a monocyte, intermediate between a monoblast and a monocyte

pro-mega-kary/o-**cyte**, a cell before the megakaryocyte, it refers to a cell that forms megakaryocytes intermediate between a megakaryoblast and a megakaryocyte

pro-mono-**cyte**, a cell before the monocyte, it refers to a cell that forms a monocyte, intermediate between a monoblast and a monocyte Syn. premonocyte

pro-myel/o-**cyte**, a precursor cell of the bone marrow that forms white blood cells of the polymorphonuclear granulocyte series

pykn/o-**cyte**, a compact cell, it refers to an abnormal compact erythrocyte with projecting spikes on its membrane

reticul/o-**cyte**, a net-like cell, it refers to an immature erythrocyte reticul/o-**cyt**-osis, abnormal condition of (too many) reticulocytes (immature erythrocytes) in blood

schist/o-**cyte**, a split cell, it refers to a fragment of a red blood cell (seen in haemolytic anaemia)

schist/o-**cyt**-osis, abnormal condition of (too many) schistocytes in blood

spermat/o-**cyte**, a sperm cell

spher/o-**cyte**, a spherical cell, it refers to a small, spherical, abnormal erythrocyte

spher/o-**cyt**-ic, pertaining to a spherocyte

spher/o-**cyt**-osis, abnormal condition of spherocytes in the blood

spongi/o-**cyte**, a sponge-like cell, it refers to vacuolated cells in the adrenal cortex or neuroglial cells

thromb/o-**cyte**, a clotting cell or platelet, it refers to a disc-like fragment of a cell that circulates in blood and plays a major role in clotting of blood

thromb/o-**cyt**-haem-ia, condition of (too many) thrombocytes in the blood

thromb/o-**cyt**/o-pen-ia, condition of deficiency (in number) of thrombocytes in the blood

thromb/o-**cyt**-osis, abnormal condition of (too many) thrombocytes in the blood

---

**Elast/o**, elastic-, elastic, elastin
From a Greek word **elaunein** meaning to drive. Here, elast/o means elastin, elastic tissue or to the quality of being elastic. Elastin is the yellow sclero-protein found in the yellow elastic fibres of connective tissues.

**elast**-ase, an enzyme that breaks down elastin

**elast**-ic, pertaining to being elastic that is able to recover size and shape after being stretched, compressed or bent

**elast**-in, the yellow scleroprotein found in the yellow elastic fibres of connective tissues

**elastic**-ity, the quality of being elastic

**elastic**-in, elastin

**elast**/o-fibr-oma, a tumour containing elements of fibrous tissue and elastin

**elast**/o-lysis, breakdown or disintegration of elastic tissue

**elast**-oma, a tumour in which elastic tissue or fibres predominates

**elast**/o-metry, technique of measuring elasticity

**elast**/o-pathy, disease of elastic tissue (deficiency of)

**elast**/o-rrhexis, rupture of elastic tissue

**elast**-osis, abnormal condition or disease of elastic tissues (degeneration of)

**elast**/o-tic, 1. pertaining to elastosis 2. of the nature of elastic tissue

---

**Endotheli/o**, endothelium
From the Greek words **endon** meaning within and **thele** meaning nipple. Here endotheli/o means endothelium, a layer of epithelial cells that line serous cavities, blood vessels and lymph vessels.

**endothelia**, plural of endothelium

**endotheli**-al, pertaining to or composed of an endothelium

**endotheli**-itis, inflammation of an endothelium

**endotheli**/o-blast-oma, a tumour of immature cells of an endothelium

**endotheli**/o-cyte, a cell of the endothelium, it refers to a phagocytic cell that arises in the endothelium of a blood vessel

**endotheli**-oid, resembling endothelium

**endotheli**/o-lyt-ic, pertaining to breaking down endothelial tissue

**endotheli**-oma, a tumour arising from the endothelium of a blood vessel

**endotheli**-omat-osis, abnormal condition of (multiple) endotheliomas

sub-**endotheli**-al, pertaining to under or below an endothelium

---

**Epitheli/o**, epithelium
From the Greek words **epi** meaning upon and **thele** meaning nipple. Here epitheli/o means epithelium, a type of tissue. Simple epith\\\\ consist of single layers of cells that cover organs and cavities. Stratified epith\\\\ consist of several layers of cells that protect surfaces liable to wear and tear. Epithelial glands are

composed of epithelial cells that secrete useful substances into ducts, onto a surface or into the blood.

**epitheli**-al, pertaining to or composed of an epithelium

**epitheli**-iz-ation, action of making an epithelium *e.g.* by growth over a damaged surface

**epitheli**al-ize, to make or cover with an epithelium

**epitheli**-itis, inflammation of an epithelium

**epitheli/o**-lysis, breakdown or destruction of an epithelium

**epitheli/o**-lyt-ic, pertaining to breakdown or destruction of an epithelium

**epitheli**-oma, a tumour derived from an epithelium

**epitheli**-omat-osis, abnormal condition of having multiple epitheliomas (epitheliomata)

**epitheli**-omat-ous, pertaining to an epithelioma

trans-**epitheli**-al, pertaining to across or through an epithelium

---

**Fibr/o, fibros-**, fibre, fibrous tissue
From a Latin word **fiber**. Here, fibr/o means fibrous connective tissue.

**fibr/o**-aden-oma, a glandular tumour in which there is formation of fibrous tissue

**fibr/o**-blast, 1. an immature cell that forms (collagen) fibres or fibrous connective tissue 2. an immature cell that forms precursor cells that produce connective tissue

**fibr/o**-blast-oma, a tumour developing from fibroblasts Syn. fibroma, fibrosarcoma

**fibr/o**-calcif-ic, pertaining to calcium salts in fibrous tissue or calcification of fibrous tissue

**fibr/o**-cartilage, cartilage containing bundles of white fibrous (collagenous) tissue

**fibr/o**-chondr-itis, inflammation of fibrocartilage

**fibr/o**-collagen-ous, pertaining to collagen fibres

**fibr/o**-cyst, a cyst or bladder-like tumour composed of fibrous tissue or fully developed connective tissue

**fibr/o**-cyst-ic, pertaining to having fibrocysts

**fibr/o**-cyte, a fibre cell, it refers to 1. an immature cell that forms (collagen) fibres or fibrous connective tissue 2. an immature cell that forms precursor cells that produce connective tissue Syn. fibroblast

**fibr/o**-elast-ic, pertaining to being elastic and fibrous

**fibr/o**-elast-osis, abnormal condition of elastic and fibrous tissue (proliferation of)

**fibr**-oid, 1. resembling fibrous tissue 2. the name for a fibroma especially in the uterus

**fibr**-oid-ectomy, removal of a fibroma especially from the uterus

**fibr**-oma, a tumour composed of fibrous or fully developed connective tissue

**fibr/o**-muscul-ar, pertaining to muscular and fibrous tissue

**fibr/o**-my-alg-ia, condition of pain in muscles and surrounding fibrous tissues

**fibr/o**-my-itis, inflammation of a muscle resulting in fibrous degeneration

**fibr/o**-my-oma, a tumour of muscle and fibrous tissue

**fibr/o**-plas-ia, condition of formation or growth of fibrous tissue

**fibr/o**-sarc-oma, a malignant fleshy tumour formed from fibroblasts

**fibr/o**-osis, abnormal condition of (formation) of fibrous tissue (in an organ)

**fibros**-itis, inflammation of fibrous tissue (especially of muscle sheaths and fascia)

**fibr/o**-tic, pertaining to or of the nature of fibrosis

**fibr**-ous, pertaining to or of the nature of fibres or fibrous tissue

**fibr/o**-vascul-ar, pertaining to (blood) vessels and fibrous tissue

---

**Hist/o**, tissues
From a Greek word **histos** meaning web. Here hist/o means the tissues of

the body. As cells become specialized, they form groups of cells known as tissues. A definition of a tissue is a group of cells similar in appearance, function and origin. There are four basic types of tissue: **epithelial**, **muscle**, **connective** and **nervous** tissue; these form the second level of organization in the body.

Note: medical terms associated with cartilage and bone, muscle and blood can be found in Section 14 The skeletal system, Section 13 The muscular system and Section 5 The blood.

**hist/o**-blast, an immature cell or embryonic cell that forms tissues

**hist/o**-chemistry, the chemistry of tissues, a branch of histology

**hist/o**-clasis, the breaking down of tissues

**hist/o**-clast-ic, pertaining to the breaking down of tissues (by cells)

**hist/o**-clin-ical, pertaining to clinical and histological assessment

**hist/o**-compatibility, the compatibility of tissues (it refers to the compatibility of human leucocyte antigens of a donor and recipient)

**hist/o**-diagnosis, diagnosis by examination of tissues (with a microscope)

**hist/o**-dialysis, breakdown of tissue (by an external agent)

**hist/o**-differentiation, the development or specialization of stem cells into the characteristic cells of a particular tissue

**hist/o**-fluorescence, fluorescence from a tissue (following administration of a dye or drug)

**hist/o**-genesis, formation of tissues (from undifferentiated tissues in the germ layers of an embryo)

**hist/o**-genet-ic, pertaining to formation of tissues (from undifferentiated tissues in the germ layers of an embryo)

**hist/o**-gen-ous, pertaining to formed by tissues

**hist/o**-graphy, 1. technique of recording tissues 2. a description of tissues

**hist/o**-haemat/o-gen-ous, pertaining to forming from the blood and tissues

**hist**-oid, 1. resembling a normal tissue 2. originating from a single tissue 3. resembling a web

**hist/o**-incompatibility, the incompatibility of tissues (it refers to the incompatibility of antigens of a donor and recipient leading to rejection of a graft)

**hist/o**-kin-esis, condition of movement that occurs in the elements of a tissue

**hist/o**-log-ic, pertaining to the study of tissues

**hist/o**-log-ical, 1. pertaining to the study of tissues 2. pertaining to histology

**hist/o**-log-ist, a specialist who studies tissues

**hist/o**-logy, the study of tissues (minute structure and function)

**hist/o**-lysis, breakdown or disintegration of tissues

**hist/o**-lyt-ic, pertaining to the breakdown or disintegration of tissues

**hist**-oma, a tissue tumour

**hist/o**-meta-plast-ic, pertaining to change in form of a tissue (one kind into another)

**hist/o**-neur/o-logy, the study of the tissues of the nervous system

**hist/o**-path/o-logy, the study of diseased tissues

**hist/o**-physi/o-logy, the study of physiology and histology, it refers to correlating the function of a part with the structure of its cells and tissues

**hist/o**-radio-graphy, technique of making a recording or X-ray picture of a tissue particularly of microscopical sections

---

**Kary/o**, nucleus of a cell

From a Greek word **karyon** meaning nut. Here, kary/o means the nucleus of a cell. The nucleus is bounded by a membranous sac called the nuclear membrane that contains nuclear pores. Within the nucleus are the genes that control the metabolism, growth, development and division of the cell. The genes are located on chromosomes visible only when the cell is undergoing division. Each gene consists of a section of DNA containing a sequence of bases (the genetic code) that enables the cell to make a specific protein.

dys-**kary**-osis, abnormal or disordered condition of the nucleus

dys-**kary**-tic, pertaining to or of the nature of an abnormal or disordered nucleus

eu-**kary**-on, a good or normal nucleus (the normal membrane-bound nucleus seen in eukaryotes, organisms whose cells have a true nucleus)

eu-**kary**-ote, an organism whose cells have a true nucleus bounded by a cell membrane. The cells of 'higher' plants and animals, protozoa, fungi and some algae are eukaryotic.

eu-**kary/o**-tic, 1. pertaining to having the characteristics of a eukaryote 2. pertaining to having a good or normal nucleus (the normal membrane-bound nucleus seen in eukaryotes)

**kary/o**-clasis, breaking of a nucleus

**kary/o**-gamy, the fusion (conjugation) of cell nuclei

**kary/o**-genesis, the formation of a cell nucleus

**kary/o**-gen-ic, pertaining to forming a cell nucleus

**kary/o**-kin-esis, the movement of the nucleus, it refers to the division of the nucleus

**kary/o**-kinet-ic, pertaining to karyokinesis

**kary/o**-lysis, breakdown or disintegration of the nucleus of a cell

**kary/o**-lyt-ic, 1. pertaining to breakdown or disintegration of the nucleus of a cell 2. pertaining to karyolysis

**kary/o**-metry, technique of measuring the nucleus of a cell

**kary/o**-morph-ism, state or shape of the cell nucleus

**kary**-on, a nucleus of a cell

**kary/o**-plasm, the material that fills the nucleus Syn. nucleoplasm

**kary/o**-pykn-osis, condition of thickening of a cell nucleus (appearance due to shrinkage and condensing of its chromatin)

**kary/o**-rrhe-tic, pertaining to karyorrhexis

**kary/o**-rrhexis, rupture of the cell nucleus

**kary/o**-some, a nuclear body (a clump of chromatin seen in the nucleus of a cell)

**kary/o**-spher-ical, pertaining to a spherical or globular nucleus

**kary/o**-type, 1. type of nucleus, it refers to the chromosome complement of the nucleus 2. a photomicrograph of a person's classified chromosomes

mega-**kary/o**-cyte, a large nucleated cell (of bone marrow from which platelets form)

pro-mega-**kary/o**-cyte, a cell before the megakaryocyte, it refers to a cell that forms megakaryocytes intermediate between a megakaryoblast and a megakaryocyte

pro-**kary**-ote, before a nucleus, it refers to 'primitive' single-celled organisms without a membrane-bound nucleus *e.g.* bacteria

pro-**kary/o**-tic, pertaining to or having the characteristics of a prokaryote, a 'primitive' single-celled organism without a membrane-bound nucleus *e.g.* bacteria

**Micro-**, small
From a Greek word **mikros** meaning small. Here micro- is used with words associated with microscopy. In order to examine cells and tissues a microscope is required. Optical microscopes have a resolving power of 0.2 μm and can be used to observe single cells including bacteria.

bio-**micro**-scope, a microscope for examining living tissue (within the body)

**micro**-analysis, 1. analysis by examination with a microscope 2. analysis of small quantities of material

**micro**-anatomy, anatomy of small structures Syn. histology

**micro**-be, a microorganism especially one causing disease

**micro**-bi-al, pertaining to or having the characteristics of a microorganism

**micro**-bi-cide, an agent that destroys microbes

**micro**-bio-log-ical, pertaining to the study of microbiology

**micro**-bio-log-ist, a specialist who studies small life (microorganisms)

**micro**-bio-logy, the study of small life (microorganisms)

**micro**-bio-phot/o-meter, an instrument that measures light passing through microbes (it detects turbidity in a bacterial culture medium)

**micro**-blast, a small immature cell (an erythroblast <5 microns in diameter)

**micro**-body, a small body, it refers to a membrane-bound structure found in the cytoplasm of cells containing enzymes and other chemicals

**micro**-cyte, an (abnormally) small cell (red blood cell)

**micro**-cyt-ic, 1. pertaining to small cells 2. pertaining to microcytes, abnormally small red blood cells

**micro**-cyt-osis, abnormal condition of microcytes (an increased number of abnormally small red blood cells)

**micro**-cyto-toxic-ity, condition or capability of being poisonous to cells in small quantities

**micro**-dissection, dissection of small things (a cell or tissue)

**micro**-environment, the small environment (at a cellular level)

**micro**-erythro-cyte, a small red cell Syn. microcyte, an abnormally small red blood cell

**micro**-fauna, small (microscopic) animals of a region

**micro**-filament, any small filament found within the cytoplasm of a cell, for example actin and myosin filaments of muscle cells

**micro**-flora, small (microscopic) plants of a region

**micro**-glia, small types of neuroglial cells (phagocytic cells that can migrate to a site of injury)

**micro**-glia-cyte, 1. a small glue cell 2. a microglial cell 3. an immature precursor cell of a microglial cell

**micro**-glio-cyte, 1. a small glue cell 2. a microglial cell 3. an immature precursor cell of a microglial cell

**micro**-graph, 1. a picture or recording of small things e.g. a picture taken using a microscope 2. an instrument that records small movements

**micro**-invasion, act of small invasion by malignant cells into adjacent tissue (seen through a microscope)

**micro**-manipulator, device for manipulating or moving small objects viewed through a microscope

**micro**-mere, a small cell of the blastula (formed by unequal cleavage)

**micro**-meter, an instrument for measuring very small distances or objects observed using a microscope

**micro**-metre, a micron or one millionth of a metre $10^{-6}$ m (µm)

**micro**-myel/o-blast, a small myeloblast or immature myelocyte

**micro**-needle, a small fine needle used in micro manipulation

**micro**-nucleus, a small nucleus

**micro**-organism, any small plant or animal visible using a microscope e.g. bacterium

**micro**-path/o-logy, 1. the study of small pathological changes 2. the study of diseases due to micro-organisms

**micro**-phage, a small phagocyte (a polymorphonuclear leucocyte)

**micro**-pino-cyt-osis, condition of forming small pinocytic vesicles (fluid-filled vesicles formed by cell membranes invaginating fluid). From a Greek word *pinein* meaning to drink

**micro**-radi/o-graphy, technique of making a recording or X-ray picture that can be used to examine small or microscopic structures

**micro**-scope, an instrument to view small objects

**micro**-scop-ic, 1. pertaining to viewing small objects with a microscope 2. extremely small

**micro**-scop-ist, a person who specializes in microscopy

**micro**-scopy, technique of viewing or examining small objects (with a microscope)

**micro**-spectr/o-scope, a spectroscope used with a microscope to view the absorption spectra of tissues

**micro**-spher/o-cyte, a small spherical cell, it refers to a small, fragile, spherical red blood cell

**micro**-some, a small body (a fragment of endoplasmic reticulum formed after homogenization of a cell)

**micro**-surgery, dissection of small structures (using a microscope)

**micro**-tome, an instrument used to cut small thin slices of tissue for microscopic examination

**micro**-tubule, a small tube (found in the cytoplasm of a cell, made of tubulin that acts to support and move substances through the cytoplasm)

**micr**-urgy, small work or micro manipulation. From a Greek word *ergon* meaning work

**micro**-zoon, a small or microscopic animal

**Nucle/o**, nucleus of a cell

From a Latin word **nucleus** meaning nut or kernel. Here, nucle/o means the nucleus of a cell. The nucleus is bounded by a membranous sac called the nuclear membrane that contains nuclear pores. Within the nucleus are genes that control the metabolism, growth, development and division of the cell. The genes are located on chromosomes visible only when the cell is undergoing division. Each gene consists of a section of DNA containing a sequence of bases (the genetic code) that enables the cell to make a specific protein.

e-**nucle**-ate, act of removing a nucleus from a cell

extra-**nucle**-ar, pertaining to outside a cell nucleus

mono-**nucle**-ar, pertaining to having one nucleus

**nucle**-ar, pertaining to a nucleus

**nucle**-ated, having one or more nuclei

**nuclei**, plural of nucleus

**nucle**-ic, pertaining to a nucleus or of the nucleus

**nucle/o**-cyto-plasm-ic, pertaining to the cytoplasm and nucleus of a cell

**nucle/o**-fug-al, pertaining to moving away from a nucleus. From a Latin word *fugare* meaning to avoid

**nucle**-oid, resembling a nucleus

**nucle**-ol-us, a small nucleus, it refers to a rounded structure within the nucleus of a cell that synthesizes rRNA

**nucle/o**-pet-al, pertaining to moving towards a nucleus. From a Latin word *petare* meaning to seek

**nucle/o**-plasm, the material that fills the nucleus

**nucle/o**-osis, abnormal condition of (too many) nuclei

**nucle/o**-tox-in, 1. an agent that is poisonous to cell nuclei 2. a poisonous substance originating in nuclei

para-**nucle**-ar, pertaining to a para-nucleus

para-**nucle**-us, a structure or body found beside the nucleus

poly-morph/o-**nucle**-ar, pertaining to having a nucleus of many forms (deeply lobed)

poly-**nucle**-ar, 1. pertaining to having many nuclei 2. polymorphonuclear

poly-**nucle**-ate, having many nuclei

pro-**nucle**-us, structure before the nucleus (the haploid nucleus of a sex cell before fusion)

**Organ/o**, organ

From a Greek word **organon**, meaning tool. Here organ/o means a body organ. Organs are formed from different tissues that interact; they form the third level of organization.

A familiar example is the heart which consists of muscle tissue, a covering of epithelium, nerve tissue and connective tissue. All these tissues interact so that the heart pumps blood.

**organ**-elle, a small specialized organ within a single cell, for example a mitochondrion

**organ/o**-genesis, the formation of organs

**organ/o**-gen-ic, 1. pertaining to forming in an organ 2. pertaining to organogenesis

**organ/o**-genet-ic, 1. pertaining to forming in an organ 2. pertaining to organogenesis

**organ/o**-geny, the formation or origin of organs

**organ**-ic, 1. pertaining to an organ 2. pertaining to having organs or an organized structure 3. pertaining to from an organism 4. in chemistry pertaining to carbon compounds

**organ**-ize, to form organs or structure

**organ**-izer, region of an embryo that organizes or determines the specialization of cells in another region

**organ/o**-fact-ion, formation and development of a body organ. From a Latin word *facere* meaning to make

**organ**-oid, resembling an organ

**organ/o**-megaly, enlargement of organs (viscera)

**organ**-on, an organ

**organ/o**-pathy, disease of organs

**organ/o**-pexy, surgical fixation of a displaced organ

**organ/o**-therapy, treatment by administration of extracts from organs

**organ/o**-troph-ic, pertaining to nourishing or stimulating organs

**organ/o**-trop-ic, pertaining to having an affinity for particular organs

**organ/o**-trop-ism, process of having an affinity for particular organs

**organ**-um, an organ

---

**-ploid-y**, the set of chromosomes in a cell

From a Greek word **eidos** meaning form. Here -ploidy means the set of chromosomes in a cell. Human body cells for example are diploid and have two sets of chromosomes; one inherited from the female parent and one from the male parent.

an-eu-**ploidy**, without good ploidy, it refers to a condition of having a chromosome number that is not a multiple of the normal haploid number of 23 *e.g.* Turner's Syndrome (45), Down's Syndrome (47)

di-**ploidy**, condition of of having two sets of chromosomes (in humans

somatic cells or body cells contain 46 chromosomes, the diploid number)

ha-**ploidy**, condition of of having one set of chromosomes (in humans the gametes contain 23 chromosomes, the haploid number)

hetero-**ploidy**, condition of of having different chromosomes, it refers to an abnormal number

hyper-**ploidy**, condition of of having above normal number of chromosomes, for example Down's Syndrome with 47 instead of 46

poly-**ploidy**, condition of of having more than two sets of chromosomes

tri-**ploidy**, condition of of having three sets of chromosomes

---

**Som/at/o**, the body

From a Greek word **soma** meaning body. Here somat/o means the body.

**som**-asthen-ia, condition of weakness of the body Syn. somatasthenia

**somat**-aesthes-ia, condition of sensation of the body (conscious or aware of the body)

**somat**-asthen-ia, condition of weakness of the body

**somat**-alg-ia, condition of pain in the body

**somat**-ic, pertaining to the body

**somat/o**-gen-ic, pertaining to originating in the body

**somat/o**-logy, the study of the body (anatomy and physiology)

**somat/o**-pathy, disease of the body (excluding mental disease)

**somat/o**-scopy, technique of examining or viewing the body

**somat/o**-troph-ic, pertaining to nourishing or stimulating the body

**somat/o**-troph-in, an agent (hormone) that stimulates growth of the body

**somat/o**-trop-ic, 1. pertaining to stimulating or having affinity for body cells 2. pertaining to somatotrophin (growth hormone) 3. pertaining to stimulating growth of the body

**somat/o**-trop-in, an agent (hormone) that stimulates growth of the body

**somat/o**-type, type of body

**System-**, system

From a Greek word **systema** meaning system. Here, system- means a system or the body as a whole. Body systems are formed from groups of organs that interact to perform a common function; they form the fourth level of organization. For example the stomach, duodenum, colon, etc. interact to form the digestive system that digests and absorbs food.

**system**a, a system

**system**-a-tic, pertaining to formed into a system

**system**-ic, 1. pertaining to the the body as a whole 2. systematic 3. in cardiology, the circulation supplied by the aorta to body systems

**system**-oid, resembling a system

# Section 2
# The digestive system

The digestive system is the collective name for the organs that interact to digest, absorb and process the food that we eat. It includes:

**The alimentary canal**
The tube which begins at the mouth and ends at the anus. It consists of:

* mouth
* pharynx
* oesophagus
* stomach
* small intestine
* large intestine
* rectum and anal canal

**Accessory organs**
* three pairs of salivary glands
* liver and biliary system
* pancreas

The alimentary canal passes through the thorax, abdomen and pelvis and ends at the anus. The canal has a general structure which is modified at different levels to digest or absorb particular components of the diet. Various secretions are poured into the alimentary canal by cells in its lining and by the accessory organs to digest the food. Digestion is necessary because many nutrients found in food such as proteins and polysaccharides are too large to enter body cells. In digestion, large, complex food molecules are broken down by chemical catalysts called enzymes into smaller, 'simpler' molecules that can cross cell membranes. Materials not absorbed into cells lining the small intestine form the faeces and leave the body through the anus.

The organs and glands of the digestive system are linked physiologically as well as anatomically in that digestion and absorption occur in stages, each stage being dependent upon the previous stage or process.

The medical specialism that includes the study of the digestive system and its associated organs is known as gastroenterology. Figure 5 shows combining forms of roots associated with the anatomy of the digestive system.

---

**Roots and combining forms**, meanings

---

**Abdomin/o**, abdomen
From the Latin word **abdomen** meaning belly. Here abdomin/o means the abdomen, the largest body cavity immediately below the thorax and separated from it by the diaphragm. The abdomen is enclosed largely by muscle and fascia and, therefore, is capable of change in shape and size. It is lined with serous membrane that forms the parietal peritoneum. The abdominal organs are surrounded with serous membranes known as visceral peritoneum.

**abdomin**-al, pertaining to the abdomen
**abdomin/o**-centesis, puncture of the abdomen (for aspiration)
**abdomin/o**-pelv-ic, pertaining to the pelvis or pelvic cavity and the abdomen
**abdomin/o**-perin-eal, pertaining to the perineum (space between the anus and scrotum or anus and vagina) and abdomen

## Quick Reference

Combining forms of roots relating to the digestive system:

| | | Page |
|---|---|---|
| **Abdomin/o** | abdomen | 20 |
| **An/o** | anus | 22 |
| **Appendic/o** | appendix | 22 |
| **Append/o** | appendix | 22 |
| **Bil/i** | bile | 23 |
| **Caec/o** | caecum | 23 |
| **Cholangi/o** | bile vessel | 24 |
| **Cholangiol/e** | fine bile vessel | 24 |
| **Chol/e** | bile | 24 |
| **Cholecyst/o** | gallbladder | 25 |
| **Choledoch/o** | common bile duct | 25 |
| **Col/o** | colon | 26 |
| **Colon/o** | colon | 26 |
| **Copr/o** | faeces | 27 |
| **Diverticul-** | diverticulum | 27 |
| **Duoden/o** | duodenum | 27 |
| **Enter/o** | intestine, s. intestine | 28 |
| **Epipl/o** | omentum | 30 |
| **Faec/o** | faeces | 30 |
| **Gastr/o** | stomach | 30 |
| **Gloss/o** | tongue | 32 |
| **Hepatic/o** | hepatic duct | 32 |
| **Hepat/o** | liver | 32 |
| **Ile/o** | ileum | 33 |
| **Jejun/o** | jejunum | 34 |
| **Lapar/o** | abdomen | 34 |
| **Lingu/o** | tongue | 34 |
| **Oesophag/o** | oesophagus | 34 |
| **Oment/o** | omentum | 35 |
| **Or/o** | mouth | 35 |
| **Pancreatic/o** | pancreatic duct | 36 |
| **Pancre/at/o** | pancreas | 36 |
| **Peps-** | digestion, pepsin | 36 |
| **Pept-** | digestion, pepsin | 36 |
| **Peritone/o** | peritoneum | 37 |
| **Port/o** | porta hepatis, portal vein | 37 |
| **Proct/o** | anus, rectum | 37 |
| **Ptyal/o** | saliva | 38 |
| **Pylor/i/o** | pylorus | 39 |
| **Rect/o** | rectum | 39 |
| **Sial/o** | saliva, salivary gland | 39 |
| **Sigmoid/o** | sigmoid colon | 40 |
| **Sphincter/o** | sphincter | 41 |
| **Splanchnic/o** | splanchnic nerve | 41 |
| **Splanchn/o** | viscera | 41 |
| **Sterc/o** | faeces | 41 |
| **Stomat/o** | mouth | 42 |
| **Typhl/o** | caecum | 42 |
| **Viscer/o** | viscera | 42 |

## Quick Reference

Common words and combining forms relating to the digestive system:

| | | Page |
|---|---|---|
| Abdomen | **abdomin/o, lapar/o** | 20 |
| Anus | **an/o, proct/o** | 22/37 |
| Appendix | **append/o, appendic/o** | 22 |
| Bile | **bil/i, chol/e** | 23/24 |
| Bile duct | **choledoch/o** | 25 |
| Bile vessel (fine) | **cholangiol/e** | 24 |
| Bile vessel | **cholangi/o** | 24 |
| Caecum | **caec/o, typhl/o** | 23/42 |
| Colon | **col/o, colon/o** | 26 |
| Common bile duct | **choledoch/o** | 25 |
| Digestion | **peps-, pept-** | 36 |
| Diverticulum | **diverticul-** | 27 |
| Duodenum | **duoden/o** | 27 |
| Entrance | **port/o** | 37 |
| Faeces | **copr/o, faec/o, sterc/o** | 27/30/41 |
| Gallbladder | **cholecyst/o** | 25 |
| Hepatic duct | **hepatic/o** | 32 |
| Ileum | **ile/o** | 33 |
| Intestine | **enter/o** | 28 |
| Jejunum | **jejun/o** | 34 |
| Liver | **hepat/o** | 32 |
| Mouth | **or/o, stomat/o** | 35/42 |
| Oesophagus | **oesophag/o** | 34 |
| Omentum | **epipl/o, oment/o** | 30/35 |
| Pancreas | **pancre/at/o** | 36 |
| Pancreatic duct | **pancreatic/o** | 36 |
| Pepsin | **peps-, pept-** | 36 |
| Peritoneum | **peritone/o** | 37 |
| Porta hepatis | **port/o** | 37 |
| Portal vein | **port/o** | 37 |
| Pylorus | **pylor/i/o** | 39 |
| Rectum | **rect/o, proct/o** | 39/37 |
| Saliva | **sial/o, ptyal/o** | 39/38 |
| Salivary gland | **sial/o, ptyal/o** | 39/38 |
| Sigmoid colon | **sigmoid/o** | 40 |
| Small intestine | **enter/o** | 28 |
| Sphincter | **sphincter/o** | 41 |
| Splanchnic nerve | **splanchnic/o** | 41 |
| Stomach | **gastr/o** | 30 |
| Tongue | **gloss/o, lingu/o** | 32/34 |
| Viscera | **splanchn/o, viscer/o** | 41/42 |

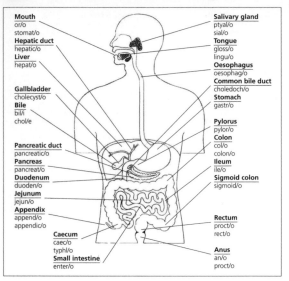

| Mouth | Salivary gland |
|---|---|
| or/o | ptyal/o |
| stomat/o | sial/o |
| **Hepatic duct** | **Tongue** |
| hepatic/o | gloss/o |
| **Liver** | lingu/o |
| hepat/o | **Oesophagus** |
| | oesophag/o |
| | **Common bile duct** |
| **Gallbladder** | choledoch/o |
| cholecyst/o | **Stomach** |
| **Bile** | gastr/o |
| bil/i | |
| chol/e | **Pylorus** |
| | pylor/o |
| | **Colon** |
| | col/o |
| **Pancreatic duct** | colon/o |
| pancreatic/o | **Ileum** |
| **Pancreas** | ile/o |
| pancreat/o | **Sigmoid colon** |
| **Duodenum** | sigmoid/o |
| duoden/o | |
| **Jejunum** | |
| jejun/o | **Rectum** |
| **Appendix** | proct/o |
| append/o | rect/o |
| appendic/o | |
| **Caecum** | **Anus** |
| caec/o | an/o |
| typhl/o | proct/o |
| **Small intestine** | |
| enter/o | |

Figure 5 The digestive system

sub-**abdomin**-al, pertaining to below the abdomen

---

**An/o**, anus
From the Latin word **anus** meaning the distal opening of the alimentary canal through which faeces leave the body. Here an/o means the anus, the opening formed by a sphincter muscle that relaxes to allow faecal matter to pass through.

**an**-al, pertaining to the anus

**an/o**-genit-al, pertaining to the genitalia and anus

**an/o**-perine-al, pertaining to the perineum and anus

**an/o**-plasty, surgical repair of anus

**an/o**-rect-al, pertaining to the rectum and anus

**an/o**-sigmoid/o-scopy, visual examination of the sigmoid colon, rectum and anus

circum-**an**-al, pertaining to around the anus

peri-**an**-al, pertaining to around the anus

---

**Append/o**, appendic/o, appendix
From the Latin word **appendix**, meaning appendage. Here appendic/o means the appendix, a blindly ending sac attached to the caecum with no known function in humans.

**append**-ectomy, removal of the appendix

**appendic**-ectomy, removal of the appendix

**appendic**-itis, inflammation of the appendix

**appendic/o**-stomy, formation of an opening into the appendix *e.g.* for drainage or the name of the opening so created

endo-**appendic**-itis, inflammation inside the appendix (the mucous membrane)

meso-**appendix**, the mesentery (peritoneal fold) of the appendix (joins the appendix to the ileum)

meso-**appendic**-itis, inflammation of the mesentery of the appendix

peri-**appendic**-itis, inflammation of the tissues around the appendix

**Bil/i**, bile

From a Latin word **bilis** meaning bile. Here bil/i means bile, a yellowish-brown liquid produced and excreted by the liver. Bile is stored in the gallbladder and excreted into the common bile duct when the gallbladder contracts eventually entering the duodenum where it acts to emulsify fat and oil.

**bil/i**-ary, pertaining to bile

**bil/i**-genesis, formation of bile

**bil/i**-gen-ic, pertaining to forming bile

**bil/i**-ous, 1. pertaining to bile 2. pertaining to biliousness

**bil/i**-ous-ness, popular term for symptoms of headache, nausea, constipation and loss of appetite formerly attributed to disordered secretion of bile

**bil/i**-rach-ia, condition of bile pigments in the spine (in spinal fluid)

**bil/i**-rub-in, a red pigment found in bile (formed from the breakdown of haemoglobin)

**bil/i**-rubin-aem-ia, condition of bilirubin in the blood

**bil/i**-rubin-ur-ia, condition of bilirubin in the urine

**bil/i**-ur-ia, condition of bile in the urine

**bil/i**-ur-ic, pertaining to bile in the urine

**bil/i**-verd-in, a green pigment found in bile (formed from the breakdown of haemoglobin and from oxidation of bilirubin)

**bil**-oma, a tumour-like swelling of bile (found encapsulated in the peritoneum)

**Caec/o**, caecum

From the Latin word **caecus** meaning blind. Here caec/o means the caecum, a blindly ending pouch attached to the vermiform appendix in the first part of the large intestine. The caecum is separated from the ileum by a valve, the ileocaecal valve.

**caec**-ectomy, removal of the caecum

**caec/o**-cele, a protrusion or hernia containing part of the caecum

**caec/o**-col/o-stomy, formation of an opening (anastomosis) between the colon and caecum or the name of the opening so created

**caec/o**-ile/o-stomy, formation of an opening (anastomosis) between the ileum and caecum or the name of the opening so created

**caec/o**-plication, act of making tucks or folds in the caecum by surgery

**caec/o**-rrhaphy, stitching or suturing of the caecum

**caec/o**-cyst/o-plasty, surgical repair or reconstruction of bladder using caecum

**caec/o**-proct/o-stomy, formation of an opening (anastomosis) between the rectum and caecum or the name of the opening so created Syn. caecorectostomy

**caec/o**-rect/o-stomy, formation of an opening (anastomosis) between the rectum and caecum or the name of the opening so created

**caec/o**-sigmoid/o-stomy, formation of an opening (anastomosis) between the sigmoid colon and caecum or the name of the opening so created

**caec/o**-stomy, formation of an opening into the caecum or the name of the opening so created

meso-**caec**-um, mesentery of the caecum (occasionally present in adults) peri-**caec**-al, pertaining to around the caecum

peri-**caec**-itis, inflammation (of structures) around the caecum

---

**Cholangi/o**, bile duct, bile vessel

From the Greek words **chole**, meaning bile, and **aggeion** meaning vessel. Here, cholangi/o means bile vessel or bile duct. The bile vessels that drain the major right and left lobes of the liver are formed by union of small bile capillaries originating between cords of liver cells. Bile vessels from the major lobes unite to form the hepatic duct which is joined by the cystic duct from the gallbladder to form the common bile duct. This joins the pancreatic duct, and the two enter the duodenum at the ampulla of Vater.

See the combining form cholangiol/e meaning a fine bile vessel.

**cholangi**-ectasis, dilation of a bile duct

**cholangi/o**-carcin-oma, a malignant tumour (cancer) of the bile duct

**cholangi/o**-enter/o-stomy, formation of an opening (anastomosis) between the small intestine and bile duct or the name of the opening so created

**cholangi/o**-gastr/o-stomy, formation of an opening (anastomosis) between the stomach and bile duct or the name of the opening so created

**cholangi/o**-gram, a recording or X-ray picture of bile vessels (hepatic duct, cystic duct and common bile duct)

**cholangi/o**-graphy, technique of making a recording or X-ray picture of bile ducts

**cholangi/o**-hepat-itis, inflammation of the liver and bile ducts

**cholangi/o**-hepat-oma, carcinoma of liver and bile ducts

**cholangi**-oma, a tumour of a bile duct (a cholangiocellular carcinoma)

**cholangi/o**-pancreat/o-graphy, technique of making a recording or X-ray of the pancreatic vessels and bile ducts e.g. ERCP endoscopic, retrograde cholangio-pancreatography

**cholangi/o**-stomy, formation of an opening into a bile duct or the name of the opening so created

**cholangi/o**-tomy, incision into a bile duct

**cholang**-itis, inflammation of bile ducts (also cholangeitis in use)

peri-**cholang**-itis, inflammation of tissues around bile ducts

---

**Cholangiol/e**, cholangiole, small bile vessels

From the Greek words **chole**, meaning bile, and **aggeion** meaning vessel. Here cholangiol/e means cholangiole, a fine termination of a bile vessel in the liver.

See the combining form cholangi/o meaning bile vessel.

**cholangiol**-ar, pertaining to cholangioles

**cholangiol**-ole, a small bile vessel

**cholangiol**-itis, inflammation of cholangioles

---

**Chol/e**, bile

From the Greek word **chole**, meaning bile. Here chol/e means bile, a yellowish-brown liquid produced and excreted by the liver. Bile is stored in the gallbladder and excreted into the common bile duct when the gallbladder contracts. Eventually, bile enters the duodenum where it acts to emulsify fat and oil.

**chol**-aem-ia, condition of blood containing bile

**chol**-agogue, an agent that promotes secretion of bile

**chol**-ia, condition of bile

**chole**-lith, a bile stone or calculus formed in the gallbladder or bile ducts, the term gallstone is in common use

**chole**-lith-iasis, presence of gallstones

**chole**-lith/o-tomy, incision of biliary tract to remove gallstones

**chole**-lith/o-tripsy, technique of crushing a gallstone

**chol**-emesis, vomiting of bile

**chole**-peritone-um, presence of bile in the peritoneum

**chole**-poiesis, formation of bile (in the liver)

**chole**-stasis, stoppage of bile flow

**chole**-steat-oma, a cyst-like mass containing cholesterol found in mastoid region behind the ear (not related to digestive system words)

**chole**-sterol, a fat-like steroid alcohol found in animal fats, bile and other tissues. Cholesterol forms a large part of most gallstones

**chole**-styram-ine, an ion-exchange resin which is used to combine with bile acids in the intestine. Used to lower cholesterol levels in the body and bring about hypocholesterolaemia

**chol**-ur-ia, condition of bile in the urine

eu-**chol**-ia, good or normal condition of bile

---

**Cholecyst/o**, gallbladder

From the Greek words **chole**, meaning bile, and **kystis** meaning bladder. Here cholecyst/o means the gallbladder, the structure that stores bile excreted by the liver. When the gallbladder contracts bile is forced through the cystic duct into the common bile duct and enters the duodenum at the ampulla of Vater.

**cholecyst**-agogue, an agent that promotes secretion of bile from the gallbladder, it evacuates the gallbladder

**cholecyst**-alg-ia, condition of pain in the gallbladder Syn. biliary colic

**cholecyst**-ectasis, dilation of the gallbladder

**cholecyst**-ectomy, removal of the gallbladder

**cholecyst**-enter/o-stomy, formation of an opening (anastomosis) between the intestine and gallbladder or the name of the opening so created

**cholecyst**-itis, inflammation of the gallbladder

**cholecyst/o**-col/o-stomy, formation of an opening (anastomosis) between the colon and gallbladder or the name of the opening so created

**cholecyst/o**-duoden-al, pertaining to the duodenum and gallbladder

**cholecyst/o**-duoden/o-stomy, formation of an opening (anastomosis) between the duodenum and gallbladder or the name of the opening so created

**cholecyst/o**-gastr/o-stomy, formation of an opening (anastomosis) between the stomach and gallbladder or the name of the opening so created

**cholecyst/o**-gram, a recording or X-ray picture of the gallbladder

**cholecyst/o**-graphy, technique of making a recording or X-ray picture of the gallbladder

**cholecyst/o**-jejun/o-stomy, formation of an opening (anastomosis) between the jejunum and gallbladder or the name of the opening so created

**cholecyst/o**-kinet-ic, pertaining to movement of the gallbladder, it refers to stimulating its contraction

**cholecyst/o**-kin-in, a hormone that stimulates gallbladder contraction (and secretion of pancreatic enzymes) Syn. pancreozymin

**cholecyst/o**-lith-iasis, presence of stones in the gallbladder (or other parts of biliary system)

**cholecyst/o**-pexy, surgical fixation of the gallbladder

**cholecyst/o**-rrhaphy, stitching or suturing of the gallbladder

**cholecyst/o**-stomy, formation of an opening into the gallbladder (for drainage) or the name of the opening so created

**cholecyst/o**-tomy, incision into the gallbladder

---

**Choledoch/o**, common bile duct

From the Greek words **chole**, meaning bile, and **dochos** meaning containing. Here choledoch/o means the common bile duct, a vessel that transfers bile from the gallbladder and hepatic ducts to the duodenum. The common bile duct joins the pancreatic duct at the ampulla of Vater and enters the duodenum.

**choledoch**-al, pertaining to the common bile duct

**choledoch**-ectomy, removal of part of the common bile duct

**choledoch**-itis, inflammation of the common bile duct

**choledoch/o**-duoden-al, pertaining to the duodenum and common bile duct

**choledoch/o**-duoden/o-stomy, formation of an opening (anastomosis) between the duodenum and common bile duct or the name of the opening so created

**choledoch/o**-enter/o-stomy, formation of an opening (anastomosis) between the small intestine and common bile duct or the name of the opening so created

**choledoch/o**-gastr/o-stomy, formation of an opening (anastomosis) between the stomach and common bile duct or the name of the opening so created

**choledoch/o**-graphy, technique of making a recording or X-ray picture of the common bile duct

**choledoch/o**-jejun/o-stomy, formation of an opening (anastomosis) between the jejunum and bile duct or the name of the opening so created

**choledoch/o**-lith-iasis, presence of stones in the common bile duct

**choledoch/o**-lith/o-tomy, incision into the common bile duct to remove stones

**choledoch/o**-plasty, surgical repair or reconstruction of the common bile duct

**choledoch/o**-rrhaphy, suturing or stitching of the common bile duct

**choledoch/o**-stomy, formation of an opening into the common bile duct (for drainage) or the name of the opening so created

**choledoch/o**-tomy, incision into the common bile duct

**choledoch**-us, the common bile duct

**Col/o, Colon/o,** colon
From a Greek word **kolon,** meaning colon. Here col/o means the colon, the large bowel extending from caecum to rectum. The colon is divided into four sections: the ascending colon, trans-

verse colon, descending colon and the sigmoid colon.

**col**-ectomy, removal of the colon

**col**-itis, inflammation of the colon

**col/o**-centesis, puncture of the colon

**col/o**-cholecyst/o-stomy, formation of an opening (anastomosis) between the gallbladder and colon or the name of the opening so created Syn. cholecystocolostomy

**col/o**-clyster, an enema injected into the colon (through the rectum)

**col/o**-col/o-stomy, formation of an opening (anastomosis) between the colon and another part of the colon or the name of the opening so created

**col/o**-cutane-ous, 1. pertaining to the skin and colon 2. communicating between the skin and colon

**col/o**-fixation, fixation or suspension of the colon e.g. for ptosis of the colon

**colon**-itis, inflammation of the colon Syn. colitis

**colon/o**-pathy, disease of the colon

**colon/o**-rrhoea, excessive flow from the colon (mucous colitis)

**colon/o**-scope, an instrument used to view the colon (a fibre-optic endoscope)

**colon/o**-scopy, technique of viewing or examining the colon with a fibre-optic endoscope

**col/o**-pexy, surgical fixation of the colon

**col/o**-plication, act of making a fold in the colon by surgery

**col/o**-proct-ectomy, removal of the rectum (anus) and colon

**col/o**-proct/o-stomy, formation of an opening (anastomosis) between the rectum and colon or the name of the opening so created Syn. colorectostomy

**col/o**-ptosis, downward displacement of the colon

**col/o**-puncture, puncture of the colon Syn. colocentesis

**col/o**-rect-al, pertaining to the rectum and colon

**col/o**-rect/o-stomy, formation of an opening (anastomosis) between the rectum and colon or the name of the opening so created

**col/o**-rectum, distal portion of colon and rectum regarded as a unit (25 cm in length)

**col/o**-rrhaphy, stitching or suturing of the colon

**col/o**-sigmoid/o-stomy, formation of an opening (anastomosis) between the sigmoid colon and colon or the name of the opening so created

**col/o**-stomy, formation of an opening into the colon (for drainage of faecal matter) to the body surface or the name of the opening so created

**col/o**-tomy, incision into the colon

**col/o**-vesic-al, pertaining to the bladder and colon

**col/o**-vesic/o-plasty, surgical repair of the bladder using colon

endo-**col**-itis, inflammation of the inside of the colon (its lining of mucous membrane)

macro-**colon**, a dilated or hypertrophied (enlarged) colon

mega-**colon**, a dilated or hypertrophied (enlarged) colon

meso-**colon**, the mesentery of the colon (it attaches the colon to the posterior abdominal wall)

pan-**col**-ectomy, removal of all of the colon

para-**col**-itis, inflammation near the colon (its outer coat)

peri-**col**-itis, inflammation around the colon (its peritoneal and sub-peritoneal coats)

## Copr/o, faeces

From a Greek word **kopros** meaning dung. Here copr/o means faeces, the residue discharged from the bowel through the anus. Faeces contains undigested plant fibres, epithelial cells, mucus, bacteria, electrolytes, stercobilin and various odour producing chemicals.

**copr/o**-lith, a faecal stone (compact faecal matter in the intestine)

**copr/o**-logy, the study of faeces (for diagnostic purposes)

**copr/o**-phagy, the eating of faeces (seen in some forms of mental illness)

**copr/o**-porphyr-ia, abnormal condition (metabolic disorder) of coproporphyrin in the faeces

**copr/o**-porphyr-in, a pyrrole, a chemical containing iron found in faeces (formed in haemopoietic organs)

**copr/o**-porphyrin-ur-ia, condition of coproporphyrin in the urine

**copr/o**-stas-ia, condition of stopping of faeces (faecal impaction or constipation)

**copr/o**-stasis, stopping of faeces (faecal impaction or constipation)

**copr/o**-zoa, animals of the faeces, it refers to organisms that digest faeces or sewage outside the body

## Diverticul-, diverticulum

From a Latin word **diverticulare** meaning to turn aside or bypass. Here diverticul- means a diverticulum, a pouch or sac protruding from the wall of a tube or hollow organ, especially the intestines. A diverticulum may be congenital or acquired.

**diverticul**-ar, pertaining to a diverticulum

**diverticul**-ectomy, removal of a diverticulum

**diverticul**-itis, inflammation of a diverticulum

**diverticul**-osis, presence of diverticula

peri-**diverticul**-itis, inflammation around a diverticulum

pre-**diverticul**-ar, pertaining to before a diverticulum, it refers to a thickening of the colon wall without the presence of a diverticulum

## Duoden/o, duodenum

From a Latin word **duodeni**, meaning twelve. Here duoden/o means the duodenum, the first 12 inches of the small intestine.

**duoden**-al, pertaining to the duodenum

**duoden**-ectomy, removal of the duodenum

27

**duoden**-itis, inflammation of the duodenum

**duoden/o**-choledoch/o-tomy, incision into the common bile duct and duodenum

**duoden/o**-duoden/o-stomy, formation of an opening (anastomosis) between the duodenum and another part of the duodenum or the name of the opening so created

**duoden/o**-enter/o-stomy, formation of an opening (anastomosis) between parts of the small intestine (jejunum or ileum) and duodenum or the name of the opening so created

**duoden/o**-gram, a recording or X-ray picture of the duodenum

**duoden/o**-hepat-ic, pertaining to the liver and duodenum

**duoden/o**-jejun-al, pertaining to the jejunum and duodenum

**duoden/o**-jejun/o-stomy, formation of an opening (anastomosis) between the jejunum and duodenum or the name of the opening so created

**duoden/o**-pancreat-ectomy, removal of the pancreas and duodenum

**duoden/o**-scope, an instrument used to view the duodenum, a fibre-optic endoscope

**duoden/o**-scopy, technique of viewing or examining the duodenum

**duoden/o**-stomy, formation of an opening into the duodenum or the name of the opening so created

meso-**duoden**-um, the mesentery of the duodenum (seen in the fetus and occasionally persists in the adult)

proto-**duoden**-um, the first part of the duodenum (from the pylorus to the duodenal papilla or ampulla of Vater)

---

**Enter/o, intestine**, usually the small intestine

From a Greek word **enteron**, meaning intestine or gut. Here enter/o means intestine or small intestine. The small intestine consists of the duodenum, jejunum and ileum that act to digest, absorb and move food towards the large intestine.

endo-**enter**-itis, inflammation inside the intestines (its mucosa)

**enter**-al, pertaining to the intestines (*e.g.* enteral feeding directly into intestines)

**enter**-alg-ia, condition of pain in the intestines

**enter**-ic, pertaining to the intestine

**enter**-itis, inflammation of the intestines

**enter/o**-anastomosis, intestinal anastomosis, it refers to an opening formed between two parts of an intestine

**enter**ob-iasis, infection with intestinal nematodes of genus *Enterobius*

**Enter**obius, a genus of intestinal nematodes (round worms)

**enter/o**-cele, a protrusion or hernia of the intestine

**enter/o**-centesis, surgical puncture of the intestine

**enter/o**-clysis, injection of liquids into the intestine

**Entero**-coccus, bacteria (streptococci) of the intestine (*e.g. Enterococcus faecalis*)

**enter/o**-col-ectomy, removal of the colon and small intestine

**enter/o**-col-itis, inflammation of the colon and small intestine

**enter/o**-col/o-stomy, formation of an opening (anastomosis) between the colon and part of the small intestine or the name of the opening so created

**enter/o**-cutane-ous, pertaining to the skin and intestine or communicating with the skin and intestine

**enter/o**-cyst, an intestinal cyst (from subperitoneal tissue)

**enter/o**-cyte, an intestinal cell

**enter/o**-enter/o-stomy, formation of an opening (anastomosis) between the two parts of the small intestine or the name of the opening so created

**enter/o**-epipl/o-cele, a protrusion or hernia of the omentum small intestine

**enter/o**-gastr-ic, pertaining to the stomach and intestine

**enter/o**-gastrone, a hormone secreted by the small intestine (duodenum) that inhibits gastric secretion

**enter/o**-gen-ous, 1. pertaining to originating in the small intestine 2. pertaining to forming from the small intestine

**enter/o**-graphy, technique of making a recording or X-ray picture of the intestines

**enter/o**-hepat-ic, pertaining to the liver and intestines

**enter/o**-hepat-itis, inflammation of the liver and intestines

**enter/o**-hepat/o-cele, a protrusion or hernia containing the liver and intestines

**enter/o**-hydr/o-cele, an intestinal protrusion or hernia with hydrocele

**enter/o**-kin-ase, an enzyme in intestinal juice that activates trypsinogen Syn. enteropeptidase

**enter/o**-kines-ia, condition of movement of the intestines (peristalsis)

**enter/o**-lith, a stone or calculus in the intestine

**enter/o**-lith-iasis, presence of calculi in the intestine

**enter/o**-log-ist, a specialist who studies the intestines

**enter/o**-logy, the study of the intestines (anatomy, diseases and treatment of)

**enter/o**-lysis, separation of intestinal adhesions (by surgery)

**enter/o**-myc-osis, abnormal condition of fungi in the intestines (fungal disease of)

**entero**n, the gut, alimentary canal or small intestine

**enter/o**-paresis, relaxation of intestine (slight paralysis)

**enter/o**-path/o-genesis, formation of a disease of the intestine

**enter/o**-pathy, disease of the intestine

**enter/o**-peptid-ase, an enzyme of intestinal juice that activates trypsinogen Syn. enterokinase

**enter/o**-pexy, surgical fixation of the intestine (to the abdominal wall)

**enter/o**-plasty, surgical repair or reconstruction of the intestine

**enter/o**-pleg-ia, condition of paralysis of intestines

**enter/o**-ptosis, downward displacement of the intestines

**enter/o**-rrhag-ia, condition of excessive flow of blood (haemorrhage) from the intestine

**enter/o**-rrhexis, rupture of the intestines

**enter/o**-scope, an instrument for viewing or examining the intestines

**enter/o**-sepsis, sepsis (infection) developed from intestinal contents

**enter/o**-staxis, slow haemorrhage (dripping) of the intestine

**enter/o**-stomy, formation of an opening into the intestines through the abdominal wall or the name of the opening so created

**enter/o**-tomy, incision into the intestines

**enter/o**-tox-aem-ia, condition of toxins (in blood) originating from the intestines

**enter/o**-tox-in, 1. a toxin arising in the intestine 2. a toxin that affects the intestine 3. an exotoxin produced by staphylococci

**enter/o**-tox-ism, process of poisoning of intestinal origin

**enter/o**-trop-ic, pertaining to affecting the intestine

**enter/o**-vagin-al, 1. pertaining to the vagina and intestine 2. pertaining to communication with the vagina and intestine

**enter/o**-ven-ous, 1. pertaining to a vein and the intestine 2. pertaining to communicating between a vein and the intestine (lumen)

**enter/o**-vesic-al, 1. pertaining to the urinary bladder and intestine 2. pertaining to communicating between the urinary bladder and intestine

**enter/o**-tribe, a metal clamp that causes necrosis of a colostomy prior to its closure

**enter/o**-virus, a virus infecting the intestines

**enter/o**-zoa, animal parasites affecting the intestines. Plural of enterozoon

**enter/o**-zoon, an animal parasite of the intestines. Singular of enterozoa

par-**enter**-al, pertaining to beyond the intestine, it refers to administering a drug in a manner other than through the intestines *e.g.* as an injection

**Epipl/o**, omentum

From a Greek word **epiploon** meaning caul. Here epipl/o means the omentum, a fold of peritoneum extending from the stomach to other adjacent viscera.

**epipl/o**-cele, a protrusion or hernia of the omentum Syn. omentocele

**epipl/o**-enter/o-cele, a protrusion or hernia containing intestines and omentum

**epipl/o**-ic, pertaining to or belonging to the omentum

**epipl**-omphal/o-cele, a protrusion or hernia of the umbilicus containing omentum

**epipl/o**-on, the omentum

**epipl/o**-pexy, surgical fixation of the omentum

**epipl/o**-plasty, 1. surgical repair or reconstruction of the omentum 2. surgical repair or reconstruction using the omentum to repair viscera

**epipl/o**-rrhaphy, stitching or suturing of the omentum

---

**Faec/a/o**, faeces

From Latin **faeces** meaning dregs. Here faec/o means faeces, the residue discharged from the bowel through the anus. Faeces contain undigested plant fibres, epithelial cells, mucus, bacteria, electrolytes, stercobilin and various odour producing chemicals.

**faec**-al, pertaining to or of the nature of faeces

**faec/a**-lith, a faecal stone (compact faecal matter in the intestine)

**faec/**-al-oid, resembling faeces or faecal matter

**faec/**-al-ur-ia, condition of urine containing faecal matter

**faec/o**-lith, a faecal stone (compact faecal matter in the intestine)

---

**Gastr/o**, stomach

From a Greek word **gaster**, meaning belly or stomach. Here gastr/o means the stomach, a dilated part of the alimentary canal situated between the oesophagus and small intestine. The stomach consists of three parts: cardia, fundus (body) and pylorus. The stomach lining (mucosa) produces gastric juice from cells lining gastric pits. The gastric juice contains hydrochloric acid and the enzyme pepsin that act to digest protein.

dextro-**gastr**-ia, condition of stomach displaced to the right

electro-**gastr/o**-graphy, technique of recording the electrical activity of the stomach

epi-**gastr**-ic, 1. pertaining to upon or above the stomach 2. pertaining to the epigastrium

epi-**gastr**-ium, the region above the stomach (the upper, middle region of the abdomen)

**gastr**-alg-ia, condition of pain in the stomach

**gastr**-ectomy, removal of the stomach

**gastr**-ic, pertaining to the stomach

**gastr**-in, a hormone secreted by gastric mucosa (stimulates the flow of gastric juice)

**gastr**-itis, inflammation of the stomach

**gastr/o**-anastomosis, formation of an opening (anastomosis) between the stomach and another remote part of the stomach or the name of the opening so created

**gastr/o**-cele, a protrusion or hernia of the stomach

**gastr/o**-col-ic, pertaining to the colon and stomach

**gastr/o**-col-itis, inflammation of the colon and stomach

**gastr/o**-col/o-stomy, formation of an opening (anastomosis) between the colon and stomach or the name of the opening so created

**gastr/o**-cnemius, belly of the tibia, a muscle in the leg (not relevant to the digestive system)

**gastr/o**-duoden-al, pertaining to the duodenum and stomach

**gastr/o**-duoden-itis, inflammation of the duodenum and stomach

**gastr/o**-duoden/o-stomy, formation of an opening (anastomosis) between the duodenum and stomach or the name of the opening so created

**gastr/o**-dyn-ia, condition of pain in the stomach

**gastr/o**-enter-alg-ia, condition of pain in the intestines and stomach

**gastr/o**-enter-itis, inflammation of the intestines and stomach

**gastr/o**-enter/o-col-itis, inflammation of the colon, small intestine and stomach

**gastr/o**-enter/o-log-ist, a specialist who studies the intestines and stomach

**gastr/o**-enter/o-logy, the study of intestines and stomach (anatomy, diseases and treatment of)

**gastr/o**-enter/o-pathy, disease of the intestines and stomach

**gastr/o**-enter/o-ptosis, displacement or prolapse of intestines and stomach

**gastr/o**-enter/o-scope, an instrument used to view the intestines and stomach (a fibre-optic endoscope)

**gastr/o**-enter/o-scopy, technique of viewing or examining the intestines and stomach

**gastr/o**-enter/o-stomy, formation of an opening (anastomosis) between the small intestine and stomach or the name of the opening so created

**gastr/o**-enter/o-tomy, incision into the intestines and stomach

**gastr/o**-**gastr/o**-stomy, formation of an opening (anastomosis) between the stomach and another remote part of the stomach or the name of the opening so created

**gastr/o**-hepat-itis, inflammation of the liver and stomach

**gastr/o**-ile-itis, inflammation of the ileum and stomach

**gastr/o**-ile/o-stomy, formation of an opening (anastomosis) between the ileum and stomach or the name of the opening so created

**gastr/o**-intestin-al, pertaining to the intestines and stomach

**gastr/o**-jejun/o-col-ic, pertaining to the colon, jejunum and stomach

**gastr/o**-jejun/o-stomy, formation of an opening (anastomosis) between the jejunum and stomach or the name of the opening so created

**gastr/o**-lien-al, pertaining to the spleen and stomach

**gastr/o**-lith-iasis, abnormal condition of stones or calculi in the stomach

**gastr/o**-logy, the study of the stomach (anatomy, diseases and treatment of)

**gastr/o**-oesophag-eal, pertaining to the oesophagus and stomach

**gastr/o**-oesophag-itis, inflammation of the oesophagus and stomach

**gastr/o**-oesophag/o-stomy, formation of an opening (anastomosis) between the oesophagus and stomach or the name of the opening so created

**gastr/o**-pathy, disease of the stomach

**gastr/o**-pexy, fixation of the stomach (by surgery)

**gastr/o**-phren-ic, pertaining to the diaphragm and stomach

**gastr/o**-plasty, surgical repair or reconstruction of stomach

**gastr/o**-plication, act of folding the stomach (wall) by surgery

**gastr/o**-ptosis, downward displacement of stomach

**gastr/o**-pylor-ectomy, removal of the pylorus and stomach

**gastr/o**-schisis, parting or splitting (incomplete closure) of the abdominal wall, the stomach and other viscera protrude

**gastr/o**-scope, an instrument used to view the stomach (a fibre-optic endoscope)

**gastr/o**-scopy, technique of viewing or examining the stomach

**gastr/o**-splen-ic, pertaining to the spleen and stomach

**gastr/o**-stomy, formation of an opening into the stomach or the name of the opening so created

**gastr/o**-tomy, incision into the stomach

hemi-**gastr**-ectomy, removal of half the stomach

hypo-**gastr**-ic, 1. pertaining to below the stomach 2. pertaining to the hypogastrium

hypo-**gastr**-ium, the region below the stomach (the lowest median region of the abdomen)

megalo-**gastr**-ia, condition of abnormally enlarged stomach tachy-**gastr**-ia, condition of fast stomach, it refers to a high frequency of electric potentials in the stomach

**Gloss/o**, tongue

From a Greek word **glossa**, meaning tongue. Here gloss/o means the tongue, the mobile muscular organ in the mouth. The tongue plays a vital role in speech, mastication (chewing of food) and swallowing. Papillae on the surface of the tongue contain nerve endings (chemoreceptors) that produce the sense of taste and are sometimes called the taste buds. The chemoreceptors detect chemicals in our food that we describe as sweet, sour, bitter or salty.

**glossa**, the tongue

**gloss**-ectomy, removal of the tongue

**gloss**-itis, inflammation of the tongue

**gloss/o**-cele, a protrusion or hernia of the tongue

**gloss/o**-dyn-ia, condition of pain in the tongue

**gloss/o**-graph, an instrument used for recording the tongue ( movements in speech)

**gloss/o**-pharyng-eal, pertaining to the pharynx and tongue

**gloss/o**-plasty, surgical repair or reconstruction of the tongue

**gloss/o**-pleg-ia, condition of paralysis of the tongue

**gloss/o**-rrhaphy, stitching or suturing of the tongue

**gloss/o**-trich-ia, condition of hairy tongue

**Hepatic/o**, hepatic duct

From a Greek word **hepatos**, meaning the liver. Here hepatic/o means the hepatic duct. The right and left hepatic ducts drain bile from the liver into the common hepatic duct.

**hepatico**-choledoch/o-stomy, formation of an opening (anastomosis) between the bile duct and hepatic duct or the name of the opening so created

**hepatic/o**-enter-ic, pertaining to the small intestine and hepatic duct

**hepatic/o**-duoden/o-stomy, formation of an opening (anastomosis) between the duodenum and hepatic duct or the name of the opening so created

**hepatic/o**-gastr/o-stomy, formation of an opening (anastomosis) between the stomach and hepatic duct or the name of the opening so created

**hepatic/o**-jejun/o-stomy, formation of an opening (anastomosis) between the jejunum and hepatic duct or the name of the opening so created

**hepatic/o**-lith/o-tomy, incision to remove a stone or calculus from the hepatic duct

**hepatic/o**-stomy, formation of an opening into the hepatic duct or the name of the opening so created

**Hepat/o**, liver

From a Greek word **hepatos**, meaning the liver. Here hepat/o means the liver, the largest organ in the body situated in the right upper section of the abdominal cavity. The liver secretes bile, stores glycogen, minerals and vitamins, and plays a major role in the metabolism of carbohydrates, proteins and lipids.

**hepat**-ectomy, removal of the liver

**hepat**-ic, pertaining to the liver

**hepat**-itis, inflammation of the liver

**hepat**-ization, a transformation into a liver-like mass

**hepat/o**-blast-oma, a malignant tumour in the liver formed from embryonic tissue, seen in children

**hepat/o**-carcin-oma, a malignant tumour of liver cells (cancer)

**hepat/o**-cele, a protrusion or hernia of the liver

**hepat/o**-cellul-ar, pertaining to or affecting liver cells

**hepat/o**-chol-angi/o-carcin-oma, a malignant tumour of bile vessels (ducts) and liver

**hepat/o**-cirrh-osis, condition of cirrhosis (orange-tawny appearance) of the liver. The liver hardens due to formation of fibrous tissue within.

**hepat/o**-cyte, a cell of the liver

**hepat/o**-gastr-ic, pertaining to the stomach and liver

**hepat/o**-gram, a recording or X-ray picture of the liver

**hepat/o**-graphy, technique of making a recording or X-ray picture of the liver

**hepat**-oid, resembling the liver

**hepat/o**-jugul-ar, pertaining to the jugular veins and liver

**hepat/o**-lith, a stone or calculus in the liver

**hepat/o**-lith-iasis, presence of stones in the liver (calculi in biliary ducts)

**hepat/o**-logy, the study of the liver (anatomy, diseases and treatment of)

**hepat/o**-lys-in, an agent that breaks down liver cells (cytolysin)

**hepat/o**-lysis, breakdown or destruction of liver cells

**hepat**-oma, a tumour of the liver (primary carcinoma). Plural hepatomata, hepatomas

**hepat/o**-megaly, enlargement of the liver

**hepat/o**-melan-osis, condition of dark pigmentation of the liver

**hepat**-omphal/o-cele, an umbilical hernia with liver protruding into the hernia sac

**hepat/o**-pancreat-ic, pertaining to the pancreas and liver

**hepat/o**-pexy, surgical fixation of the liver

**hepat/o**-pneumon-ic, 1. pertaining to the lungs and liver 2. affecting or communicating with the lungs and liver

**hepat/o**-port-al, pertaining to the portal system and liver

**hepat/o**-ren-al, pertaining to the kidneys and liver

**hepat/o**-rrhexis, rupture of the liver

**hepat**-osis, abnormal condition of the liver

**hepat/o**-splen-ic, pertaining to the spleen and liver

**hepat/o**-splen-itis, inflammation of the spleen and liver

**hepat/o**-splen/o-megaly, enlargement of the spleen and liver

**hepat/o**-tox-aem-ia, condition of blood poisoning originating in the liver

**hepat/o**-tox-ic, pertaining to poisoning of the liver

**hepat/o**-tox-in, an agent poisonous to the liver, it destroys the liver

post-**hepat**-ic, pertaining to behind the liver

post-**hepat**-itic, pertaining to after hepatitis

sub-**hepat**-ic, pertaining to below the liver

---

**Ile/o**, ileum

From a Latin word **ilia**, meaning intestines. Here ile/o means the ileum, the distal three-fifths of the small intestine lying between the jejunum and caecum and connected to the caecum at the ileocaecal valve. The ileum is approximately 3.6 m long and has a large surface area to absorb nutrients across its surface (mucosa).

**ile**-itis, inflammation of the ileum

**ile/o**-caec-al, pertaining to the caecum and ileum

**ile/o**-caec/o-stomy, formation of an opening (anastomosis) between the caecum and ileum or the name of the opening so created

**ile/o**-col-ic, pertaining to the colon and ileum

**ile/o**-col-itis, inflammation of the colon and ileum

**ile/o**-col/o-stomy, formation of an opening (anastomosis) between the colon and ileum or the name of the opening so created

**ile/o**-cutane-ous, pertaining to or communicating with the skin and ileum

**ile/o**-cyst/o-plasty, surgical repair or reconstruction of the bladder using ileum

**ile/o**-cyst/o-stomy, formation of an opening (anastomosis) between the bladder and abdominal wall using ileum

**ile/o**-ile/o-stomy, formation of an opening (anastomosis) between the ileum and another remote part of the ileum or the name of the opening so created

**ile/o**-proct/o-stomy, formation of an opening (anastomosis) between the anus and ileum or the name of the opening so created

**ile/o**-rect-al, pertaining to the rectum and ileum

**ile/o**-rrhaphy, stitching or suturing of the ileum

**ile/o**-sigmoid/o-stomy, formation of an opening (anastomosis) between the sigmoid colon and ileum or the name of the opening so created

**ile/o**-stomy, formation of an opening into the ileum through the abdominal wall (for drainage of faecal matter) or the name of the opening so created

**ile/o**-tomy, incision into the ileum

**ile/o**-ureter/o-stomy, formation of an opening (anastomosis) between the ureters and ileum or the name of the opening so created

**ile**-us, intestinal obstruction in the ileum

---

**Jejun/o**, jejunum

From a Latin word **jejunus**, meaning empty. Here jejun/o means the jejunum, part of the intestine between the duodenum and ileum approximately 2.4 m. in length. The jejunum acts to digest and absorb food.

**jejun**-al, pertaining to the jejunum

**jejun**-ectomy, removal of the jejunum

**jejun/o**-caec/o-stomy, formation of an opening (anastomosis) between the caecum and jejunum or the name of the opening so created

**jejun/o**-ile-itis, inflammation of the ileum and jejunum

**jejun/o-jejun/o**-stomy, formation of an opening (anastomosis) between two parts of the jejunum or the name of the opening so created

**jejun/o**-stomy, formation of an opening into the jejunum or the name of the opening so created

**jejun/o**-tomy, incision into the jejunum

---

**Lapar/o**, abdominal wall, flank

From a Greek word **lapara**, meaning loin. Here lapar/o means flank, the soft part between the ribs and hips but by common usage it has come to mean the abdominal wall.

**lapar**-ectomy, removal of tissue from the wall of the abdomen

**lapar/o**-enter/o-stomy, formation of an opening between the intestine and the abdominal wall (for drainage) or the name of the opening so created

**lapar/o**-enter/o-tomy, incision into the intestine through the abdominal wall

**lapar/o**-scope, an instrument (endoscope) used to view the abdomen (peritoneal cavity) through the abdominal wall

**lapar/o**-scop-ic, pertaining to viewing or examining the abdomen (peritoneal cavity) with an endoscope through the abdominal wall

**lapar/o**-scopy, technique of viewing or examining the abdomen (peritoneal cavity) with an endoscope through the abdominal wall

**lapar/o**-tomy, incision into the abdominal wall

---

**Lingu/o**, tongue

From a Latin word **lingua** meaning tongue. Here lingu/o means the tongue, the mobile muscular organ in the mouth. The tongue plays a vital role in speech, mastication (chewing of food) and swallowing. Papillae on the surface of the tongue contain nerve endings (chemoreceptors) that produce the sense of taste and are sometimes called the taste buds. The chemoreceptors detect chemicals in our food that we describe as sweet, sour, bitter or salty.

**lingu**a, the tongue

**lingu**-al, pertaining to the tongue

**lingu/o**-dist-al, pertaining to the lingual and distal surfaces *e.g.* of a tooth or tooth cavity

**lingu/o**-papill-itis, inflammation of the papillae of the tongue

---

**Oesophag/o**, oesophagus

From a Greek word **oisophagos**, meaning gullet. Here, oesophag/o means the oesophagus, a musculo-membranous canal 23 cm in length extending from the pharynx to the stomach, it acts to transfer food from the mouth to the stomach.

oesophag-eal, pertaining to the oesophagus

oesophag-ectasis, dilation of the oesophagus

oesophag-ectomy, removal of the oesophagus

oesophag-itis, inflammation of the oesophagus

oesophag/o-cele, a protrusion or hernia of the oesophagus

oesophag/o-col/o-plasty, surgical repair or reconstruction of the oesophagus using colon

oesophag/o-duoden/o-stomy, formation of an opening (anastomosis) between the duodenum and oesophagus or the name of the opening so created

oesophag/o-gastr-ectomy, removal of the stomach and oesophagus

oesophag/o-gastr/o-duoden/o-scopy, technique of viewing or examining the duodenum, stomach and oesophagus (with a fibre-optic endoscope)

oesophag/o-gastr/o-stomy, formation of an opening (anastomosis) between the stomach and oesophagus or the name of the opening so created

oesophag/o-jejun/o-stomy, formation of an opening (anastomosis) between the jejunum and oesophagus or the name of the opening so created

oesophag/o-my/o-tomy, incision through the muscular coat of the oesophagus

oesophag/o-oesophag/o-stomy, formation of an opening (anastomosis) between the oesophagus and another remote part of the oesophagus or the name of the opening so created

oesophag/o-plication, act of making tucks or folds in the oesophagus by surgery

oesophag/o-scope, an instrument used to view the oesophagus (endoscope)

oesophag/o-scopy, technique of viewing or examining the oesophagus

oesophag/o-sten-osis, abnormal condition of narrowing of the oesophagus

oesophag/o-stomy, formation of an opening into the oesophagus (*e.g.* for feeding) or the name of the opening so created

oesophag/o-tomy, incision into the oesophagus

---

**Oment/o**, omentum
From a Latin word **omentum**. Here oment/o means the omentum, a fold of peritoneum extending from the stomach to other adjacent viscera.

oment-al, pertaining to the omentum

oment-ectomy, removal of the omentum

oment-itis, inflammation of the omentum

oment/o-pexy, surgical fixation of the omentum

oment/o-rrhaphy, stitching or suturing of the omentum

oment/o-cele, a protrusion or hernia of the omentum Syn. epiplocele

oment/o-plasty, 1. surgical repair or reconstruction of the omentum 2. using the omentum to repair viscera

oment/o-splen/o-pexy, surgical fixation of the spleen and omentum

oment/o-tomy, incision of the omentum

---

**Or/o**, mouth
From a Latin word **oris**, meaning mouth. Here or/o means the mouth, a cavity bounded by the closed lips and facial muscles, the hard and soft palate and lower jaw. The mouth contains the upper and lower teeth and the tongue. Three pairs of salivary glands (parotid, submaxillary and sublingual) secrete saliva into the mouth.

or-al, pertaining to the mouth

or-al-ity, 1. state or condition pertaining to the mouth 2. all aspects of the mouth (sucking, mouthing, and the oral stage of psychosexual development)

**or/o**-genit-al, pertaining to the genitalia and mouth

**or/o**-lingu-al, pertaining to the tongue and mouth

**or/o**-nas-al, pertaining to the nose and mouth

**or/o**-pharynx, part of pharynx between the soft palate and upper epiglottis

---

**Pancreatic/o**, pancreatic duct

From a Greek word **pankreas**, meaning the pancreas. Here pancreatic/o means the pancreatic duct, a vessel that transfers pancreatic juice containing digestive enzymes from the pancreas to the duodenum.

**pancreatic/o**-duoden-al, pertaining to the duodenum and pancreatic duct

**pancreatic/o**-duoden-ectomy, removal of the duodenum and pancreatic duct or pancreas. Whipple's procedure

**pancreatic/o**-duoden-ostomy, formation of an opening (anastomosis) between the duodenum and pancreatic duct or the name of the opening so created

**pancreatic/o**-enter/o-stomy, formation of an opening (anastomosis) between the small intestine and pancreatic duct or the name of the opening so created

**pancreatic/o**-gastr/o-stomy, formation of an opening (anastomosis) between the stomach and pancreatic duct or the name of the opening so created

**pancreatic/o**-jejun/o-stomy, formation of an opening (anastomosis) between the jejunum and pancreatic duct or the name of the opening so created

---

**Pancre/a/t/o**, pancreas

From the Greek word **pankreas**, **pan** meaning all and **kreas** meaning flesh. Here pancreat/o means the pancreas, a large gland situated below and behind the stomach approximately 18 cm long. The exocrine part of the gland secretes pancreatic juice into the duodenum via the pancreatic duct. The juice contains enzymes that digest fats, proteins and carbohydrates. The pancreas also con-

tains patches of endocrine tissue called the Islets of Langerhan's that secrete the hormones insulin and glucagon.

**pancreat**-ectomy, removal of the pancreas

**pancreat**-ic, pertaining to or belonging to the pancreas

**pancreat**-in, a mixture of enzymes from the pancreas

**pancreat**-itis, inflammation of the pancreas

**pancreat/o**-duoden-ectomy, removal of the duodenum and (head of) the pancreas

**pancreat/o**-gen-ous, pertaining to forming or arising in the pancreas

**pancreat/o**-graphy, technique of making a recording or X-ray picture of the pancreas

**pancreat/o**-lith-ectomy, removal of a stone from the pancreas

**pancreat/o**-lith-iasis, presence of stones in the pancreas, in the duct system or parenchyma of the pancreas

**pancreat/o**-lith-tomy, incision into the pancreas to remove a stone

**pancreat/o**-lysis, breakdown or disintegration of the pancreas

**pancreat/o**-lyt-ic, pertaining to the breakdown or disintegration of the pancreas

**pancreat/o**-megaly, enlargement of the pancreas

**pancreat/o**-tomy, incision into the pancreas

**pancreat/o**-trop-ic, pertaining to having an affinity for the pancreas

**pancrea**-troph-ic, pertaining to nourishing or having an influence on the pancreas

**pancreo**-priv-ic, pertaining to lacking a pancreas

**pancreo**-zym-in, a hormone secreted by the duodenum that stimulates the flow of pancreatic juice

---

**Peps-, pept-**, digestion, pepsin

From a Greek word **peptein** meaning to digest. Here, peps- and pept- mean digestion, pepsin or the action of gastric juice in the stomach.

dys-**peps**-ia, condition of difficult or bad digestion (usually applied to epigastric pain)

dys-**pept**-ic, 1. pertaining to having dyspepsia 2. pertaining to difficult or bad digestion (usually applied to epigastric pain)

eu-**peps**-ia, 1. condition of good digestion 2. secreting the normal amount of pepsin

eu-**pept**-ic, 1. pertaining to having eupepsia 2. pertaining to secreting the normal amount of pepsin

**pept**-ic, 1. pertaining to digestion 2. pertaining to pepsin

**peps**-in, an agent (enzyme) that digests protein to peptides in the stomach

**peps**in/o-gen, an agent that forms pepsin (a precursor of pepsin secreted by the stomach)

---

**Peritone/o**, peritoneum

From a Greek word **peri**, meaning around, and **teinein**, meaning to stretch. Here peritone/o means the peritoneum, the serous membrane that lines the abdominal and pelvic cavities and covers abdominal organs. Parietal peritoneum lines the walls of cavities and visceral peritoneum covers organs. These membranes secrete a lubricating serous fluid that allows abdominal organs to slide over each other as they move.

endo-**periton**-itis, inflammation inside or within the peritoneum (its serous lining)

hydro-**peritone**-um, accumulation of water in the peritoneal cavity (ascites)

pachy-**periton**-itis, inflammation and thickening of the peritoneum

**peritone**-al, pertaining to the peritoneum

**peritone**-alg-ia, condition of pain in the peritoneum

**peritone/o**-centesis, puncture of the abdominal cavity through the peritoneum

**peritone/o**-clysis, injection of fluid into the peritoneal cavity

**peritone/o**-scopy, technique of viewing or examining the peritoneum Syn. laparoscopy

**peritone/o**-tomy, incision into the peritoneum

**peritone/o**-ven-ous, pertaining to or communication between the venous system and peritoneum

**periton**-itis, inflammation of the peritoneum

retro-**peritone**-al, pertaining to behind the peritoneum

retro-**periton**-itis, inflammation of the retroperitoneum

retro-**peritone**-um, the space behind the peritoneum

---

**Port/o**, entrance, porta hepatis, portal vein

From a Latin word **porta** meaning gateway or entrance. Here, port/o means an entrance through which blood vessels supply or drain an organ. The porta hepatis is a transverse fissure on the underside of the liver through which the portal vein passes.

**porta**-hepat-itis, inflammation of the liver porta (transverse fissure)

**port**-al, pertaining to a porta especially porta hepatis

**port/o**-cav-al, pertaining to the inferior vena cava and portal vein

**port/o**-enter/o-stomy, formation of an opening (anastomosis) between the small intestine and porta hepatis or the name of the opening so created

**port/o**-gram, a recording or X-ray picture of the portal vein

**port/o**-graphy, technique of making a recording or X-ray picture of the portal vein

**port/o**-system-ic, pertaining to or communicating with the systemic venous and portal circulation

---

**Proct/o**, anus, rectum

From a Greek word **proktos**, meaning anus. Here proct/o means the anus or rectum. The rectum is the distal canal through which faeces leave the body, the anus is the opening of the rectum.

peri-**proct**-itis, inflammation (of tissues) around the rectum and anus

**proct**-alg-ia, condition of pain in the rectum

**proct**-atres-ia, condition of absence of anus or imperforate anus

**proct**-ectas-ia, condition of dilation of rectum or anus

**proct**-ectomy, removal of the rectum

**proct**-eurynter, a bag-like device used to dilate the anus

**proct**-itis, inflammation of the rectum

**proct/o**-cele, a protrusion or hernia of the rectum *e.g.* into the vaginal wall

**proct/o**-clysis, injection of liquid into the rectum, an enema

**proct/o**-col-ectomy, removal of the colon and rectum

**proct/o**-col-itis, inflammation of the colon and rectum

**proct/o**-colp/o-plasty, surgical repair or reconstruction of the vagina and rectum *e.g.* of a fistula between the vagina and rectum

**proct/o**-cyst/o-plasty, surgical repair or reconstruction of the bladder and rectum *e.g.* of a fistula between the bladder and rectum

**proct/o**-cyst/o-tomy, incision of the bladder through the rectum

**proct/o**-deum, depression in the caudal end of the embryo which forms the anus. From a Greek word *hodaios* meaning concerning a way

**proct/o**-logy, the study of the rectum and anus (anatomy, diseases and treatment of)

**proct/o**-paralysis, paralysis of the rectal and anal muscles

**proct/o**-pexy, surgical fixation of the rectum

**proct/o**-plasty, surgical repair or reconstruction of the rectum

**proct/o**-pleg-ia, condition of paralysis of the rectum

**proct/o**-ptosis, displacement or prolapse of the rectum

**proct/o**-rrhaphy, stitching or suturing of the rectum

**proct/o**-rrhoea, excessive discharge or flow from the anus or rectum

**proct/o**-scope, an instrument used to view the rectum

**proct/o**-scop-ic, pertaining to viewing with a proctoscope

**proct/o**-scopy, technique of viewing or examining the rectum

**proct/o**-sigmoid-itis, inflammation of the sigmoid colon and rectum

**proct/o**-sigmoid/o-scope, an instrument used to view the sigmoid colon and rectum

**proct/o**-sigmoid/o-scopy, technique of viewing or examining the sigmoid colon and rectum

**proct/o**-sten-osis, condition of narrowing of the rectum

**proct/o**-stomy, formation of an opening into the rectum from body surface or the name of the opening so created

**proct/o**-tomy, incision into the rectum

**Ptyal/o**, saliva

From a Greek word **ptyalon**, meaning saliva. Here ptyal/o means saliva, a secretion produced by the three pairs of salivary glands (parotid, submaxillary and sublingual) in the mouth. Saliva contains water, mucin and the enzyme amylase (ptyalin) that can digest starch into maltose sugar.

**ptyal**-agogue, an agent which stimulates or induces flow of saliva Syn. sialagogue

**ptyal**-ectasis, dilation of a salivary duct or vessel

**ptyal**-in, an agent in saliva, it refers to the salivary enzyme (amylase)

**ptyal**-ism, process of excessive secretion of saliva

**ptyal/o**-cele, a protrusion or swelling containing saliva *e.g.* cystic tumour

**ptyal/o**-gen-ic, pertaining to forming from the action of saliva

**ptyal/o**-lith, a stone in or calculus in the saliva Syn. sialolith

**ptyal/o**-react-ion, a reaction occurring in or performed on saliva

**ptyal/o**-rrhoea, excessive flow of saliva Syn. ptyalism, sialorrhoea and sialismus

**Pylor/o**, pylor/i/o

From a Greek word **pylouros**, meaning gate-keeper. Here pylor/o means the pylorus, the opening of the stomach into the duodenum encircled by a sphincter muscle. The pylorus opens periodically to allow partially digested food to leave the stomach.

**pylor**-alg-ia, condition of pain in the pylorus

**pylor**-ectomy, removal of the pylorus

**pylor/i**-sten-osis, condition of narrowing of the pylorus Syn. pyloric stenosis

**pylor**-ic, pertaining to the pylorus

**pylor/o**-diosis, dilation of the pylorus with a finger during operation. From a Greek word *diosis* meaning a pushing apart

**pylor/o**-duoden-al, pertaining to the duodenum and pylorus

**pylor/o**-duoden-itis, inflammation of the duodenum and pylorus

**pylor/o**-gastr-ectomy, removal of the stomach and pylorus

**pylor/o**-my/o-tomy, incision of the muscles (circular and longitudinal) of the pylorus

**pylor/o**-plasty, surgical repair or reconstruction of the pylorus

**pylor/o**-scopy, technique of viewing or examining the pylorus *e.g.* with an endoscope

**pylor/o**-spasm, spasm of pyloric muscle

**pylor/o**-stomy, formation of an opening into the pylorus from the surface of the body or the name of the opening so created

**pylor/o**-tomy, incision into the pylorus

**Rect/o**, rectum

From a Latin word **rectus**, meaning straight. Here rect/o means the rectum, the straight distal part of the large intestine. The rectum lies between the sigmoid flexure and anal canal.

mega-**rect**-um, an abnormally enlarged rectum

**rect**-alg-ia, condition of pain in the rectum

**rect**-ectomy, removal of the rectum Syn. proctectomy

**rect**-itis, inflammation of the rectum Syn. proctitis

**rect/o**-abdomin-al, pertaining to the abdomen and rectum

**rect/o**-cele, a protrusion or hernia of rectum (into the vagina)

**rect/o**-col-itis, inflammation of the colon and rectum Syn. coloproctitis

**rect/o**-cutane-ous, pertaining to the skin and rectum

**rect/o**-labi-al, pertaining to the labia majus and rectum

**rect/o**-pexy, surgical fixation of the rectum Syn. proctopexy

**rect/o**-plasty, surgical repair or reconstruction of the rectum Syn. proctoplasty

**rect/o**-scope, an instrument used to view the rectum

**rect/o**-sigmoid, pertaining to the sigmoid colon and rectum *e.g.* the rectosigmoid junction

**rect/o**-sigmoid-ectomy, removal of the sigmoid colon and rectum

**rect/o**-stomy, formation of an opening into the rectum from body surface or the name of the opening so created Syn. proctostomy

**rect/o**-urethr-al, 1. pertaining to the urethra and rectum 2. communicating with the urethra and rectum

**rect/o**-uter-ine, 1. pertaining to the uterus and rectum 2. communicating with the uterus and rectum

**rect/o**-vagin-al, 1. pertaining to the vagina and rectum 2. communicating with the vagina and rectum

**rect/o**-vesic-al, 1. pertaining to the bladder and rectum 2. communicating with the bladder and rectum

**rect**-us, a straight structure, the rectum

**Sial/o**, saliva, salivary gland

From a Greek word **sialon**, meaning saliva. Here sial/o means saliva, salivary glands or salivary duct. Saliva is the secretion produced by the salivary glands in the mouth. It contains water, mucin and the enzyme amylase (ptyalin) that can digest starch into maltose sugar. There are three pairs of salivary glands in the mouth, parotid, submaxillary and sublingual.

poly-**sial**-ia, condition of too much saliva

**sial**-aden-itis, inflammation of a salivary gland

**sial**-aden-osis, abnormal condition of a salivary gland Syn. sialadenitis

**sial**-agogue, an agent that stimulates or induces flow of saliva

**sial**-ectas-ia, condition of dilation of a salivary duct

**sial**-ine, pertaining to saliva

**sial**-ismus, excessive secretion of saliva Syn. ptyalism

**sial**-itis, inflammation of a salivary gland

**sial**/o-aden-ectomy, removal of a salivary gland

**sial**/o-aden-itis, inflammation of a salivary gland

**sial**/o-aden/o-tomy, incision into a salivary gland (often for drainage)

**sial**/o-aer/o-phag-ia, condition of swallowing air and saliva

**sial**/o-angi-ectasis, condition of dilated salivary vessels or ducts Syn. sialectasia

**sial**/o-angi-itis, inflammation of salivary vessels or ducts

**sial**/o-angi/o-graphy, technique of making a recording or X-ray picture of salivary vessels or ducts

**sial**/o-cele, a swelling of the salivary gland *e.g.* salivary cyst

**sial**/o-doch-itis, inflammation of a salivary duct

**sial**/o-doch/o-plasty, surgical repair or reconstruction of a salivary duct

**sial**/o-duct-itis, inflammation of a salivary duct Syn. sialoangiitis

**sial**/o-gen-ous, pertaining to producing or forming saliva

**sial**/o-gram, a recording or X-ray picture of the salivary glands and ducts

**sial**/o-graphy, technique of making a recording or X-ray picture of saliva (*i.e.* salivary vessels) Syn. sialangiography

**sial**/o-lith, a stone in a salivary gland or duct

**sial**/o-lith-iasis, presence of stones or calculi in saliva

**sial**/o-lith/o-tomy, incision to remove a salivary stone or calculus

**sial**/o-meta-plas-ia, condition of transformation of normal adult cells of the salivary glands to abnormal cells

**sial**/o-rrhoea, excessive flow of saliva Syn. ptyalism or sialismus

**sial**/o-schesis, suppression of secretion of saliva

**sial**-osis, abnormal condition of of saliva, it refers to abnormal flow of saliva

**sial**/o-sten-osis, condition of narrowing of the salivary ducts

**sial**/o-syrinx, 1. an abnormal opening (fistula) in a salivary gland or duct 2. a drainage tube for the salivary ducts

---

**Sigmoid/o**, sigmoid colon

From a Greek word **sigma** – meaning the letter S. Here sigmoid/o means the sigmoid colon, the distal part of the descending colon (large bowel) that resembles an S-shape. The sigmoid colon connects the descending colon to the rectum.

**sigm**-oid, resembling an S, used to refer to the S-shaped sigmoid colon

**sigmoid**-ectomy, removal of the sigmoid colon

**sigmoid**-itis, inflammation of the sigmoid colon

**sigmoid**/o-pexy, surgical fixation of the sigmoid colon

**sigmoid**/o-proct/o-stomy, formation of an opening (anastomosis) between the rectum and sigmoid colon or the name of the opening so created

**sigmoid**/o-scope, an instrument used to view the sigmoid colon

**sigmoid**/o-scop-ic, pertaining to viewing or examining the sigmoid colon

**sigmoid**/o-scopy, technique of viewing or examining the sigmoid colon

**sigmoid**/o-sigmoid/o-stomy, formation of an opening (anastomosis) between two parts of the sigmoid colon or the name of the opening so created

**sigmoid/o**-stomy, formation of an opening into the sigmoid colon (for drainage to the body surface) or the name of the opening so created

**sigmoid/o**-tomy, incision into the sigmoid colon

**sigmoid/o**-vesic-al, 1. pertaining to the bladder and sigmoid colon 2. communicating with the bladder and sigmoid colon

---

**Sphincter/o**, sphincter

From a Greek word **sphigkter** meaning one who binds. Here sphincter/o means a sphincter, a circular band of muscle that contracts to close an orifice, for example the anal sphincter and pyloric sphincter.

**sphincter**-al, pertaining to a sphincter

**sphincter**-alg-ia, condition of pain in a sphincter (muscle)

**sphincter**-ectomy, removal of a sphincter

**sphincter**-ic, pertaining to a sphincter

**sphincter**-ismus, spasm of a sphincter (muscle)

**sphincter**-itis, inflammation of a sphincter

**sphincter/o**-plasty, surgical reconstruction of a sphincter

**sphincter/o**-tomy, incision into a sphincter

---

**Splanchnic/o**, splanchn/o, viscera

From a Greek word **splagchna** meaning viscera. Here splanchn/o means viscera, the internal organs of the body cavities especially those of the abdomen. Splanchnic/o from the same root means the splanchnic nerve.

Note viscus is the singular of viscera.

**splanchn**-aesthes-ia, condition of sensation from the viscera

**splanchn**-aesthe-tic, pertaining to sensation from the viscera

**splanchn**-ec-top-ia, condition of of displacement of viscera

**splanchn**-emphraxis, blocking or obstruction of a viscus (particularly an intestinal obstruction)

**splanchn**-ic, pertaining to the viscera

**splanchnic**-ectomy, removal of the splanchnic nerve

**splanchnic/o**-tomy, incision into the splanchnic nerve

**splanchn/o**-cele, a protrusion or hernia of a viscus

**splanchn/o**-diastasis, displacement or separation of viscera. From a Greek word *diastasis* meaning a standing apart

**splanchn/o**-dyn-ia, condition of pain in the viscera (usually an abdominal viscus)

**splanchn/o**-graphy, technique of recording the viscera, here a written description of

**splanchn/o**-lith, a stone or calculus in a viscus (an intestinal calculus)

**splanchn/o**-lith-iasis, presence of stones or calculi in the viscera (intestinal calculi)

**splanchn/o**-logy, the study of viscera (anatomy, diseases and treatment of)

**splanchn/o**-megaly, enlargement of a viscus Syn. visceromegaly

**splanchn/o**-pathy, disease of the viscera

**splanchn/o**-ptosis, falling or downward displacement of the viscera

**splanchn/o**-scler-osis, abnormal condition of hardening of the viscera

**splanchn/o**-staxis, dripping of blood from the viscera (from splanchnic vessels)

**splanchn/o**-tomy, incision of the viscera

**splanchn/o**-tribe, a device for crushing a viscus (the intestine to temporarily occlude its lumen)

---

**Sterc/o**, stercor/o, faeces

From a Latin word **stercus** meaning dung. Here sterc/o means faeces, the residue discharged from the bowel through the anus. Faeces contains undigested plant fibres, epithelial cells, mucus, bacteria, electrolytes, stercobilin and various odour producing chemicals.

**sterc/o**-bil-in, a (brown-coloured) chemical derived from bile found in the faeces

**sterc/o**-bilin/o-gen, an agent that forms stercobilin

**sterc/o**-lith, a faecal stone (compact faecal matter in the intestine) Syn. faecalith

**stercor**-aceous, 1. pertaining to resembling faeces 2. faecal 3. containing faeces

**stercor**-al, 1. pertaining to resembling faeces 2. faecal

**stercor**-oma, tumour-like hardened faeces in the rectum

**stercor**-ous, pertaining to faeces

**sterc**-us, faeces

---

**Stom/at/o**, mouth

From a Greek word **stomatos**, meaning mouth. Here stomat/o means the mouth, a cavity bounded by the closed lips and facial muscles, the hard and soft palate and lower jaw. The mouth contains the upper and lower teeth and the tongue. Three pairs of salivary glands (parotid, submaxillary and sublingual) secrete saliva into the mouth.

**stom**a, 1. the mouth 2. a mouth-like opening made by surgery and kept open for drainage

**stomat**-alg-ia, condition of pain in the mouth

**stomat**-itis, inflammation of the mouth

**stomat/o**-dyn-ia, condition of pain in the mouth

**stomat/o**-gnath-ic, pertaining to the jaws and mouth

**stomat/o**-log-ic, pertaining to the study of the mouth

**stomat/o**-logy, the study of the mouth (anatomy, diseases and treatment of)

**stomat/o**-malac-ia, condition of softening of the mouth (parts)

**stomat/o**-men-ia, condition of bleeding (menses) from the mouth at the time of menstruation

**stomat/o**-myc-osis, abnormal condition of fungi in the mouth (fungal infection)

**stomat/o**-pathy, disease of the mouth

**stomat/o**-plasty, surgical repair or reconstruction of the mouth

**stomat/o**-rrhag-ia, condition of excessive flow of blood from the mouth

**stom/o**-cephal-us, a fetus with head and mouth (showing rudimentary development)

**stom**-ode-al, pertaining to a stomodeum

**stom**-ode-um, a structure (depression) at the head of embryo which becomes the mouth

---

**Typhl/o**, caecum

From a Greek word **typhlos** meaning blind. Here typhl/o means the caecum, a blindly ending pouch attached to the vermiform appendix in the first part of the large intestine. The caecum is separated from the ileum by a valve, the ileocaecal valve.

**typhl**-ectas-ia, condition of dilation of the caecum

**typhl**-ectasis, dilation of the caecum

**typhl**-ectomy, removal of the caecum

**typhl/o**-cele, a protrusion or hernia of the caecum

**typhl/o**-diclid-itis, inflammation of the valve of the caecum (ileocaecal valve). From a Greek word *diklis* meaning valve

**typhl/o**-lith-iasis, condition or presence of stones or calculi in the caecum (faecal concretions)

**typhl/o**-megaly, enlargement of the caecum

**typhl/o**-pexy, surgical fixation of the caecum

**typhl/o**-ptosis, falling or displacement of the caecum

**typhl/o**-rrhaphy, stitching or suturing of the caecum

**typhl/o**-sten-osis, condition of narrowing of the caecum

**typhl/o**-stomy, formation of an opening into the caecum or the name of the opening so created

**typhl/o**-tomy, incision into the caecum

---

**Viscer/o**, internal organs of body cavities, viscera

From a Latin word **viscus** meaning internal organ. Here viscer/o means

42

viscera, the internal organs of a body cavity particularly the abdominal cavity. Note viscus is the singular of viscera.

e-**viscer**-ation, action of removing abdominal viscera

e-**viscer**-ate, to remove abdominal viscera

**viscer**a, internal organs. Plural of viscus

**viscer**-ad, towards the viscera

**viscer**-al, pertaining to viscera (internal organs)

**viscer**-alg-ia, condition of pain in the viscera

**viscer/o**-gen-ic, pertaining to originating in the viscera

**viscer/o**-megaly, enlargement of the viscera Syn. splanchnomegaly

**viscer/o**-motor, action (movements) of the viscera

**viscer/o**-pariet-al, pertaining to the wall of the abdomen and the viscera

**viscer/o**-peritone-al, pertaining to the peritoneum and the viscera

**viscer/o**-pleur-al, pertaining to the pleura and viscera

**viscer/o**-ptosis, falling or displacement of viscera

**viscer/o**-skelet-al, pertaining to the visceral skeleton

**viscer/o**-trop-ic, pertaining to having an affinity for the viscera

**visc**-us, an internal organ. Singular of viscera

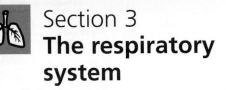

# Section 3
# The respiratory system

The respiratory system consists of a group of organs that interact to provide body cells with a continuous supply of oxygen. As oxygen enters the body, carbon dioxide, a waste product of cell metabolism, is removed. The organs that form the respiratory system include:

- **nose**
- **pharynx**
- **larynx**
- **trachea**

- **bronchioles and smaller passages**
- **two lungs and the pleura**
- **intercostal muscles and diaphragm.**

Air enters the paired lungs through the upper respiratory tract during breathing. Breathing is the mechanism that ventilates the lungs and consists of two movements, inspiration and expiration. During inspiration, the intercostal muscles and diaphragm contract to expand the lungs, increasing

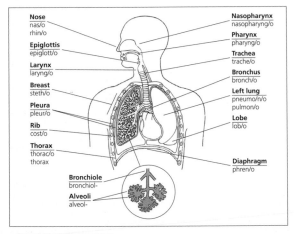

Figure 6 The respiratory system

their volume. As volume increases, the pressure within decreases, causing air to move from the nose into the body. During expiration the intercostal muscles and diaphragm relax and elastic recoil returns the lungs to their original volume. As volume decreases, pressure increases forcing air out of the body.

While air is in the lungs gaseous exchange takes place across the surface of the microscopic alveoli or air sacs. In this process oxygen is exchanged for carbon dioxide. Oxygen diffuses into the blood from inspired air and is used by body cells for aerobic respiration to release energy from food. Carbon dioxide, a waste product of aerobic respiration, diffuses out of the blood into the alveoli and leaves the body in expired air.

Figure 6 shows the anatomy of the respiratory system and combining forms associated with its components.

## Roots and combining forms, meanings

**Alveo/l-,** alveolus, air sac

From a Latin word **alveus** meaning hollow cavity. Here alveol- means the alveoli, microscopic air sacs found at the end of the smallest bronchioles. Alveoli form a large surface area of the lungs across which the gases oxygen and carbon dioxide are exchanged and therefore play an essential role in maintaining life.

Note: alveol- can also refer to cavities in teeth, dental alveoli.

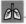 

**alveo**-bronchiol-itis, inflammation of (terminal) bronchioles and alveoli

**alveol**-ar, pertaining to alveoli or air sacs

**alveol**-itis, inflammation of alveoli or air sacs

**alveol**-us, an air sac or alveolus (anatomical part, meaning hollow cavity)

---

**Bronch/i/o**, bronchi, bronchus

From a Greek word **brogchos**, meaning windpipe. Here bronch/i/o means the bronchi, the two large air passages formed by the bifurcation of the trachea. Each bronchus conveys air into a lung and divides within it delivering air to smaller branches called bronchioles. In a few words bronch/i/o means a bronchiole, a small division of a bronchus.

**bronch/i**-al, pertaining to the bronchi

**bronch/i**-ectasis, excessive dilation of the bronchi

**bronchi/o**-cele, a dilation or hernia of a bronchiole

**bronchi/o**-crisis, a bronchial crisis

**bronch/i**-ole, a small bronchus, it terminates in an alveolus. See the combining form bronchiol/o

**bronchi/o**-lith, a stone or calculus in a bronchus

**bronchi/o**-spasm, sudden contraction of bronchi (the muscles in the bronchial wall)

**bronchi/o**-sten-osis, abnormal condition of narrowing of bronchi

**bronch**-itic, pertaining to having bronchitis

**bronch**-itis, inflammation of bronchi

**bronch/o**-aden-itis, inflammation of glands in the bronchi

**bronch/o**-alveol-ar, pertaining to alveoli and bronchi

**bronch/o**-alveol-itis, inflammation of the alveoli and bronchioles Syn. bronchopneumonia

**bronch/o**-aspergill-osis, abnormal condition of *Aspergillus* (a species of fungi) in the bronchi

**bronch/o**-blast/o-myc-osis, abnormal condition of *Blastomyces* (a species of fungi) in the bronchi

**bronch/o**-blenn/o-rrhoea, excessive discharge of mucus from bronchi

**bronch/o**-candid-iasis, presence of *Candida* (a species of fungi) in the bronchi

**bronch/o**-cele, a protrusion or hernia of a bronchus

**bronch/o**-constrict-ion, narrowing of bronchi

**bronch/o**-constrict-or, an agent that constricts the bronchi

**bronch/o**-dilat-ion, procedure of widening a constricted bronchus

**bronch/o**-dilat-or, an agent that dilates bronchi, it causes smooth muscle of bronchi to relax

**bronch/o**-fibre-scope, an instrument used for viewing bronchi that utilizes a flexible fibre-optic tube

**bronch/o**-gen-ic, 1. pertaining to forming the bronchi 2. pertaining to originating in the bronchi

**bronch/o**-gram, a recording or X-ray picture of the bronchi

**bronch/o**-graphy, technique of making recording or X-ray picture of the bronchi

**bronch/o**-lith, a stone or calculus in a bronchus

**bronch/o**-lith-iasis, presence of calculi or stones in a bronchus

**bronch/o**-log-ical, 1. pertaining to the study of bronchi 2. pertaining to bronchology

**bronch/o**-logy, the study of the bronchi (anatomy, diseases and treatment of)

**bronch/o**-malac-ia, condition of softening of the bronchi, it refers to softening of cartilage in the bronchial wall

**bronch/o**-muc/o-trop-ic, pertaining to stimulating the (secretion of) bronchial mucus

**bronch/o**-myc-osis, abnormal condition of fungi in the bronchi

**bronch/o**-oesophag-eal, pertaining to the oesophagus and a bronchus

**bronch/o**-oesophag/o-scopy, technique of viewing or examining the oesophagus and bronchus

**bronch/o**-pancreat-ic, pertaining to the pancreas and a bronchus *e.g.* a bronchopancreatic fistula

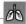

**bronch/o**-pathy, disease of the bronchi

**bronch/o**-phon-ic, pertaining to sounds of the bronchi (heard in a stethoscope)

**bronch/o**-phon-y, process of listening to sounds from bronchi (using a stethoscope)

**bronch/o**-plasty, surgical repair or reconstruction of a bronchus

**broncho**-pleg-ia, condition of paralysis of the bronchi

**bronch/o**-pleur-al, 1. pertaining to the pleura and a bronchus 2. communicating with the pleural cavity and bronchus

**bronch/o**-pleur/o-pneumon-ia, condition of pneumonia, pleurisy and bronchitis (co-existing)

**bronch/o**-pneumon-ia, condition of inflammation of bronchioles and other lung tissue

**bronch/o**-pulmon-ary, pertaining to the lungs and bronchi

**bronch/o**-radi/o-graphy, technique of making a recording or X-ray picture of the bronchi and bronchioles

**bronch/o**-rrhag-ia, condition of bursting forth of blood from bronchi (haemorrhage)

**bronch/o**-rrhaphy, suturing or stitching of the bronchi

**bronch/o**-rrhoea, excessive flow or discharge from the bronchi

**bronch/o**-scope, an instrument used to view or examine the bronchi (a fibreoptic endoscope)

**bronch/o**-scopy, technique of viewing or examining the bronchi

**bronch/o**-sinus-itis, inflammation of (paranasal) sinuses and bronchi (upper bronchi)

**bronch/o**-spasm, involuntary contraction of smooth muscle in the bronchi

**bronch/o**-spiro-metry, technique of measuring breathing (the capacity of the bronchi in a lung or one of its lobes)

**bronch/o**-staxis, haemorrhage or bleeding from the bronchi

**bronch/o**-sten-osis, abnormal condition of narrowing of the bronchi

**bronch/o**-stomy, formation of an opening into a bronchus or the name of the opening so created

**bronch/o**-trache-al, pertaining to the trachea and bronchi

**bronch/o**-tome, an instrument used to cut a bronchus (or the trachea)

**bronch/o**-tomy, incision into a bronchus (or the trachea)

**bronch/o**-trache-al, pertaining to the trachea and bronchi

**bronch/o**-vesicul-ar, pertaining to alveoli and bronchi. From a Latin word *vesicula* meaning small bladder, here referring to an alveolus

**bronch**-us, a bronchus (-us meaning an anatomical part)

endo-**bronch**-ltis, inflammation within a bronchus (its epithelial lining)

---

**Bronchiol-**, bronchiole

From a Latin word **bronchiolus** meaning little bronchus. Here bronchiol- means bronchiole, a microscopic subdivision of a bronchus that terminates in an alveolus within the lungs.

**bronchi-ole**, a small bronchus, a microscopic subdivision of a bronchus

**bronchiol**-ectasis, dilation of the bronchioles

**bronchiol**-itis, inflammation of bronchioles

**bronchiol**-us, a bronchiole (-us meaning an anatomical part)

peri-**bronchiol**-itis, inflammation of tissues around bronchioles

---

**Cost/o**, rib

From a Latin word **costa**, meaning rib. Here cost/o means rib, one of the 12 pairs of curved bones that form part of the thorax.

**cost**-al, pertaining to a rib

**cost**-alg-ia, condition of pain in the ribs

**cost/o**-cervic-al, pertaining to the neck and ribs

**cost/o**-chondr-al, pertaining to the cartilage of a rib

**cost/o**-chondr-itis, inflammation of a rib cartilage

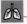 

**cost/o**-clavicul-ar, pertaining to the clavicle and ribs

**cost/o**-coracoid, pertaining to the coracoid process (of scapula) and ribs

**cost/o**-gen-ic, 1. pertaining to forming a rib 2. pertaining to originating in a rib

**cost/o**-phren-ic, pertaining to the diaphragm and ribs

**cost/o**-pleur-al, pertaining to the pleura and ribs

**cost/o**-pulmon-ary, pertaining to the lungs and ribs

**cost/o**-scapul-ar, pertaining to the scapula and ribs

**cost/o**-stern-al, pertaining to the sternum and ribs

**cost/o**-stern/o-plasty, surgical repair or reconstruction of sternum and ribs (a segment of a rib is used to support the sternum)

**cost/o**-tome, an instrument used to cut a rib (or costal cartilage)

**cost/o**-tomy, technique of cutting ribs

**cost/o**-transvers-ectomy, removal of transverse process (of a vertebra) and rib

**cost/o**-vertebr-al, pertaining to vertebrae and ribs

**cost/o**-xiphoid, pertaining to the xiphoid process (of sternum) and ribs

inter-**cost**-al, pertaining to between ribs

pre-**cost**-al, pertaining to before or in front of the ribs

sub-**cost**-al, pertaining to below the ribs

supra-**cost**-al, pertaining to above the ribs

---

**Epiglott/o**, epiglottid-, epiglottis

From the Greek words **epi-** meaning above or on and **glossa** meaning tongue. Here epiglott/o means the epiglottis, the leaf-shaped cartilage that covers the entrance to the larynx on swallowing.

**epiglott**-ectomy, removal of the epiglottis

**epiglott**-ic, 1. pertaining to the epiglottis 2. pertaining to connected to the epiglottis

**epiglottid**-ectomy, removal of the epiglottis

**epiglottid**-itis, inflammation of the epiglottis

**epiglott**-itis, inflammation of the epiglottis

**epiglott/o**-hyoid-ean, pertaining to the hyoid bone and epiglottis

---

**Laryng/o**, larynx, voice box

From a Greek word **larynx** meaning the voice box. Here laryng/o means the larynx, the organ containing the vocal cords that produces the voice.

endo-**laryng**-eal, pertaining to within the larynx

hemi-**laryng**-ectomy, removal of one (lateral) half of the larynx

**laryng**-alg-ia, condition of pain in the larynx

**laryng**-eal, pertaining to the larynx

**laryng**-ectomy, removal of the larynx

**laryng**-emphraxis, blocking up or closing of the larynx

**laryng**-ismus, process or state of the larynx, it refers to laryngismus striulus, a sudden spasm with closure of the glottis

**laryng**-itic, pertaining to having laryngitis

**laryng**-itis, inflammation of the larynx

**laryng/o**-cele, a protrusion or hernia of the larynx (an air-containing cavity)

**laryng/o**-centesis, puncture of the larynx (short incision)

**laryng/o**-epiglott-itis, inflammation of the epiglottis and larynx (a form of croup in children)

**laryng/o**-gram, a recording or X-ray picture of the larynx

**laryng/o**-graph, an instrument that records the larynx (its movements in speech)

**laryng/o**-graphy, technique of making a recording or X-ray picture of the larynx

**laryng/o**-log-ist, a specialist who studies the larynx (anatomy, diseases and treatment of)

**laryng/o**-logy, the study of the larynx (anatomy, diseases and treatment of)

**laryng/o**-metry, technique of measuring the larynx

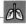

**laryng/o**-paralysis, paralysis of the larynx

**laryng/o**-pathy, disease of the larynx

**laryng/o**-pharyng-eal, 1. pertaining to the pharynx and larynx 2. pertaining to the laryngopharynx

**laryng/o**-pharyng-ectomy, removal of the pharynx (lower part and larynx)

**laryng/o**-pharyng-itis, 1. inflammation of the pharynx and larynx 2. inflammation of the laryngopharynx

**laryng/o**-pharynx, the pharynx closer to the larynx (lower portion)

**laryng/o**-phon-y, process of listening to sounds from larynx (using a stethoscope held over the larynx)

**laryng/o**-phthisis, wasting away of the larynx (seen in tuberculosis of the larynx)

**laryng/o**-plasty, surgical repair or reconstruction of the larynx

**laryng/o**-pleg-ia, condition of paralysis of the larynx

**laryng/o**-ptosis, downward displacement or falling of the larynx

**laryng/o**-py/o-cele, 1. a protrusion or hernia of the larynx containing pus 2. a laryngocele containing pus

**laryng/o**-rhin/o-logy, the study of the nose and larynx (anatomy, diseases and treatment of)

**laryng/o**-rhin/o-scopy, technique of viewing or examining the nose and larynx

**laryng/o**-rrhag-ia, condition of bursting forth of blood or haemorrhage from the larynx

**laryng/o**-rrhaphy, stitching or suturing of the larynx

**laryng/o**-rrhoea, excessive discharge (of mucus) from the larynx

**laryng/o**-scler-oma, swelling of hard tissue in the larynx

**laryng/o**-scope, an instrument used to view or examine the larynx

**laryng/o**-scop-ic, 1. pertaining to viewing or examining the larynx 2. pertaining to laryngoscopy

**laryng/o**-scopy, technique of viewing or examining the larynx

**laryng/o**-spasm, involuntary muscular contraction of the larynx (obstructs air flow)

**laryng/o**-stasis, cessation of movement of the larynx (croup)

**laryng/o**-sten-osis, abnormal condition of narrowing of the larynx (aperture)

**laryng/o**-stomy, formation of an opening into the larynx or the name of the opening so created

**laryng/o**-tomy, incision into the larynx

**laryng/o**-trache-al, pertaining to the trachea and larynx

**laryng/o**-trache-itis, inflammation of the trachea and larynx

**laryng/o**-trache/o-bronch-itis, inflammation of the bronchi, trachea and larynx

**laryng/o**-trache/o-bronch/o-scopy, technique of viewing the bronchi, trachea and larynx, using a fibre-optic bronchoscope

**laryng/o**-trache/o-plasty, surgical repair or reconstruction of the trachea and larynx (usually to widen a stenosed airway)

**laryng/o**-trache/o-tomy, incision into the trachea and larynx

peri-**laryng**-itis, inflammation of tissue around the larynx

---

**Lob/o**, lobe of the lung
From a Greek word **lobos**, meaning lobe, a rounded section of an organ. Here, lob/o means a lobe of a lung formed by fissures or septa that divide the right lung into three lobes and the left lung into two. Note that other organs in the body are lobar.

inter-**lob**-ar, pertaining to between lobes

inter-**lob**-itis, inflammation between lobes (interlobular pleurisy)

**lob**-ation, having the condition of lobes

**lob**-ectomy, removal of a lobe

**lob**/o-tomy, incision into a lobe

**lob**-ule, a small lobe (a subdivision of a lobe)

---

**Nas/o**, nose
From a Latin word **nasus** meaning nose. Here nas/o means nose, the organ that acts to warm, filter and moisten air entering the respiratory system. The

nose is the the organ of the sense of smell (olfaction). Nerve endings that detect odours are located in the roof of the nose in the area of the cribriform plate of the ethmoid bone and nasal conchae.

See the combining form rhin/o also meaning nose.

**nas**-al, pertaining to the nose

**nas**-endo-scope, an instrument used to view or examine inside the nose (nasal passages, post nasal space and larynx)

**nas**-endo-scopy, technique of viewing or examining inside the nose (nasal passages, post nasal space and larynx) using a fibre-optic endoscope

**nas**-itis, inflammation of the nose

**nas/o**-antr-al, pertaining to the Antrum of Highmore (maxillary sinus) and nose

**nas/o**-antr-itis, inflammation of the Antrum of Highmore (maxillary sinus) and nose

**nas/o**-antr/o-stomy, formation of an opening between the Antrum of Highmore (maxillary sinus) and the nose or the name of the opening so created

**nas/o**-aur-al, pertaining to the ears and nose

**nas/o**-bucc-al, pertaining to the mouth cavity and nose

**nas/o**-bucc/o-pharyng-eal, pertaining to the pharynx, mouth cavity and nose

**nas/o**-cili-ary, pertaining to the eyelids and nose

**nas**-ocul-ar, pertaining to the eyes and nose

**nas/o**-duoden-al, pertaining to the duodenum and nose

**nas/o**-endo-scope, an instrument used to view or examine inside the nose (nasal passages, post nasal space and larynx)

**nas/o**-endo-scopy, technique of viewing or examining inside the nose (nasal passages, post nasal space and larynx) using a fibre-optic endoscope

**nas/o**-front-al, pertaining to the frontal bones and nose

**nas/o**-gastr-ic, pertaining to the stomach and nose

**nas/o**-graph, an instrument used to record the nose, it is used to determine the patency of the nasal passages

**nas/o**-jejun-al, pertaining to the jejunum and nose

**nas/o**-labi-al, pertaining to the lips and nose

**nas/o**-lacrim-al, pertaining to the lacrimal apparatus and nose

**nas/o**-logy, the study of the nose (anatomy, diseases and treatment of)

**nas/o**-man/o-meter, an instrument used to measure pressure in the nose (during breathing)

**nas/o**-occipt-al, pertaining to the occiput and nose

**nas/o**-oesophag-eal, pertaining to the oesophagus and nose

**nas/o**-palat-ine, pertaining to the palate and nose

**nas/o**-palpebr-al, pertaining to the eyelids and nose

**nas/o**-pharyng-eal, pertaining to the nasopharynx

**nas/o**-pharyng-itis, inflammation of the nasopharynx

**nas/o**-pharyng/o-laryng/o-scope, an instrument used for viewing or examining the larynx, and nasopharynx (a fibre-optic endoscope)

**nas/o**-pharyng/o-scope, an instrument used for viewing or examining the nasopharynx (a fibre-optic endoscope)

**nas/o**-pharynx, part of the pharynx above the soft palate near the nose. See the combining form nasopharyng/o

**nas/o**-rostr-al, pertaining to the rostrum (of the sphenoid bone) and the nose

**nas/o**-scope, an instrument used to view or examine the nose

**nas/o**-sept-al, pertaining to the septum of the cavity of the nose

**nas/o**-sinus-itis, inflammation of the (paranasal) sinuses and the nose

**nas**-us, the nose (-us meaning an anatomical part)

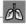

### Nasopharyng/o, nasopharynx

From a Latin word **nasus**, meaning nose and a Greek word **pharynx** meaning throat. Here nasopharyng/o means the nasopharynx, the nasal portion of the pharynx behind the nose and above the soft palate.

**nasopharyng**-eal, pertaining to the nasopharynx

**nasopharyng**-itis, inflammation of the nasopharynx

**nasopharyng**/o-laryng/o-scope, an instrument used for viewing or examining the larynx, and nasopharynx (a fibre-optic endoscope)

**nasopharyng**/o-scope, an instrument used for viewing or examining the nasopharynx (a fibre-optic endoscope)

**nasopharynx**, part of the pharynx above the soft palate near the nose

### Pharyng/o, pharynx

From a Greek word **pharynx** meaning throat. Here pharyng/o means the pharynx, the cone-shaped cavity at the back of the mouth lined with mucous membrane. The pharynx varies in length (average 75 mm) and has three parts, the nasopharynx, oropharynx and laryngopharynx. At its lower end the pharynx opens into the oesophagus.

epi-**pharyng**-eal, 1. pertaining to above the pharynx 2. pertaining to the epipharynx (nasopharynx)

epi-**pharynx**, above or upon the pharynx Syn. nasopharynx

**pharyng**-alg-ia, condition of pain in the pharynx

**pharyng**-eal, pertaining to the pharynx

**pharyng**-ectas-ia, condition of widening or dilation of the pharynx

**pharyng**-ectomy, removal of the pharynx

**pharyng**-emphraxis, stopping up or obstruction of the pharynx

**pharyng**-ismus, process or state of the pharynx (sudden spasm)

**pharyng**-itic, pertaining to having pharyngitis

**pharyng**-itis, inflammation of the pharynx

**pharyng**/o-cele, a protrusion or hernia of the pharynx

**pharyng**/o-dyn-ia, condition of pain in the pharynx

**pharyng**/o-epiglott-ic, pertaining to the epiglottis and pharynx

**pharyng**/o-gloss-al, pertaining to the tongue and pharynx

**pharyng**/o-laryng-eal, pertaining to the larynx and pharynx

**pharyng**/o-laryng-itis, inflammation of the larynx and pharynx

**pharyng**/o-lith, a stone or calculus in the pharynx

**pharyng**/o-logy, the study of the pharynx (anatomy, diseases and treatment of)

**pharyng**/o-maxill-ary, pertaining to the maxilla (jaw) and pharynx

**pharyng**/o-myc-osis, abnormal condition of fungi in the pharynx

**pharyng**/o-nas-al, pertaining to the nose and pharynx

**pharyng**/o-oesophag-eal, pertaining to the oesophagus and pharynx

**pharyng**/o-or-al, pertaining to the mouth and pharynx

**pharyng**/o-palat-ine, pertaining to the palate and pharynx

**pharyng**/o-paralysis, paralysis (of muscles) of the pharynx

**pharyng**/o-plasty, surgical repair of the pharynx

**pharyng**/o-pleg-ia, condition of paralysis of the pharynx

**pharyng**/o-rhin-itis, 1. inflammation of the nose and pharynx 2. inflammation of the nasopharynx

**pharyng**/o-rhin/o-scopy, technique of viewing or examining the nose and pharynx (with a rhinoscope)

**pharyng**/o-rrhag-ia, condition of bursting forth of blood from the pharynx (haemorrhage)

**pharyng**/o-rrhoea, excessive flow or discharge from the pharynx

**pharyng**/o-salping-itis, inflammation of the Eustachian tube (auditory tube) and pharynx

**pharyng**/o-scler-oma, a hard tumour or swelling in the pharynx

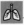 

**pharyng/o**-scope, an instrument used to view or examine the pharynx

**pharyng/o**-scopy, technique of viewing or examining the pharynx

**pharyng/o**-spasm, involuntary contraction (of muscles) in the pharynx

**pharyng/o**-sten-osis, abnormal condition of narrowing of the pharynx

**pharyng/o**-tomy, incision into the pharynx

**pharyng/o**-tonsill-itis, inflammation of the tonsils and the pharynx

**pharyng/o**-tympan-ic, pertaining to the middle ear and pharynx

**pharyng/o**-xer-osis, abnormal condition of dry pharynx (due to lack of secretions)

retro-**pharyng**-itis, inflammation behind the pharynx (involving the posterior part of the pharynx)

sub-**pharyng**-eal, pertaining to under or beneath the pharynx

vel/o-**pharyng**-eal, pertaining to the pharynx and soft palate

---

**Phren/o**, diaphragm

From a Greek word **phren**, meaning midriff. Here phren/o means the diaphragm, the muscular septum separating the thorax and abdomen that acts as the main respiratory muscle. Phrenic/o refers to the phrenic nerve that controls the diaphragm.

Note: phren/o is also used as an old fashioned term meaning the mind.

**phren**-ic, pertaining to the diaphragm

**phren/ic**-clas-ia, condition of breaking the phrenic nerve (by clamping)

**phren/ic**-ectomy, removal of the phrenic nerve

**phren/ic/o**-exeresis, removal of the phrenic nerve

**phren/ic/o**-neur-ectomy, removal of the phrenic nerve (part or whole)

**phren/ic/o**-tomy, incision into the phrenic nerve

**phren/ic/o**-tripsy, crushing of phrenic nerve (by surgery)

**phren**-itis, inflammation of the diaphragm

**phren/o**-col-ic, pertaining to the colon and diaphragm

**phren/o**-cost-al, pertaining to the ribs and diaphragm

**phren/o**-dyn-ia, condition of pain in the diaphragm

**phren/o**-gastr-ic, pertaining to the stomach and diaphragm

**phren/o**-glott-ic, pertaining to the glottis and diaphragm

**phren/o**-graph, an instrument that records the diaphragm (movements of)

**phren/o**-hepat-ic, pertaining to the liver and diaphragm

**phren/o**-paralysis, paralysis of the diaphragm

**phren/o**-pleg-ia, condition of paralysis of the diaphragm

**phren/o**-ptosis, downward displacement of the diaphragm

**phren/o**-spasm, involuntary contraction of diaphragm (muscles)

**phren/o**-splen-ic, pertaining to the spleen and diaphragm

sub-**phren**-ic, pertaining under or beneath to the diaphragm

---

**Pleur/a/o**, pleura, pleural membranes

From a Greek word **pleura**, meaning rib. Here pleur/o means the pleura, the shiny membranes covering the lungs and internal surfaces of the thorax. The space between the membranes is known as the pleural cavity.

pachy-**pleur**-itis, inflammation and thickening of the pleura Syn. fibrothorax

**pleur/a**-centesis, puncture of the pleura (by surgery to drain the cavity of the pleura)

**pleur**-al, pertaining to the pleura

**pleur**-alg-ia, condition of pain in the pleura (caused by inflammation of intercostal muscles)

**pleur**-alg-ic, 1. pertaining to having pleuralgia 2. pertaining to pain in the pleura

**pleur**-ectomy, removal of the pleura

**pleur**-isy, inflammation of the pleura

**pleur**-itic, pertaining to having pleuritis or pleurisy (inflammation of the pleura)

**pleur**-itis, inflammation of the pleura

**pleur/o**-bronch-itis, inflammation of the bronchi and pleura (simultaneously)

**pleur/o**-cele, a protrusion or hernia of the pleura (and/or lung)

**pleur/o**-centesis, puncture of the pleura

**pleur/o**-cholecyst-itis, inflammation of the gallbladder and pleura (simultaneously)

**pleur/o**-clysis, infusion or injection of fluid into the pleura

**pleur/o**-cutane-ous, pertaining to the skin and pleura

**pleur/o**-desis, fixation of the pleura

**pleur/o**-dyn-ia, condition of pain in the pleura

**pleur/o**-gen-ic, pertaining to originating in or forming in the pleura

**pleur/o**-gram, a recording or X-ray picture of the pleura

**pleur/o**-graphy, technique of making a recording or X-ray picture of the pleura

**pleur/o**-hepat-itis, inflammation of the liver and pleura

**pleur/o**-lith, a stone or calculus in the pleura

**pleur/o**-lysis, separating the pleura (by surgery)

**pleur/o**-oesophag-eal, pertaining to the oesophagus and pleura

**pleur/o**-pariet/o-pexy, fixation of the parietal pleura to the pulmonary pleura

**pleur/o**-pericard/i-al, pertaining to the pericardium and pleura

**pleur/o**-pericard-itis, inflammation of the pericardium and pleura

**pleur/o**-peritone-al, pertaining to the peritoneum and pleura

**pleur/o**-peritone-um, the peritoneum and pleura (as a structure, one membrane)

**pleur/o**-periton-itis, inflammation of the peritoneum and pleura

**pleur/o**-pneumon-ia, condition of (inflammation of) the lungs and pleura

**pleur/o**-pulmon-ary, pertaining to the lungs and pleura

**pleur/o**-py-esis, abnormal condition of pus in the pleura (pleurisy with a septic effusion)

**pleur/o**-rrhag-ia, condition of bursting forth of blood from the pleura (haemorrhage)

**pleur/o**-scopy, technique of viewing or examining the pleura

**pleur/o**-tome, an instrument used to cut the pleura

**pleur/o**-tomy, technique of cutting the pleura

**pleur/o**-viscer-al, pertaining to the visceral pleura

sub-**pleur**-al, pertaining to under or beneath the pleura

---

**pne/o**, breathing

From a Greek word **pnoe** meaning breath. Here pne/o means breathing, a muscular movement that ventilates the lungs; it consists of inspiration (the intake of air) and expiration (the output of air).

**pne/o**-gram, a recording or tracing made by a spirograph (an instrument that records breathing movements)

**pne/o**-meter, instrument that measures breathing (capacities or changes in volume)

**pne/o**-dynam-ics, 1. the science studying the force or power of breathing movements 2. the mechanics of breathing

---

**Pneumat/o**, pneum/o, air, gas, breathing, lung

From a Greek word **pneuma**, meaning air. Here, pneumat/o means mean gas, air, lungs or breathing.

See the combining forms pneumon/o and pulmon/o also meaning lung.

**pneumat**-ic, 1. pertaining to gas or air 2. pertaining to respiration

**pneumat/o**-card-ia, condition of gas or air in the the heart

**pneumat/o**-cele, 1. a protrusion or hernia of the lung 2. a benign, air-containing cyst in the lung

**pneumat/o**-gram, 1. a recording of respiratory movements (*i.e.* of air or gas in and out of the lungs) 2. an X-ray picture of the lungs

**pneumat/o**-graph, an instrument for recording respiratory movements (*i.e.* of air or gas in and out of the lungs)

**pneumat/o**-graphy, technique of recording respiratory movements (*i.e.* of air or gas in and out of the lungs)

**pneumat/o**-logy, 1. the study of gases 2. the study of respiration

**pneumat/o**-meter, an instrument used to measure amount of air inhaled and exhaled

**pneumat/o**-metry, technique of measuring the amount of air inhaled and exhaled

**pneumat/o**-osis, abnormal condition of gas or air (in an abnormal position *e.g.* in the pleural cavity)

**pneumat/o**-therapy, treatment using air or gas

**pneumat/o**-thorax, presence of air or gas in the thorax

**pneumo/o**-alveoli/o-graphy, technique of making a recording or X-ray picture of pulmonary alveoli

**pneumo/o**-cardi-al, pertaining to the heart and lungs

**pneumo/o**-cele, 1. a protrusion or hernia of the lung 2. a benign, air-containing cyst in the lung

**pneumo/o**-centesis, puncture of the lungs (to aspirate a cavity)

**pneumo/o**-cirrh-osis, abnormal condition of yellow lungs (pulmonary fibrosis)

**pneumo/o**-cocc-al, pertaining to pneumococci (berry-like bacteria that infect the lung)

**pneumo/o**-cocc-us, a berry-like bacterium that infects the lung, it refers to a gram-positive diplococcus that causes pneumonia and meningitis, *Streptococcus pneumoniae*

**pneumo/o**-coni/i-osis, abnormal condition of dust in the lungs (coal dust, asbestos etc.)

**Pneumo**cystis, a micro-organism (considered to be a protozoan) causing pneumonia (in individuals who are immunologically compromised)

**pneumo/o**-cyte, a lung cell (Type 1 cells that line the alveoli, Type 2 cells that secrete surfactant)

**pneumo/o**-dynam-ics, 1. the science studying the force or power of movement of the lungs 2. the mechanics of respiration

**pneumo/o**-dyn-ia, condition of pain in the lungs

**pneumo/o**-em-py-ema, a swelling of pus and gas (in the pleural space)

**pneumo/o**-dynam-ics, 1. the science studying the force or power of breathing movements 2. the mechanics of breathing

**pneumo/o**-gastr-ic, pertaining to stomach and lungs

**pneumo/o**-gram, 1. a recording of respiratory movements *i.e.* of air or gas in and out of the lungs 2. a recording or X-ray picture of the lungs

**pneumo/o**-graph, an instrument used to record respiratory movements *i.e.* of air or gas in and out of the lungs

**pneumo/o**-graphy, technique of recording respiratory movements *i.e.* of air or gas in and out of the lungs

**pneumo/o**-haem-ia, condition of blood containing air (the presence of air in arteries or veins)

**pneumo/o**-haem/o-thorax, blood and air in the thorax (in the pleural cavity between the wall of the thorax and lungs as in a stabbing injury)

**pneumo/o**-lith, a stone or calculus in the lungs

**pneumo/o**-lith-iasis, presence of stones or calculi in the lungs

**pneumo/o**-logy, the study of the lungs and respiration

**pneumo/o**-lysis, separating the lung and (parietal) pleura (by surgery to collapse the lung)

**pneumo/o**-malac-ia, condition of softening of the lung

**pneumo/o**-melan-osis, abnormal condition of dark pigment in the lungs *e.g.* coal dust

**pneumo/o**-meter, an instrument used to measure the amount of air inhaled and exhaled

**pneumo/o**-metry, technique of measuring the amount of air inhaled and exhaled

**pneum/o**-monil-iasis, presence of *Monilia* species in the lungs (now known as Candida)

**pneum/o**-myc-osis, abnormal condition of fungi in the lungs

**pneum/o**-myc/o-tic, pertaining to fungi in the lungs

**pneum/o**-peritone•um, air or gas in the peritoneal cavity

**pneum/o**-tax-ic, pertaining to ordered movement of lungs

**pneum/o**-thorax, air in the thorax (in the pleural cavity between the visceral and parietal pleura as in a stabbing injury or intentional introduction of air that results in collapse of a lung).

**Pneumon/o**, lung

From a Greek word **pneumon**, meaning lung. Here pneumon/o means lung, the organ of respiration. The lungs are two conical organs occupying most of the thoracic cavity; they are separated from each other by the heart and other components of the mediastinum. Within each lung is a bronchial tree, the fine terminations of which end in tiny sacs called alveoli. Gaseous exchange in the alveoli oxygenates the blood and allows carbon dioxide to be excreted.

See the combining forms pulmon/o and pneum/o also meaning lung.

**pneumon**-aem-ia, condition of blood in the lungs (excess)

**pneumon**-alg-ia, condition of pain in the lungs

**pneumon**-ectas-ia, condition of dilation of the lungs (pulmonary emphysema)

**pneumon**-ectasis, dilation of the lungs (pulmonary emphysema)

**pneumon**-ectomy, removal of a lung

**pneumon**-ia, abnormal condition of the lung (inflammation due to infection)

**pneumon**-ic, 1. pertaining to the lung 2. pertaining to pneumonia

**pneumon**-itis, inflammation of the lungs

**pneumon/o**-cele, a protrusion or hernia of a lung

**pneumon/o**-centesis, puncture of the lungs (by surgery for aspiration)

**pneumon/o**-cirrh-osis, abnormal condition of yellow lungs (pulmonary fibrosis)

**pneumon/o**-cocc-us, a berry like bacterium that infects the lungs, it refers to a gram-positive diplococcus that causes pneumonia and meningitis, *Streptococcus pneumoniae*

**pneumon/o**-con/i-osis, abnormal condition of dust in the lungs (coal dust, asbestos etc.)

**pneumon/o**-cyte, a lung cell (the term includes Type 1 cells that line the alveoli, Type 2 cells that secrete surfactant and alveolar macrophages)

**pneumon/o**-graph, an instrument that records lungs (chest movements during respiration)

**pneumon/o**-graphy, technique of recording lungs (chest movements during respiration)

**pneumon/o**-lysis, breakdown or disintegration of lungs (causes collapse of lungs)

**pneumon/o**-melan-osis, abnormal condition of dark pigment in the lungs *e.g.* coal dust

**pneumon/o**-meter, an instrument that measures the lungs (volume of inhaled and exhaled air)

**pneumon/o**-metry, technique of measuring the lungs (volume of inhaled and exhaled air)

**pneumon/o**-monil-iasis, presence of *Monilia* species in the lungs (now known as Candida)

**pneumon/o**-myc-osis, abnormal condition of fungi in the lungs

**pneumon/o**-paresis, slight paralysis of the lung (due to an inelastic condition)

**pneumon/o**-pathy, disease of a lung

**pneumon/o**-pexy, fixation of a lung (by surgery to thoracic wall)

**pneumon/o**-pleur-itis, inflammation of the pleura and lungs (pleurisy and pneumonia)

**pneumon/o**-rrhag-ia, condition of bursting forth of blood from the lungs (haemorrhage and haemoptysis)

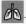 

**pneumon/o**-rrhaphy, stitching or suturing of a lung

**pneumon/o**-osis, abnormal condition of the lung (any diseased, morbid condition of the lungs)

**pneumon/o**-therapy, 1. the treatment of lung (disorders) 2. the treatment of the lungs using air

**pneumon/o**-tomy, incision into a lung

---

**-pnoea**, breathing

From a Greek word **pnoia** meaning breath or **pnein** meaning to breathe. Here, -pnoea means breathing, a muscular movement that ventilates the lungs; it consists of inspiration (the intake of air) and expiration (the output of air).

a-**pnoea**, without breathing

brady-**pnoea**, slow breathing

dys-**pnoea**, difficult or painful breathing

eu-**pnoea**, good or normal breathing

hyper-**pnoea**, above normal breathing (depth and rate of)

hypo-**pnoea**, below normal breathing (depth and rate of)

ortho-**pnoea**, straight breathing, it refers to difficult breathing unless in the upright position

poly-**pnoea**, too much breathing Syn. hyperpnoea

tachy-**pnoea**, fast breathing

trepo-**pnoea**, breathing when turned, it refers to breathing more easily when turned into a particular position or lying down. From a Greek word *trepein* meaning to turn

---

**Pulm/o**, pulmon/o, lung

From a Latin word **pulmonis**, meaning lung. Here pulmon/o means the lung, the organ of respiration. The lungs are two conical organs occupying most of the thoracic cavity; they are separated from each other by the heart and other components of the mediastinum. Within each lung is a bronchial tree, the fine terminations of which end in tiny sacs called alveoli. Gaseous exchange in the alveoli oxygenates the blood

and allows carbon dioxide to be excreted.

See the combining forms pneum/o and pneumon/o also meaning lung.

extra-**pulmon**-ary, pertaining to outside (not connected to) the lungs

**pulm/o**-aort-ic, pertaining to the aorta and lungs

**pulm/o**-meter, an instrument used to measure the lungs (a type of spirometer used to determine volume of inhaled and exhaled air)

**pulm/o**-metry, technique of measuring the lungs (to determine the volume of inhaled and exhaled air using a type of pulmometer)

**pulmon**-ary, pertaining to the lungs

**pulmon**-ectomy, removal of a lung Syn. pneumonectomy

**pulmon**-ic, pertaining to the lungs

**pulmon**-itis, inflammation of the lungs

**pulmon/o**-aort-ic, 1. pertaining to the aorta and lungs 2. pertaining to the aorta and pulmonary arteries

**pulmon/o**-hepat-ic, pertaining to the liver and lungs

**pulmon/o**-lith, a stone or calculus in a lung

**pulmon/o**-periton-eal, pertaining to the peritoneum and lungs

sub-**pulmon**-ary, pertaining to under or beneath the lungs

---

**Rhin/o**, nose

From a Greek word **rhinos**, meaning nose. Here rhin/o means nose, the organ that acts to warm, filter and moisten air entering the respiratory system. The nose is the the organ of the sense of smell (olfaction). Nerve endings that detect odours are located in the roof of the nose in the area of the cribriform plate of the ethmoid bone and nasal conchae.

See the combining form nas/o also meaning nose.

**rhin**-aesthes-ia, condition of sensation in the nose (the sense of smell or olfaction)

**rhin**-al, pertaining to the nose

**rhin**-alg-ia, condition of pain in the nose

**rhin**-eurynter, a device to distend or widen the nose (the nostrils)

**rhin**-iatry, 1. treatment of the nose by a doctor 2. speciality of treatment of the nose

**rhin**-ic, pertaining to the nose

**rhin**-itis, inflammation of the nose

**rhin/o**-anem/o-meter, an instrument used for measuring air in the nose (during respiration)

**rhin/o**-antr-itis, inflammation of the Antrum of Highmore (maxillary sinus) and nose (nasal cavity)

**rhin/o**-blenn/o-rrhoea, excessive discharge of mucus from the nose

**rhin/o**-canth-ectomy, removal of the inner canthus of the eye (nearest to the nose)

**rhin/o**-cheil/o-plasty, surgical repair or reconstruction of the lips and nose

**rhin/o**-cleisis, obstruction of the nose (its nasal passages)

**rhin/o**-dacry/o-lith, a stone or calculus in the nasal duct of the lacrimal (tear) apparatus

**rhin/o**-dyn-ia, condition of pain in the nose

**rhin/o**-gen-ous, pertaining to forming or arising in the nose

**rhin/o**-kyph-ectomy, removal of a hump on the nose (cosmetic surgery)

**rhin/o**-kyph-osis, abnormal condition of hump on the nose (ridge)

**rhin/o**-lal-ia, condition of speaking with a nasal voice

**rhin/o**-laryng-itis, inflammation of the larynx and nose

**rhin/o**-laryng/o-logy, the study of the larynx and nose (anatomy, diseases and treatment of)

**rhin/o**-lith, a stone or calculus in the nose

**rhin/o**-lith-iasis, presence of stones or calculi in the nose

**rhin/o**-log-ical, 1. pertaining to the study of the nose 2. pertaining to rhinology

**rhin/o**-log-ist, a specialist who studies the nose (anatomy, diseases and treatment of)

**rhin/o**-logy, the study of the nose (anatomy, diseases and treatment of)

**rhin/o**-man/o-metry, technique of measuring pressure in the nose (air flow)

**rhin/o**-meiosis, shortening or reduction in the size of the nose (by surgery)

**rhin/o**-miosis, shortening or reduction in the size of the nose (by surgery)

**rhin/o**-myc-osis, abnormal condition of fungi in the nose

**rhin/o**-necr-osis, 1. abnormal condition of dead tissue in the nose 2. destruction of nasal bones

**rhin/o**-neur-osis, 1. abnormal nervous condition or neurosis characterized by nasal symptoms 2. abnormal condition of the nerves in the nose

**rhin/o**-path-ia, condition of disease of the nose (any morbid condition)

**rhin/o**-pathy, disease of the nose

**rhin/o**-pharyng-eal, pertaining to the pharynx and nose (nasal part of the pharynx or nasopharynx)

**rhin/o**-pharyng-itis, 1. inflammation of the nasopharynx 2. inflammation of the pharynx and nose

**rhin/o**-pharyng/o-cele, a protrusion or hernia of the nasal part of the pharynx (an air-filled cyst)

**rhin/o**-pharyng/o-lith, a stone or calculus in the nasal part of the pharynx

**rhin/o**-pharynx, the nasal part of the pharynx

**rhin/o**-phon-ia, condition of having a nasal sound to the voice (speech through the nose)

**rhin/o**-phyma, swelling of the nose (nodular enlargement of the skin)

**rhin/o**-plast-ic, 1. pertaining to plastic surgery of the nose 2. pertaining to rhinoplasty

**rhin/o**-plasty, surgical repair or reconstruction of the nose

**rhin/o**-polyp-us, a nasal polyp

**rhin**-ops-ia, condition of nasal site (it refers to eyes converging towards the nose, a convergent squint)

**rhin/o**-rrhag-ia, condition of excessive flow of blood from the nose (a nosebleed or epistaxis)

**rhin/o**-rrhaphy, 1. stitching or suturing of the nose 2. an operation to remove an epicanthus, a fold of skin on the side of the nose that may cover the inner canthus of the eye

**rhin/o**-rrhoea, excessive flow or discharge from the nose

**rhin/o**-salping-itis, inflammation of the Eustachian tube (auditory tube) and nose

**rhin/o**-scler-oma, a hard tumour or swelling in the nose (due to infection with *Klebsiella*)

**rhin/o**-scope, an instrument used to view or examine the nose

**rhin/o**-scop-ic, 1. pertaining to viewing or examining the nose 2. pertaining to rhinoscopy

**rhin/o**-scopy, technique of viewing or examining the nose

**rhin/o**-sinus-itis, inflammation of the sinuses and nose

**rhin/o**-sinus/o-path-ia, condition of disease of the sinuses and nose

**rhin/o**-sten-osis, abnormal condition of narrowing of the nose (the nasal passage)

**rhin/o**-tomy, incision into the nose

**rhin/o**-virus, a virus that affects the nose (*e.g.* picornavirus that causes a cold)

---

**Spir/o**, breathing

From a Greek word **spirare** meaning to breathe. Here spir/o means breathing, a muscular movement that ventilates the lungs; it consists of inspiration (the intake of air) and expiration (the output of air).

**spir/o**-gram, 1. a recording or tracing made by a spirograph 2. a recording or tracing of breathing (movements of lungs)

**spir/o**-graph, an instrument that records breathing (movements of lungs)

**spir/o**-graphy, technique of recording breathing (movements of the lungs)

**spir/o**-meter, an instrument that measures breathing (capacities or changes in volume)

**spir/o**-metr-ic, 1. pertaining to measuring breathing (capacities or changes

in volume) 2. pertaining to measurement with a spirometer

**spir/o**-metry, technique of measuring breathing (capacities or changes in volume)

---

**Stern/o**, breast bone, sternum

From a Greek word **sternon** meaning chest. Here stern/o means the sternum, a long, flat bone forming the anterior wall of the thorax in the median line.

meso-**stern**-um, the middle (body) of the sternum

**stern**-al, pertaining to the sternum

**stern**-alg-ia, condition of pain in the sternum

**stern/o**-clavicul-ar, pertaining to the clavicle and sternum

**stern/o**-cleid/o-mastoid, pertaining to or belonging to the mastoid process, clavicle and sternum

**stern/o**-coracoid, pertaining to or belonging to the coracoid process and sternum

**stern/o**-cost-al, pertaining to the ribs and sternum

**stern/o**-hyoid, pertaining to or belonging to the hyoid bone and sternum

**stern**-oid, resembling the sternum

**stern/o**-mastoid, pertaining to or belonging to the mastoid process and sternum

**stern/o**-pericardi-al, pertaining to the pericardium and sternum

**stern/o**-scapul-ar, pertaining to the scapula and sternum

**stern/o**-schisis, cleaving or splitting of the sternum (a congenital fissure)

**stern/o**-thyroid, pertaining to or belonging to the thyroid cartilage or gland and the sternum

**stern/o**-tomy, incision into the sternum

**stern/o**-trache-al, pertaining to the trachea and sternum

**stern/o**-xiphoid, pertaining to or belonging to the xiphoid process and sternum

sub-**stern**-al, pertaining to under or beneath the sternum

supra-**stern**-al, pertaining to above the sternum

**Steth/o**, chest
From a Greek word **stethos** meaning breast. Here steth/o means the chest.

**steth**-alg-ia, condition of pain in the chest

**steth/o**-goni/o-meter, an instrument used to measure the angle (curvature) of the chest

**steth/o**-meter, an instrument used to measure the chest (circular dimension and expansion)

**steth/o**-scopy, technique of examining the chest (listening with a stethoscope)

**steth/o**-scope, an instrument used to examine (listen to) the chest

**steth/o**-scop-ic, 1. pertaining to examining (listening to) the chest 2. pertaining to examination with a stethoscope

**steth/o**-spasm, involuntary contraction of the chest (muscles)

---

**Thorac/ic/o**, chest cavity, thorax
From a Greek word **thorax**, meaning chest. Here thorac/o means the thorax or chest cavity. The chest cavity contains the heart, lungs and great vessels.
See the suffix -thorax also meaning the thorax.

intra-**thorac**-ic, pertaining to inside or within the thorax

**thorac**-alg-ia, condition of pain in the thorax

**thorac**-ectomy, removal of the thorax, it refers to an incision into the thorax and removal of part of a rib

**thorac**-ic, pertaining to the thorax

**thoracic/o**-abdomin-al, pertaining to the abdomen and thorax

**thoracic/o**-acromi-al, pertaining to the acromion (point of the shoulder) and thorax

**thoracic/o**-humer-al, pertaining to the humerus and thorax

**thorac/o**-abdomin-al, pertaining to the abdomen and thorax

**thorac/o**-acromi-al, pertaining to the acromion (point of the shoulder) and thorax

**thorac/o**-bronch/o-tomy, incision into the bronchi through the thorax

**thorac/o**-cel/o-schisis, fissure or splitting of the abdomen and thorax (congenital)

**thorac/o**-centesis, puncture of the thorax

**thorac/o**-coel/o-schisis, fissure or splitting of the abdomen and thorax (congenital)

**thorac/o**-dyn-ia, condition of pain in the thorax

**thorac/o**-gastr/o-schisis, fissure or splitting of the stomach (abdomen) and thorax (congenital)

**thorac/o**-graph, an instrument that records the thorax (its expansion and contraction)

**thorac/o**-lapar/o-tomy, incision into the abdomen through the thorax

**thorac/o**-lumb-ar, pertaining to the lumbar regions and thorax

**thorac/o**-lysis, separation of the thorax (stripping of pleural adhesions by surgery)

**thorac/o**-meter, an instrument used for measuring the thorax (dimensions)

**thorac/o**-my/o-dyn-ia, condition of pain in muscles of the thorax

**thorac/o**-pathy, disease of the thorax

**thorac/o**-plasty, surgical repair or reconstruction of the thorax (removal of ribs to allow chest wall to collapse and diseased lung to rest)

**thorac/o**-pneum/o-graph, an instrument that records the lungs and thorax (respiratory movements)

**thorac/o**-pneum/o-plasty, surgical repair or reconstruction of the lungs and thorax (in tuberculosis to secure a permanent collapsed lung)

**thorac/o**-schisis, fissure or splitting of the thorax (congenital)

**thorac/o**-scope, an instrument used to view or examine the thorax

**thorac/o**-scopy, technique of viewing or examining the thorax

**thorac/o**-sten-osis, abnormal condition of narrowing of the thorax (due to contraction)

**thorac/o**-stomy, formation of an opening into the thorax or the name of the opening so created

**thorac/o**-tomy, incision into the thorax

---

**-thorax**, chest

From a Greek word **thorax**, meaning chest. Here -thorax is used as a suffix to mean the thorax or chest cavity. The chest cavity contains the heart, lungs and great vessels.

See the combining form thorac/o also meaning thorax.

blenn/o-**thorax**, accumulation of mucus in the thorax or chest

fibr/o-**thorax**, fibrous tissue in the thorax, the pleura adhere and the lung is covered with thick fibrous tissue

haem/o-pneum/o-**thorax**, air or gas and blood in the thorax (in the pleural cavity)

haem/o-**thorax**, blood in the thorax (in the pleural cavity)

hydr/o-pneum/o-**thorax**, gas and water (serous fluid) in the thorax (in the pleural cavity)

hydr/o-**thorax**, water (serous fluid) in the thorax (in the pleural cavity)

pneum/o-haem/o-**thorax**, blood and air or gas in the thorax (in the pleural cavity)

pneum/o-**thorax**, air or gas in the thorax (in the pleural cavity)

schist/o-**thorax**, cleaving or splitting of the thorax or sternum (a congenital fissure)

---

**Trache/o**, trachea, windpipe

From a Greek word **tracheia**, meaning rough. Here trache/o means the trachea, or the windpipe, a structure containing rings of cartilage that give it a rough appearance. The trachea transfers air between the larynx and lungs and its lining cleans inspired air. Cleaning is achieved when dust and bacteria become trapped in its mucus secretion and are transported away from the lungs by the action of ciliated cells in its lining epithelium.

endo-**trache**-al, pertaining to inside the trachea

intra-**trache**-al, pertaining to inside the trachea

**trache**-al, pertaining to the trachea

**trache**-alg-ia, condition of pain in the trachea

**trache**-itis, inflammation of the trachea

**trache/o**-aer/o-cele, a protrusion or hernia of the trachea containing air

**trache/o**-blenn/o-rrhoea, excessive flow of mucus from the trachea

**trache/o**-bronch/i-al, pertaining to the bronchi and trachea

**trache/o**-bronch-itis, inflammation of the bronchi and trachea

**trache/o**-bronch/o-gram, a recording or X-ray picture of the bronchi and trachea (upper respiratory tract)

**trache/o**-bronch/o-scopy, technique of viewing or examining the bronchi and trachea (upper respiratory tract)

**trache/o**-cele, a protrusion or hernia of the trachea (its mucous membrane)

**trache/o**-fissure, a fissure (groove or furrow) in the trachea

**trache/o**-laryng-eal, pertaining to the larynx and trachea

**trache/o**-laryng/o-tomy, incision into the larynx and trachea

**trache/o**-malac-ia, condition of softening of the trachea (its tracheal cartilages)

**trache/o**-oesophag-eal, pertaining to the oesophagus and trachea

**trache/o**-path-ia, condition of disease of the trachea (any morbid condition)

**trache/o**-pathy, disease of the trachea

**trache/o**-pharyng-eal, pertaining to the pharynx and trachea

**trache/o**-phon-y, sound of the trachea (heard by auscultation over the trachea)

**trache/o**-plasty, surgical repair or reconstruction of the trachea

**trache/o**-py-osis, abnormal condition of pus in the trachea (seen in tracheitis)

**trache/o**-rrhag-ia, condition of bursting forth of blood from the trachea (haemorrhage)

**trache/o**-rrhaphy, stitching or suturing of the trachea

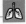

**trache/o**-schisis, splitting of the trachea (a fissure)

**trache/o**-scop-ic, 1. pertaining to viewing or examining the trachea 2. pertaining to tracheoscopy

**trache/o**-scopy, technique of viewing or examining the trachea

**trache/o**-sten-osis, abnormal condition of narrowing of the trachea

**trache/o**-stome, an artificial opening into the trachea (made by tracheostomy)

**trache/o**-stomy, formation of an opening into the trachea (temporary or permanent) or the name of the opening so created

**trache/o**-tomy, incision into the trachea

**trach**-itis, inflammation of the trachea

# Section 4
# The cardiovascular system

The cardiovascular system continuously circulates blood around the body. This act sustains the life of all cells by providing them with oxygen and nutrients and removing their wastes. The organs that form the cardiovascular system are:

- **heart**
  a four-chambered muscular pump that circulates blood through vessels
- **vessels**
  a network of tubes that transport blood to the tissues and return it to the heart. There are three main types: arteries, veins and capillaries.

## The heart

The heart is a four-chambered muscular pump that continuously forces blood into arteries. The right and left atria (singular: atrium) form its top chambers, and the right and left ventricles the lower chambers. The pumping action consists of a series of events known as the cardiac cycle. During each heartbeat or cardiac cycle, the chambers of the heart contract and relax alternately. The period of contraction is known as systole and that of relaxation when the heart refills, diastole. Figure 7 shows the anatomy of the heart and the combining forms associated with its components.

## The vessels

Humans have a closed circulation. By closed we mean that blood never leaves the vessels unless they are damaged. Blood leaves the heart in arteries that divide into smaller arterioles and then into the smallest vessels called capil-

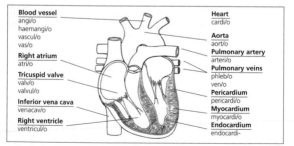

| | |
|---|---|
| **Blood vessel** | **Heart** |
| angi/o | cardi/o |
| haemangi/o | |
| vascul/o | **Aorta** |
| vas/o | aort/o |
| **Right atrium** | **Pulmonary artery** |
| atri/o | arteri/o |
| **Tricuspid valve** | **Pulmonary veins** |
| valv/o | phleb/o |
| valvul/o | ven/o |
| **Inferior vena cava** | **Pericardium** |
| venacav/o | pericardi/o |
| **Right ventricle** | **Myocardium** |
| ventricul/o | myocardi/o |
| | **Endocardium** |
| | endocardi- |

Figure 7 The heart and major blood vessels

laries. In the capillaries materials are exchanged between the blood and tissue cells, oxygen and nutrients leave the blood while carbon dioxide and other metabolic wastes are picked up. Upon leaving the capillaries blood enters small vessels called venules that unite to form larger veins. These return blood to the heart. Unlike arteries, veins contain valves that prevent the back flow of blood.

The heart pumps blood into two anatomically separate systems of blood vessels. First, the right side of the heart pumps blood to the lungs and back to the heart through vessels that form the pulmonary circulation. Then oxygenated blood returning to the left side of the heart from the lungs is pumped into vessels that form the systemic circulation supplying the rest of the body with blood.

**Roots and combining forms**, meanings

**Aneurysm/o**, aneurysm

From a Greek word **aneurysma**, meaning a dilatation. Here aneurysm/o means an aneurysm, a dilated vessel usually an artery. An aneurysm is caused by a local fault in a vessel wall through defect, disease or injury. It appears as a pulsating swelling that can rupture.

**aneurysm/o**-plasty, surgical repair or reconstruction of an aneurysm

**aneurysm/o**-rrhaphy, stitching or suturing of an aneurysm

endo-**aneurysm/o**-rrhaphy, stitching or suturing of the inside of an aneurysm once it has been opened and drained

micro-**aneurysm**, a very small aneurysm

pseudo-**aneurysm**, a false aneurysm, it refers to a dilated, twisted vessel with the appearance of an aneurysm

---

**Angi/o**, vessel

From a Greek word **angeion**, meaning vessel. Here angi/o means a blood vessel.

See the combining forms haemangi/o, vascul/o and vas/o also meaning blood vessel.

**angi**-asthen-ia, condition of weakness (lack of tone) of blood vessels

**angi**-ectas-ia, condition of dilation of blood vessels

**angi**-ectasis, dilation of blood vessels

**angi**-ectomy, removal of a blood vessel

**angi**-ec-top-ia, condition of abnormal position or displacement of a blood vessel Syn. angioectopia

**angi**-itis, inflammation of blood vessels

**angi/o**-blast, an immature cell or embryonic cell that forms blood vessels

**angi/o**-blast-ic, 1. pertaining to cells that forms blood vessels 2. pertaining to angioblasts

**angi/o**-blast-oma, a tumour that arises from cells that form blood vessels *e.g.* an angioblastic meningioma

**angi/o**-cardi/o-gram, a recording or X-ray picture of the heart and major vessels

**angi/o**-cardi/o-graphy, technique of making a recording or X-ray picture of the heart and major vessels

**angi/o**-cardi/o-kinet-ic, pertaining to the movement of the heart and blood vessels

**angi/o**-card-itis, inflammation of the heart and blood vessels

**angi/o**-chondr-oma, a cartilage tumour with presence of blood vessels

**angi/o**-dys-plas-ia, condition of poor growth of blood vessels (vessel abnormalities)

**angi/o**-dys-troph-ia, condition of poor nourishment of blood vessels

**angi/o**-ec-top-ia, condition of abnormal position or displacement of a blood vessel Syn. angiectopia

**angi/o**-endotheli-oma, a tumour (benign) in which endothelial cells from the walls of blood vessels are a main component Syn. haemangioendothelioma

**angi/o**-fibr-oma, a tumour of (cells of) blood vessels containing fibrous tissue

**angi/o**-follicul-ar, pertaining to a (lymph) follicle (within a lymph node) and its blood vessels

**angi/o**-genesis, formation or development of blood vessels

**angi/o**-gen-ic, 1. pertaining to forming blood vessels 2. pertaining to originating in blood vessels

**angi/o**-gli-oma, a glioma containing blood (or lymph) vessels

**angi/o**-gram, a recording or X-ray picture of blood vessels (often arteries)

**angi/o**-graph, an instrument that records blood vessels (movements of the arterial pulse)

**angi/o**-graphy, technique of making a recording or X-ray picture of blood vessels (often arteries)

**angi/o**-hyalin-osis, abnormal condition of glass-like blood vessels (due to amyloid degeneration in the walls of vessels)

**angi**-oid, resembling blood vessels

**angi/o**-kerat-oma, swelling of the epidermis containing blood vessels in which dilated red blood vessels (telangiectasis) are visible

**angi/o**-kinet-ic, pertaining to the movement of vessels (dilation and constriction) Syn. vasomotor

**angi/o**-lei/o-my-oma, a tumour of the smooth muscle of a blood vessel

**angi/o**-lip/o-lei/o-my-oma, a (benign) tumour containing smooth muscle, fat and blood vessels Syn. angiomyolipoma angi/o-lith, a stone or calculus in a blood vessel (wall)

angi/o-logy, the study of blood vessels (anatomy, diseases and treatment of)

angi/o-lup-oid, resembling lupus vulgaris with blood vessels, it refers to a granuloma that consists of small red plaques covered with dilated vessels often on the nose

angi/o-lysis, breakdown of blood vessels

angi-oma, a tumour or swelling formed from blood vessels (a non-malignant naevus)

angi/o-malac-ia, condition of softening of (the walls) of blood vessels

angi-omat-a, plural of angioma, it refers to multiple angiomas

angi-omat-osis, abnormal condition of the presence of multiple angiomas (angiomata)

angi-omat-ous, pertaining to or of the nature of angioma

angi/o-megaly, enlargement of a blood vessel

angi/o-meter, an instrument used to measure blood vessels (diameter and tension)

angi/o-myo-lip-oma, a (benign) tumour containing fat, muscle and blood vessels Syn. angiolipoleiomyoma

angi/o-my-oma, a tumour of (smooth) muscle of a blood vessel

angi/o-my/o-sarc-oma, a tumour composed of connective tissue, muscle and blood vessels

angi/o-necr-osis, abnormal condition of decaying or dead blood vessels

angi/o-neur-oma, a tumour of nerves and blood vessels (Syn. glomangioma, a tumour of a glomus, a knot of fine arterioles with a rich nerve supply)

angi/o-neur/o-my-oma, a tumour of muscle, nerves and blood vessels (Syn. glomangioma, a tumour of a glomus, a knot of fine arterioles with a rich nerve supply)

angi/o-neur/o-pathy, 1. disease of nerves of blood vessels 2. disease of vasomotor system

angi/o-neur/o-path-ic, 1. pertaining to angioneuropathy 2. pertaining to disease of vasomotor system

angi/o-neur-osis, abnormal condition of the nerves of blood vessels (due to injury to vasomotor nerves or the vasomotor centre in the brain)

angi/o-neur/o-tic, pertaining to angioneurosis

angion-oma, swelling (ulceration) of blood vessels

angi/o-oedema, swelling due to fluid leaking from dilated blood vessels with increased permeability

angi/o-paralysis, paralysis of blood vessels (vasomotor paralysis)

angi/o-paresis, slight paralysis of blood vessels (vasomotor paralysis)

angi/o-path/o-logy, the study of diseases of blood (and lymph) vessels

angi/o-pathy, disease of blood vessels

angi/o-plasty, surgical repair or reconstruction of blood vessels

angi/o-poiesis, formation of blood vessels

angi/o-poie-tic, 1. pertaining to angiopoiesis 2. pertaining to formation of blood vessels

angi/o-rrhaphy, stitching or suturing of a blood vessel

angi/o-sarc-oma, a malignant tumour formed from fibroblastic tissue and blood vessels (endothelial tissue) Syn. haemangiosarcoma

angi/o-scler-osis, abnormal condition of hardening of blood vessels

angi/o-scope, an instrument used to view blood vessels

angi/o-scot-oma, a scotoma (dark spot in the retina) caused by the shadow of blood vessels

angi/o-scot/o-metry, technique of measuring scotomas (dark spots in the retina) caused by blood vessels. Used to diagnose glaucoma

angi/o-spasm, sudden contraction of the smooth muscle in the walls of a blood vessel

angi/o-staxis, dripping of blood from vessels, it refers to a tendency to bleed as in haemophilia

angi/o-sten-osis, abnormal condition of narrowing of blood vessels

angi-oste-osis, abnormal condition of ossification or calcification of a vessel

**angi/o**-tel-ectasis, dilation of a web of blood vessels (minute arteries and veins)

**angi/o**-tens-in-ase, enzyme that inactivates angiotensin

**angi/o**-tens-in, an agent (hormone) that increases tension or tone in blood vessels (responsible for renal hypertension)

**angi/o**-ot-itis, inflammation of ear vessels

**angi/o**-ton-ic, pertaining to increased tone or tension in blood vessels (vasoconstriction)

**angi/o**-tribe, a device formerly used to arrest haemorrhage by crushing tissue containing an artery

**angi/o**-troph-ic, pertaining to nutrition of blood vessels

tel-**angi**-ectas-ia, condition formed by dilation of a web of blood vessels

tel-**angi**-ectasis, dilation of a web of blood vessels

tel-**angi**-osis, abnormal condition of a web of blood vessels

---

**Aort/o**, aorta

From a Greek word **aorte**, meaning great vessel. Here aort/o means the aorta, the largest artery in the body. The aorta leaves the left ventricle of the heart and divides into smaller arteries that supply all body systems with oxygenated blood.

**aort**-ic, pertaining to the aorta

**aort**-itis, inflammation of the aorta

**aort/o**-graphy, technique of making a recording or X-ray picture of the aorta

**aort/o**-pathy, disease of the aorta

**aort/o**-rrhaphy, stitching or suturing of the aorta

**aort/o**-scler-osis, abnormal condition of hardening of the aorta

**aort/o**-tomy, incision into the aorta

end-**aort**-itis, inflammation inside the aorta (its lining membrane)

---

**Arter/i/o**, artery

From a Greek word **arteria**, meaning artery. Here arteri/o means artery, the

vessels that move blood away from the heart. Arteries divide into smaller arterioles and then into capillaries that exchange materials with the tissue cells.

**arter**-ectomy, removal of an artery or portion of an artery Syn. arteriectomy

**arter/i**-al, pertaining to arteries

**arter/i**-ectomy, removal of an artery (section of) Syn. arterectomy

**arteri/o**-graphy, technique of making a recording or X-ray picture of arteries

**arter/i**-ola, a small artery, an arteriole. See the combining form arteriol/o

**arter/i**-ol-ar, pertaining to an arteriole. See the combining form arteriol/o

**arter/i**-ole, a small artery (microscopic). See the combining form arteriol/o

**arteri/o**-lith, a stone or calculus in an artery

**arteri/o**-motor, having an action on arteries (causing dilation or constriction)

**arteri/o**-my-omat-osis, abnormal condition of myomas (thickening and overgrowth of muscle fibres) in the walls of arteries

**arteri/o**-necr-osis, abnormal condition of decay of arteries

**arteri/o**-plasty, surgical repair or reconstruction of an artery

**arteri/o**-rrhaphy, stitching or suturing of an artery

**arteri/o**-rrhexis, breaking or rupture of an artery

**arteri/o**-scler-osis, abnormal condition of hardening of arteries (the arterial walls become thick and inelastic)

**arteri/o**-scler/o-tic, 1. pertaining to having arteriosclerosis 2. pertaining to hardening of arteries

**arteri/o**-sten-osis, abnormal condition of narrowing of arteries

**arteri/o**-sympath-ectomy, removal of sympathetic pathway or plexus from around arteries

**arteri/o**-tomy, incision of an artery

**arteri/o**-ven-ous, pertaining to a vein and artery

**arter**-itis, inflammation of an artery

dys-**arteri/o**-ton-y, condition of poor tone in arterioles, results in abnormal high or low blood pressure

end-**arter**-ectomy, removal of the lining (inside) of an artery

peri-**arteri**-al, pertaining to around an artery

peri-**arter**-itis, inflammation around an artery, its outer coat and surrounding tissues

---

**Arteriol/o**, arteriole

From a Lain word **arteriole** meaning little artery. Here arteriol/o means arteriole, a microscopic vessel that joins an artery to a capillary.

**arteriol**-a, arteriole. Plural arteriolae

**arteriol**-ar, pertaining to an arteriole

**arteriol**/o-necr-osis, abnormal condition of destruction or death of arterioles

**arteriol**/o-scler-osis, abnormal condition of hardening (narrowing) of arterioles

---

**Ather/o**, atheroma

From a Greek word **adhere**, meaning porridge. Here ather/o means atheroma, a fatty plaque that forms on the walls of blood vessels. Build-up of atheroma in a vessel may eventually obstruct the flow of blood to a tissue.

**ather/o**-embolus, an embolus formed from atheroma, it refers to a blockage in a vessel

**ather/o**-gen-ic, pertaining to formation of atheroma

**ather/o**-genesis, formation of atheroma in blood vessel walls

**ather**-oma, a swelling caused by a fatty plaque in the wall of a blood vessel

**ather**-omat-osis, abnormal condition of diffuse atheroma in blood vessels

**ather/o**-scler-osis, abnormal condition of hardening of the arteries and atheroma (co-existing)

---

**Atri/o**, atrium

From a Latin word **atrium** word meaning a hall, entrance or passage. Here

atri/o means the right or left atrium of the heart. The atria form the two upper chambers of the heart, their function is to accept blood returning through veins and pass it to the lower chambers (ventricles). The right atrium receives deoxygenated blood from the venae cavae and the left atrium receives oxygenated blood from the pulmonary veins.

**atri**-a, the two upper chambers of the heart. Plural of atrium

**atri**-al, pertaining to an atrium or atria

**atri/o**-megaly, enlargement of an atrium

**atri/o**-sept/o-pexy, surgical fixation of the inter-atrial septum (to correct a defect)

**atri/o**-sept/o-plasty, surgical repair or reconstruction of the inter-atrial septum

**atri/o**-ventricul-ar, pertaining to a ventricle and an atrium or to the ventricles and atria

**atri**-um, one of the upper chambers of the heart that receives blood

---

**Card/i/o**, heart

From a Greek word **kardia** meaning heart. Here cardi/o means the heart, a four chambered muscular pump that continuously pushes blood into arteries. The right and left atria (singular – atrium) form the top chambers and the right and left ventricles the lower chambers.

The atria receive blood from veins and push it into the ventricles. The right ventricle then forces blood through the pulmonary artery to the lungs where it is oxygenated. Simultaneously, oxygenated blood that has returned to the left side of the heart is forced by the left ventricle through the aorta into the systemic circulation.

brady-**card**-ia, condition of slow heart beat

brady-tachy-**card**-ia, condition of (alternating) slow and fast heart beat

dextro-**card**-ia, condition of right heart (heart displaced to the right) diplo-**card**-ia, condition of separation of two halves of the heart (by a fissure)

echo-**card/o**-graphy, technique of recording (ultrasound) echoes of the heart

ecto-**card**-ia, condition of (congenital) displacement of the heart

electro-**cardi/o**-graph, an instrument that records the electrical activity of the heart

electro-**cardi/o**-gram, a recording or tracing of the electrical activity of the heart, the ECG

electro-**cardi/o**-graphy, technique of recording the electrical activity of the heart

endo-**cardi**-al, 1. pertaining to within the heart 2. pertaining to the endocardium

endo-**card**-itis, inflammation of the endocardium (the inside lining of the heart)

epi-**cardi**-ectomy, removal of the epicardium

epi-**cardi**-um, structure upon the heart, it refers to the visceral layer of pericardium that covers the heart

**cardi**-ac, pertaining to the heart

**cardi**-alg-ia, condition of pain in the heart

**cardi**-ectasis, dilation of the heart

**cardi/o**-accelerat-or, an agent that accelerates the heart's rhythm

**cardi/o**-angi/o-logy, the study of the blood vessels and heart (anatomy, diseases and treatment of)

**cardi/o**-cele, a protrusion or hernia of the heart (through a wound or the diaphragm)

**cardi/o**-centesis, puncture of the heart (by surgery)

**cardi/o**-cirrh-osis, abnormal condition of cirrhosis (inflammation and fibrosis of the liver) affecting the heart

**cardi/o**-dynam-ics, the science of studying the force of movement of the heart

**cardi/o**-dyn-ia, condition of pain in the heart

**cardi/o**-gen-ic, 1. pertaining to originating in the heart 2. pertaining to forming the heart

**cardi/o**-gram, a tracing or recording made by a cardiograph

**cardi/o**-graph, an instrument that records the heart (beat, force and form of)

**cardi/o**-inhibit-or, an agent that inhibits the heart's rhythm

**cardi/o**-kinet-ic, pertaining to movement of the heart (stimulating or exciting)

**cardi/o**-kym/o-graph-ic, pertaining to making a recording of the movement of the heart (using an electrokymograph)

**cardi/o**-kym/o-graphy, technique of making a recording of the movement of the heart (using an electrokymograph)

**cardi/o**-log-ist, a specialist who studies the heart (anatomy, diseases and treatment of)

**cardi/o**-logy, the study of the heart (anatomy, diseases and treatment of)

**cardi/o**-malac-ia, condition of softening of the heart (muscle)

**cardi/o**-megaly, enlargement of the heart

**cardi/o**-melan-osis, abnormal condition of darkening of heart muscle

**cardi/o**-motil-ity, state or condition of the heart's movement

**cardi/o**-my/o-lip-osis, abnormal condition of fat in the heart muscle (fatty degeneration of heart muscle)

**cardi/o**-my/o-pexy, fixation of (pectoral) muscle to the heart (by surgery as a means of improving the blood supply to the myocardium)

**cardi/o**-my/o-pathy, disease of heart muscle

**cardi/o**-oment/o-pexy, surgical fixation of the omentum to the heart

**cardi/o**-palud-ism, state or condition of heart disease due to malaria. From a Latin word *palus* meaning stagnant water, used to mean malaria which is endemic in marshy areas

**cardi/o**-pathy, disease of the heart

**cardi/o**-pericardi/o-pexy, surgical fixation of the pericardium to the heart (a treatment for coronary heart disease)

**cardi/o**-plasty, surgical repair or reconstruction of the heart

**cardi/o**-pleg-ia, condition of paralysis of the heart (induced during surgical procedures)

**cardi/o**-pleg-ic, pertaining to paralysis of the heart (induced during surgical procedures)

**cardi/o**-pneumat-ic, pertaining to breathing or respiration and the heart

**cardi/o**-ptosis, downward displacement or falling of the heart

**cardi/o**-pulmon-ary, pertaining to the lungs and heart

**cardi/o**-puncture, puncture of the heart (by surgery) Syn. cardiocentesis

**cardi/o**-ren-al, pertaining to the kidneys and heart

**cardi/o**-respirat-ory, pertaining to the respiratory system and heart

**cardi/o**-rrhaphy, stitching or suturing of the heart

**cardi/o**-rrhexis, rupture of the heart

**cardi/o**-scler-osis, abnormal condition of hardening of the heart (due to formation of fibrous tissue)

**cardi/o**-selective, having an affinity for heart tissue

**cardi/o**-sphygm/o-graph, an instrument that records the pulse and (movement of) the heart

**cardi/o**-splen/o-pexy, surgical fixation of the spleen to the heart (for revascularization)

**cardl/o**-tach/o-meter, an instrument that measures (and records) the speed of the heart while subject is active over an extended period

**cardi/o**-therapy, treatment of diseases of the heart

**cardi/o**-thorac-ic, pertaining to the thorax and heart

**cardi/o**-toc/o-graph, an instrument that records the fetal heart beat during birth (may record and monitor a range of parameters simultaneously during labour)

**cardi/o**-toc/o-graphy, technique of making a recording of the fetal heart beat during birth

**cardi/o**-ton-ic, 1. an agent that affects the tone of the heart 2. pertaining to stimulating the tone of the heart

**cardi/o**-top/o-metry, technique of measuring an area of the heart (showing cardiac dullness)

**cardi/o**-tox-ic, pertaining to poisonous to the heart

**cardi/o**-valv/o-tome, an instrument to cut a heart valve

**cardi/o**-vascul-ar, pertaining to blood vessels and the heart

**cardi/o**-version, turning of the heart, it refers to restoration of normal rhythm by electric shock

**cardi/o**-verter, an instrument that restores the normal rhythm of the heart by electric shock

**card**-itis, inflammation of the heart Syn. myocarditis

**cardi**-valvul-itis, inflammation of heart valves

intra-**cardi**-ac, pertaining to within the heart

meso-**card**-ia, condition in which the apex of the heart is in the median line of the thorax

meso-**cardi**-um, the embryonic mesentery of the heart ( it connects the heart to the body wall)

micro-**card**-ia, condition of having a small heart

my/o-**cardl**-um, the heart muscle

pan-**card**-itis, inflammation of all of the heart

phono-**cardi/o**-graphy, technique of recording heart sounds

presby-**card**-ia, condition of the heart due to old age (impaired function due to aging)

tachy-**card**-ia, condition of a fast heart rate

**Coron/ar**-, coronary
From a Latin word **corona** meaning crown. Here, coron- means the coronary system of blood vessels that are in the form of a crown or circlet. The coronary arteries encircle the heart muscle and supply it with oxygenated blood.

**coronar**-itis, inflammation of coronary arteries

**coronar**-ism, condition of the coronary arteries (spastic contraction)

**coron**-ary, pertaining to the coronary arteries or coronary system

---

**Diastol-**, diastole
From the Greek words **dia** meaning between and **stellein** meaning to set. Here diastol- means diastole, the period in the cardiac cycle when the heart refills.

brady-**diastole**, slow diastole (an abnormally prolonged diastole)
**diastol**-ic, pertaining to or belonging to diastole
post-**diastol**-ic, pertaining to after diastole
pre-**diastole**, before diastole, it refers to the interval in the cardiac cycle immediately before diastole
pre-**diastol**-ic, pertaining to before diastole
proto-**diastol**-ic, pertaining to first or early diastole (follows the second heart sound)

---

**Embol/o**, embolus
From a Greek word **embolos** meaning a plug. Here embol/o means an embolus, the sudden blocking of an artery by a clot. An embolus can be caused by a blood clot as well as fat, air and infective material.

**embol**-ectomy, removal of an embolus
**embol**-i, plural of embolus
**embol**-ic, pertaining to or belonging to an embolus
**embol**-ism, process of the sudden formation of an embolus
**embol**-oid, resembling an embolus
**embol/o**-myc/o-tic, pertaining to a fungal embolism (embolism caused by an infection)
**embol**-us, thing or structure that forms a sudden blockage in a vessel *e.g.* a blood clot, fat, air or infective material.

---

**Endocardi-**, endocardium
From the Greek words **endo-** meaning inside and **kardi-** meaning heart. Here

endocardi- means the endocardium, the smooth endothelial tissue lining the heart and covering the valves.

**endocardi**-al, pertaining to the endocardium
**endocard**-itic, pertaining to having endocarditis
**endocard**-itis, inflammation of the endocardium
**endocardi**-um, the structure inside the heart (the smooth endothelial tissue lining the inside of the heart and covering the valves)
sub-**endocardi**-al, pertaining to beneath the endocardium

---

**Endotheli/o**, endothelium
From the Greek words **endon** meaning within and **thele** meaning nipple. Here endotheli/o means endothelium, a layer of epithelial cells that lines cavities, blood vessels and lymph vessels.

**endothelia**, plural of endothelium
**endotheli**-al, pertaining to or composed of an endothelium
**endotheli**-itis, inflammation of an endothelium
**endotheli/o**-blast-oma, a tumour of immature cells or embryonic cells that form an endothelium
**endotheli/o**-cyte, a cell of the endothelium, it refers to a phagocytic cell that arises in the endothelium of a blood vessel
**endotheli**-oid, resembling endothelium
**endotheli/o**-lyt-ic, pertaining to breaking down endothelial tissue
**endotheli**-oma, a tumour arising from the endothelium of a blood vessel
**endotheli**-omat-a, plural of endothelioma, it refers to multiple endotheliomas
**endotheli**-omat-osis, abnormal condition of having (multiple) endotheliomas
sub-**endotheli**-al, pertaining to under or below an endothelium

---

**Haemangi/o**, blood vessel
From the Greek words **haima** meaning blood and **angeion** meaning vessel.

Here haemangi/o means a blood vessel.

Note words referring specifically to blood are listed in Section 5 on The blood.

**haemangi**-ectas-ia, condition of dilation of blood vessels

**haemangi/o**-blast, an immature cell or embryonic cell that forms the endothelium of blood vessels and haemocytoblasts

**haemangi/o**-blast-oma, a tumour of immature cells that form blood vessels, it refers to a capillary haemangioma of the brain containing angioblasts

**haemangi/o**-endotheli/o-blast-oma, a tumour of immature cells that form the endothelial cells that line blood vessels

**haemangi/o**-endotheli-oma, a swelling formed by the overgrowth of endothelial cells that line blood vessels

**haemangi/o**-endotheli/o-sarc-oma, a malignant tumour formed from fibroblastic tissue and endothelial tissue of blood vessels Syn. haemangiosarcoma

**haemangi/o**-fibr-oma, a fibroma combined with a haemangioma

**haemangi**-oma, a benign swelling composed of (dilated blood) vessels

**haemangi/o**-peri-cyt-oma, a tumour of blood vessels containing pericytes (elongated contractile cells that surround arterioles)

**haemangi/o**-sarc-oma, a malignant tumour formed from fibroblastic tissue and blood vessels (endothelial tissue) Syn. angiosarcoma

---

**Myocard/i/o**, myocardium
From the Greek words **mys** meaning muscle and **kardi** meaning heart. Here myocardi/o means the myocardium, the middle, thickest layer of the heart wall consisting of highly specialized cardiac muscle fibres.

**myocardi**-al, pertaining to the myocardium or heart muscle

**myocardi/o**-gram, a recording of (movement of) the myocardium (made by a myocardiograph)

**myocardi/o**-graph, an instrument that records the myocardium (movements of)

**myocardi/o**-pathy, disease of myocardium (non inflammatory)

**myocardi/o**-rrhaphy, stitching or suturing of the myocardium

**myocardi**-osis, abnormal condition of the myocardium (any non inflammatory, degenerative condition) Syn. myocardiopathy

**myocard**-ism, abnormal condition of the myocardium (a tendency to develop degeneration of)

**myocard**-itic, 1. pertaining to having myocarditis 2. pertaining to of the nature of myocarditis

**myocard**-itis, inflammation of the myocardium

**myocardi**-um, the heart muscle

**myocard**-osis, abnormal condition of the myocardium (any non-inflammatory, degenerative condition) Syn. myocardiopathy

---

**Pericard/i/o**, pericardium
From the Greek words **peri** meaning around and **kardi** meaning heart. Here pericardi/o means the pericardium, the double, serous, membranous sac around the heart. The visceral layer (epicardium) forms the inside and the parietal layer the outside. Between the two is the pericardial space containing a small amount of serous fluid that prevents friction as the heart contracts.

cardi/o-**pericardi**-pexy, fixation of the pericardium to the heart

endo-**pericard**-itis, inflammation of the pericardium and endocardium

**pericard**-ectomy, removal of the pericardium

**pericardi**-al, pertaining to the pericardium

**pericardi/o**-centesis, puncture of the pericardium by surgery

**pericardi/o**-lysis, breaking up of the pericardium, it refers to surgical freeing of adhesions between the parietal and visceral layers

**pericardi/o**-phren-ic, pertaining to the diaphragm and pericardium

**pericardi/o**-rrhaphy, stitching or suturing of the pericardium

**pericardi/o**-stomy, formation of an opening into the pericardium (usually for drainage) or the name of the opening so created

**pericard**-itis, inflammation of the pericardium (the membrane around the heart)

**pericard**-um, the structure around the heart (the double membranous sac)

**pericard/o**-tomy, incision into the pericardium

haem/o-**pericardi**-um, structure or thing of blood in the pericardium, it refers to an accumulation of blood in the pericardial sac

hydro-**pericard**-itis, inflammation of the pericardium with an accumulation of water (a serous effusion)

---

**Phleb/o**, vein

From a Greek word **phlebos**, meaning vein. Here phleb/o means a vein, a blood vessel that transfers blood back to the heart. Small veins called venules that drain capillaries join to form the larger veins. Unlike arteries, veins contain valves that prevent the back flow of blood.

See the combining form ven/o also meaning vein.

meso-**phleb**-itis, inflammation of the middle layer of a vein

peri-**phleb**-itis, inflammation around a vein, its outer coat or surrounding tissues

**phleb**-angi-oma, swelling of a vein (a venous aneurysm)

**phleb**-arteri-ectas-ia, condition of dilation of arteries and veins

**phleb**-arteri-ectasis, dilation of arteries and veins

**phleb**-ectomy, removal of a vein (or section of a vein)

**phleb**-emphraxis, stopping up or blockage of a vein (by a clot)

**phleb**-ismus, condition of veins (obstruction and over distension)

**phleb**-itic, pertaining to having or of the nature of phlebitis

**phleb**-itis, inflammation of a vein

**phleb/o**-clysis, injection or infusion into a vein

**phleb/o**-graphy, 1. technique of making a recording or X-ray picture of veins 2. technique of recording the venous pulse

**phleb/o**-lith, a stone or calculus within a vein

**phleb/o**-lith-iasis, presence of stones or calculi in a vein

**phleb/o**-man/o-meter, an instrument used to measure the pressure within a vein

**phleb/o**-rrhaphy, stitching or suturing of a vein

**phleb/o**-scler-osis, abnormal condition of hardening of veins (fibrous induration)

**phleb/o**-stasis, cessation (of movement of blood) in a vein

**phleb/o**-thromb-osis, abnormal condition of thrombi (clots) in veins (in the absence of inflammation)

**phleb/o**-tom-ist, a specialist (technician) who makes an incision into veins (for collection of blood )

**phleb/o**-tomy, incision into a vein Syn. venotomy and venesection

---

**Rhythm/o**, rrhythm/o, rhythm

From a Greek word **rrhythmos** meaning rhythm. Here rrhythm/o means the cardiac rhythm. The beating of the heart or cardiac rhythm results from the regular electrical discharge of the sinoatrial node or 'pacemaker'.

a-**rrhythm**-ia, condition of without a normal rhythm of the heart

a-**rrhythm**-ic, pertaining to without a normal rhythm

a-**rrhythm/o**-gen-ic, pertaining to forming an arrhythmia

brady-a-**rrhythm**-ia, condition of without normal rhythm and presence of bradycardia (a slow heart beat)

eu-**rrhythm**-ia, condition of good (regular) rhythm of the heart

**rhythm**-ic, pertaining to a rhythm or having rhythmical contractions

**rhythm**-ical, pertaining to a rhythm or having rhythmical contractions

**rhythm**-ic-ity, condition or ability of the heart to contract rhythmically without external stimulation

---

**Sphygm/o**, pulse

From a Greek word **sphygmos**, meaning pulsation. Here sphygm/o means the pulse, the rhythmical throbbing that can be felt wherever an artery is near to the surface of the body. The pulsation is due to the heart forcing blood into the arterial system at ventricular systole (contraction); the pulse rate is therefore a measure of heart rate.

brady-**sphygm**-ia, condition of slow pulse Syn. bradycardia

micro-**sphygm**-ia, condition of small pulse, one difficult to detect with the finger

post-**sphygm**-ic, pertaining to after the pulse wave

pre-**sphygm**-ic, pertaining to before the pulse wave

**sphygm/o**-cardi/o-graph, an instrument that records the heart beat and pulse

**sphygm/o**-dynam/o-meter, an instrument that measures the force of the pulse (pressure and volume)

**sphygm/o**-gram, a tracing or recording of the pulse

**sphygm/o**-graph, an instrument that records the pulse

**sphygm/o**-oid, resembling the pulse

**sphygm/o**-man/o-meter, an instrument that measures the pressure of the pulse (arterial blood pressure)

**sphygm/o**-meter, an instrument that measures the pulse

**sphygm/o**-metry, technique of measuring the pulse

**sphygm/o**-scope, an instrument to view the pulse (it makes the movement visible)

**sphygm/o**-ton/o-meter, an instrument that measures the tone of the pulse, it refers to measuring the elasticity of the arterial walls

---

**Systol-**, systole

From a Greek word **systole** meaning contraction. Here -systol- means systole, the period in the cardiac cycle when the chambers of the heart contract. Atrial systole results in blood being forced into the ventricles, ventricular systole forces blood out of the heart into the vessels.

para-**systole**, wrong or near systole, it refers to a cardiac irregularity caused by two foci discharging cardiac impulses at different rates

post-**systol**-ic, pertaining to after systole

pre-**systole**, before systole, it refers to the interval in the cardiac cycle immediately before systole

pre-**systol**-ic, 1. pertaining to before systole 2. pertaining to presystole

**systol**-ic, pertaining to or belonging to systole

---

**Thromb/o, clot**, thrombus

From a Greek word **thrombos**, meaning a clot. Here thromb/o means a thrombus or blood clot. Clots are composed mainly of platelets, fibrin and blood cells. They can block blood vessels, restricting or stopping the flow of blood.

**thromb/o**-angi-itis, inflammation of a blood vessel with clot formation (thrombosis)

**thromb/o**-arter-itis, inflammation of an artery with clot formation (thrombosis)

**thromb**-ectomy, removal of a blood clot

**thrombi-**, blood clots. Plural of thrombus

**thromb**-in, an enzyme that catalyses clot formation (it converts fibrinogen to fibrin)

**thromb/o**-cyte, a cell concerned with clotting (also known as a platelet)

**thromb/o**-cyt-haem-ia, condition of blood with thrombocytes (too many)

**thromb/o**-cyt/o-pen-ia, condition of blood with few thrombocytes (deficiency)

**thromb/o**-cyt-osis, abnormal condition of thrombocytes (too many)

**thromb/o**-embol-ic, pertaining to a thrombosis producing an embolism that plugs another vessel

**thromb/o**-embol-ism, condition of a thrombosis producing an embolism that plugs another vessel

**thromb/o**-end-arter-ectomy, removal of the lining of an artery and a thrombus

**thromb/o**-genesis, formation of blood clots

**thromb/o**-gen-ic, pertaining to formation of clots

**thromb/o**-lysis, disintegration or breakdown of clots

**thromb/o**-lyt-ic, 1. pertaining to disintegration or breakdown of clots 2. an agent that breaks down clots

**thromb/o**-phleb-itis, inflammation of a vein with clot formation (thrombosis)

**thromb/o**-plast-in, a chemical that forms a clot (a lipoprotein released from damaged tissue that triggers the extrinsic coagulation pathway)

**thromb/o**-poiesis, 1. formation of blood clots 2. formation of thrombocytes (platelets)

**thromb**-osis, 1. abnormal condition of blood clots 2. the presence of a thrombus

**thromb/o**-tic, pertaining to or having a thrombosis

**thromb**-us, a clot (primarily fibrin threads with platelets, trapped cells and other blood factors)

---

**Valv/o**, valvul/o, valve
From a Latin word **valva**, meaning a fold. Here valv/o means a valve, especially a heart valve. Valves are formed from folds in membranes within vessels and passageways and permit the flow of fluid in one direction only. There are four valves in the heart, the tricuspid and bicuspid valves between the atria and ventricles, and the pulmonary and aortic valves (semilunar valves) in the vessels that leave the heart. The bicuspid valve is also called the mitral valve.

cardi/o-**valvul/o**-tome, instrument for cutting a heart valve

**valv**-ectomy, removal of a valve

**valv/o**-plasty, surgical repair or reconstruction of a valve

**valv/o**-tomy, incision into a valve

**valv**-ula, a small valve

**valvul**-ar, pertaining to a valve

**valvul**-itis, inflammation of a valve (especially a heart valve)

**valvul/o**-plasty, surgical repair or reconstruction of a valve (especially a heart valve)

**valvul/o**-tome, an instrument for cutting a valve (especially a heart valve)

**valvul/o**-tomy, incision into a valve

---

**Varic/i/o**, varix, a dilated twisted vein
From a Latin word **varix** meaning dilated vein. Here varic/o means a varix, a dilated twisted vein.

**varic**-ation, 1. action of forming a varix 2. a varicosity

**varic**-eal, pertaining to a varix or of the nature of a varix

**varices**, dilated twisted veins. Plural of varix

**varic/i**-form, 1. having the form of a varix 2. varicose

**varic/o**-blephar-on, an eyelid with a varicosity

**varic/o**-cele, a swelling or protrusion of a dilated vein, it refers to a testicular vein producing swelling of the scrotum

**varic/o**-cel-ectomy, removal of a varicocele

**varic/o**-phleb-itis, a varicosity with inflammation, it refers to an inflamed varicose vein

**varic**-ose, having the nature of a varix or swollen vein

**varic**-osis, abnormal condition of varicosity of veins

**varic**-os-ity, 1. condition of being varicose 2. a varicose vein

**varic/o**-tomy, incision (to remove) a varicose vein

**varix**, a dilated twisted vein

---

**Vascul/o**, blood vessel, vessel
From a Latin word **vasculum**, meaning

small vessel. Here vascul/o means a blood vessel of any type.

See the combining forms angi/o, haemangi/o and vas/o also meaning blood vessel

a-**vascul**-ar, pertaining to without blood vessels

**vascul**-ar, pertaining to blood vessels

**vascul**-ar-ization, process of making blood vessels

**vascul**-itis, inflammation of blood vessels

**vascul**/o-gen-ic, pertaining to forming blood vessels (vascularization)

**vascul**/o-pathy, disease of blood vessels (any disorder)

---

**Vas/i/o**, blood vessel, vessel

From a Latin word **vas** meaning a vessel. Here, vas/o means a blood vessel of any type.

See the combining forms angi/o, haemangi/o and vascul/o also meaning blood vessel.

Note the combining form vas/o is also used to mean the vas deferens or sperm duct, see Section 15 The male reproductive system.

**vas**/I-form, having the form of or resembling a blood vessel

**vas**/o-active, having an action on blood vessels (diameter of)

**vas**/o-constrict-ion, the process of constricting (narrowing) blood vessels (raising blood pressure)

**vas**/o-constrict-or, an agent that constricts (narrows) blood vessels (raising blood pressure)

**vas**/o-depress-ion, the process of depressing blood pressure

**vas**/o-depress-or, 1. an agent that depresses blood pressure 2. having the effect of depressing blood pressure

**vas**/o-dilat-ion, the process of dilating blood vessels

**vas**/o-dilat-or, an agent that dilates (widens) blood vessels

**vas**/o-format-ive, pertaining to forming blood vessels

**vas**/o-graphy, technique of making a recording or X-ray of blood vessels

**vas**/o-hyper-ton-ic, 1. pertaining to increased tone or tension in blood vessels (vasoconstriction) 2. an agent that causes increased tone or tension in blood vessels (vasoconstrictor)

**vas**/o-hypo-ton-ic, 1. pertaining to decreased tone or decreased tension in blood vessels (vasodilation) 2. an agent that causes decreased tone or decreased tension in blood vessels (a vasodilator)

**vas**/o-inhibit-or, an agent that inhibits vasomotor nerves

**vas**/o-motor, movement or action of blood vessels, it refers to the nerves and muscles that control the diameter of blood vessels

**vas**/o-paresis, slight paralysis of vasomotor nerves (the nerves that control blood vessels)

**vas**/o-reflex, a reflex action affecting a blood vessel

**vas**/o-spasm, sudden contraction of a blood vessel (due to contraction of smooth muscle in the vessel wall, decreasing its diameter)

**vas**/o-spas-tic, pertaining to sudden contraction of a blood vessel (due to contraction of smooth muscle in the vessel wall, decreasing its diameter)

**vas**/o-stimul-ant, having the characteristic of stimulating blood vessels or having a vasomotor action

**vas**/o-ton-ia, condition of tone or tension of blood vessels

**vas**/o-ton-ic, pertaining to tone or tension of blood vessels

**vas**/o-troph-ic, 1. pertaining to nourishing blood vessels 2. pertaining to affecting the nutrition of a part by controlling the blood supply

**vas**/o-trop-ic, pertaining to stimulating or acting on blood vessels

**vas**/o-vag-al, pertaining to the vagus nerve and blood vessels

---

**Venacav/o**, venae cavae

From a Latin word **vena cavum**, meaning hollow vein. Here venacav/o

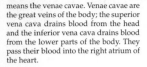 

means the venae cavae. Venae cavae are the great veins of the body; the superior vena cava drains blood from the head and the inferior vena cava drains blood from the lower parts of the body. They pass their blood into the right atrium of the heart.

**venacav/o**-gram, a recording or X-ray picture of the venae cavae

**venacav/o**-graphy, technique of making a recording or X-ray picture of the venae cavae

---

**Ven/e/i/o**, vein

From a Latin word **vena**, meaning vein. Here ven/o means vein, a blood vessel that transfers blood back to the heart. Small veins called venules that drain capillaries join to form the larger veins. Unlike arteries, veins contain valves that prevent the back flow of blood.

See the combining form phleb/o also meaning vein.

**ven**-ectas-ia, condition of dilation of a vein

**ven**-ectasis, dilation of a vein

**ven**-ectomy, removal of a vein or section of a vein Syn. phlebectomy

**ven/e**-puncture, puncture of a vein (by surgery)

**ven/e**-sect-ion, action to cut a vein Syn. phlebotomy

**ven/i**-puncture, puncture of a vein (by surgery)

**ven/i**-suture, stitching or suturing a vein Syn. phleborrhaphy

**ven/o**-clysis, injection or infusion into a vein

**ven/o**-gram, a recording or X-ray picture of a vein

**ven/o**-graphy, technique of making a recording or X-ray picture of veins

**ven/o**-occlusive, tendency to obstruct a vein

**ven/o**-peritone/o-stomy, formation of an opening (anastomosis) between the peritoneum and a vein (the saphenous vein for drainage) or the name of the opening so created

**ven/o**-press-or, 1. an agent that constricts veins 2. pertaining to venous blood pressure

**ven/o**-scler-osis, abnormal condition of hardening of veins (fibrous thickening) Syn. phlebosclerosis

**ven/o**-stasis, stopping or cessation of flow of veins (venous outflow from a part)

**ven/o**-tomy, incision into a vein Syn. phlebotomy

**ven**-ous, pertaining to a vein

**ven/o-ven/o**-stomy, formation of an opening (anastomosis) between a vein and another remote vein or the name of the opening so created

---

**Ventricul/o**, ventricle

From a Latin word **ventriculum** meaning a small, belly-like cavity. Here ventricul/o means a ventricle, one of the two lower chambers of the heart. When the right ventricle contracts blood is pumped into the pulmonary circulation; when the left ventricle contracts, blood is pumped into the systemic circulation.

**atri/o-ventricul**-ar, pertaining to a ventricle and an atrium or to the ventricles and atria

**ventricul**-ar, pertaining to a ventricle or the ventricles

**ventricul/o**-atri/o-stomy, formation of an opening between an atrium and a ventricle or the name of the opening so created

**ventricul/o**-graphy, technique of making a recording or X-ray picture of the ventricles

**ventricul/o**-tomy, incision into a ventricle

# Section 5
# The blood

Blood is a complex fluid classified as a connective tissue because it contains cells, plus an intercellular matrix known as plasma. The components of whole blood include:

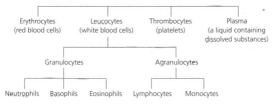

The blood cells carry out a variety of functions: erythrocytes transport gases while leucocytes defend the body against invasion by micro-organisms and foreign antigens. Thrombocytes, or platelets, are fragments of large cells called megakaryocytes. Platelets play a major role in the formation of blood clots following injury.

The plasma carries nutrients, wastes, hormones, antibodies, and blood-clotting proteins. While in the capillaries, some components of the plasma cross the capillary wall and form the tissue fluid or extra-cellular fluid. This fluid forms the immediate environment of the cells in a tissue and maintains their existence by providing nutrients and oxygen and removing metabolic wastes.

Haematology, the study of blood, is very important in medicine for the diagnosis of disease.

Figure 8 shows combining forms associated with the formed elements (cells and cell fragments) of blood and

plasma. Figure 8a shows the origin and types of blood cell.

---

**Roots and combining forms**, meanings

**Agglutin/o**, agglutination, agglutinin
From a Latin word **agglutinare** meaning to glue. Here agglutin/o means agglutination, a process in which bacteria or red blood cells clump together when exposed to specific antibodies called agglutinins. Agglutin/o also means agglutinin, an antibody that develops in the blood serum of a previously infected or sensitized person.

**agglutin**-ation, 1. action or process of cells clumping together *e.g.* red blood cells 2. the action or process of wound healing

**agglutin**-in, an agent (antibody) in blood serum that causes cells or antigens to clump together

**agglutin/o**-gen, an agent that stimulates the formation of agglutinin

## Quick Reference

Combining forms relating to the blood:

| | | Page |
|---|---|---|
| -aem- | blood (see haemat/o) | 83 |
| **Agglutin/o** | agglutinin, agglutination | 77 |
| **Bas/o** | alkaline, basic | 80 |
| -chrom- | colour, haemoglobin | 80 |
| **Cyan/o** | blue | 80 |
| -cytosis | condition of cells | 80 |
| **Embol/o** | embolus | 81 |
| **Eosin/o** | eosin dye | 81 |
| **Erythr/o** | erythrocyte, red, red blood cell | 81 |
| **Granul/o** | granule, granulocyte | 83 |
| **Haemat/o** | blood | 83 |
| **Haem/o** | blood | 83 |
| **Haemoglobin/o** | haemoglobin | 86 |
| **Leuc/o** | leucocyte,white, white blood cell | 87 |
| **Leuk/o** | leucocyte,white, white blood cell | 87 |
| **Lymph/o** | lymph, lymphocyte | 88 |
| **Macro-** | large | 89 |
| **Mega, megalo-** | large | 89 |
| **Monocyt/o** | monocyte | 90 |
| **Myel/o** | bone marrow, myelocyte | 90 |
| **Neutr/o** | neutral, neutrophil | 91 |
| **Norm/o** | normal | 91 |
| -ox- | oxygen | 92 |
| **Phag/o** | phagocyte | 92 |
| **Plasm/a** | plasma | 92 |
| **Py/o** | pus | 93 |
| **Reticul/o** | reticulocyte | 93 |
| **Sanguin/o** | blood | 93 |
| **Thromb/o** | blood clot, thrombus | 93 |
| **Thrombocyt/o** | platelet, thrombocyte | 95 |

## Quick Reference

Common words and combining forms relating to the blood:

| | | Page |
|---|---|---|
| Agglutination | **agglutin/o** | 77 |
| Agglutinin | **agglutin/o** | 77 |
| Alkaline | **bas/o** | 80 |
| Basic | **bas/o** | 80 |
| Blood | **-aem-, haemat/o,** | 83 |
| | **haem/o** | 83 |
| | **sanguin/o** | 93 |
| Blood clot | **thromb/o** | 93 |
| Blue | **cyan/o** | 80 |
| Bone marrow | **myel/o** | 90 |
| Clot | **thromb/o** | 93 |
| Clotting cell | **thrombocyt/o** | 95 |
| Colour | **-chrom-** | 80 |
| Condition of cells | **-cytosis** | 80 |
| Embolus | **embol/i/o** | 81 |
| Eosin dye | **eosin/o** | 81 |
| Erythrocyte | **erythr/o** | 81 |
| Granule | **granul/o** | 83 |
| Granulocyte | **granul/o** | 83 |
| Haemoglobin | **-chrom-,** | 80 |
| | **haemoglobin/o** | 86 |
| Large | **macro-, mega-,** | |
| | **megalo-** | 89 |
| Leucocyte | **leuc/o, leuk/o** | 87 |
| Lymph | **lymph/o** | 88 |
| Lymphocyte | **lymph/o** | 88 |
| Marrow | **myel/o** | 90 |
| Monocyte | **monocyt/o** | 90 |
| Myelocyte | **myel/o** | 90 |
| Neutral | **neutr/o** | 91 |
| Neutrophil | **neutr/o** | 91 |
| Normal | **norm/o** | 91 |
| Oxygen | **-ox-** | 92 |
| Phagocyte | **phag/o** | 92 |
| Plasma | **plasm/a** | 92 |
| Platelet | **thrombocyt/o** | 95 |
| Pus | **py/o** | 93 |
| Red | **erythr/o** | 81 |
| Red blood cell | **erythr/o** | 81 |
| Reticulocyte | **reticul/o** | 93 |
| Thrombocyte | **thrombocyt/o** | 95 |
| Thrombus | **thromb/o** | 93 |
| White | **leuc/o, leuk/o** | 87 |
| White blood cell | **leuc/o,** | |
| | **leuk/o** | 87 |

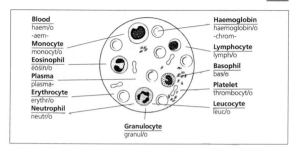

Figure 8a  The blood

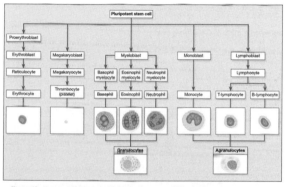

Figure 8b  Haemopoiesis: stages in the development of blood cells
(from Ross and Wilson, Figure 4.2, p. 62)

**agglutin/o**-gen-ic, pertaining to the formation of agglutinin

**agglutin/o**-phil-ic, pertaining to loving agglutination or agglutinating easily

auto-**agglutin**-ation, 1. action or process of cells clumping together of an individual's cells by his/her own serum

2. clumping together of cells or antigens by themselves (in the absence of specific antibodies)

auto-**agglutin**-in, an agent (antibody) in blood serum that causes cells or antigens to clump together in the same individual

79

**Bas/o**, alkaline, basic

From a Greek word **basis** meaning base. Here bas/o means having the characteristic of a base, in chemistry this means able to neutralize an acid or showing an alkaline reaction. In the blood are basophils, types of granulo-cytic, polymorphonuclear leucocyte that stain readily with basic dyes; these cells are involved in inflammation.

**bas/o**-erythr/o-cyte, a red cell or erythro-cyte taking up a basophilic stain (it contains basophilic granules)

**bas/o**-erythr/o-cyt-osis, abnormal con-dition of basoerythrocytes, it refers to red cells taking up basic stains (they contain basophilic granules)

**bas/o**-pen-ia, condition of reduction (virtual absence) of basophils in blood

**bas/o**-phil, 1. a cell with an affinity (love) for basic dyes 2. a granulocytic, poly-morphonuclear leucocyte with an affinity for basic dyes

**bas/o**-phil-ia, condition of (increase) of basophils in the blood

**bas/o**-phil-ic, pertaining to an affinity (love) for basic dyes or staining with basic dye

**bas/o**-phil-ism, abnormal condition of (increase) in basophilic cells

---

**-chrom-**, colour, haemoglobin

From a Greek word **chroma** meaning colour. Here **-chrom-** means haemo-globin, the red iron-containing protein found in red blood cells that associates with oxygen to form oxyhaemoglobin and with carbon dioxide to form carbaminohaemoglobin. Haemoglobin acts to transport oxygen and carbon dioxide around the body in the blood.

See the combining form haemo-globin/o also meaning haemoglobin.

hyper-**chrom**-ia, condition of abnormal increase in haemoglobin in erythro-cytes, it shows as an increase in their colour

hyper-**chrom**-ic, 1. pertaining to an abnormal increase in colour 2. per-

taining to an abnormal increase in colour of erythrocytes due to an increase in synthesis of haemoglobin

hypo-**chrom**-ia, condition of abnormal decrease in haemoglobin in erythro-cytes, it shows as a decrease in their colour

hypo-**chrom**-ic, 1. pertaining to an abnor-mal decrease in colour 2. pertaining to an abnormal decrease in colour of erythrocytes due to a decrease in synthesis of haemoglobin

norm/o-**chrom**-ia, condition of normal colour or normal haemoglobin content of erythrocytes

norm/o-**chrom**-ic, pertaining to normal colour of erythrocytes (normal mean corpuscular haemoglobin concen-tration of erythrocytes)

---

**Cyan/o**, blue

From a Greek word **kyanos** meaning blue. Here cyan/o means blue and is used in words referring to the colour of haemoglobin. Without oxygen haemoglobin takes on a bluish tinge. Nail beds, lips and skin show signs of cyanosis (*i.e.* look blue) when oxygenation of the blood is deficient.

**cyan**-aem-ia, condition of bluish blood

**cyan**-osed, pertaining to having a blue coloration of skin and mucous mem-branes (due to poor oxygenation of the blood)

**cyan**-osis, abnormal condition of blue coloration of skin and mucous membranes (due to poor oxygenation of the blood)

**cyan/o**-tic, 1. pertaining to having a blue coloration of skin and mucous membranes (due to poor oxygenation of the blood) 2. pertaining to having cyanosis

---

**-cytosis**, condition of cells

From the Greek words **kytos** meaning cell and **osis** condition of. Here -cytosis means the condition of red cells (erythrocytes) in the blood, usually the presence of too many of a particular type.

an-iso-**cytosis**, condition of cells (erythrocytes) of unequal size (without equality)

ellipto-**cytosis**, condition of elliptical cells (elliptical erythrocytes)

iso-**cytosis**, condition of equal cells (erythrocytes of equal size)

macro-**cytosis**, condition of abnormally large cells (large erythrocytes)

micro-**cytosis**, condition of small cells (small erythrocytes or microcytes)

norm/o-**cytosis**, condition of normal cells (normal erythrocytes)

poikilo-**cytosis**, condition of irregular-shaped cells (irregular erythrocytes)

schist/o-**cytosis**, condition of an accumulation of schistocytes (split erythrocytes) in the blood

---

**Embol/i/o**, embolus
From a Greek word **embolos** meaning plug. Here embol/o means an embolus, a foreign body that can plug a blood vessel. An embolus can suddenly form from a blood clot, mass of tumour cells, globule of fat, a bubble of gas or infectious material.

**embol**-aem-ia, condition of emboli in the blood

**embol**-ectomy, removal of an embolus (from a vessel)

**emboli**, plural of embolus

**embol**-ic, pertaining to an embolus

**embol**-i-form, having the form of an embolus

**embol**-ism, sudden obstruction of a blood vessel by an embolus (undissolved material such as a thrombus [clot], clump of bacteria or other foreign body).

**embol**-iz-ation, 1. the process of making or forming an embolus 2. the deliberate occlusion of a vessel by introduction of a substance that acts as a plug

**embol/o**-gen-ic, pertaining to producing an embolus

**embol**-oid, resembling an embolus

**embol**-us, a thrombus (clot) or other foreign body transported in the circulation that suddenly blocks a smaller vessel

---

**Eosin/o**, eosin
From a Greek word **eos** meaning dawn. Here eosin/o means an acidic red dye used for staining histological specimens. Types of granular leucocyte known as eosinophils stain readily with acid dyes and can be clearly seen in blood smears. Eosinophils combat the effects of histamine in allergic reactions, phagocytose antigen–antibody complexes and help destroy parasitic worms.

**eos**-in, a red, acidic dye used for staining histological specimens such as blood smears

**eosin/o**-blast, an immature cell (found in bone marrow) that forms an eosinophil

**eosin/o**-pen-ia, condition of deficiency of eosinophils in the blood

**eosin/o**-phil, a granular leucocyte that has an affinity for eosin (loves eosin)

**eosin/o**-phil-ia, condition of abnormal increase of eosinophils in the blood

**eosin/o**-phil-ic, pertaining to (loving) eosin, it refers to staining with or taking up eosin

**eosin/o**-phil/o-tact-ic, pertaining to an ordered movement or arrangement of eosinophils (attracting eosinophils). From a Greek word taxis meaning arrangement

---

**Erythr/o**, red, erythrocyte, red blood cell
From a Greek word **erythros**, meaning red. Here erythr/o means red and is used in words referring to red blood cells (erythrocytes).

**erythr**-aem-ia, condition of blood containing red cells (an increase in red cell mass) Syn. polycythaemia vera

**erythr/o**-blast, an immature cell or embryonic cell that gives rise to erythrocytes

**erythr/o**-blast-ic, pertaining to or belonging to erythroblasts

**erythr/o**-blast-oma, a tumour composed of cells that resemble erythroblasts

**erythr/o**-blast-osis, abnormal condition of erythroblasts in the blood

**erythr/o**-blast/o-tic, 1. pertaining to erythroblastosis 2. pertaining to having an abnormal condition of erythroblastis in the blood

**erythr/o**-clasis, breaking up of erythrocytes

**erythr/o**-clast-ic, pertaining to breaking up of erythrocytes

**erythr/o**-cyt-apheresis, process of withdrawal of blood, removal of red cells and transfusion of the remainder into the donor

**erythr/o**-cyte, a red cell (of the blood)

**erythr/o**-cyt-haem-ia, condition of erythrocytes in the blood (too many red blood cells)

**erythr/o**-cyt-ic, pertaining to or of the nature of erythrocytes

**erythro**-cyt/o-lysis, breakdown of erythrocytes

**erythr/o**-cyt/o-meter, an instrument used to measure (count) erythrocytes

**erythr/o**-cyt/o-metry, technique of measuring (counting) erythrocytes

**erythr/o**-cyt/o-pen-ia, condition of deficiency in the number of erythrocytes Syn. erythropenia

**erythr/o**-cyt/o-rrhexis, rupture of erythrocytes (with loss of cytoplasm)

**erythr/o**-cyt/o-schisis, splitting of erythrocytes (into disc-like plaques)

**erythr/o**-cyt-osis, abnormal condition of erythrocytes (too many)

**erythr/o**-cyt/o-trop-ic, pertaining to having an affinity for erythrocytes

**erythr/o**-cyt-ur-ia, condition of erythrocytes in the urine Syn. haematuria

**erythr/o**-genesis, formation of red blood cells

**erythr/o**-gen-ic, pertaining to forming erythrocytes

**erythr**-oid, red or reddish in colour

**erythr/o**-kinet-ics, the science of studying the movement of erythrocytes, it refers to the quantitative study of the rates of production and destruction of erythrocytes in the blood

**erythr/o**-leuk-aem-ia, condition of the blood containing a large number of atypical leucocytes and erythrocytes (a malignant blood dyscrasia)

**erythr**-on, a term used to describe the circulating erythrocytes their precursors and all the cells concerned with erythropoiesis

**erythr/o**-neo-cyt-osis, abnormal condition of new erythrocytes (immature red blood cells) in the blood

**erythr/o**-pathy, disease of erythrocytes

**erythr/o**-pen-ia, condition of reduction in number of erythrocytes

**erythr/o**-phage, a phagocyte that ingests erythrocytes (a phagocyte is a cell that 'eats' or engulfs particles)

**erythr/o**-phag-ia, condition of ingesting erythrocytes (by phagocytosis)

**erythr/o**-phag/o-cyt-osis, abnormal condition of ingesting erythrocytes (by phagocytosis)

**erythr/o**-phag-ous, pertaining to ingestion of erythrocytes (by phagocytosis)

**erythr/o**-phthisis, wasting away of erythrocyte forming tissue

**erythr/o**-poiesis, formation of erythrocytes

**erythr/o**-poie-tic, pertaining to the formation of erythrocytes

**erythr/o**-poie-tin, an agent (hormone) secreted by the kidney in adults and liver in the fetus, it stimulates the formation of erythrocytes from stem cells

**erythr/o**-rrhexis, rupture of erythrocytes (with loss of cytoplasm) Syn. erythrocytorrhexis

**erythr**-osis, abnormal condition (of too many cells) in the tissue in which erythrocytes are formed

**erythr/o**-stasis, the stopping or cessation of flow of erythrocytes in the capillaries

micro-**erythr/o**-cyte, an (abnormally) small cell red blood cell, less than 5 microns in diameter

pro-**erythr/o**-blast, an immature cell or embryonic cell before the erythroblast, it refers to an immature cell that

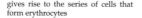

gives rise to the series of cells that form erythrocytes

**Granul/o, granular, granule**
From a Latin word **granulum** meaning little grain. Here granul/o means granule and is used in words relating to the granular series of white blood cells known as polymorphonuclear leucocytes. These cells contain granules and have multi-lobed nuclei; there are three main types found in the blood, neutrophils, eosinophils and basophils. These cells play an important role in defending the body against microbes and other foreign agents.

a-**granul/o**-cyte, a cell without granules (nongranular leucocyte)

a-**granul/o**-cyt-osis, abnormal condition of cells without granules (a decrease in the number of granulocytes)

a-**granul/o**-plast-ic, 1. pertaining to forming cells without granules 2. pertaining to lack of formation of granular cells

**granul**-ar, pertaining to or composed of granules

**granul/o**-blast, an immature cell or embryonic cell that forms the granular series of leucocytes Syn. myeloblast

**granul/o**-cyte, a cell containing granules, a granular leucocyte

**granul/o**-cyt-ic, pertaining to granulocytes or cells containing granules

**granul/o**-cyt/o-pen-ia, condition of reduction in the number of granulocytes Syn. agranulocytosis

**granul/o**-cyt/o-poiesis, formation of granulocytes

**granul/o**-cyt/o-poie-tic, pertaining to the formation of granulocytes

**granul/o**-cyt-osis, abnormal condition of (too many) granulocytes in the blood

**granul/o**-pen-ia, condition of reduction in the number of granulocytes Syn. agranulocytosis

**granul/o**-plast-ic, pertaining to forming granules

**granul/o**-poiesis, formation of granulocytes

**granul/o**-poie-tic, pertaining to the formation of granulocytes

**Haemat/o,** haem/a/o, -aem-, blood
From a Greek word **haima**, meaning blood. Here haem/o means blood.
See the combining form sanguin/o also meaning blood.

an-**aem**-ia, condition of without blood, it refers to a reduced number of red cells and/or quantity of haemoglobin

auto-**haem**-agglutin-ation, action or process of blood cells (erythrocytes) clumping together, caused by factors in an individual's own serum

auto-**haem**-agglutin-in, an agent produced in an individual that agglutinates his/her own red blood cells

auto-**haem/o**-lys-in, an agent found in serum that lyses one's own red blood cells

auto-**haem/o**-lysis, breakdown of one's own red blood cells, caused by agents in the patient's serum

auto-**haem/o**-ly-tic, pertaining to auto-haemolysis

dys-**haemat/o**-poie-tic, pertaining to bad or defective formation of blood

electro-**haem/o**-stasis, stopping of bleeding by electrocautery

**haem/a**-cyt/o-meter, an instrument used to measure blood cells (numbers of) Syn. haemocytometer

**haem**-agglutin-in, an agent (antibody in serum) that agglutinates red blood cells

**haem**-al, pertaining to the blood or the blood vascular system

**haem**-analysis, the process of analysing the blood (splitting into its components for analysis)

**haem**-apheresis, process of withdrawal of blood, removal of red cells, leucocytes or platelets and transfusion of the remainder into the donor

**haem**-arthr-osis, abnormal condition of discharge of blood into a joint

**haemat**-emesis, vomiting of blood

**haemat**-ic, 1. pertaining to blood 2. acting on the blood 3. containing blood

**haemat/o**-idr-osis, abnormal condition of sweat containing blood. From a Greek word *hidros* meaning sweat.

**haemat/o**-cele, a swelling or cyst containing blood

**haemat/o**-colp/o-metra, blood (accumulation) in the uterus and vagina

**haemat/o**-colpos, blood (accumulation) in the vagina

**haemat/o**-crit, 1. an instrument that measures the volume of erythrocytes in a sample 2. the actual value of the measured volume of erythrocytes in a sample of blood

**haemat/o**-cyt-ur-ia, condition of blood cells (erythrocytes) in the urine

**haemat/o**-gen-ic, 1. pertaining to the formation of blood cells Syn. haematopoietic 2. originating in the blood

**haemat/o**-gen-ous, 1. pertaining to the formation of blood cells 2. originating in the blood

**haemat/o**-log-ist, a specialist who studies blood (composition, diseases and treatment of)

**haemat/o**-logy, the study of blood (composition, diseases and treatment of)

**haemat/o**-lymph-angi-oma, a tumour of lymph vessels and blood vessels

**haemat**-oma, a swelling containing blood

**haemat/o**-mediastin-um, effusion of blood into the mediastinum and its spaces

**haemat/o**-metra, blood (accumulation) in the uterus

**haemat/o**-metry, technique of measuring the percentages of blood cells and haemoglobin concentration in blood samples

**haemat/o**-myel-ia, condition of blood in the spinal cord, it refers to haemorrhage into the substance of the spinal cord

**haemat/o**-myel-itis, inflammation of the spinal cord containing an effusion of blood

**haemat/o**-myel/o-pore, formation of pores or channels in the spinal cord by blood (haemorrhage)

**haemat/o**-path/o-logy, the study of disease of the blood

**haemat/o**-phag-ia, condition of eating or feeding off blood

**haemat/o**-phag-ous, pertaining to eating or feeding off blood

**haemat/o**-poiesis, formation of blood

**haemat/o**-poie-tic, pertaining to formation of blood

**haemat/o**-rrhachis, condition of blood in the spine, it refers to haemorrhage into the substance of the spinal cord Syn. haematomyelia

**haemat/o**-rrhoea, excessive flow of blood or haemorrhage

**haemat/o**-salpinx, blood in the uterine tube

**haemat/o**-spermat/o-cele, a swelling or hernia of the epididymis or rete testis (a spermatocele) containing blood

**haemat**-oste-on, blood (haemorrhage) into a bone marrow cavity

**haemat/o**-tox-ic, 1. pertaining to blood poisoning 2. pertaining to poisonous to blood and the blood forming system

**haemat/o**-trop-ic, pertaining to having an affinity for or affecting blood or blood cells

**haemat**-ur-ia, condition of blood in the urine

**haem/o**-blast, an immature cell or embryonic cell that forms all the cellular elements of blood Syn. haemocytoblast

**haem/o**-blast-osis, 1. an abnormal condition of (too many) haemoblasts 2. an increase in blood forming tissue

**haem/o**-cather-esis, the breakdown (haemolysis) of red blood cells. From a Greek word *kathairein* meaning to bring down

**haem/o**-cathere-tic, 1. pertaining to the breakdown (haemolysis) of red blood cells. From a Greek word *kathairein* meaning to bring down 2. pertaining to or of the nature of haemocatheresis

**haem/o**-coel-ia, condition of blood in the peritoneal cavity

**haem/o**-concentration, increase in concentration of formed elements of the blood relative to the amount of fluid

haem/o-cyte, a blood cell

haem/o-cyt/o-blast, an immature cell or embryonic cell that forms all the cellular elements of blood

haem/o-cyt/o-blast-oma, a tumour containing haemocytoblasts (all cells typical of bone marrow)

haem/o-cyt/o-cather-esis, the breakdown (haemolysis) of red blood cells. From a Greek word kathairein meaning to bring down

haem/o-cyt/o-meter, an instrument used to measure blood cells (numbers of) Syn. haemacytometer

haem/o-cyt/o-tripsis, breakdown of blood cells by heavy pressure. From a Greek word tripsis meaning a rubbing

haem/o-dia-filtration, process of using filtration and haemodialysis, it refers to a type of renal replacement therapy that removes waste products from the blood

haem/o-diagnosis, using blood tests to diagnose disease

haem/o-dialyzer, device that performs haemodialysis

haem/o-dialysis, separation of waste products from the blood, it refers to a process that enables metabolic wastes to diffuse out of the blood across a differentially permeable membrane into a rinsing solution or diasylate; as in a haemodialysis machine or artificial kidney

haem/o-dilution, decrease in concentration of formed elements of the blood relative to the amount of fluid

haem/o-dynam-ic, pertaining to the force and movement of blood

haem/o-dynam-ics, the science of studying the force and movement of the blood

haem/o-filtration, filtration of the blood (to remove waste products)

haem/o-globin, a blood protein found in red blood cells that transports oxygen and carbon dioxide.

haem/o-histi/o-blast, an immature cell or embryonic cell that forms all the tissue (cellular elements) of blood

haem-oid, resembling blood

haem/o-kinesis, the movement or flow of blood

haem/o-lymph, lymph and blood

haem/o-lys-in, an agent that lyses or splits red blood cells

haem/o-lysis, breakdown or disintegration of red blood cells (with liberation of haemoglobin into the plasma)

haem/o-lyt-ic, 1. pertaining to haemolysis 2. an agent that lyses or splits red blood cells

haem/o-lyse, to cause or produce haemolysis

haem/o-mediastin-um, effusion of blood into the mediastinum and its spaces

haem/o-metra, blood (accumulation) in the uterus Syn. haematometra

haem/o-path-ic, pertaining to disease of the blood

haem/o-path/o-logy, the study of diseases of the blood

haem/o-pathy, disease of the blood

haem/o-perfusion, process of perfusing blood (passing blood through an absorbent material to remove poisons)

haem/o-peri-card/i-um, an effusion of blood in the pericardial sac (around the heart)

haem/o-peritone-um, an effusion of blood into the peritoneal cavity

haem/o-pexis, fixation or coagulation of blood

haem/o-phag/o-cyte, a phagocyte that ingests and destroys blood cells

haem/o-phil, blood loving, it refers to microorganisms that thrive in blood or culture media containing blood

haem/o-phil-ia, condition of loving blood, a sex-linked inherited condition in which clotting factors are deficient causing the sufferer to bleed excessively from minor wounds

haem/o-phil-ic, 1. pertaining to loving or having an affinity for blood 2. pertaining to or of the nature of haemophilia

haem/o-phillias, name for the group of inherited sex-linked diseases with blood coagulation defects Haemophilia A, Haemophilia B *etc.*

**haem/o**-phili-oid, resembling classical haemophilia

**haem/o**-phob-ia, irrational fear of blood, bleeding or losing blood

**haem/o**-plast-ic, pertaining to the formation of blood Syn. haematopoietic

**haem/o**-pneum/o-peri-cardi-um, an effusion of air and blood in the pericardium

**haem/o**-pneum/o-thorax, an effusion of air and blood in the thorax (pleural cavity)

**haem/o**-poiesis, formation of blood

**haem/o**-ptysis, spitting up of blood

**haem/o**-rrhage, bursting forth of blood

**haem/o**-rrhag-ic, pertaining to bursting forth of blood or haemorrhage

**haem/o**-rrhoea, excessive flow of blood or excessive haemorrhage

**haem/o**-rrhoe-logy, the study of the flow properties of the components of blood in vessels

**haem/o**-rrhoid, a swelling of blood (varicose dilation) at the anal margin. From a Greek word *haimorrhois* meaning a vein liable to discharge blood

**haem/o**-rrhoid-ectomy, removal of a haemorrhoid

**haem/o**-stasis, cessation of blood flow or stopping of bleeding by clotting

**haem/o**-stat, an agent or instrument used to stop blood flow or prevent haemorrhage

**haem/o**-stat-ic, pertaining to stopping blood flow or preventing haemorrhage

**haem/o**-therapy, treatment of disease using blood

**haem/o**-thorax, effusion of blood into the thorax (pleural cavity)

**haem/o**-tox-ic, 1. pertaining to blood poisoning 2. pertaining to poisonous to blood and the blood forming system Syn haematotoxic

**haem/o**-tox-in, an agent poisonous to red blood cells, it refers to an agent with haemolytic activity

olig-**aem**-ia, condition of little blood (diminished total quantity)

para-**haem/o**-phil-ia, condition of near haemophilia (a congenital haemorrhagic disease resembling haemophilia associated with deficiency of Factor V)

poly-cyt-**haem**-ia, condition of too many blood cells (usually an increase in number of red cells)

pseudo-an-**aem**-ia, condition of false anaemia, it refers to the appearance of pallor without evidence of anaemia

septic-**aem**-ia, condition of decay of blood (due to infection)

xanth-**aem**-ia, condition of yellow blood, due to excessive amounts of carotene Syn. carotenaemia

---

**Haemoglobin/o**, haemoglobin

From the Greek words **haima** meaning blood and Latin **globus** meaning ball. Here, haemoglobin/o means haemoglobin, the red iron-containing protein found in red blood cells that associates with oxygen to form oxyhaemoglobin and with carbon dioxide to form carbaminohaemoglobin. Haemoglobin acts to transport oxygen and carbon dioxide around the body in the blood.

See the root -chrom- also meaning haemoglobin.

**haemoglob**-in, a blood protein found in red blood cells that transports oxygen and carbon dioxide

**haemoglobin**-aem-ia, condition of haemoglobin in the blood (excessive amounts free in blood plasma)

**haemoglobin/o**-lysis, breakdown of haemoglobin

**haemoglobin/o**-meter, an instrument that measures haemoglobin

**haemoglobin/o**-path-ic, 1. pertaining to disease of haemoglobin 2. pertaining to haemoglobinopathy

**haemoglobin/o**-pathy, disease of haemoglobin, due to a mutation in the gene that determines the molecular structure of haemoglobin

**haemoglobin**-ur-ia, condition of haemoglobin in the urine

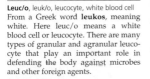

**Leuc/o**, leuk/o, leucocyte, white blood cell
From a Greek word **leukos**, meaning white. Here leuc/o means a white blood cell or leucocyte. There are many types of granular and agranular leucocyte that play an important role in defending the body against microbes and other foreign agents.

**leuc/o**-agglutin-in, an agglutinin (antibody) that acts on leucocytes

**leuc**-apheresis, process of withdrawal of blood, removal of leucocytes and transfusion of the remainder into the donor

**leuc/o**-blast, an immature cell or embryonic cell that gives rise to leucocytes

**leuc/o**-blast-osis, abnormal condition of too many leucoblasts, it results in a proliferation of leucocytes

**leuc/o**-cid-in, an agent that kills leucocytes (produced by some pathogenic bacteria)

**leuc/o**-crit, 1. an instrument that measures the volume of leucocytes in a sample 2. the actual value of the measured volume of leucocytes in a sample of blood

**leuc/o**-cyt-haem-ia, condition of leucocytes in the blood (too many) Syn. leukaemia

**leuc/o**-cyt-ic, pertaining to or of the nature of leucocytes

**leuc/o**-cyt/o-blast, an immature cell or embryonic cell that gives rise to leucocytes

**leuc/o**-cyt/o-clasis, breaking or disintegration of leucocytes

**leuc/o**-cyt/o-clast-ic, 1. pertaining to breaking or disintegration of leucocytes 2. pertaining to leucocytoclasis

**leuc/o**-cyt/o-genesis, formation of white blood cells

**leuc/o**-cyt-oid, resembling a leucocyte

**leuc/o**-cyt/o-lysis, breakdown or disintegration of leucocytes

**leuc/o**-cyt-o-lyt-ic, 1. pertaining to breakdown or disintegration of leucocytes 2. pertaining to leucocytolysis

**leuc/o**-cyt-oma, a tumour-like mass of leucocytes

**leuc/o**-cyt/o-pen-ia, condition of reduction of leucocytes Syn. leucopenia

**leuc/o**-cyt/o-plan-ia, condition of wandering or migration of leucocytes (from the blood)

**leuc/o**-cyt/o-poiesis, formation of leucocytes Syn. leucopoiesis

**leuc/o**-cyt-osis, abnormal condition of white cells (an increase in the number of white blood cells, usually transient in response to infection)

**leuc/o**-cyt/o-tax-ia, condition of ordered movement of leucocytes (away or towards a focus e.g. towards a site of damaged or infected tissue)

**leuc/o**-cyt/o-taxis, condition of ordered movement of leucocytes (away or towards a focus e.g. towards a site of damaged or infected tissue) Syn. leucotaxis

**leuc/o**-cyt/o-tic, pertaining to a leucocytosis

**leuc/o**-cyt/o-toxic-ity, state or condition of poisonous to leucocytes Syn. lymphocytotoxicity

**leuc/o**-depleted, depletion or reduction of leucocytes, describes donated blood from which leucocytes have been removed

**leuc/o**-erythr/o-blast-osis, condition of immature red cells and white (myeloid cells) cells in the blood

**leuc/o**-gen-ic, pertaining to forming leucocytes

**leuc/o**-path-ia, condition of disease of leucocytes

**leuc/o**-pathy, 1. disease of leucocytes 2. a condition caused by accumulation of dead leucocytes

**leuc/o**-pedesis, outward movement of leucocytes through the walls of a blood vessel. From a Greek word *pedesis* meaning an oozing

**leuc/o**-pen-ia, condition of deficiency or reduced number of white blood cells

**leuc/o**-pen-ic, 1. pertaining to a deficiency of leucocytes 2. pertaining to or affected by leucopenia

**leuc/o**-pheresis, process of withdrawal of blood, removal of leucocytes and transfusion of the remainder into the donor

**leuc/o**-poiesis, formation of white blood cells

**leuc/o**-sarc-oma, a well-differentiated, malignant lymphocytic lymphoma. Syn. lymphoma

**leuc/o**-sarc-omat-osis, abnormal condition of multiple sarcomas (sarcomata) composed of leukaemic cells

**leuc**-osis, abnormal condition of tissue from which leucocytes form, it refers to an abnormal increase

**leuc/o**-taxis, condition of ordered movement of leucocytes (away or towards a focus *e.g.* towards a site of damaged or infected tissue

**leuc/o**-thromb/o-pen-ia, condition of reduction in thrombocytes (platelets) and leucocytes (in the blood)

**leuc/o**-tox-ic, pertaining to poisonous to white cells

**leuk**-aem-ia, condition of white blood, it refers to a malignant cancer of haemopoietic tissue showing an abnormal increase in the number of leucocytes Syn. leukocythaemia

**leuk**-aem-ic, 1. pertaining to leuk-aemia 2. pertaining to having leukaemia

**leuk**-aem/o-gen, an agent that forms leukaemia

**leuk**-aem/o-genesis, formation of leukaemia

**leuk**-aem/o-gen-ic, pertaining to to forming or causing leukaemia

**leuk**-aem-oid, resembling leukaemia

**leuk/o**-lymph/o-sarc-oma, a malignant tumour of lymph cells (lympho-sarcoma) forming a leukaemia

pre-**leuk**-aem-ia, condition before leukaemia, it refers to a bone marrow disorder before the onset of acute myelogenous leukaemia

pre-**leuk**-aem-ic, 1. pertaining to before the onset of leukaemia 2. pertaining to before to having a bone marrow disorder before the onset of acute myelo-genous leukaemia

---

**Lymph/o**, lymphocyte
From a Greek word **lympha**, meaning water. Here lymph/o means

lymphocyte, a type of agranular leucocyte. These cells form in lymphoid tissue in lymph nodes, spleen, gastrointestinal tract and bone marrow, they defend the body against foreign agents by producing antibodies and T-cells.

Note: Other words associated with the lymph and the lymphatic system are listed in Section 6 The lymphatic system and immunity.

---

**lymph**-apheresis, process of withdrawal of blood, removal of lymphocytes and transfusion of the remainder into the donor Syn. lymphocytopheresis, lymphocytapheresis

**lymph/o**-blast, an immature cell or embryonic cell that forms into a mature lymphocyte

**lymph/o**-blast-ic, 1. pertaining to or forming immature cells or embryonic cells that develop into mature lymphocytes 2. pertaining to lymphoblasts

**lymph/o**-blast-oma, a (malignant) tumour that arises from lympho-blasts

**lymph/o**-blast-osis, abnormal condition of (excess) lymphoblasts (in the blood)

**lymph/o**-cyt-apheresis, process of withdrawal of blood, removal of lymphocytes and transfusion of the remainder into the donor Syn. lymphocytopheresis, lympha-pheresis

**lymph/o**-cyte, a lymph cell

**lymph/o**-cyt-ic, pertaining to lympho-cytes

**lymph/o**-cyt/o-blast, an immature cell or embryonic cell that forms into a mature lymphocyte Syn. lympho-blast

**lymph/o**-cyt-oma, a (malignant) tumour composed of lymphocytes, it refers to a lymphocytic lymphoma

**lymph/o**-cyt/o-pen-ia, condition of reduction in the number of lymphocytes (in the blood)

**lymph/o**-cyt/o-pheresis, process of withdrawal of blood, removal

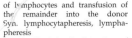

of lymphocytes and transfusion of the remainder into the donor Syn. lymphocytapheresis, lymphapheresis

**lymph/o**-cyt/o-poiesis, the formation of lymphocytes

**lymph/o**-cyt-osis, abnormal condition of (excess) lymphocytes (in the blood or other effusion)

**lymph/o**-cyt/o-tox-ic-ity, condition or state of being poisoned to lymphocytes

**lymph/o**-cyt/o-tox-in, an agent that poisons lymphocytes

**lymph/o**-pen-ia, condition of reduction in the number of lymphocytes in the blood

**lymph/o**-plasm-apheresis, process of withdrawal of blood, selective removal of lymphocytes and plasma followed by transfusion of the remainder into the donor

**lymph/o**-poiesis, the formation of lymphocytes or lymph tissue

**lymph/o**-poie-tic, 1. pertaining to the formation of lymphocytes or lymph tissue 2. pertaining to lymphopoiesis

**lymph/o**-taxis, ordered movement of lymphocytes (attraction or repulsion)

**lymph/o**-tox-in, 1. an agent poisonous to lymph cells 2. an agent released by sensitized lymphocytes poisonous to cells

pro-**lymph/o**-cyte, a cell before the lymphocyte, it refers to an immature cell between the lymphoblast and lymphocyte in the lymphocytic series

---

**Macro-**, abnormally large, large
From a Greek word **macros** meaning large. Here, macro- means large or abnormally large and is used as a prefix, often to indicate a large atypical blood cell.

**macro**-blast, an immature, abnormally large nucleated, red blood cell, it gives rise to an abnormal erythrocyte series

**macro**-cyte, an abnormally large red blood cell

**macro**-cyt-haem-ia, condition of macrocytes in the blood

**macro**-cyt-ic, pertaining to or of the nature of macrocytes

**macro**-cyt-osis, abnormal condition of macrocytes in the blood

**macro**-mono-cyte, an abnormally large monocyte

**macro**-myelo-blast, an abnormally large myeloblast

**macro**-normo-blast, an abnormally large normoblast

**macro**-phage, a large eater, it refers to large phagocytic cells of the monocyte-macrophage system derived from monocytes

**macro**-poly-cyte, an abnormally large leucocyte with many lobes in its nucleus

---

**Mega-**, megal/o, large
From a Greek word **megas** meaning large. Here megal/o means large or abnormally large.

**mega**-kary/o-blast, an immature cell or embryonic cell that forms the thrombocyte series (matures to form a promegakaryocyte)

**mega**-kary/o-cyte, a large cell of bone marrow with a (lobed) nucleus (fragments break off the cell to form platelets)

**mega**-kary/o-cyt/o-pen-ia, condition of reduction of megakaryocytes in the blood

**mega**-kary/o-cyt-osis, abnormal condition of megakaryocytes in the blood

**mega**-kary/o-phthisis, wasting away of the megakaryocytes (deficiency in the marrow)

**megal/o**-blast, a large immature cell, it refers to a cell that forms a series of abnormally large erythrocytes

**megal/o**-blast-ic, pertaining to or of the nature of megaloblasts

**megal/o**-cyte, a very large erythrocyte

**megal/o**-cyt-osis, abnormal condition of megalocytes in the blood

pro-**mega**-kary/o-cyte, a cell before the megakaryocyte, it refers to a precursor of the thrombocyte series of cells intermediate between a megakaryoblast and a megakaryocyte

---

**Monocyt/o**, monocyte

From the Greek words **monos** meaning single and **kytos** meaning cell. Here monocyt/o means monocyte, a large, nucleated leucocyte seen in normal blood. The monocyte is phagocytic and is transported to tissues such as the lungs where it develops into a macrophage.

macro-**monocyte**, a large monocyte

**monocyt**-ic, pertaining to or of the nature of monocytes

**monocyt/o**-pen-ia, condition of reduction or deficiency of monocytes in the blood

**monocyt/o**-poiesis, the formation of monocytes (in the bone marrow)

**monocyt**-osis, abnormal condition of an increase in monocytes in the blood

pro-**monocyte**, a cell before the monocyte, it refers to a cell intermediate between a monoblast and monocyte

---

**Myel/o**, bone marrow, bone marrow cell, myelocyte

From a Greek word **myelos**, meaning marrow. Here myel/o means bone marrow, the substance that fills the medullary cavity and spaces in cancellous bone containing the haemopoietic tissue that produces blood cells. Myel/o also means myelocyte, a precursor cell of the polymorphonuclear series of granulocytes found in bone marrow.

Note: myel/o also means spinal cord, see Section 8 The nervous system and for more words on bone marrow Section 14 The skeletal system.

meta-**myel/o**-cyte, an intermediate myelocyte, it refers to an immature myelocyte in a stage of development between a promyelocyte and granular leucocyte

micro-**myel/o**-blast, 1. a small immature cell or embryonic cell of the marrow 2. a small immature myelocyte

**myel**-itic, pertaining to having myelitis

**myel**-itis, inflammation of the bone marrow

**myel/o**-blast, an immature cell or embryonic cell of the marrow, a precursor of the granular series of leucocyte

**myel/o**-blast-aem-ia, condition of myeloblasts in the blood

**myel/o**-blast-oma, a malignant tumour composed of myeloblasts, seen in myelocytic leukaemia

**myel/o**-blast-osis, abnormal condition of myeloblasts in the blood, seen in myeloblastic leukaemia

**myel/o**-cyte, a marrow cell, a precursor cell of the polymorphonuclear series of granulocytes

**myel/o**-cyt-haem-ia, condition of myelocytes in the blood as in myeloid leukaemia

**myel/o**-cyt-ic, pertaining to or of the nature of myelocytes

**myel/o**-cyt-oma, a tumour of myelocytes Syn. myeloma

**myel/o**-cyt-osis, abnormal condition of myelocytes in the blood

**myel/o**-fibr-osis, condition of fibres in marrow, it refers to replacement of bone marrow by fibrous tissue

**myel/o**-genet-ic, pertaining to originating or forming in bone marrow

**myel/o**-gen-ous, pertaining to originating or forming in bone marrow

**myel/o**-gone, a primitive leucocyte of the myeloid series

**myel/o**-gon-ic, pertaining to a myelogone

**myel/o**-gram, a picture or recording of cells found in bone marrow (used in haematology)

**myel**-oid, 1. resembling myelocytes 2. resembling bone marrow or derived from bone marrow

**myel**-oid-osis, abnormal condition (hyperplasia) of myeloid tissue

**myel/o**-lip-oma, a tumour of fatty tissue and myeloid cells (a benign tumour of the adrenal gland)

**myel**-oma, a tumour of myeloid tissue or bone marrow cells

**myel**-omat-oid, resembling a myeloma

**myel**-omat-osis, abnormal condition of multiple myelomas Syn. multiple myeloma

**myel**-omat-ous, pertaining to myelomas

**myelo**-path-ic, pertaining to disease of the bone marrow

**myelo**-pathy, disease of the bone marrow

**myel/o**-phthisis, wasting of the bone marrow caused by the depression of cell-forming actions of bone-marrow

**myel/o**-plast, a marrow cell, it refers to any leucocyte found in bone marrow

**myel/o**-poiesis, formation of bone marrow or bone marrow cells

**myel/o**-poie-tic, pertaining to formation of bone marrow or bone marrow cells

**myel/o**-proliferative, increase in one or more of the cellular components of bone marrow

**myel/o**-sarc-oma, a malignant tumour composed of myeloid tissue or bone marrow cells

**myel/o**-scler-osis, abnormal condition of hardening of bone marrow (the marrow cavity fills with bony tissue)

**myel**-osis, abnormal condition of (increase) in bone marrow tissue leading to myelocytic leukaemia

**myel/o**-suppressive, 1. inhibition of bone marrow activity 2. an agent that inhibits bone marrow activity

**myel/o**-therapy, treatment with bone marrow preparations

**myel/o**-tox-ic, pertaining to poisonous to bone marrow

**myel/o**-toxic-osis, abnormal condition of poisoning of bone marrow

**myel/o**-tox-in, an agent that is poisonous to bone marrow

pan-**myel/o**-phthisis, wasting of all bone marrow cells Syn. aplastic anaemia

pre-**myel/o**-blast, a cell before the myeloblast (a precursor cell of the myeloblast)

pro-**myel/o**-cyte, a cell before the myelocyte, it refers to an immature precursor cell of the myelocyte that produces the granulocytic series of leucocytes

**Neutr/o**, neutral, neutrophil

From a Latin word **neuter** meaning neither. Here neutr/o means neutral or neutrophil. Neutrophils are types of granular leucocyte that are only weakly stained with acid or basic dyes. Neutrophils are phagocytic functioning in the destruction of pathogenic organisms and other foreign matter.

**neutr**-al, pertaining to neutral *i.e.* neither acid nor basic

**neutr/o**-pen-ia, condition of a reduction in the number of neutrophils

**neutr/o**-phil, loving neutral (dyes), it refers to a granular leucocyte only weakly stained with acid or basic dyes

**neutr/o**-phil-ia, condition of neutrophils (increase) in the blood

**neutr/o**-phil-ic, 1. pertaining to or of the nature of neutrophils 2. pertaining to stainable with neutral dyes

**neutr/o**-phil/o-pen-ia, condition of reduction in numbers of neutrophils in the blood

**neutr/o**-taxis, pertaining to an ordered movement or arrangement of neutrophils (attracting or repulsing neutrophils) From a Greek word *taxis* meaning arrangement

**Norm/o**, normal

From a Latin word **norma** meaning rule. Here norm/o means normal with respect to erythrocytes of normal colour, size and shape.

**norm/o**-blast, an immature cell or embryonic cell of the erythrocyte series

**norm/o**-blast-osis, abnormal condition of normoblasts, it refers to excessive production of normoblasts by bone marrow

**norm/o**-chrom-ia, 1. condition of the normal colour of erythrocytes 2. condition of the normal haemoglobin content of erythrocytes

**norm/o**-chrom-ic, pertaining to normal colour of erythrocytes (the normal mean corpuscular haemoglobin concentration of erythrocytes)

**norm/o**-cyte, a normal erythrocyte (of typical colour, size and shape)

**norm/o**-cyt-ic, pertaining to or of the nature of normocytes

**norm/o**-cyt-osis, condition of normal erythrocytes in the blood

pro-**norm/o**-blast, an immature cell before the normoblast, it refers to the earliest erythrocyte precursor

---

**-ox-**, oxygen

From the Greek words **oxys** meaning sharp and **genein** meaning to produce. Here -ox- means the gas oxygen.

an-**ox**-aem-ia, condition of blood without oxygen

an-**ox**-aem-ic, 1. pertaining to blood without oxygen 2. pertaining to having anoxaemia

an-**ox**-ia, condition of without oxygen supply to a tissue

an-**ox**-ic, pertaining to without oxygen supply to a tissue

hyp-**ox**-aem-ia, condition of below normal oxygenation of the blood

hyp-**ox**-ia, condition of below normal oxygen supply to a tissue

hyp-**ox**-ic, pertaining to below normal oxygen supply to a tissue

---

**Phag/o**, phagocyte

From a Greek word **phagein** meaning to eat. Here, phag/o refers to a phagocyte, a cell that eats. Phagocytes can engulf and digest particulate matter and micro-organisms that have entered the body; they fall into two main groups, microphages and macrophages.

Neutrophils and monocytes are phagocytes present in the blood. The neutrophil (a granulocyte) is a type of microphage whereas the monocyte (an agranulocyte) is a blood cell that can enlarge and develop into a macrophage, a large phagocytic cell

that can leave the blood and migrate to areas of infection.

macro-**phag**e, a large eater, it refers to a large, highly phagocytic cell of the reticulo-endothelial system that forms from a monocyte

micro-**phag**e, small eater, it refers to a small, mobile phagocytic cell, a polymorphonuclear leucocyte

**phag/o**-cyte, 1. a cell that eats or ingests foreign organisms and particles 2. a cell that performs phagocytosis

**phag/o**-cyt-ic, 1. pertaining to phagocytosis 2. pertaining to or of the nature of phagocytes

**phag/o**-cyt-in, a (bactericidal) agent secreted by phagocytes (neutrophils)

**phag/o**-cyt/o-blast, an immature cell that forms phagocytes

**phag/o**-cyt/o-lysis, breakdown or destruction of phagocytes

**phag/o**-cyt/o-lyt-ic, pertaining to breakdown or destruction of phagocytes

**phag/o**-cyt-ose, to perform the act of engulfing or ingesting foreign organisms and particles

**phag/o**-cyt-osis, condition of engulfing or ingesting foreign organisms and particles by phagocytes

**phag/o**-cyt/o-tic, pertaining to phagocytosis

**phag/o**-some, a body (membrane bound vesicle) found inside a phagocyte, it contains ingested material

---

**Plasm/a/o**, plasma

From a Greek word **plassein** meaning to mould. Here plasm/a means plasma, the fluid portion of blood in which the blood cells are suspended.

Note: the combining form also refers to plasmacytes, cells of the immune system derived from B-lymphocytes that manufacture antibodies. See Section 6 The lymphatic system and immunology for words referring to these cells.

auto-**plasm/o**-therapy, treatment using one's own blood plasma

**plasma**-globul-in, a globulin (protein) found in plasma *e.g.* immunoglobulin IgG

**plasm**-apheresis, process of withdrawal of blood, removal of plasma and transfusion of the remaining cells in an isotonic solution or fresh plasma into the donor

**plasma**-therapy, treatment with blood plasma

**plasma**-tic, pertaining to plasma

**plasm**-ic, pertaining to plasma

---

**Py/o**, pus

From a Greek word **pyon**, meaning pus. Here py/o means pus, a yellow, protein-rich liquid, composed of tissue fluids containing bacteria and leucocytes formed in infected wounds. When a wound is forming or discharging pus it is said to be suppurating. Pus is formed in response to certain types of infection.

**py**-aem-ia, condition of pus (septic emboli) in the blood (a septicaemia causing multiple abscesses)

**py/o**-coccus, a berry-like bacterium (coccus) that forms pus

**py/o**-cyst, a cyst containing pus

**py/o**-genesis, the formation of pus

**py/o**-gen-ic, pertaining to forming pus

**py**-oid, resembling pus

**py/o**-poiesis, the formation of pus Syn. pyogenesis

**py/o**-ptysis, the expectoration (spitting) of pus

**py/o**-rrhoea, excessive discharge or flow of pus

**py/o**-rrhoe-al, pertaining to the excessive discharge or flow of pus

**py**-osis, the formation of pus or suppuration

**py/o**-stat-ic, pertaining to an agent that stops pus or suppuration

---

**Reticul/o**, reticulocyte

From a Latin word **reticulum**, meaning small net. Here, reticul/o is mainly used to mean a reticulocyte, a very young erythrocyte lacking a nucleus; its cytoplasm has a net-like appearance when stained with basic dyes.

**reticul**-ar, 1. pertaining to or belonging to a reticulum 2. pertaining to resembling a net

**reticul**-ation, process of forming a network or presence of a network

**reticul/o**-cyte, an immature erythrocyte

**reticul/o**-cyt/o-gen-ic, pertaining to the formation of reticulocytes

**reticul/o**-cyt/o-pen-ia, condition of deficiency of reticulocytes

**reticul/o**-cyt-osis, abnormal condition of too many reticulocytes in the blood

**reticul/o**-cyt-pen-ia, condition of deficiency or reduction of reticulocytes

**reticul/o**-plasm/o-cyt-oma, a tumour formed from plasmacytes and reticulocytes

---

**Sanguin/e/o**, blood

From a Latin word **sanguis** meaning blood. Here **sanguin**/o means blood.

See the combining form haem/o also meaning blood.

ex-**sanguin**-ation, act of losing blood, by internal or external haemorrhage

**sangui**-fer-ous, pertaining to carrying blood

**sanguin/e**-ous, 1. pertaining to blood 2. containing blood 3. bloody

**sanguin/o**-poie-tic, pertaining to the formation of blood Syn. haematopoietic

---

**Thromb/o**, blood clot, thrombus

From a Greek word **thrombos**, meaning a clot. Here throm/o means a thrombus or blood clot. Blood clots consist mainly of platelets, fibrin fibres and blood cells and they form when blood coagulates. Clots can block blood vessels and restrict or stop the flow of blood.

anti-**throm/o**-plast-in, an agent that acts against or prevents the action of thromboplastin

**thromb**-asthen-ia, condition of weakness of clots (a platelet abnormality characterized by defective clot

**thromb**-ectomy, removal of a clot (from a vessel)

**thrombi**, clots. Plural of thrombus

**thromb**-in, an agent (enzyme) concerned with clotting (thrombin catalyses conversion of fibrinogen to fibrin)

**thromb/o**-angi-itis, inflammation of blood vessels associated with clots

**thromb/o**-arter-itis, inflammation of arteries associated with clots

**thromb/o**-clasis, breaking up or dissolution of clots Syn. thrombolysis

**thromb/o**-clast-ic, pertaining to breaking up or dissolution of clots Syn. thrombolytic

**thromb/o**-cyst, a cyst (formed by a membrane) surrounding a thrombus

**thromb/o**-cyst-is, a cyst (formed by a membrane) surrounding a thrombus

**thromb/o**-cyte, a clotting cell or platelet. See thrombocyt/o below

**thromb/o**-cyt-ic, pertaining to a thrombocyte or platelet

**thromb/o**-embol-ic, pertaining to an embolism produced by a clot

**thromb/o**-embol-ism, an embolism (obstruction of a vessel) by a clot carried in the circulation

**thromb/o**-embol-ization, the process of making or forming an embolus from a detached clot in the circulation

**thromb/o**-end-arter-ectomy, removal of the inner lining of an artery and an associated clot

**thromb/o**-end-arter-itis, inflammation of the inner lining of an artery with an associated thrombosis

**thromb/o**-endo-card-itis, inflammation of the inner lining of the heart (endocardium) with the formation of a thrombus (on a heart valve)

**thromb/o**-gen-ic, 1. pertaining to thrombogenesis 2. pertaining to capable of clotting blood

**thromb/o**-genesis, clot formation

**thromb**-oid, resembling a clot

**thromb/o**-kin-ase, an enzyme that forms clots, it is released from damaged tissue and initiates the extrinsic coagulation pathway Syn. thromboplastin

**thromb/o**-kinet-ics, the science of studying the dynamics of blood clotting or coagulation

**thromb/o**-lymph-ang-itis, inflammation of a lymph vessel associated with a thrombus or clot

**thromb/o**-lysis, breakdown or dissolution of a thrombus

**thromb/o**-lyt-ic, pertaining to breakdown or dissolution of a thrombus

**thromb/o**-phil-ia, condition of loving clots, it refers to a tendency to form thrombi

**thromb/o**-phleb-itis, inflammation of a vein associated with a thrombus

**thromb/o**-plast-ic, pertaining to forming clots or coagulating blood

**thromb/o**-plast-in, an agent that forms a blood clot, it refers to an enzyme released from damaged tissue that initiates the extrinsic coagulation pathway, it aids the conversion of prothrombin to thrombin Syn. thrombokinase

**thromb/o**-poiesis, 1. formation of thrombi or clots Syn. thrombogenesis 2. formation of thrombocytes or platelets Syn. thrombocytopoiesis

**thromb/o**-poie-tic, 1. pertaining to thrombopoiesis 2. pertaining to formation of thrombocytes or platelets Syn. thrombocytopoietic

**thromb**-osed, affected with thrombosis

**thromb**-osis, abnormal condition of or formation of thrombi

**thromb/o**-stasis, stopping or cessation of flow of blood due to an associated thrombus

**thromb**-ox-anes, a group of lipids released from platelets that cause a clot, they act by inducing vasoconstriction and platelet aggregation during platelet plug formation

**thromb**-us, a blood clot

pro-**thromb**-in, an agent before thrombin, it refers to a plasma protein that forms thrombin (Factor II) essential for the normal coagulation of blood

**Thrombocyt/o**, clotting cell, platelet, thrombocyte

From the Greek words **thrombos**, meaning a clot and **kytos** meaning cell. Here thrombocyt/o means a thrombocyte or platelet, a disc-shaped fragment of a larger cell called a megakaryocyte that plays an important role in the clotting of blood. In damaged tissue platelets aggregate to form a platelet plug and release chemicals that participate in blood coagulation.

**thrombocyt**-haem-ia, condition of blood with thrombocytes (abnormal increase)

**thrombocyt**-ic, pertaining to thrombocytes or platelets

**thrombocyt/o**-crit, 1. an instrument that measures the volume of thrombocytes in a sample 2. the actual value of the measured volume of thrombocytes in a sample of blood

**thrombocyt/o**-lysis, breakdown or disintegration of thrombocytes

**thrombocyt/o**-pathy, disease of thrombocytes

**thrombocyt/o**-pen-ia, condition of reduction in the number of thrombocytes

**thrombocyt/o**-poiesis, formation of thrombocytes

**thrombocyt/o**-poie-tic, pertaining to formation of thrombocytes

**thrombocyt**-osis, abnormal condition of thrombocytes, it refers to an increase in number in the circulation

# Section 6
# The lymphatic system and immunology

The lymphatic system consists of:

- lymph
- lymph vessels
- lymph nodes
- lymph organs *e.g.* spleen and thymus
- diffuse lymphoid tissue, *e.g.* tonsils
- bone marrow.

All tissue cells are bathed in tissue fluid (or extracellular fluid) that consists of the diffusible constituents of blood and waste materials from cells. Some tissue fluid returns to the blood circulation through capillaries at their venous ends and the remainder diffuses into the lymphatic capillaries and becomes lymph.

Lymph is a clear, watery fluid similar in composition to blood plasma but lacking plasma proteins. It passes through vessels of increasing size, from lymph capillaries to vessels and ducts, and through a varying number of lymph nodes before returning to the blood near the heart. The lymphatic system performs three important functions: (i) transportation of lymphocytes that defend the body against infection and foreign antigens, (ii) transportation of lipids, and (iii) by its formation, the drainage of excess fluid from the tissues.

Figure 9 shows the anatomy of the lymphatic system and the combining forms associated with its components.

## Structure and function of lymph nodes

Lymph nodes consist of lymphatic channels held in place by fibrous connective tissue that forms a capsule. The nodes contain **lymphocytes**, and special cells called **macrophages** (large

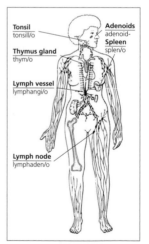

**Tonsil**
tonsill/o

**Adenoids**
adenoid-

**Spleen**
splen/o

**Thymus gland**
thym/o

**Lymph vessel**
lymphangi/o

**Lymph node**
lymphaden/o

Figure 9 The lymphatic system

## Quick Reference

Combining forms relating to the lymphatic system and immunology:

| | | Page |
|---|---|---|
| **Aden/o** | gland | 99 |
| **Adenoid-** | adenoids | 99 |
| **Chyl/o** | chyle | 100 |
| **Clon/ō** | clone of cells | 100 |
| **Histi/o** | histiocyte | 100 |
| **Immun/o** | immune, immunity | 101 |
| **Lymphaden/o** | lymph node | 102 |
| **Lymphangi/o** | lymph vessel | 103 |
| **Lymphat/o,**<br>**lymph/o** | lymph | 103 |
| **Phag/o** | phagocyte | 105 |
| **Plasma-** | plasma cell | 106 |
| **Reticuloendotheli-** | reticuloendothelial system | 106 |
| **Ser/o** | serum | 106 |
| **Splen/o** | spleen | 107 |
| **Thymic/o,**<br>**thym/o** | thymus gland | 108 |
| **Tonsill/o** | tonsil | 109 |

## Quick Reference

Common words and combining forms relating to the lymphatic system and Immunology:

| | | Page |
|---|---|---|
| Adenoids | **adenoid-** | 99 |
| Chyle | **chyl/o** | 100 |
| Clone | **clon/o** | 100 |
| Gland | **aden/o** | 99 |
| Histiocyte | **histi/o** | 100 |
| Immune | **immun/o** | 101 |
| Immunity | **immun/o** | 101 |
| Lymph | **lymphat/o,**<br>**lymph/o** | 103 |
| Lymph node | **lymphaden/o** | 102 |
| Lymph vessel | **lymphangi/o** | 103 |
| Phagocyte | **phag/o** | 105 |
| Plasma cell | **plasma-** | 106 |
| Reticuloendothelial system | **reticuloendotheli-** | 106 |
| Serum | **ser/o** | 106 |
| Spleen | **splen/o** | 107 |
| Thymus gland | **thymic/o,**<br>**thym/o** | 108 |
| Tonsil | **tonsill/o** | 109 |

eaters) which, like neutrophils, can engulf foreign substances and micro-organisms by phagocytosis. Lymph nodes often trap malignant cells as well as micro-organisms. During infection lymphocytes and macrophages multiply rapidly, causing the nodes to swell; they may become inflamed and sore. Lymphocytes and macrophages leave the nodes in lymph that eventually drains through ducts into blood vessels near the heart. These cells then circulate in the blood and form a proportion of the white blood cell population.

If disease in the lymphatic system is suspected, a **nodal biopsy** may be performed. In this procedure a node is removed for examination by a histopathologist. Distinct patches of lymphatic tissue have been given specific names; the familiar ones mentioned here include the spleen, tonsils, adenoids, and thymus.

## The reticuloendothelial system

The macrophages that line the lymph organs are part of a large system of cells known as the reticuloendothelial system or monocyte–macrophage system. Cells that form this network have a common ancestry and carry out phagocytosis in the liver, bone marrow, lymph nodes, spleen, nervous system, blood, and connective tissues. Macrophages found in connective tissues are known as **histiocytes** (tissue cells). If there is an increase in the number of histiocytes without infection this is known as a histiocytosis.

## Immunology

Understanding the meaning of the following terms will help you understand definitions of words associated with the immune response.

### Antigen

An antigen is any foreign substance that enters the body and stimulates antibody production or a response associated with sensitized T-cells or both.

Note: antigens present on the surface of any foreign cell that enters the body will provoke a response from the immune system.

## Antibody

An antibody is a chemical that circulates in the blood destroying or precipitating specific foreign substances (antigens) that have entered the body. (*Anti-* means against, *-body* is an Anglo-Saxon word, in this case referring to a foreign body.)

Two basic types of cell are involved in the immune response:

## B-cells

B-cells are types of lymphocyte named for historical reasons after the site where they were first seen in birds, the Bursa of Fabricius. In humans, B-cells first differentiate in the fetal liver and transform into large **plasma cells** when confronted with specific antigens. Once sensitized by an antigen, the plasma cell multiplies to form a large clone of similar cells (**plasmacytosis**). Each cell in the clone secretes the same antibody to the sensitizing antigen; this is known as the **humoral response**. Some antibodies activate a protein in the blood known as **complement** that aids the antibody in destroying antigen.

## T-cells (thymic cells)

Some lymphocytes formed in the bone marrow of the embryo move to the thymus to be processed into thymic cells or T-cells. The T-cells then move to other parts of the lymphatic system where they are responsible for the **cell-mediated response**. Once sensitized to a specific antigen, these cells multiply rapidly and produce various cell types that play a role in the immune response. One type, the **cytotoxic (killer) T-cell**, attacks and kills infectious microorganisms containing the specific antigen directly. These cells are particularly effective against slowly growing bacteria and fungi, cancer cells and skin grafts.

The immune response not only resists the invasion by infective organisms but also acts to identify and destroy everything described as 'non-self', for example foreign antigens that have entered the body or, body cells that have changed their form and become malignant.

Patients infected with microorganisms, for example those who present with tonsillitis, experience swollen lymph nodes and their blood counts indicate an increase in circulating white blood cells. The nodes swell because they contain plasma cells and T-cells forming clones of cells to 'fight' the infection. Once the foreign cells have been destroyed, the nodes return to their normal size. The response of the body to the initial sensitization with the antigen is called the *primary response*.

An important feature of the immune response is that some activated B-cells develop into **memory B-cells** rather than plasma cells. These remain in the nodes and other lymphoid tissue ready to respond should the same antigen enter the body again. If the same antigen is contacted the memory B-cells divide rapidly to produce plasma cells, these release large amounts of antibody, destroying the antigen before symptoms appear.

In a similar way some **memory T-cells** remain in the lymphoid tissue, and can be rapidly activated in response to another contact with the same antigen. The accelerated and increased response of the memory cells is called the *secondary response*, and it endows us with immunity.

Immunology is the scientific study of immunity and related disciplines such as immunotherapy and immunochemistry. Immunological research has intensified recently because of the spread of the immunodeficiency virus (HIV) that causes AIDS. Many pharmaceutical companies are actively engaged in the search for vaccines and new treatments based on our increased knowledge of the immune process.

## Roots and combining forms, meanings

**Aden/o**, gland

From a Greek word **aden** meaning gland. Here, aden/o refers to glands in general and in some words to lymphoid tissue. A patch of lymphoid tissue is sometimes called a lymph gland, but the term lymph node is preferred. Unlike true glands lymph nodes do not produce secretions, instead they produce cells that act to defend the body against noxious agents such as microorganisms and toxins.

See the combining form lymphaden/o that refers specifically to a lymph node.

**aden**-alg-ia, condition of pain in a gland

**aden**-ectomy, removal of a gland

**aden**-ia, condition of a gland, it refers to enlargement of lymph nodes

**aden**-itis, inflammation of a gland

**aden**-iz-ation, action of becoming gland-like in appearance

**aden/o**-blast, an embryonic cell or immature cell that forms gland tissue

**aden/o**-carcin-oma, a malignant tumour formed from gland tissue

**aden/o**-gen-ous, pertaining to originating in a gland or gland tissue

**aden**-oid, 1. resembling a gland 2. resembling lymphoid tissue 3. the pharyngeal tonsil (adenoids). See the combining form adenoid/o

**aden/o**-lymph-itis, inflammation of the lymph glands (nodes) Syn. lymphadenitis

**aden/o**-lymph-oma, a cystic tumour containing lymphoid tissue and glandular tissue usually found in salivary glands

**aden**-oma, a tumour containing glandular tissue or derived from glandular tissue

**aden/o**-malac-ia, condition of softening of a gland

**aden**-omat-oid, resembling an adenoma

**aden**-omat-osis, abnormal condition of having multiple adenomas (adenomata)

**aden**-onc-us, a tumour or swelling of a gland

**aden/o**-pathy, disease of glands, especially enlargement of lymph nodes

**aden/o**-pharyng-itis, inflammation of the pharynx and adenoids

**aden/o**-scler-osis, abnormal condition of hardening of a gland

**aden**-osis, abnormal condition of glands or lymph nodes

**aden/o**-tome, an instrument used to cut into a gland or the adenoids (for removal)

**aden/o**-tomy, incision into a gland or into the adenoids (for removal)

**aden/o**-tonsill-ectomy, removal of the tonsils and adenoids

hyper-**aden**-osis, abnormal condition of above normal enlargement of a gland

peri-**aden**-itis, inflammation of tissues around a gland

poly-**aden**-osis, abnormal condition of many glands

---

**Adenoid-**, adenoids

From a Greek word **aden** meaning gland and **eidos** meaning form. Here adenoid- means the adenoids, a single enlarged pharyngeal tonsil that extends into the nasopharynx of children. Sometimes it obstructs the passage of air or interferes with hearing when it blocks the entrance to the auditory tube.

Note: although ending with an 's', adenoids is used to mean the single enlarged pharyngeal tonsil.

**adenoid**-al, pertaining to the adenoids

**adenoid**-ectomy, removal of the adenoids (the pharyngeal tonsil)

**adenoid**-itis, inflammation of the adenoids (the pharyngeal tonsil)

**adenoid**-ism, process of describing the presence of enlarged adenoids (giving characteristic adenoid face, facial pallor and breathing through the mouth)

**adenoids**, the condition of having an enlarged pharyngeal tonsil (formed by hypertrophy of lymphoid tissue into the nasopharynx)

---

**Chyl/i/o**, chyle

From a Greek word **chylos** meaning juice. Here, chyl/o means chyle, the milky fluid transported by the microscopic lacteal vessels in the intestinal mucosa. Chyle consists of lymph and digested fat droplets (chylomicrons) in a stable emulsion.

**chyl**-aem-ia, condition of chyle in the blood

**chyl**-angi-oma, a tumour of intestinal lymph vessels filled with chyle

**chyl**-ectas-ia, condition of dilation of a vessel containing chyle such as a lacteal

**chyl/i**-facient, chyle-forming. From a Latin word *facere* meaning to make

**chyli**-fer-ous, 1. pertaining to carrying chyle 2. pertaining to forming chyle

**chyl/i**-form, having the form of or resembling chyle

**chyl/o**-cyst, the cisterna chyli, the dilated part of the thoracic duct

**chyl/o**-derma, skin with chyle, it refers to swelling of the scrotum due to blockage, dilation and rupture of lymph vessels in the scrotal skin with a fluid discharge (caused by filarial worms blocking lymph vessels)

**chyl**-oid, resembling chyle

**chyl/o**-micron, a small fat droplet approximately 1 nm in diameter, formed from triglycerides, cholesterol and lipoproteins within the intestinal mucosa. Chylomicrons enter the lymphatic system through the lacteals in the intestine.

**chyl/o**-micron-aem-ia, condition of (excess) chylomicrons in the blood

**chyl/o**-pericardi-um, an effusion of chyle in the pericardium

**chyl/o**-peritone-um, an effusion of chyle in the peritoneum

**chyl/o**-phor-ic, pertaining to carrying chyle

**chyl/o**-pneumo-thorax, an effusion of air and chyle in the thorax

**chyl/o**-poiet-ic, pertaining to forming chyle

**chyl/o**-rrhoea, excessive flow of chyle, due to rupture of lymph vessels

**chyl/o**-thorax, an effusion of chyle in the thorax

**chyl**-ous, pertaining to or of the nature of chyle

**chyl**-ur-ia, condition of chyle in the urine (due to rupture of renal lymphatics)

---

**Clon/o**, clone

From a Greek word **klon** meaning a cutting used for propagation. Here clon/o means a clone of cells. Cells that form a clone are similar genetically and are derived by cell division from a single cell.

**clon**-al, pertaining to a clone

**clon**-al-ity, state or ability to form a clone

mono-**clon**-al, pertaining to a clone from a single cell

poly-**clon**-al, pertaining to many clones (derived from different cells)

**clon/o**-gen-ic, pertaining to forming a clone of cells

---

**Histi/o**, histiocyte

From a Greek word **histos**, meaning web. Here, histi/o is used in a set of words referring to histiocytes (tissue cells), large phagocytic cells of the reticulo-endothelial system. These cells usually remain in connective tissue of the skin, and subcutaneous layer and are called fixed macrophages.

Note: words containing the combining form hist/o meaning tissue are listed in Section 1 Cells, tissues organs and systems.

**histi/o**-blast, a tissue-forming cell

**histi/o**-cyte, a tissue cell (a large phagocytic cell of the reticulo-endothelial system, a macrophage)

**histi/o**-cyt-oma, a tumour containing histiocytes

**histi/o**-cyt-osis, abnormal condition of histiocytes (in the blood)

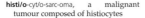

**histi/o**-cyt/o-sarc-oma, a malignant tumour composed of histiocytes

---

**Immun/o**, immunity

From a Latin word **immunis**, meaning exempt from public burden. Here immun/o means the state of being immune or having immunity (exemption from disease). In some words, immun/o means antibody or the antigen–antibody reaction.

auto-**immun**e, state in which the immune response is directed towards oneself, it refers to the production of immunoglobulins or a cell-mediated response directed against the body's own tissues

auto-**immun**-ity, condition in which the immune response is directed towards oneself, it refers to the production of immunoglobulins or a cell-mediated response directed against the body's own tissues

auto-**immun**-iz-ation, action or process of producing an immune response directed towards oneself it refers to the production of immunoglobulins or a cell-mediated response directed against the body's own tissues

heter/o-**immun**-ity, condition or state of immunity induced in an individual by antigens from a different species

**Immune**, 1. having immunity or protection against a particular disease 2. state of having an intrinsic or acquired state of resistance to an infectious agent due to the formation of humoral antibodies and/or the development of a cell-mediated immune response

**immun**-ity, 1. condition or state of having protection against a particular disease 2. an intrinsic or acquired state of resistance to an infectious agent due to the formation of humoral antibodies and/or the development of a cell-mediated immune response

**immun**-iz-ation, process or action of initiating immunity

**immun**-ize, to make immune or to produce immunity

**immun/o**-adjuv-ant, an agent injected with an antigen that enhances the immune response. From a Latin word *juvare* meaning to help

**immun/o**-assay, technique of measuring antigens using the antigen–antibody reaction

**immun/o**-bio-logy, branch of biology that studies the effects of the immune system on biological processes

**immun/o**-blast, an immature cell or embryonic cell that forms lymphoid tissue

**immun/o**-blast-ic, pertaining to or of the nature of immunoblasts

**immun/o**-chemistry, the science or study of the chemical basis of the immune response

**immun/o**-chemo-therapy, treatment involving chemotherapy and immunotherapy

**immun/o**-competence, ability to develop an immune response to an antigen

**immun/o**-complex, an antigen combined with its specific antibody

**immun/o**-compromised, state of having a defective immune response (due to immunosuppressive drugs, irradiation, malnutrition or disease)

**Immun/o**-cyte, a cell concerned with immunity, it refers to any lymphoid cell that reacts with an antigen

**immun/o**-deficiency, state of a deficient immune response due to a reduction in the number of lymphoid cells

**immun/o**-dermato-logy, the study of immune responses in relation to skin disorders

**immun/o**-diagnosis, the use of immune reactions to diagnose disease

**immun/o**-electr/o-phoresis, technique that uses electrophoresis (movement of charged particles in an electric field) and immunodiffusion (diffusion of antibodies in a gel) to identify proteins

**immun/o**-fluorescence, fluorescence detected when a specimen is exposed to antibody or antigen labelled with a fluorochrome, a technique that uses fluorescent dyes to locate antibodies or antigens

**immun/o**-gen, an agent that produces a specific immune response

**immun/o**-genesis, formation or production of immunity

**immun/o**-genet-ic, pertaining to the transmission of genes or genetic factors associated with the immune response

**immun/o**-genet-ics, the science of studying the transmission of genes or genetic factors associated with the immune response

**immun/o**-gen-ic, pertaining to the ability of a substance to produce a specific immune response

**immun/o**-gen-ic-ity, 1. ability of a substance to produce a specific immune response 2. the degree to which a substance produces a specific immune response

**immun/o**-globul-in, a protein associated with immunity, it refers to a protein with antibody activity found in the blood plasma, there are five classes IgA, IgD, IgE, IgG and IgM

**immun/o**-haemat/o-logy, the study of immune responses (antigen–antibody reactions) and their association with blood disorders

**immun/o**-incompetent, inability to develop an immune response to an antigen

**immun/o**-log-ical, 1. pertaining to immunity 2. pertaining to immunology

**immun/o**-log-ist, person who specializes in the study of immunity

**immun/o**-logy, 1. the study of immunity 2. the study of the reactions of immune system tissues to antigens

**immun/o**-path/o-genesis, formation of a disease in which the immune response is involved

**immun/o**-path/o-logy, the study of diseases associated with the immune response

**immun/o**-radi/o-metry, technique of measuring radioactive (labelled) antibody, a radio immunoassay technique

**immun/o**-stimul-ation, action of stimulating or inducing the immune response

**immun/o**-suppress-ant, an agent or drug that reduces the immune response

**immun/o**-suppression, deliberate inhibition of the immune response by means of drug, radiation or anti-lymphocyte immunoglobulin

**immun/o**-suppressive, an agent or drug that reduces the immune response

**immun/o**-therapy, treatment of the immune system, it refers to the administration of antibodies or immunocompetent tissue produced in another individual. The term has also come to include treatment with immunostimulants and immunosuppressants

**immun/o**-tox-in, an agent (antibody) produced in response to a toxin Syn. antitoxin

**immun/o**-transfusion, transfusion of blood from a donor who is immune to a disease affecting the recipient

---

**Lymphaden/o**, lymph gland, lymph node

From the Latin word **lympha** meaning water and Greek word **aden** meaning gland. Here, lymphaden/o means lymph node rather than lymph gland because the structure referred to is no longer considered a true gland. A lymph node is a mass of lymphoid tissue containing cells that defend the body against noxious agents such as microorganisms and toxins, it does not produce a secretion.

**lymphaden**-ectasis, dilation of a lymph node

**lymphaden**-ectomy, removal of a lymph node

**lymphaden**-hyper-trophy, above normal nourishment (enlargement) of the lymph nodes

**lymphaden**-ia, condition of the lymph nodes (hypertrophy or enlargement)

**lymphaden**-itis, inflammation of the lymph nodes

**lymphaden/o**-cele, a swelling (cyst) of a lymph node

**lymphaden/o**-gram, a recording or X-ray picture of the lymph nodes

**lymphaden/o**-graphy, technique of recording or making an X-ray picture of the lymph nodes

**lymphaden**-oma, a malignant tumour forming from lymphoid tissue Syn. lymphoma

**lymphaden**-oid, resembling lymph nodes

**lymphaden/o**-path-ic, pertaining to disease of lymph nodes

**lymphaden/o**-pathy, disease of lymph nodes

**lymphaden**-osis, abnormal condition of disease of lymph nodes (hypertrophy of lymph tissue)

**lymphaden**-tomy, incision into a lymph node (for removal)

---

**Lymphangi/o**, lymph vessel

From the Latin word **lympha** meaning water and Greek word **aggeion** meaning vessel. Here lymphangi/o means a lymph vessel, a structure that transports lymph from lymph capillaries towards the larger thoracic duct or towards the right lymphatic duct.

**lymphangi/-al**, pertaining to a lymph vessel

**lymphangi**-ectas-ia, condition of dilation of a lymph vessel

**lymphangi**-ectasis, dilation of a lymph vessel

**lymphangi**-ecta-tic, pertaining to dilation of a lymph vessel

**lymphangi**-ectomy, removal of a lymph vessel

**lymphangi/o**-endotheli-oma, a malignant tumour originating in the endothelial cells lining lymphatic vessels

**lymphangi/o**-fibr-oma, a tumour composed of fibrous tissue and lymph vessels (benign)

**lymphangi/o**-gram, a recording or X-ray picture of lymph vessels

**lymphangi/o**-graphy, technique of recording or making an X-ray picture of lymph vessels

**lymphangi/o**-logy, the study of lymph vessels or the lymphatic system

**lymphangi**-oma, a tumour of lymph vessels, similar to an angioma but filled with lymph (it contains new lymph spaces and channels)

**lymphangi/o**-my-oma, a tumour of smooth muscle and lymph vessels

**lymphangi/o**-my-omat-osis, abnormal condition of multiple lymphangiomyomas (seen in women in lymph nodes, thoracic duct and lungs)

**lymphangi/o**-phleb-itis, inflammation of veins and lymph vessels

**lymphangi/o**-plasty, surgical repair or reconstruction of lymph vessels

**lymphangi/o**-sarc-oma, a malignant tumour of lymph vessels

**lymphangi/o**-tomy, incision into a lymph vessel

**lymphang**-itis, inflammation of lymph vessels

peri-**lymphang**-itis, inflammation around lymph vessels

---

**Lymphat/o**, lymph/o, lymph

From a Greek word **lympha**, meaning water. Here lymph/o means the fluid lymph or lymphatic tissue. Lymph is a clear, colourless fluid derived from tissue fluid. It is similar in composition to blood plasma but without the plasma proteins. Unlike blood, lymph contains only one main type of cell, the lymphocyte.

**lymph**-apheresis, process of withdrawal of blood, removal of lymphocytes and transfusion of the remainder into the donor Syn. lymphocytopheresis, lymphocytapheresis

**lymphat**-ic, 1. pertaining to a lymphatic vessel or lymph 2. the name for a lymph vessel

**lymphatic/o**-splen-ic, pertaining to the spleen and lymph (nodes)

**lymphat**-ism, process of (excessive growth of) lymph tissue

**lymphat**-itis, inflammation of the lymphatic system (any part of)

**lymphat/o**-lysis, breakdown or destruction of lymph tissue

**lymphat/o**-lyt-ic, pertaining to the breakdown or destruction of lymph tissue

**lymph**-ectas-ia, condition of dilation of lymph vessels

**lymph**-nod-itis, inflammation of a lymph node

**lymph/o**-blast, an immature cell or embryonic cell that forms into a mature lymphocyte

**lymph/o**-blast-ic, 1. pertaining to or forming lymphoblasts 2. pertaining to or of the nature of lymphoblasts

**lymph/o**-blast-oma, a (malignant) tumour that arises from lymphoblasts

**lymph/o**-blast-osis, abnormal condition of (excess) lymphoblasts (in the blood)

**lymph/o**-cele, a swelling or cyst containing lymph

**lymph/o**-cyt-apheresis, process of withdrawal of blood, removal of lymphocytes and transfusion of the remainder into the donor Syn. lymphocytopheresis, lymphapheresis

**lymph/o**-cyte, a lymph cell

**lymph/o**-cyt-ic, pertaining to or of the nature of lymphocytes

**lymph/o**-cyt/o-blast, an immature cell or embryonic cell that forms into a mature lymphocyte Syn. lymphoblast

**lymph/o**-cyt-oma, a (malignant) tumour composed of lymphocytes Syn. lymphocytic lymphoma

**lymph/o**-cyt/o-pen-ia, condition of reduction in the number of lymphocytes (in the blood)

**lymph/o**-cyt/o-pheresis, process of withdrawal of blood, removal of lymphocytes and transfusion of the remainder into the donor Syn. lymphocytapheresis, lymphapheresis

**lymph/o**-cyt/o-poiesis, the formation of lymphocytes

**lymph/o**-cyt-osis, abnormal condition of (excess) lymphocytes (in the blood or in an effusion)

**lymph/o**-cyt/o-toxic-ity, condition or state of being poisonous to lymphocytes

**lymph/o**-cyt/o-tox-in, an agent that poisons lymphocytes

**lymph/o**-duct, a lymphatic vessel

**lymph**-oedema, a swelling due to lymph

**lymph/o**-epitheli-oma, a malignant tumour (carcinoma) arising from the epithelium covering lymph tissue (found in the nasopharynx)

**lymph/o**-genesis, the formation of lymph

**lymph/o**-gen-ic, 1. pertaining to originating in lymph tissue 2. pertaining to producing lymph

**lymph/o**-gen-ous, 1. pertaining to originating in lymph tissue 2. pertaining to producing lymph

**lymph/o**-glandula, a lymph node

**lymph/o**-gram, a recording or X-ray picture of the lymphatic system

**lymph/o**-granul-oma, 1. a granular tumour of the lymphatic tissue, Hodgkin's disease 2. a granular tumour caused by infection

**lymph/o**-granul-omat-osis, 1. abnormal condition of granular tumours of the lymphatic tissue, Hodgkin's disease 2. abnormal condition of granulomas caused by infection

**lymph/o**-graphy, technique of recording or making an X-ray of the lymphatic system

**lymph**-oid, resembling lymph or lymphatic tissue

**lymph**-oid-ectomy, removal of lymphatic tissue

**lymph/o**-kin-esis, the movement of lymph, it refers to the circulation of lymph in the body

**lymph/o**-logy, the study of the lymphatic system (anatomy, diseases and treatment of)

**lymph**-oma, a malignant tumour forming from lymphoid tissue

**lymph**-omat-oid, resembling a lymphoma

**lymph**-omat-osis, abnormal condition of forming or having multiple lymphomas (lymphomata)

**lymph**-omat-ous, pertaining to or having the characteristics of a lymphoma

**lymph/o**-myel-oma, a tumour of bone marrow containing cells that resemble lymphocytes

**lymph/o**-myx-oma, a tumour of lymphoid tissue, it refers to any benign, soft growth of adenoid tissue

**lymph/o**-nod-us, a lymph node

**lymph/o**-path-ia, 1. condition of disease of lymph vessels or nodes 2. an old term for lymphogranuloma venereum

**lymph/o**-pathy, disease of the lymph vessels or nodes

**lymph/o**-pen-ia, condition of reduction in the number of lymphocytes in the blood

**lymph/o**-plasm-apheresis, process of withdrawal of blood, removal of lymphocytes and plasma followed by transfusion of the remainder into the donor

**lymph/o**-poiesis, the formation of lymphocytes or lymph tissue

**lymph/o**-poie-tic, pertaining to lympho-poiesis

**lymph/o**-proliferative, pertaining to the proliferation (increase) of lymphoid tissue

**lymph/o**-reticul-ar, pertaining to the reticuloendothelial cells of lymph nodes

**lymph/o**-reticul-osis, abnormal condition (increase) in the reticuloendothelial cells of lymph nodes

**lymph/o**-rrhag-ia, condition of bursting forth of lymph Syn. lymphorrhoea

**lymph/o**-rrhoea, excessive flow or discharge of lymph (from a cut or ruptured lymph vessel)

**lymph/o**-rrhoid, dilation of a (perianal) lymph vessel, it resembles a haemorrhoid

**lymph/o**-sarc-oma, a malignant tumour of lymphoid tissue (not including Hodgkin's disease), an old term for some types of non-Hodgkin's lymphoma

**lymph/o**-stasis, stopping or cessation of flow of lymph

**lymph/o**-taxis, ordered movement of lymphocytes (attraction or repulsion)

**lymph/o**-tox-ic, pertaining to poisonous to lymph tissue

**lymph/o**-tox-in, 1. an agent poisonous to lymph cells 2. an agent (chemical mediator) released by lymphocytes that is poisonous to cells

---

**Phag/o**, phagocyte

From a Greek word **phagein** meaning to eat. Here, phag/o refers to a phago-cyte, a cell that eats. Phagocytes can engulf and digest particulate matter and micro-organisms that have entered the body; they fall into two main groups, microphages and macrophages.

Neutrophils and monocytes are phagocytes present in the blood. The neutrophil (a granulocyte) is a type of microphage whereas the monocyte (an agranulocyte) is a blood cell that can enlarge and develop into a macrophage, a large phagocytic cell that can leave the blood and migrate to areas of infection.

macro-**phage**, a large eater, it refers to a large, highly phagocytic cell of the reticulo-endothelial system that forms from a monocyte

micro-**phage**, small eater, it refers to a small, mobile phagocytic cell, a poly-morphonuclear leucocyte

**phag/o**-cyte, 1. a cell that eats or ingests foreign organisms and particles 2. a cell that performs phagocytosis

**phag/o**-cyt-ic, 1. pertaining to phago-cytosis 2. pertaining to or of the nature of phagocytes

**phag/o**-cyt-in, a (bactericidal) agent secreted by phagocytes (neutrophils)

**phag/o**-cyt/o-blast, an immature cell that forms phagocytes

**phag/o**-cyt/o-lysis, breakdown or destruction of phagocytes

**phag/o**-cyt/o-lyt-ic, pertaining to break-down or destruction of phagocytes

**phag/o**-cyt-ose, to perform the act of engulfing or ingesting foreign organisms and particles

**phag/o**-cyt-osis, condition of engulfing or ingesting foreign organisms and particles by phagocytes

**phag/o**-cyt/o-tic, pertaining to phago-cytosis

**phag/o**-some, a body (membrane bound vesicle) found inside a phagocyte (contains ingested material)

---

**Plasma-**, plasma

From a Greek word **plassein** meaning to mould. Here plasm/a refers to plasmacytes, cells of the immune system derived from B-lymphocytes that manufacture antibodies.

**plasma**-blast, an immature cell that forms plasma cells or plasmacytes

**plasma**-cyte, a plasma cell, an antibody-secreting cell that develops from a B-lymphocyte

**plasma**-cyt-ic, pertaining to or of the nature of plasmacytes

**plasma**-cyt-oma, a malignant tumour composed of plasmacytes *e.g.* multiple myeloma

**plasma**-cyt-osis, abnormal condition of plasmacytes (excess in the blood)

---

**Reticuloendotheli-**, reticul/o, reticuloendothelial system

From a Latin word **reticulum**, meaning small net, and the Greek words **endon** meaning within and **thele** meaning nipple. Here, reticul/o and reticulo-endotheli- refer to the cells of the reticuloendothelial system. This system, also known as the monocyte–macrophage system, is a network of connective tissue cells that perform phagocytosis.

**reticuloendotheli**-al, pertaining to the reticulo-endothelial system or monocyte–macrophage system (a network of cells with a common ancestry that carry out phagocytosis in the liver, bone marrow, lymph nodes, spleen and other tissues.)

**reticuloendotheli**-oma, a tumour formed from cells of the reticuloendothelial system (a malignant lymphoma)

**reticuloendotheli**-osis, abnormal condition of the reticuloendothelial system (abnormal increase in cells of the reticuloendothelial system)

**reticuloendotheli**-um, the tissue of the reticuloendothelial system

**reticul**-oma, a tumour of cells of the reticulo-endothelial system

**reticul/o**-sarc-oma, a malignant tumour formed from monocytes of the reticulo-ndothelial system

**reticul**-osis, abnormal condition of the reticuloendothelial system (an abnormal increase in reticulo-endothelial cells)

---

**Ser/o**, serum

From a Latin word **serum**, meaning whey. Here ser/o means the clear portion of any liquid separated from its more solid elements. Blood serum is the supernatant liquid formed when blood clots; it can be used as a source of antibodies.

Serum investigations can lead to a patient being diagnosed seronegative or seropositive for the presence of a particular antibody. Seronegative means showing a lack of antibody and seropositive the presence of a high level of antibody *e.g.* HIV positive means antibodies to the human immuno-deficiency virus are present in a patient's blood.

**ser/o**-conversion, conversion of a seronegative test from negative to positive (indicates the development of antibodies to an antigen)

**ser/o**-culture, culturing or growing bacteria in blood serum

**ser/o**-diagnosis, use of sera to diagnose disease

**ser/o**-diagnost-ic, pertaining to the use of sera to diagnose disease

**ser/o**-fibrin-ous, pertaining to or composed of fibrin and serum (used when referring to an exudate)

**ser/o**-group, group of bacteria containing a common antigen

**ser/o**-immun-ity, condition of immunity conferred by administration of an antiserum (passive immunization)

**ser/o**-log-ic, 1. pertaining to the study of sera 2. pertaining to serology

**ser/o**-log-ical, 1. pertaining to the study of sera 2. pertaining to serology

**ser/o**-log-ist, a person who specializes in the study of sera to diagnose and treat disease

**ser/o**-logy, the study of sera (antigen–antibody reactions *in vitro*)

**ser**-oma, a swelling of serum (a collection of serum in a tissue)

**ser/o**-muc-ous, pertaining to or consisting of mucus and serum

**ser/o**-negative, giving a negative result to a serological test (indicating an absence of an antibody)

**ser/o**-positive, giving a positive result to a serological test (indicating presence of an antibody)

**ser/o**-purulent, pertaining to or composed of pus and serum

**ser/o**-pus, an exudate containing pus and serum

**ser/o**-reaction, a reaction that involves serum or occurs in serum

**ser/o**-sanguin-ous, pertaining to or composed of blood and serum

**ser/o**-survey, screening of serum to determine susceptibility to disease

**ser/o**-synov-itis, inflammation of synovial membranes with the effusion of serum

**ser/o**-therapy, treatment of infection using an immune serum (antitoxin)

**ser/o**-type, type of micro-organism identified and classified by its antigens

**ser/o**-typing, technique of identifying types of micro-organisms by their antigens

**ser**-ous, 1. pertaining to producing or containing serum 2. pertaining to resembling serum

**ser/o**-vaccin-ation, action of vaccinating with bacteria (active immunization) and serum (passive immunization) at the same time

**ser**-um, the yellow fluid that remains after whole blood or plasma has been allowed to clot (blood serum). Immune serum is the blood serum from an animal immunized against a particular antigen, it contains antibodies used for passive immunization

**serum**-al, 1. pertaining to serum 2. formed from serum

---

**Splen/o**, spleen

From a Greek word **splen** meaning spleen. Here splen/o means the spleen, an organ with four main functions: destruction of old blood cells, blood storage, blood filtration and participation in the immune response.

hyper-**splen**-ism, process of increased activity of an enlarged spleen, especially increased haemolytic activity

micro-**splen**-ia, condition of having a small spleen

**splen**-aden-oma, a tumour or swelling of the spleen (an increase in cells of the spleen pulp)

**splen**-alg-ia, condition of pain in the spleen

**splen**-a-trophy, 1. without nourishment or wasting away of the spleen 2. atrophy of the spleen

**splen**-ectasis, dilation of the spleen

**splen**-ectom-ize, to remove the spleen

**splen**-ectomy, removal of the spleen

**splen**-ectop-ia, condition of displacement of the spleen (a floating spleen)

**splen**-elc-osis, abnormal condition of ulceration of the spleen

**splen**-ic, pertaining to or belonging to the spleen

**splen**-itis, inflammation of the spleen

**splen**-ization, action of making spleen-like tissue

**splen/o**-cav-al, pertaining to the (inferior) vena cava and spleen

**splen/o**-cele, a hernia or swelling of the spleen

**splen/o**-col-ic, pertaining to the colon and spleen

**splen/o**-cyte, a spleen cell (a monocyte found in splenic tissue)

**splen/o**-dyn-ia, condition of pain in the spleen

**splen/o**-gen-ic, pertaining to forming or originating in the spleen

**splen/o**-gen-ous, pertaining to forming or originating in the spleen

**splen/o**-gram, 1. a recording or X-ray picture of the spleen 2. a recording of the number and type of cells found in the spleen following splenic puncture

**splen/o**-graphy, technique of making a recording or X-ray picture of the spleen

**splen/o**-hepat/o-megaly, enlargement of the liver and spleen

**splen**-oid, resembling the spleen

**splen/o**-logy, the study of the spleen (anatomy, diseases and treatment of)

**splen//o**-lys-in, an agent that breaks down the spleen

**splen/o**-lysis, breakdown or destruction of the spleen

**splen**-oma, a tumour or swelling of the spleen

**splen/o**-malac-ia, condition of softening of the spleen

**splen/o**-medull-ary, pertaining to bone marrow and the spleen

**splen/o**-megaly, enlargement of the spleen

**splen/o**-myel/o-gen-ous, pertaining to originating in the bone marrow and spleen

**splen/o**-myel/o-malac-ia, condition of softening of the bone marrow and spleen

**splen**-onc-us, a tumour or swelling of the spleen

**splen/o**-pancreat-ic, pertaining to or belonging to the pancreas and spleen

**splen/o**-pathy, disease of the spleen

**splen/o**-pexy, surgical fixation of the spleen

**splen/o**-phren-ic, pertaining to the diaphragm and spleen

**splen/o**-pneumon-ia, condition of the lung (infection and inflammation) resembling the appearance of the spleen (splenization of lung tissue)

**splen/o**-port-al, pertaining to the hepatic portal vein and spleen

**splen/o**-port/o-gram, a recording or X-ray picture of the hepatic portal vein and spleen

**splen/o**-port/o-graph-ic, pertaining to recording or making an X-ray of the hepatic portal vein and spleen

**splen/o**-ptosis, falling or downward displacement of the spleen

**splen/o**-ren-al, pertaining to the kidney and spleen

**splen/o**-rrhag-ia, condition of bursting forth of blood (haemorrhage) from the spleen

**splen/o**-rrhaphy, stitching or suturing of the spleen

**splen/o**-tomy, incision into the spleen

---

**Thymic/o**, thym/o, thymus gland
From a Greek word **thymos**, meaning soul or emotion. Here thym/o means the thymus gland, a structure that lies behind the breast above the aorta and extends upward as far as the thyroid gland. The thymus controls the development of the immune system in early life reaching its greatest size towards puberty.

Note thym/o is also used to mean the mind, soul or emotions.

**thym**-ectomy, removal of the thymus gland

**thym**-ectom-ize, action of removing the thymus gland

**thym**-elc-osis, abnormal condition of ulceration of the thymus gland

**thym**-ic, pertaining to the thymus gland

**thymic/o**-lympha-tic, pertaining to lymph nodes and the thymus gland

**thym**-in, an agent (hormone) produced by the thymus gland that stimulates differentiation of precursor lymphocytes into thymocytes Syn. thymopoietin

**thym**-itis, inflammation of the thymus gland

**thym/o**-cele, a hernia or protrusion of the thymus gland

**thym/o**-cyte, a thymus cell, it refers to a lymphocyte originating in the thymus gland

**thym/o**-cyt-ic, 1. pertaining to cells of the thymus 2. pertaining to or of the nature of thymocytes

**thym/o**-kinet-ic, pertaining to movement of the thymus gland, it refers to stimulating the thymus gland

**thym/o**-lysis, breakdown or lysis of the thymus gland

**thym/o**-lyt-ic, 1. pertaining to breakdown or lysis of the thymus gland 2. pertaining to thymolysis

**thym**-oma, a tumour of the thymus gland

**thym/o**-metastasis, a metastasis or spread of cells from the thymus to other tissues

**thym/o**-path-ic, pertaining to disease of the thymus gland

**thym/o**-pathy, disease of the thymus gland

**thym/o**-pexy, surgical fixation of the thymus gland

**thym/o**-poiet-in, an agent (hormone) that forms the thymus, it refers to a hormone that stimulates differentiation of precursor lymphocytes into thymocytes

**thym/o**-priv-ic, pertaining to or caused by lack of the thymus gland (due to removal or atrophy)

**thym/o**-priv-ous, pertaining to or caused by lack of the thymus gland (due to removal or atrophy)

**thymos**-in, an agent (hormone) secreted by the thymus gland that promotes the maturation of T-cells

**thym/o**-tox-ic, pertaining to poisoning of the thymus gland

**thym**-us-ectomy, removal of the thymus gland

---

**Tonsill/o**, tonsil

From a Latin word **tonsillae**, meaning tonsils. Here, tonsill/o means a tonsil, a patch of lymphoid tissue located in the mouth or nasopharynx. The pharyngeal tonsil (or adenoids) is found in the posterior wall of the nasopharynx, and the palatine tonsils in the folds formed by the soft palate and oropharynx. The palatine tonsils are known more commonly as the 'tonsils'. The lingual tonsils are found at the base of the tongue. Tonsils are important in the formation of antibodies and lymphocytes that defend against infection.

**tonsilla**, a tonsil (plural -tonsillae)

**tonsill**-ar, pertaining to the tonsils

**tonsill**-ectomy, removal of a tonsil

**tonsill**-itic, pertaining to or having tonsillitis

**tonsill**-itis, inflammation of the tonsils

**tonsill**-lith, a stone or calculus in a tonsil

**tonsill/o**-monil-iasis, condition of the fungus Monilia (Candida) in the tonsils

**tonsill/o**-myc-osis, abnormal condition of fungi in the tonsils

**tonsill/o**-pathy, disease of the tonsils

**tonsill/o**-pharyng-eal, pertaining to the pharynx and tonsils

**tonsill/o**-scope, an instrument used to view or examine the tonsils

**tonsill/o**-scopy, technique of viewing or examining the tonsils

**tonsill/o**-tome, an instrument used to cut the tonsils

**tonsill/o**-tomy, incision into a tonsil

**tonsil**-sector, an instrument used to cut a tonsil (a type of tonsillotome)

# Section 7
# The urinary system

The urinary system plays a major role in homeostasis by regulating the composition and pH of the internal environment of the body. The organs that interact to form the urinary system are the:

- **two kidneys**
- **two ureters**
- **bladder**
- **urethra.**

The kidneys remove metabolic wastes from the blood by ultrafiltration and form them into urine. This yellow liquid is passed from the kidneys through the ureters to the urinary bladder where it is stored. Periodically urine is excreted from the body through the urethra during urination.

Besides removing waste substances that could be toxic to tissue cells, the kidneys maintain blood volume and regulate its electrolyte concentration and pH. They also produce the hormone eythropoietin, which regulates the rate of production of red blood cells and renin, an enzyme that helps to control blood pressure.

To maintain homeostasis the kidneys continuously excrete metabolic waste and adjust the composition of the blood. They are therefore essential to life.

Figure 10 shows the anatomy of the urinary system and the combining forms associated with its components.

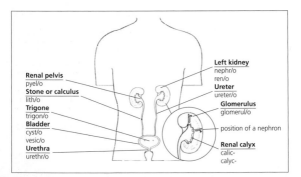

**Renal pelvis**
pyel/o
**Stone or calculus**
lith/o
**Trigone**
trigon/o
**Bladder**
cyst/o
vesic/o
**Urethra**
urethr/o

**Left kidney**
nephr/o
ren/o
**Ureter**
ureter/o
**Glomerulus**
glomerul/o
position of a nephron
**Renal calyx**
calic-
calyc-

Figure 10 The urinary system

## Quick Reference

Combining forms of roots relating to the urinary system:

## Quick Reference

Common words and combining forms relating to the urinary system:

## Roots and combining forms, meanings

**Albumin/o**, albumin

From a Latin word **albus** meaning white. Here albumin/o means albumin, a protein found in blood plasma and produced in the liver.

**albumin/o**-chol-ia, condition of albumin in the bile

**albumin/o**-gen-ous, pertaining to forming albumin

**albumin/o**-oid, resembling albumin

**albumin/o**-lysis, breakdown of albumin

**albumin/o**-osis, abnormal condition of excess albumin (in blood)

**albumin**-uret-ic, 1. pertaining to forming albuminuria 2. pertaining to characterized by albuminuria 3. an agent that stimulates excretion of albumin in the urine

**albumin**-ur-ia, condition of the urine containing albumin (excess)

**albumin**-ur-ic, 1. pertaining to urine containing albumin (excess) 2. pertaining to having albuminuria

**Azot/o**, urea, nitrogen compounds

From a French word **azote** meaning nitrogen. Here, azot/o means urea and/or other nitrogenous compounds found in the human body. Urea is the main waste product of protein metabolism and is formed in the liver from the breakdown of amino acids in a process called deamination.

**azot**-aem-ia, condition of the blood with (excess) urea or nitrogenous compounds

**azot/o**-rrhoea, excessive flow or discharge of urea or other nitrogenous compounds (in the urine or faeces)

**azot**-ur-ia, condition of the urine with (excess) urea or other nitrogenous compounds

**azot**-ur-ic, 1. pertaining to having azoturia 2. pertaining to urine with (excess) urea or other nitrogenous compounds

**Cali/c/x**, caly/c/x, calix, calyx, cup-shaped

From a Greek word **kalyx** meaning shell. Here calic- mean a renal calyx or calix, one of the cup-shaped cavities that form subdivisions of the renal pelvis enclosing the pyramids.

**calic**-ectasis, dilation of a renal calix

**calic**es, plural of calix

**calic**-ul-us, a small calix

**calix**, a cup-shaped cavity

**calyc**es, plural of calyx

**calyc**-ul-us, a small calyx

**calyx**, a cup-shaped cavity

mega-**calyc**-osis, abnormal condition of large or dilated renal calyces

micro-**calix**, a very small renal calix

micro-**calyx**, a very small renal calyx

peri-**calic**-eal, pertaining to around a renal calix

---

**Cyst/o**, bladder

From a Greek word **kystis**, meaning a bladder. Here, it means the urinary bladder, an organ that stores urine prior to its excretion from the body.

**cyst**-alg-ia, condition of pain in the urinary bladder

**cyst**-a-troph-ia, condition of without nourishment (growth) of the bladder

**cyst**-ectas-ia, condition of dilation of the bladder

**cyst**-ectomy, removal of the urinary bladder

**cyst**-elc-osis, abnormal condition of ulceration of the bladder

**cyst**-ic, pertaining to the bladder

**cyst**-itis, inflammation of the urinary bladder

**cyst/o**-cele, a protrusion or hernia of the urinary bladder (into the vagina)

**cyst/o**-col/o-stomy, formation of an opening between the colon and urinary bladder or the name of the opening so created

**cyst/o**-dia-thermy, process of heating through the urinary bladder (to remove tumours)

**cyst/o**-dyn-ia, condition of pain in the urinary bladder

**cyst/o**-elytr/o-plasty, surgical repair or reconstruction of the vagina and bladder (to a vaginal injury or vesico-vaginal fistula)

**cyst/o**-enter/o-cele, a protrusion or hernia of the intestine and urinary bladder

**cyst/o**-epipl/o-cele, a protrusion or hernia of the omentum and urinary bladder

**cyst/o**-gram, a recording or X-ray picture of the urinary bladder

**cyst/o**-graphy, technique of making a recording or X-ray picture of the urinary bladder

**cyst/o**-lith, a bladder stone or calculus

**cyst/o**-lith-ectomy, removal of stones or calculi from the urinary bladder Syn. cystolithotomy

**cyst/o**-lith-iasis, condition of stones or calculi in the urinary bladder

**cyst/o**-lith-ic, 1. pertaining to a bladder stone or calculus 2. pertaining to having a bladder stone or calculus

**cyst/o**-lith/o-tomy, incision to remove a stone or calculus from the urinary bladder Syn. cystolithectomy

**cyst/o**-meter, an instrument to measure the urinary bladder (the capacity or pressure within)

**cyst/o**-metr/o-gram, a recording or tracing of the measured volume and pressure of the urinary bladder

**cyst/o**-metr/o-graphy, technique of measuring the volume and pressure of the urinary bladder

**cyst/o**-metry, technique of measuring the urinary bladder (capacity and pressure)

**cyst/o**-paralysis, paralysis of the urinary bladder

**cyst/o**-pexy, surgical fixation of the urinary bladder (to the abdominal wall)

**cyst/o**-plasty, surgical repair or reconstruction of the urinary bladder

**cyst/o**-pleg-ia, condition of paralysis of the urinary bladder

**cyst/o**-proct/o-stomy, formation of an opening between the rectum and urinary bladder or the name of the opening so created

**cyst/o**-ptosis, falling or displacement of the urinary bladder

**cyst/o**-pyel-itis, inflammation of the renal pelvis and urinary bladder

**cyst/o**-pyel/o-graphy, technique of making a recording or X-ray picture of the renal pelvis and urinary bladder

**cyst/o**-pyel/o-nephr-itis, inflammation of the kidney, renal pelvis and urinary bladder

**cyst/o**-radi/o-graphy, technique of making a recording or X-ray picture of the urinary bladder

**cyst/o**-rect/o-stomy, formation of an opening between the rectum and urinary bladder or the name of the opening so created

**cyst/o**-rrhag-ia, condition of bursting forth of blood from the urinary bladder (haemorrhage)

**cyst/o**-rrhaphy, stitching or suturing of the urinary bladder

**cyst/o**-rrhexis, rupture of the urinary bladder

**cyst/o**-rrhoea, 1. a discharge from the urinary bladder 2. flow of blood from the urinary bladder 3. excessive flow (of urine) from the urinary bladder

**cyst/o**-schisis, splitting of the bladder (a congenital fissure)

**cyst/o**-scope, an instrument used to view or examine the urinary bladder

**cyst/o**-scop-ic, 1. pertaining to cystoscopy 2. pertaining to viewing or examining the urinary bladder

**cyst/o**-scopy, technique of viewing or examining the urinary bladder (with an endoscope)

**cyst/o**-spasm, sudden contraction or spasm of the urinary bladder

**cyst/o**-stomy, formation of an opening into the urinary bladder or the name of the opening so created

**cyst/o**-tomy, incision into the urinary bladder

**cyst/o**-trachel/o-tomy, incision into the neck of the urinary bladder

**cyst/o**-ureter-itis, inflammation of the ureters and urinary bladder

**cyst/o**-ureter/o-gram, a recording or X-ray picture of the ureters and urinary bladder

**cyst/o**-ureter/o-pyel-itis, inflammation of the renal pelvis, ureters and urinary bladder

**cyst/o**-urethr-itis, inflammation of the urethra and urinary bladder

**cyst/o**-urethr/o-gram, a recording or X-ray picture of the urethra and urinary bladder

**cyst/o**-urethr/o-graphy, technique of making a recording or X-ray picture of the urethra and urinary bladder

**cyst/o**-urethr/o-pexy, surgical fixation of the urethra and urinary bladder

**cyst/o**-urethr/o-scope, an instrument used to view or examine the urethra and urinary bladder

**cyst/o**-urethr/o-scopy, technique of viewing or examining the urethra and urinary bladder

endo-**cyst**-itis, inflammation within the bladder (its mucosa)

intra-**cyst**-ic, 1. pertaining to within a bladder 2. pertaining to within a cyst

pan-**cyst**-itis, inflammation of all of the bladder (its entire wall)

---

**Glomerul/o**, glomerulus
From a Latin word **glomus** meaning ball. Here glomerul/o means a glomerulus, a ball of capillaries surrounded by porous membranes that filters metabolic wastes from the blood. A glomerulus can be found invaginating the entrance of every nephron in the cortex of a kidney. Each kidney contains about one million nephrons or uriniferous tubules that do the work of ultrafiltration and selective reabsorption.

**glomerul**-ar, pertaining to a glomerulus

**glomeruli**, plural of glomerulus

**glomerul**-itis, inflammation of the glomeruli

**glomerul/o**-nephr-itis, inflammation of the kidney glomeruli

**glomerul/o**-pathy, disease of glomeruli

**glomerul/o**-scler-osis, abnormal condition of hardening of the glomeruli (fibrosis)

juxta-**glomerul**-ar, pertaining to near or adjoining a glomerulus

---

**Kal/i/o**, potassium

From a Greek word **kali** meaning potash. Here, kal/i means potassium and it refers to the presence of potassium ions in the blood or urine.

hyper-**kal**-aem-ia, condition of excess of potassium (in the blood)

hyper-**kal**-aem-ic, 1. pertaining to an excess of potassium (in the blood) 2. pertaining to having hyperkalaemia

hypo-**kal**-aem-ia, condition of deficiency of potassium (in the blood)

hypo-**kal**-aem-ic, 1. pertaining to having hypokalaemia 2. an agent that promotes the lowering of potassium in the blood

**kal**/i-aem-ia, condition of potassium in the blood

**kali**/o-pen-ia, condition of deficiency of potassium (in the blood)

**kal**/i-ur-esis, condition of excretion of excess potassium in the urine

---

**Lith/o**, stone

From a Greek word **lithos**, meaning stone. Here, lith/o means a stone or calculus, an abnormal concretion composed chiefly of mineral substances that forms within the passages of the urinary system.

Note: stones can form in cavities and passages that transmit secretions in other parts of the body.

anti-**lith**-ic, 1. pertaining to against stones or calculi (preventing their formation) 2. an agent that prevents the formation of stones

**lith**-ectas-y, process of dilating (the urethra) for removal of a stone or calculus

**lith**-iasis, abnormal condition or presence of stones or calculi

**lith/o**-clast, an instrument that breaks stones or calculi Syn. lithotrite

**lith/o**-cyst/o-tomy, incision into the bladder to remove a stone or calculus

**lith/o**-dialysis, 1. the breakdown of stones or calculi *in situ* (using drugs) 2. the breakdown of stones or calculi followed by washing away of the fragments (litholapaxy)

**lith/o**-genesis, the formation of stones or calculi

**lith/o**-gen-ic, pertaining to the formation of stones or calculi

**lith/o**-gen-ous, pertaining to the formation of stones or calculi

**lith**-oid, resembling a stone or calculus

**lith/o**-lapaxy, washing of stones from the bladder following crushing

**lith/o**-lysis, breakdown of stones or calculi *in situ* (using drugs)

**lith/o**-lyt-ic, 1. pertaining to breakdown of stones or calculi (*in situ* using drugs) 2. pertaining to litholysis

**lith/o**-malac-ia, condition of softening of a stone or calculus

**lith/o**-nephr-itis, inflammation of the kidney due to stones

**lith/o**-nephr-osis, abnormal condition of stones or calculi in the kidney

**lith/o**-nephr/o-tomy, incision into the kidney to remove a stone or calculus

**lith/o**-scope, an instrument used to view or examine stones or calculi *in situ*

**lith/o**-tomy, incision into a duct or organ to remove a stone or calculus

**lith/o**-tripsy, the process of fragmenting stones *e.g.* using shockwaves from a lithotriptor

**lith/o**-tript-ic, 1. pertaining to breakdown of stones or calculi *in situ* using drugs 2. a chemical agent used to breakdown of stones or calculi

**lith/o**-tript/o-scope, an instrument used to view or examine stones or calculi while they are fragmented

**lith/o**-tript/o-scopy, technique of viewing or examining stones or calculi while they are fragmented with a lithotriptor

**lith/o**-tript-er, an instrument that fragments stones using shockwaves

**lith/o**-tript-or, an instrument that fragments stones using shock waves

**lith/o**-trite, an instrument for crushing stones

**lith/o**-trit-y, the process of fragmenting stones *e.g.* using shockwaves from a lithotriptor

**lith**-ous, pertaining to or of the nature of stones or calculi

**lith**-ur-esis, abnormal condition of stones in the urine

---

**Natr/i**, sodium

From a Latin word **natrium** meaning sodium. Here natr/i means sodium and it refers to the presence of sodium ions in the blood or urine.

hyper-**natr**-aem-ia, condition of excess sodium in the blood

hyper-**natr**-aem-ic, 1. pertaining to excess sodium in the blood 2. pertaining to having hypernatraemia

hypo-**natr**-aem-ia, condition of deficiency of sodium in the blood (salt depletion)

**natr/i**-ur-esis, condition of excretion of (excess) sodium in the urine

**natr/i**-uret-ic, 1. pertaining to or promoting natriuresis 2. an agent that promotes excretion of (excess) sodium in the urine

---

**Nephr/o**, nephr

From a Greek word **nephros**, meaning kidney. Here, nephr/o means the kidney, the organ that filters the blood and forms waste products into urine.

hydro-**nephr**-osis, abnormal condition of water in the kidney (producing a swelling)

**nephr**-alg-ia, condition of pain in the kidney

**nephr**-alg-ic, 1. pertaining to having pain in the kidney 2. pertaining to nephralgia

**nephr**-ectas-ia, condition of dilation of a kidney

**nephr**-ectom-ize, act of removing a kidney

**nephr**-ectomy, removal of a kidney

**nephr**-elc-osis, abnormal condition of ulceration in a kidney

**nephr**-ic, pertaining to a kidney

**nephr**-itic, pertaining to having nephritis

**nephr**-itis, inflammation of a kidney

**nephr/o**-abdomin-al, pertaining to the abdomen or abdominal wall and kidney

**nephr/o**-blast-oma, a malignant tumour of immature cells or embryonic cells of the kidney (Wilm's tumour)

**nephr/o**-calcin-osis, abnormal condition of calcium (phosphate) in the kidneys (causes renal insufficiency)

**nephr/o**-capsul-ectomy, removal of a renal capsule (the fibrous covering of a kidney)

**nephr/o**-capsul/o-tomy, incision into a renal capsule (the fibrous covering of a kidney)

**nephr/o**-cele, a protrusion or hernia of the kidney

**nephr/o**-col-ic, 1. pertaining to the colon and a kidney 2. pertaining to renal colic (pain)

**nephr/o**-col/o-pexy, surgical fixation of the colon and kidney (to appropriate positions)

**nephr/o**-col/o-ptosis, downward displacement or falling of the colon and a kidney

**nephr/o**-cyst-itis, inflammation of the urinary bladder and kidneys

**nephr/o**-cyst-osis, abnormal condition of cysts in a kidney

**nephr**-oedema, 1. a swelling due to fluid in a kidney 2. hydronephrosis

**nephr/o**-gen-ic, pertaining to forming or originating in a kidney

**nephr/o**-gen-ous, pertaining to forming or originating in a kidney

**nephr/o**-gram, a recording or X-ray picture of the kidneys

**nephr/o**-graphy, technique of making a recording or X-ray picture of the kidneys

**nephr/o**-hyper-trophy, above normal development or nourishment of a kidney, it results in enlargement of the kidney

**nephr/o**-lith, a kidney stone or calculus

**nephr/o**-lith-iasis, abnormal condition of stones or calculi in the kidney

**nephr/o**-lith-ic, pertaining to having a kidney stone or calculus

**nephr/o**-lith/o-tomy, incision to remove a kidney stone or calculus

**nephr/o**-logy, the study of the kidneys (anatomy, diseases and treatment of)

**nephr/o**-lysis, 1. breakdown or disintegration of a kidney 2. a surgical procedure to separate a kidney from adhesions

**nephr/o**-lyt-ic, pertaining to nephrolysis

**nephr**-oma, a tumour of a kidney

**nephr/o**-malac-ia, condition of softening of a kidney

**nephr/o**-megaly, enlargement of a kidney

**nephr/o**-meiosis, reduction in size or shrinkage of a kidney

**nephr/o**-n, the microscopic structural and functional unit of a kidney that forms urine. Each nephron consists of a knot of capillaries called a glomerulus and a renal tubule. The renal tubule consists of a Bowman's capsule, proximal convoluted tubule, Loop of Henle, distal convoluted tubule and a collecting duct that drains urine from several nephrons into the renal pelvis.

**nephr**-onc-us, a tumour of a kidney

**nephron/o**-phthisis, wasting away of nephrons (kidney tissue)

**nephr/o**-path-ic, pertaining to kidney disease

**nephr/o**-pathy, disease of the kidneys

**nephr/o**-pexy, fixation of a kidney (by surgery)

**nephr/o**-plasty, surgical repair or reconstruction of a kidney

**nephr/o**-poie-tic, pertaining to the formation of kidney tissue

**nephr/o**-ptosis, a falling kidney (downward displacement)

**nephr/o**-pyel-itis, inflammation of a renal pelvis and kidney

**nephr/o**-pyel/o-graphy, technique of making a recording or X-ray picture of a renal pelvis and kidney

**nephr/o**-pyel/o-lith/o-tomy, incision to remove a stone from the renal pelvis Syn. pyelolithotomy

**nephr/o**-pyel/o-plasty, surgical repair or reconstruction of the renal pelvis, to improve ureteral drainage in hydronephrosis

**nephr/o**-py-osis, abnormal condition of pus in a kidney

**nephr/o**-rrhag-ia, condition of flow of blood (haemorrhage) from a kidney

**nephr/o**-rrhaphy, stitching or suturing of a kidney

**nephr/o**-scler-osis, abnormal condition of hardening of a kidney

**nephr/o**-scope, an instrument used to view or examine the kidney (inside) of a kidney

**nephr**-osis, abnormal condition or disease of the kidney (especially degenerative disease of renal tubules)

**nephr/o**-splen/o-pexy, surgical fixation of the spleen and kidney (in appropriate positions)

**nephr/o**-stomy, formation of an opening into a kidney (into a renal pelvis) or the name of the opening so created

**nephr/o**-tic, 1. pertaining to having nephrosis 2. pertaining to like a nephrosis

**nephr/o**-tom/o-gram, a recording or X-ray picture of a slice or section through a kidney

**nephr/o**-tom/o-graphy, technique of making a recording or X-ray picture of a slice or section through a kidney

**nephr/o**-tomy, incision into a kidney

**nephr/o**-tox-ic, pertaining to poisonous to a kidney

**nephr/o**-tox-in, a chemical agent that is poisonous to a kidney

**nephr/o**-troph-ic, pertaining to nourishing or stimulating a kidney

**nephr/o**-trop-ic, pertaining to having an affinity for or pertaining to stimulating a kidney

**nephr/o**-tubercul-osis, abnormal condition of the kidneys caused by tuberculosis (*Mycobacterium tuberculosis*)

**nephr/o**-ureter-ectomy, removal of a ureter and its kidney

**nephr/o**-ureter/o-cyst-ectomy, removal of (a portion of) the bladder, a ureter and its kidney

para-**nephr**-ic, pertaining to near the kidney

para-**nephr**-itis, pertaining to inflammation near a kidney (in its surrounding tissues)

---

**Pelvi/o**, renal pelvis

From a Latin word **pelvis** meaning a basin. Here, pelvi/o means the space inside the kidney called the renal pelvis, the funnel-shaped dilation at the upper end of the ureter in which urine collects after its formation.

See the combining form pyel/o also meaning renal pelvis.

Note: pelvi/o is also used to mean the basin-shaped bony ring at the lower end of the trunk formed by the two innominate bones, the sacrum and coccyx, see Section 14 The skeletal system.

**pelvi**-calic-eal, pertaining to the calices and renal pelvis

**pelvi**-calyc-eal, pertaining to the calyces and renal pelvis

**pelvi/o**-lith/o-tomy, incision into the renal pelvis to remove a stone

**pelvi/o**-tomy, incision into the renal pelvis Syn. pyelotomy

---

**Pyel/o**, renal pelvis

From a Greek word **pyelos**, meaning pelvis (a basin). Here, pyel/o means the space inside the kidney called the renal pelvis, the funnel-shaped dilation at the upper end of the ureter in which urine collects after its formation.

(Do not confuse this word with py/o – meaning pus.)

See the combining form pelvi/o also meaning renal pelvis.

**pyel**-ectasis, dilation of a renal pelvis

**pyel**-itic, pertaining to having pyelitis

**pyel**-itis, inflammation of a renal pelvis

**pyel/o**-cali-ectasis, dilation of a calix and renal pelvis (a calix is a cup-shaped recess a subdivision of the renal pelvis))

**pyel/o**-cyst-itis, inflammation of the bladder and renal pelvis

**pyel/o**-fluor/o-scopy, technique of viewing or examining the renal pelvis using fluoroscopic methods

**pyel/o**-gram, a recording or X-ray picture of the renal pelvis

**pyel/o**-graphy, technique of making a recording or X-ray picture of the renal pelvis

*ante-grade pyelography*, technique of making a recording or X-ray picture of the renal pelvis by injecting dye in front of the renal pelvis through a percutaneous puncture

*intra-ven-ous pyelography*, technique of making a recording or X-ray picture of the renal pelvis by injecting dye into a vein

*retro-grade pyelography*, technique of making a recording or X-ray picture of the renal pelvis by injecting dye back into the ureter

**pyel/o**-interstit-ial, pertaining to interstitial tissue of the renal pelvis

**pyel/o**-lith/o-tomy, incision to remove a stone from the renal pelvis

**pyel/o**-lympha-tic, pertaining to lymphatic drainage of the renal pelvis and the renal pyramids

**pyel/o**-nephr-itic, pertaining to having pyelonephritis

**pyel/o**-nephr-itis, inflammation of the kidney and renal pelvis

**pyel/o**-nephr-osis, abnormal condition of the kidney and renal pelvis (other than acute inflammation)

**pyel/o**-pathy, disease of a renal pelvis

**pyel/o**-phleb-itis, inflammation of the veins of the renal pelvis

**pyel/o**-plasty, surgical repair or reconstruction of the renal pelvis

**pyel/o**-plic-ation, act of making tucks or folds in a dilated renal pelvis

**pyel/o**-ren-al, pertaining to the kidney (tubules) and renal pelvis

**pyel/o**-stomy, formation of an opening into the renal pelvis or the name of the opening so created

**pyel/o**-tomy, incision into the renal pelvis

**pyel/o**-tubul-ar, pertaining to the renal tubules and renal pelvis

**pyel/o**-ureter-ectasis, dilation of a ureter and its renal pelvis

**pyel/o**-ureter/o-plasty, surgical repair or reconstruction of a ureter and its renal pelvis

**pyel/o**-ven-ous, pertaining to the venous circulation (of the kidney) and renal pelvis

---

**Ren/i/o,** kidney

From a Latin word **ren**, meaning kidney. Here, ren/o means kidney, the organ that filters the blood and forms its waste products into urine.

**ren**-al, pertaining to a kidney

**ren/i**-pelv-ic, pertaining to the pelvis of the kidney

**ren/i**-port-al, pertaining to the portal system of the kidney

**ren/o**-gastr-ic, pertaining to the stomach and kidney

**ren/o**-gram, a recording or X-ray picture of the kidneys

**ren/o**-graphy, technique of making a recording or X-ray picture of the kidneys

**ren/o**-intestin-al, pertaining to the intestine and kidney

**ren/o**-pathy, disease of the kidneys Syn. nephropathy

**ren/o**-priv-al, pertaining to loss of function of the kidneys

**ren/o**-pulmon-ary, pertaining to the lungs and kidneys

**ren/o**-troph-ic, pertaining to nourishment or stimulation of the kidneys

**ren**-ule, small kidney, it refers to a small section supplied by a renal arteriole

supra-**ren**-al, pertaining to above a kidney

---

**Trigon/o,** trigone

From a Greek word **trigonos** meaning three cornered. Here trigon/o means the trigone, the triangular area in the bladder between the openings of the ureters and the urethra.

**trigon**-al, pertaining to the trigone

**trigon**-ectomy, removal of of the trigone of the bladder

**trigon**-itis, inflammation of the trigone of the bladder

**trigon/o**-tome, an instrument to cut the trigone of the bladder

---

**Ureter/o,** ureter

From a Greek word **oureter,** meaning the ureter. Here ureter/o means ureter, the narrow tube that connects each kidney to the bladder. Urine flows through the ureters assisted by waves of contraction produced by smooth muscle.

hydro-**ureter,** a ureter dilated with water, it refers to dilation with urine caused by an obstruction

inter-**ureter**-al, pertaining to between ureters

inter-**ureter**-ic, pertaining to between ureters

megalo-**ureter,** a large dilated ureter (congenital)

**ureter**-al, pertaining to a ureter

**ureter**-alg-ia, condition of pain in a ureter

**ureter**-ectas-ia, condition of dilation of a ureter

**ureter**-ectasis, dilation of a ureter

**ureter**-ectomy, removal of a ureter

**ureter**-ic, pertaining to a ureter

**ureter**-itis, inflammation of a ureter

**ureter/o**-cele, a protrusion or hernia of the ureter

**ureter/o**-cel-ectomy, removal of a ureterocele

**ureter/o**-cervic-al, pertaining to the cervix and a ureter

**ureter/o**-col-ic, pertaining to the colon and ureters

**ureter/o**-col/o-stomy, formation of an opening between the colon and ureter or the name of the opening so created

**ureter/o**-cyst-ic, pertaining to the bladder and ureters

**ureter/o**-cyst/o-scope, an instrument used to view or examine the bladder and ureters, used for inserting a catheter into a ureter

**ureter/o**-cyst/o-stomy, formation of an opening between the bladder and ureter (an alternative opening) or the name of the opening so created

**ureter/o**-dialysis, the separation or rupture of a ureter

**ureter/o**-enter-ic, pertaining to the intestine and ureter

**ureter/o**-enter/o-stomy, formation of an opening between the intestine and ureter or the name of the opening so created

**ureter/o**-gram, a recording or X-ray picture of a ureter

**ureter/o**-graphy, technique of making a recording or X-ray picture of a ureter

**ureter/o**-hydr/o-nephr-osis, abnormal condition of a kidney and ureter dilated with water (due to obstruction)

**ureter/o**-lle-al, pertaining to the ileum and ureters

**ureter/o**-ile/o-stomy, formation of an opening between the ileum (an isolated section connected to the abdominal wall) and ureters or the name of the opening so created

**ureter/o**-lith, a stone or calculus in a ureter

**ureter/o**-lith-iasis, condition of or presence of stones or calculi in a ureter

**ureter/o**-lith/o-tomy, incision to remove a stone or calculus from a ureter

**ureter/o**-lysis, 1. disintegration or rupture of a ureter 2. an operation to free a ureter from adhesions

**ureter/o**-neo-cyst/o-stomy, formation of a new opening between the bladder and ureters (at a different site) or the name of the opening so created

**ureter/o**-neo-pyel/o-stomy, formation of a new opening between the renal pelvis and a ureter or the name of the opening so created Syn. uretero-pyeloneostomy

**ureter/o**-nephr-ectomy, removal of a kidney and a ureter

**ureter/o**-pathy, disease of a ureter

**ureter/o**-pelvi/o-plasty, surgical repair or reconstruction of the renal pelvis and ureter

**ureter/o**-plasty, surgical repair or reconstruction of a ureter

**ureter/o**-proct/o-stomy, formation of an opening between the rectum and ureter or the name of the opening so created

**ureter/o**-pyel-itis, inflammation of a renal pelvis and ureter

**ureter/o**-pyel/o-graphy, technique of making a recording or X-ray picture of a renal pelvis and ureter

**ureter/o**-pyel/o-neo-stomy, formation of a new opening between the renal pelvis and a ureter or the name of the opening so created Syn. uretero-neopyelostomy

**ureter/o**-pyel/o-nephr-itis, inflammation of a kidney, renal pelvis and ureter

**ureter/o**-pyel/o-plasty, surgical repair or reconstruction of a renal pelvis and ureter

**ureter/o**-pyel/o-stomy, formation of an opening between the renal pelvis and a ureter or the name of the opening so created Syn. uretero-pyeloneostomy

**ureter/o**-py-osis, abnormal condition of pus in a ureter

**ureter/o**-rect/o-stomy, formation of an opening between the rectum and ureter or the name of the opening so created, it acts as an outlet for urine from the ureter

**ureter/o**-ren/o-scope, an instrument used to view or examine kidneys and ureters (a fibre-optic endoscope)

**ureter/o**-ren/o-scopy, technique of viewing or examining the kidneys and ureters

**ureter/o**-rrhag-ia, condition of excessive flow of blood from a ureter

**ureter/o**-rrhaphy, stitching or suturing of a ureter

**ureter/o**-sigmoid/o-stomy, formation of an opening between the sigmoid colon and a ureter or the name of the opening so created

**ureter/o**-sten-osis, abnormal condition of narrowing of a ureter

**ureter/o**-stomy, formation of an opening into a ureter (a new outlet) or the name of the opening so created

**ureter/o**-tomy, incision into a ureter

**ureter/o**-ureter/o-stomy, formation of an opening between one part of a ureter and another part of the ureter or the name of the opening so created

**ureter/o**-uter-ine, pertaining to the uterus and ureter

**ureter/o**-vagin-al, pertaining to the vagina and ureters

**ureter/o**-vesic-al, pertaining to the bladder and ureters

**ureter/o**-vesic/o-stomy, formation of an opening between the bladder and a ureter (a new opening) or the name of the opening so created

---

**Urethr/o**, urethra

From a Greek word **ourethro** meaning urethra. Here, urethr/o means the urethra, the tube through which urine leaves the body from the bladder.

trans-**urethr**-al, pertaining to through the urethra

**urethr**-al, pertaining to the urethra

**urethr**-alg-ia, condition of pain in the urethra

**urethr**-atres-ia, condition of absence of opening of the urethra, an imperforate urethra

**urethr**-ectomy, removal of the urethra

**urethr**-emphraxis, stopping up or obstruction of the urethra

**urethr**-ism, process (of sudden spasm or irritability) of the urethra

**urethr**-ismus, process (of sudden spasm or irritability) of the urethra

**urethr**-itis, inflammation of the urethra

**urethr/o**-blenn/o-rrhoea, excessive flow or discharge of mucus from the urethra (usually a purulent discharge)

**urethr/o**-bulb-ar, pertaining to the bulb of the penis and urethra

**urethr/o**-cele, a protrusion or hernia of the urethra

**urethr/o**-cyst-itis, inflammation of the bladder and urethra

**urethr/o**-cyst/o-graphy, technique of making a recording or X-ray picture of the urinary bladder and urethra

**urethr/o**-cyst/o-pexy, surgical fixation of the urinary bladder and urethra (a treatment for incontinence in women)

**urethr/o**-dyn-ia, condition of pain in the urethra

**urethr/o**-gram, a recording or X-ray picture of the urethra

**urethr/o**-graphy, technique of making a recording or X-ray picture of the urethra

**urethr/o**-metry, technique of measuring the urethra

**urethr/o**-pen-ile, pertaining to the penis and the urethra

**urethr/o**-perine-al, pertaining to the perineum and the urethra

**urethr/o**-perine/o-scrot-al, pertaining to the scrotum, perineum and urethra

**urethr/o**-pexy, fixation (by surgery) of the urethra (to the symphysis pubis and rectus abdominis muscle, a treatment for incontinence in women)

**urethr/o**-phraxis, blocking or obstruction of the urethra

**urethr/o**-phyma, a tumour or boil in the urethra

**urethr/o**-plasty, surgical repair or reconstruction of the urethra

**urethr/o**-prostat-ic, pertaining to the prostate gland and the urethra

**urethr/o**-rect-al, pertaining to the rectum and urethra

**urethr/o**-rrhag-ia, condition of excessive flow of blood from the urethra

**urethr/o**-rrhaphy, stitching or suturing of the urethra

**urethr/o**-rrhoea, excessive flow or discharge from the urethra

**urethr/o**-scope, an instrument used to view or examine the urethra

**urethr/o**-scop-ic, 1. pertaining to viewing or examining the urethra 2. pertaining to urethroscopy

**urethr/o**-scopy, technique of viewing or examining the urethra

**urethr/o**-spasm, sudden contraction of muscle in the urethra

**urethr/o**-staxis, dripping of blood from the urethra

**urethr/o**-sten-osis, abnormal condition of narrowing of the urethra

**urethr/o**-stomy, formation of an opening into the urethra or the name of the opening so created

**urethr/o**-tome, an instrument used for cutting the urethra

**urethr/o**-tomy, incision into the urethra

**urethr/o**-trigon-itis, inflammation of the trigone and urethra

**urethr/o**-ureter-al, pertaining to the ureters and urethra

**urethr/o**-vagin-al, pertaining to the vagina and urethra

**urethr/o**-vesic-al, pertaining to the bladder and urethra

---

**Uric/o/s**, uric acid

From a Latin word **urina**, meaning urine. Here uric/o means uric acid, a substance formed from the breakdown of nucleoproteins in the tissues. Uric acid is the end-product of purine metabolism and is a normal constituent of urine.

hyper-**uric**-aem-ia, condition of blood with an excess of uric acid

hypo-**uric**-aem-ia, condition of blood with a deficiency of uric acid

**uric**-acid-aem-ia, condition of blood containing (excess) uric acid Syn. hyperuricaemia

**uric**-acid-ur-ia, condition of urine containing (excess) uric acid

**uric**-aem-ia, condition of blood containing (excess) uric acid Syn. hyperuricaemia

**uric/o**-chol-ia, condition of bile containing uric acid

**uric/o**-lyt-ic, 1. pertaining to the breakdown of uric acid 2. an agent that destroys uric acid

**uric/o**-meter, an instrument that measures uric acid (in urine)

**uricos**-ur-ia, condition of excretion of uric acid in urine

**uricos**-ur-ic, 1. pertaining to uricosuria 2. an agent that promotes the excretion of uric acid in the urine (used as a treatment for gout)

---

**Urin/a/i/o**, urine

From a Latin word **urina**, meaning urine. Here urin/o means urine, the excretory product of the kidneys.

**urin/a**-lysis, splitting or separating urine for analysis

**urin**-ary, pertaining to urine

**urin**-ate, to pass urine

**urin**-ation, process of passing or discharging urine

**urin/i**-fer-ous, pertaining to carrying urine

**urin/i**-par-ous, pertaining to producing (passing) urine

**urin/o**-genit-al, pertaining to the genital organs and urinary organs

**urin/o**-gen-ous, 1. pertaining to formation of urine 2. pertaining to originating in the urinary tract

**urin**-oma, a tumour or swelling (cyst) containing urine

**urin/o**-meter, an instrument that measures urine (its specific gravity)

**urin/o**-metry, technique of measuring urine (its specific gravity using a urinometer)

**urin/o**-sanguin-ous, pertaining to blood and urine

**urin**-ous, pertaining to or of the nature of urine

---

**Ur/o**, urine, urinary tract

From a Greek word **ouron**, meaning urine. Here ur/o means the urinary tract or urine.

albumin-**ur**-ia, condition of albumin in urine

azot-**ur**-ia, condition of urea (too much) in urine

dys-**ur**-ia, condition of painful or difficult flow of urine

enur-esis, condition of urinating (involuntarily, usually at night). From a Greek word enourein meaning to urinate

haemat-**ur**-ia, condition of blood in the urine

hyper-calc/i-**ur**-ia, condition of too much calcium in the urine olig-**ur**-ia, condition of little urine (diminished excretion of)

poly-**ur**-ia, condition of much urine, it refers to producing too much

py-**ur**-ia, condition of pus in the urine

**ur**-aem-ia, condition of urine in the blood, it refers to the retention of urea and nitrogenous substances in the blood

**ur**-aem-ic, pertaining to having uraemia

**ur**-aem-i-gen-ic, pertaining to forming uraemia

**ur**-elc-osis, abnormal condition of ulceration of the urinary tract

**ur**-esis, process of passing urine or urination

**ur**-etic, pertaining to passing urine or urination

**ur/o**-cele, a swelling or protrusion due to urine discharged into the scrotum

**ur/o**-ches-ia, condition of discharge of urine through the rectum. From a Greek word *chezein* – to defecate

**ur/o**-chez-ia, condition of discharge of urine through the rectum. From a Greek word *chezein* – to defecate

**ur/o**-chrome, a coloured pigment of urine (a yellow breakdown product of haemoglobin)

**ur/o**-cyst, the urinary bladder

**ur/o**-cyst-ic, pertaining to the urinary bladder

**ur/o**-cyst-itis, inflammation of the urinary bladder

**ur/o**-dynam-ics, the science of studying the movement (propulsion and flow) of urine

**ur/o**-dyn-ia, condition of pain on passing urine

**ur/o**-flo-metry, technique of measuring the flow of urine

**ur/o**-genit-al, pertaining to the genitalia and urinary tract

**ur/o**-gen-ous, pertaining to the formation of urine or derived from urine

**ur/o**-gram, a recording or X-ray picture of the urinary tract

**ur/o**-graphy, technique of making a recording or X-ray picture of the urinary tract

**ur/o**-lith, a stone or calculus in the urine

**ur/o**-lith-iasis, presence of stones or calculi in the urine

**ur/o**-lith-ic, 1. pertaining to stones or calculi in the urine 2. pertaining to urolithiasis

**ur/o**-log-ic, pertaining to the study of the urinary system

**ur/o**-log-ist, a specialist who studies urology

**ur/o**-logy, the study of the urinary tract (anatomy, diseases and treatment of)

**ur/o**-metry, technique of measuring urine (pressure changes due to ureteal peristalsis)

**ur**-onc-us, swelling or mass caused by urine (urinary cyst)

**ur/o**-nephr-osis, abnormal condition of urine in the kidney (distention of the renal pelvis with urine)

**ur/o**-oedema, oedema due to urine

**ur/o**-pathy, disease of the urinary tract

**ur/o**-phan-ic, pertaining to appearing in the urine. From a Greek word *phanein* meaning to appear

**ur/o**-poiesis, formation of urine

**ur/o**-poiet-ic, pertaining to the formation of urine

**ur/o**-psammus, a sand-like sediment in the urine or urinary gravel. From a Greek word *psammos* meaning sand

**ur/o**-pyo-nephr-osis, abnormal condition of pus and urine in the kidney

**ur/o**-radi/o-logy, the study of the urinary tract using radiation, X-rays *etc.*

**ur/o**-rrhag-ia, condition of excessive flow of urine

**ur/o**-rrhoea, 1. excessive flow of urine Syn. polyuria 2. (involuntary) discharge of urine as in bed wetting

**ur/o**-schesis, 1. involuntary retention of urine 2. stopping of urinary excretion

**ur/o**-scop-ic, pertaining to viewing or examining urine (for diagnostic purposes)

**ur/o**-scopy, technique of viewing or examining urine (for diagnostic purposes)

**ur/o**-sepsis, an infection or septic poisoning from retained urine

**ur/o**-stomy, formation of an opening to drain urine or the name of the opening so created

**ur/o**-ureter, a ureter distended with urine

---

**Vesic/o**, vesic

From a Latin word **vesica**, meaning bladder. Here, vesic/o means the urinary bladder, an organ that stores urine prior to its excretion from the body.

pre-**vesic**-al, pertaining to in front of or anterior to the urinary bladder

retro-**vesic**-al, pertaining to behind or at the back of the urinary bladder

trans-**vesic**-al, pertaining to through the urinary bladder

**vesic**-al, pertaining to the urinary bladder

**vesic/o**-abdomin-al, pertaining to the abdominal wall and bladder

**vesic/o**-cele, a protrusion or hernia of the bladder

**vesic/o**-cervic-al, pertaining to the cervix uteri and the urinary bladder

**vesic/o**-clysis, infusion or injection into the urinary bladder

**vesic/o**-enter-ic, pertaining to the intestine and urinary bladder

**vesic/o**-intestin-al, pertaining to the intestine and urinary bladder

**vesic/o**-prostat-ic, pertaining to the prostate gland and the urinary bladder

**vesic/o**-pub-ic, pertaining to the pubes (pubic region) and urinary bladder

**vesic/o**-rect-al, pertaining to the rectum and urinary bladder

**vesic/o**-sigmoid, pertaining to the sigmoid flexure and urinary bladder

**vesic/o**-sigmoid/o-stomy, formation of an opening between the sigmoid colon and urinary bladder (to drain urine) or the name of the opening so created

**vesic/o**-spin-al, pertaining to the spine and urinary bladder

**vesic/o**-stomy, formation of an opening into the urinary bladder (from the abdominal wall) or the name of the opening so created

**vesic/o**-tomy, incision into the urinary bladder

**vesic/o**-umbilic-al, pertaining to the umbilicus and urinary bladder

**vesic/o**-ureter-al, pertaining to the ureters and urinary bladder

**vesic/o**-ureter-ic, pertaining to a ureter and the urinary bladder

**vesic/o**-uter-ine, pertaining to the uterus and urinary bladder

**vesic/o**-uter/o-vagin-al, pertaining to the vagina, uterus and urinary bladder

**vesic/o**-vagin-al, pertaining to the vagina and urinary bladder

**vesic/o**-vagin/o-rect-al, pertaining to the rectum, vagina and urinary bladder

# Section 8
# The nervous system

Humans have a complex nervous system with a brain that is large in proportion to their body size. The brain and spinal cord are estimated to contain at least $10^{10}$ cells, with vast numbers of connections between them. The nervous system performs three basic functions:

- It receives, stores and analyses information from sense organs such as the eyes and ears, making us aware of our environment. This awareness enables us to think and make responses that will aid our survival in changing conditions.
- It controls the physiological activities of the body systems and maintains constant conditions

(homeostasis) within the body.

- It controls our muscles, enabling us to move and speak.

The major components of the nervous system are grouped as follows;

- **The central nervous system (CNS)** consisting of the brain and spinal cord
- **The peripheral nervous system (PNS)** consisting of 12 pairs of cranial nerves and 31 pairs of spinal nerves that connect the central nervous system to sense organs, muscles and glands.

The peripheral nervous system can be subdivided on the basis of how its parts function:

- **The somatic nervous system (SNS)** consists of neurons that convey information from the receptors in the head, body wall and skin to the CNS, and motor neurons that control skeletal muscles. The motor activities are under conscious voluntary control
- **The autonomic nervous system** consists of sensory neurons that convey information from receptors in viscera to the CNS and motor neurons that control

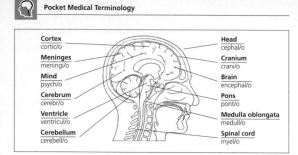

| | | | |
|---|---|---|---|
| **Cortex** cortic/o | | **Head** cephal/o | |
| **Meninges** meningi/o | | **Cranium** crani/o | |
| **Mind** psych/o | | **Brain** encephal/o | |
| **Cerebrum** cerebr/o | | **Pons** pont/o | |
| **Ventricle** ventricul/o | | **Medulla oblongata** medull/o | |
| **Cerebellum** cerebell/o | | **Spinal cord** myel/o | |

Figure 11 Sagittal section through the head showing the central nervous system

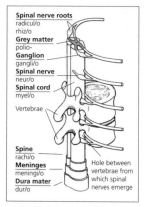

**Spinal nerve roots** radicul/o rhiz/o

**Grey matter** polio-

**Ganglion** gangli/o

**Spinal nerve** neur/o

**Spinal cord** myel/o

Vertebrae

**Spine** rachi/o

**Meninges** meningi/o

**Dura mater** dur/o

Hole between vertebrae from which spinal nerves emerge

Figure 12 Section through the spine

smooth muscle, cardiac muscle and glands. The responses of the ANS are involuntary. The autonomic system can be subdivided into the sympathetic and parasympathetic subsystems.

Figures 11 and 12 show the structure of the central nervous system and combining forms related to its anatomy.

**Roots and combining forms**, meanings

**Aesthe/s/i/o/t**, sensation
From a Greek word **aisthesis**, meaning perception or sensation. Here aethesi/o means sensation or feeling.

**aesthes**-ia, condition of sensation or feeling

**aesthesi**-od-ic, pertaining to conducting sensory impulses to the brain. From a Greek word *hodos* meaning way

**aesthesi/o**-logy, the study of sensation or sensory organs

**aesthesi/o**-neur-osis, abnormal condition of sensory nerves

an-**aesthes**-ia, 1. condition of without sensation or feeling 2. condition of loss of consciousness produced by a general anaesthetic

an-**aesthesi/i**-meter, 1. an instrument that measures the degree of anaesthesia 2. an instrument that measures amount of anaesthetic administered to a patient

an-**aesthesi/o**-log-ist, a specialist who studies anaesthesiology

an-**aesthesi/o**-logy, 1. the study of anaesthesia and anaesthetics 2. the science dealing with the administration and effect of anaesthetics

an-**aesthe**-tic, 1. pertaining to without sensation or feeling 2. an agent that produces anaesthesia

**an**-aesthet-ist, a specialist (medically qualified) who administers anaesthetics to patients

brady-**aesthes**-ia, condition of slow perception with dullness of intellect

cry-**aesthes**-ia, condition of abnormal sensitivity to cold

cry-an-**aesthes**-ia, condition of without sensitivity to cold

dys-**aesthes**-ia, 1. condition of a painful or unpleasant sensation 2. condition of poor sensation especially of touch

hemi-an-**aesthes**-ia, condition of without sensation on one side (half) of the body

hemi-hyper-**aesthes**-ia, condition of above normal sensitivity to stimulation of one side (half) of the body

hyper-**aesthes**-ia, condition of increased or above normal sensitivity to stimulation

hypo-**aesthes**-ia, condition of decreased or below normal sensitivity to stimulation

para-an-**aesthes**-ia, condition of without sensation or feeling in the lower part of the body

par-**aesthes**-ia, condition of abnormal sensation or feeling

par-an-**aesthes**-ia, condition of without sensation or feeling in the lower part of the body

post-an-**aesthes**-ia, following or after anaesthesia

pre-an-**aesthes**-ia, before anaesthesia

pseud-**aesthes**-ia, 1. condition of false sensation, a sensation occurring without an objective stimulus 2. an imaginary sensation

syn-**aesthes**-ia, condition of associated sensation, it refers to a condition in which a stimulus produces a normal sensation and an accompanying sensation *e.g.* a sound may produce a sensation of colour

thigm-**aesthes**-ia, condition of sensation of touch

---

**Alges/i**, sense of pain

From a Greek word **algesis**, meaning pain. Here, alges/i means having a sense of pain.

**alg**-aesth-esis, condition of sensation of pain

**alges**-ia, condition of pain (excessive sensitivity to)

**alges**-ic, pertaining to pain (excessive sensitivity to)

**alges/i**-meter, an instrument that measures sensitivity to pain

an-**alges**-ia, condition of without pain

an-**alges**-ia, 1. pertaining to without pain 2. an agent that reduces pain

an-**alg**-ia, condition of without pain

an-**alg**-ic, pertaining to without pain (insensitivity to pain)

cry/o-an-**alges**-ia, condition of reduced pain brought about by cooling nerves with a cryoprobe

hyper-**alges**-ia, condition of above normal sensitivity to pain

hypo-**alges**-ia, condition of below normal sensitivity to pain

top-**alg**-ia, condition of pain in a particular place or location

---

**ax/i/o**, **axon/o**, axon

From a Greek word **axon** word meaning axle. Here ax/o means an axon, a thread-like process of a neuron that conducts impulses away from the cell body. Many axons are covered with a myelin sheath that increases the speed of nerve impulse transmission.

**ax/i**-fug-al, pertaining to extending away from an axon

**ax/i**-pet-al, pertaining to towards an axon

**ax/o**-dendrit-ic, pertaining to a synapse between an axon of a neuron and a dendrite of another neuron

**ax/o**-fug-al, pertaining to extending away from an axon

**ax/o**-lemma, the outer membrane of an axon

**ax/o**-lysis, breakdown of an axon (degeneration)

**axon**-al, 1. pertaining to an axon 2. having an effect on an axon

**axon**-tmesis, damage caused to an axon by prolonged pressure or crushing rather than compete severance, the axon may regenerate.

From a Greek word *tmesis* meaning to cut apart

ax/o-pet-al, pertaining to extending toward an axon

ax/o-phage, cell that 'eats' axons, it refers to a glial cell that digests myelin (in myelitis)

ax/o-plasm, the cytoplasm of an axon

ax/o-plasm-ic, pertaining to axoplasm

ax/o-somat-ic, pertaining to a synapse between an axon of a neuron and the cell body of another neuron

---

## Cephal/o, head

From a Greek word **kephale**, meaning head. Here cephal/o means the head.

a-**cephal**-ous, pertaining to without a head (an embryological defect)

**cephal**-alg-ia, condition of pain in the head or headache

**cephal**-haemat/o-cele, a protrusion or blood-filled swelling in the head, it refers to a blood-filled swelling communicating through the bones of the skull with a dural sinus

**cephal**-haemat-oma, swelling of blood within the head, it refers to a collection of blood in sub-periosteal space

**cephal**-hydr/o-cele, a protrusion or hernia of a watery swelling in the head (under the pericranium)

**cephal**-ic, pertaining to the head

**cephal**-in, a chemical found in the head (a brain phosphoglyceride)

**cephal/o**-cele, a protrusion or hernia (of the brain) from the head

**cephal/o**-centesis, surgical puncture of the head

**cephal/o**-gram, a recording or X-ray picture of the head

**cephal/o**-gyr-ic, pertaining to a turning motion of the head

**cephal/o**-meter, an instrument that measures the head

**cephal/o**-metry, technique of measuring the head

**cephal/o**-motor, action or motion of the head

**cephal/o**-pathy, disease of the head

dorso-**cephal**-ad, towards the back of the head

dys-**cephal**-ic, pertaining to dyscephaly

dys-**cephal**-y, condition of poor or bad head, it refers to malformation of the head and facial bones

eury-**cephal**-ic, pertaining to having a wide head

hydro-**cephal**-us, thing (baby) with water in the head, it refers to an abnormal amount of cerebro-spinal fluid in the ventricles of the brain

hydro-micro-**cephal**-y, condition of a small head containing water, it refers to a condition of having a small head containing an abnormal amount of fluid in the ventricles of the brain

lepto-**cephal**-us, thing (person) with a thin head (tall and narrow)

macro-**cephal**-ic, pertaining to having an abnormally large head

macro-**cephal**-us, thing (fetus) with a large head

micro-**cephal**-ic, pertaining to having an abnormally small head

pachy-**cephal**-ic, pertaining to having an abnormally thick head, it refers to having a thick skull

pachy-**cephal**-y, condition of having an abnormally thick head, it refers to having a thick skull

pro-**cephal**-ic, pertaining to the front of the head, its anterior or ventral part

---

## Cerebell/i/o, cerebellum

From a Latin word **cerebellum** meaning small brain. Here cerebell/o means the cerebellum, the part of the brain that lies behind and below the cerebrum. Its chief functions are the co-ordination of fine voluntary movements and the maintenance of posture.

**cerebell**-ar, pertaining to the cerebellum

**cerebell/i**-fug-al, pertaining to extending away from the cerebellum

**cerebell/i**-pet-al, pertaining to extending towards the cerebellum

**cerebell**-itis, inflammation of the cerebellum

**cerebell/o**-pont-ine, pertaining to the pons and the cerebellum

**cerebell/o**-spin-al, pertaining to the spinal cord and cerebellum

**Cerebr/o**, cerebrum, cerebral hemisphere

From a Latin word **cerebrum**, meaning brain. Here cerebr/o means the cerebral hemispheres or cerebrum of the brain.

**cerebr**-al, pertaining to the cerebrum

**cerebr**-ation, action or activity of the cerebrum

**cerebr**-itis, inflammation of the cerebrum

**cerebr**-oma, a tumour or swelling of the cerebrum

**cerebr/o**-macul-ar, pertaining to the macula lutea (in the retina of the eye) and the cerebrum

**cerebr/o**-malac-ia, condition of softening of the cerebrum

**cerebr/o**-mening-eal, pertaining to the meninges and the cerebrum

**cerebr/o**-mening-itis, inflammation of the meninges and cerebrum Syn. meningoencephalitis

**cerebr/o**-ocul-ar, pertaining to the eye and cerebrum

**cerebr/o**-path-ia, condition of disease of the cerebrum

**cerebr/o**-pathy, disease of the cerebrum

**cerebr/o**-physi/o-logy, the study of the physiology of the cerebrum

**cerebr/o**-pont-ile, pertaining to the pons and cerebrum

**cerebr/o**-scler-osis, abnormal condition of hardening of the cerebrum

**cerebr**-osis, abnormal condition or disease of the cerebrum

**cerebr/o**-spin-al, pertaining to the spinal cord and cerebrum

**cerebr/o**-spin-ant, an agent that affects the spinal cord and cerebrum

**cerebr/o**-tomy, incision into the cerebrum

**cerebr/o**-vascul-ar, pertaining to the vessels of the cerebrum (arteries and veins)

dextro-**cerebr**-al, pertaining to the right cerebrum

sinistro-**cerebr**-al, pertaining to the left cerebrum

**Cistern/o, cistern, cisterna magna**

From a Latin word **cistern** meaning a vessel serving as a reservoir for fluid. Here cistern/o means the cisterna magna, the subarachnoid space in the cleft between the cerebellum and medulla oblongata containing cerebrospinal fluid.

**cistern**-al, 1. pertaining to a cistern 2. pertaining to the cisterna magna

**cistern/o**-gram, 1. a recording or X-ray picture of a cistern 2. a recording or X-ray picture of the cisterna magna

**cistern/o**-graphy, 1. technique of making a recording or X-ray picture of a cistern 2. technique of making a recording or X-ray picture of the cisterna magna

**Cortic/o**, cortex

From a Latin word **cortex** meaning bark as in the outer bark of a tree. Here cortic/o means the cerebral cortex, the outer layer of grey matter on the surface of the cerebral hemispheres in the brain.

**cortic**-al, pertaining to or composed of cerebral cortex

**cortic**-ate, having a cortex

**cortic/o**-bulb-ar, pertaining to the medulla oblongata and cerebral cortex

**cortic/o**-pont-ine, pertaining to the pons and cerebral cortex

**cortic/o**-pont/o-cerebell-ar, pertaining to the cerebellum, pons and cerebral cortex (the nerve pathway that connects the cerebellum to the cerebral cortex via the pons)

**cortic/o**-spin-al, pertaining to or belonging to the spinal cord and cerebral cortex

**cortic/o**-thalam-ic, pertaining to the thalamus and cerebral cortex

electro-**cortic/o**-graphy, technique of recording the electrical activity of the brain using electrodes placed on the cerebral cortex

trans-**cortic**-al, 1. pertaining to across a cortex 2. connecting two parts of the cerebral cortex

**Cran/i/o**, cranium, skull

From a Greek word **kranion** meaning skull. Here crani/o means the cranium, the part of the skull enclosing the brain. It consists of eight bones: the occipital, two parietals, frontal, two temporals, sphenoid and ethmoid.

**cran/i-al**, pertaining to the cranium

**crani/o-aur-al**, pertaining to the ear and cranium

**crani/o-cele**, a protrusion or hernia (of brain substance) through the cranium

**crani/o-clasis**, breaking or crushing of the cranium (of a dead fetus to make delivery possible)

**crani/o-clasty**, process of breaking or crushing of the cranium (of a dead fetus to make delivery possible) Syn. cranioclasis

**crani/o-faci-al**, pertaining to the face and cranium

**crani/o-fenestr-ia**, condition of windows in the cranium, it refers to points where bone has failed to develop. From a Latin word *fenestra* meaning window

**crani/o-graph**, an instrument that records the cranium (its outline and its diameters to scale)

**crani/o-graphy**, technique of making a recording or tracing of the cranium (its outline and diameters to scale)

**crani/o-lacun-ia**, condition of hollows, depressions on the inner surface of the cranium, it refers to defective development of the fetal cranium. From a Latin word *lacuna* meaning hollow

**crani/o-malac-ia**, condition of softening of the cranium

**crani/o-mandibul-ar**, pertaining to the mandible and cranium

**crani/o-mening/o-cele**, a protrusion or hernia of the meninges through the cranium

**crani/o-meter**, an instrument that measures the cranium (its diameters)

**crani/o-metr-ic**, 1. pertaining to measuring the cranium (its diameters) 2. pertaining to craniometry

**crani/o-metry**, technique of measuring the cranium (its diameters)

**crani/o-pathy**, disease of the cranium

**crani/o-pharyng-eal**, pertaining to the pharynx and cranium

**crani/o-pharyng/i-oma**, a tumour of the pharynx and cranium (a pituitary tumour seen in children)

**crani/o-plasty**, surgical repair or reconstructive surgery of the cranium

**crani/o-rachi-schisis**, splitting or fissure of the spinal column and cranium (a congenital defect)

**crani/o-sacr-al**, pertaining to the sacrum and cranium

**crani/o-schisis**, splitting or fissure of the cranium (a congenital defect)

**crani/o-scler-osis**, abnormal condition of hardening (thickening) of the cranium

**crani/o-spin-al**, pertaining to the spine and cranium

**crani/o-sten-osis**, abnormal condition of narrowing of the cranium (due to premature closure of cranial sutures)

**cran/i-ost-osis**, abnormal condition of ossification (bone formation) in the cranium. A congenital defect in which cranial sutures are closed

**crani/o-syn-ost-osis**, abnormal condition of bones of the cranium fusing together (due to premature closure of cranial sutures)

**crani/o-tabes**, thinning or wasting away of the cranium in infancy. From a Latin word *tabes* meaning a wasting away

**crani/o-tomy**, 1. incision into the cranium 2. process of cutting the cranium of a dead fetus to make delivery possible

**endo-crani/i-um**, 1. the inner structure of the cranium 2. the structure within the cranium, it refers to the outer layer of the cerebral dura mater on the inner surface of the cranium

**intra-crani-al**, pertaining to within the cranium

**macro-cran-ia**, condition of enlarged cranium

**peri-cran-itis**, inflammation of the pericranium

peri-**cran/i**-um, the structure around the cranium, it refers to the connective tissue membrane (periostium) that covers the cranium

sub-**cran/i**-al, pertaining to under the cranium

---

**Dendr/i/o**, dendrit-, dendrite, dendron
From a Greek word **dendron** meaning tree. Here dendr/o means a dendrite, a small tree-like filament branching from the body of a nerve cell. Dendrites transmit impulses towards the nerve cell body. The term dendron is used synonymously with dendrite.

**dendr/i**-form, having the form of a tree, branched

**dendr/o-dendrit**-ic, pertaining to a synapse between dendrites of two neurons

**dendr**-oid, resembling a tree, branched like a tree

**dendr/o**-phag/o-cyt-osis, condition or process of a cell 'eating' dendrites, it refers to a microglial cell breaking down degenerating astrocytes

---

**Dolor/i/o**, pain
From a Latin word **dolor** meaning pain. Here dolor/o means pain. Note: pain is measured in units of pain intensity called dols.

**dolor/i**-fic, pertaining to causing pain. From a Latin word *facere* to make

**dolor/i**-meter, an instrument used for measuring pain (in units called dols)

**dolor/i**-metry, technique of measuring pain (in units called dols)

**dolor/o**-gen-ic, pertaining to producing pain

---

**Dur/o**, dura mater
From the Latin words **dura** meaning hard and **mater** meaning mother. Here dur/o means the dura mater, the outer fibrous meningeal membrane. This is the thickest of the three meninges, it is dense and inelastic and lines the interior of the skull. The dura mater is two layered, the outer endosteal layer is in contact with the skull and the inner layer protects the brain and spinal cord.

epi-**dur**-al, pertaining to above or upon the dura mater

epi-**dur/o**-graphy, technique of making a recording or X-ray picture following injection of dye above the dura (into the epidural space)

**dur**-al, pertaining to the dura mater

**dur**-itis, inflammation of the dura mater Syn. pachymeningitis

**dur/o**-arachn-itis, inflammation of the arachnoid mater and dura mater

intra-**dur**-al, pertaining to within or inside the dura mater

sub-**dur**-al, pertaining to under the dura mater

---

**Encephal/o**, brain
From a Greek word **encephalos**, meaning brain. Here, encephal/o means the brain or encephalon.

an-**encephal**-ic, pertaining to without a brain (an embryological defect)

echo-**encephal/o**-gram, a picture or tracing of the brain made using reflected ultrasound echoes

electro-**encephal/o**-graph, an instrument that records the electrical activity of the brain

electro-**encephal/o**-graphy, technique of recording the electrical activity of the brain

**encephal**-alg-ia, condition of pain within the brain (head)

**encephal**-a-trophy, 1. without nourishment or wasting away of the brain 2. atrophy of the brain

**encephal**-ic, 1. pertaining to the brain 2. pertaining to within the head

**encephal**-itic, pertaining to having encephalitis

**encephal**-itis, inflammation of the brain

**encephal/o**-cele, a protrusion or hernia of the brain (through the cranium)

**encephal/o**-cyst/o-cele, a protrusion or hernia of the brain (through the cranium) caused by a cyst of fluid

131

**encephal/o**-gram, a recording or X-ray picture of the brain

**encephal/o**-graphy, technique of making a recording or X-ray picture of of the brain

**encephal/o**-oid, resembling the brain or brain tissue

**encephal/o**-lith, a stone or calculus in the brain

**encephal/o**-logy, the study of the brain (anatomy, diseases and treatment of)

**encephal/o**-oma, a tumour of the brain

**encephal/o**-malac-ia, condition of softening of the brain

**encephal/o**-mening-itis, inflammation of the meninges and brain Syn. meningo-encephalitis

**encephal/o**-mening/o-cele, a protrusion or hernia of the meninges and brain (through the cranium) Syn. meningo-encephalocele

**encephal/o**-mening/o-pathy, disease of the meninges and brain

**encephal/o**-meter, an instrument used to measure the brain (to determine positions of centres and regions within the brain)

**encephal/o**-myel-ic, pertaining to the spinal cord and brain

**encephal/o**-myel-itis, inflammation of the spinal cord and brain

**encephal/o**-myel/o-neur/o-pathy disease of the (peripheral) nerves, spinal cord and brain

**encephal/o**-myel/o-pathy, disease of the spinal cord and brain

**encephal/o**-myel/o-radicul-itis, inflammation of spinal nerve roots, spinal cord and brain

**encephal/o**-myel/o-radicul/o-neur-itis, inflammation of (peripheral) nerves, spinal nerve roots, spinal cord and brain. Guillain-Barré Syndrome

**encephal/o**-myel/o-radicul/o-pathy, disease of spinal nerve roots, spinal cord and brain

**encephalon**, the brain

**encephal/o**-onc-us, a tumour in the brain

**encephal/o**-path-ic, pertaining to disease of the brain

**encephal/o**-pathy, disease of the brain

**encephal/o**-py-osis, abnormal condition of pus in the brain

**encephal/o**-rrhag-ia, condition of bursting forth of blood (haemorrhage) from the brain (capillaries)

**encephal/o**-sepsis, infection of the brain

**encephal/o**-osis, abnormal condition or disease of the brain (degenerative)

**encephal/o**-tomy, incision into the brain

macr-**encephal**-y, condition of abnormal enlargement of the brain

mes-**encephal**-on, the middle brain

micro-**encephal**-y, condition of having a small brain

pan-**encephal**-itis, inflammation of all of the brain, it refers to a fatal degeneration of brain cells of viral origin seen in children

polio-**encephal**-itis, inflammation of the grey matter of the brain

---

**Epilept/i/o**, epilepsy
From a Greek word **epileptikos**, meaning a seizure. Here epilept/o means epilepsy, the disordered electrical activity of the brain that produces a 'fit' and unconsciousness.

**epileps**-ia, condition of epilepsy

**epilept**-ic, 1. pertaining to epilepsy 2. one who is liable to attacks of epilepsy

**epilept/i**-form, having the form of epilepsy

**epilept/o**-gen-ic, pertaining to formation of epilepsy or an epileptic seizure

**epilept/o**-gen-ous, pertaining to formation of epilepsy or an epileptic seizure

**epilept**-oid, resembling epilepsy Syn. epileptiform

**epilept**-osis, any mental disorder that belongs to the epilepsy group

post-**epilept**-ic, pertaining to following or after an epileptic fit or seizure

---

**Gangli/o**, ganglion-, ganglion
From a Greek word **ganglion**, meaning swelling. Here gangli/o means a

ganglion, a knot of nerve cell bodies located outside the central nervous system (plural ganglia).

**gangli**-a, plural of ganglion

**gangli**-al, pertaining to a ganglion

**gangli**-ate, having ganglia

**gangli**-form, having the form or appearance of a ganglion

**gangli**-itis, inflammation of a ganglion Syn. ganglionitis

**gangli/o**-blast, an immature cell or embryonic cell that gives rise to a (spinal) ganglion

**gangli/o**-cyte, a ganglion cell

**gangli/o**-cyt-oma, a tumour of ganglion cells

**gangli/o**-form, having the form or appearance of a ganglion

**gangli/o**-gli/o-neur-oma, a glioneuroma containing ganglion cells

**gangli**-oid, resembling a ganglion

**gangli**-oma, a tumour of a ganglion

**ganglion**-ate, having ganglia

**ganglion**-ectomy, removal of a ganglion

**gangli/o**-neur-oma, a tumour of ganglion cells of the sympathetic nervous system

**ganglion**-ic, pertaining to or of the nature of a ganglion

**gangli/o**-pathy, disease of a ganglion

**gangli/o**-pleg-ia, condition of paralysis of a ganglion, it refers to a failure to transmit impulses normally

**gangli/o**-pleg-ic, pertaining to paralysis of a ganglion, it refers to a failure to transmit impulses normally

**gangli/o**-plex-us, a network of nerves within a ganglion

**gangli/os**-ide, a chemical (cerebroside) found in nervous tissue of the central nervous system. Accumulation may occur in some inherited disorders, for example Tay-Sachs disease

**gangli/o**-sympath-ectomy, removal of a sympathetic ganglion

pre-**ganglion**-ic, pertaining to before a ganglion

post-**ganglion**-ic, pertaining to after a ganglion

**Gli/o**, glial cell, neurogliocyte

From a Greek word **glia** meaning glue. Here, gli/o is used on its own or with -cyte to mean a gliacyte (glue cell) or neurogliocyte. Glial cells support (hold together) the neurons of the central nervous system; there are four types: astrocytes, microglia, oligodendrocytes and ependymocytes.

**glia**-cyte, 1. a glial cell or neurogliocyte 2. a cell of the neuroglia, the supporting structure of nervous tissue

**gli**-al, pertaining to glial cells or neuroglia

**gli/o**-blast-oma, a tumour of immature cells or embryonic germ cells that contain neuroglia

**gli/o**-cyte, 1. a glial cell or neurogliocyte 2. a cell of the neuroglia, the supporting structure of nervous tissue Syn. gliacyte

**gli**-oma, a tumour composed of glial cells or neurogliocytes, a primary tumour of the brain

**gli**-omat-ous, 1. pertaining to or of the nature of a glioma 2. pertaining to having a glioma

**gli/o**-my-oma, a tumour of muscle and glial cells

**gli/o**-neur-oma, a tumour of nerve cells (neuroma) and elements of their supporting connective tissue (glioma)

macro-**glia**, the large types of glial cell considered together (astrocytes and oligodendrocytes)

micro-**glia**, the small types of glial cell, they are phagocytic and can migrate to a site of injury

micro-**gli**-al, pertaining to microglia

micro-**gli/o**-cyte, a small gliocyte (an immature gliocyte)

---

**-mania**, man-ic, mania

From a Greek word **mania**, here it means: 1. a disordered mental state of extreme excitement 2. an obsessive preoccupation with something e.g. a homicidal mania

Note: These terms have complex meanings in psychiatry.

anti-**man**-ic, a drug that acts against mania, it is used to control acute attacks of mania and prevent their reoccurrence

**mania**, a condition that forms a phase of manic depressive psychosis in which the mood is one of extreme excitement and often accompanied by pronounced psychomotor activity

**mani**-ac, one afflicted with mania or insanity

**mani**-ac-al, pertaining to or affected with mania

**man**-ic, pertaining to mania (in manic depression the mood alternates between phases of mania and depression)

megalo-**mania**, a large mania, it refers to a mental condition in which the patient has grandiose delusions about himself including an unwarranted belief in his/her own goodness, power or greatness

nymph/o-**mania**, an exaggerated sexual desire in women

nymph/o-**mani**-ac, a woman with an exaggerated sexual desire

---

**Medull/o**, medulla oblongata, spinal cord, myelin sheath

From a Latin word **medulla** meaning marrow. Medulla means a soft marrow-like central part of a structure. Here it refers to the medulla oblongata, the spinal cord or the myelin sheath of nerve fibres. The medulla oblongata forms the lowest part of the brain stem where it passes through the foramen magnum to become the spinal cord; it contains the cardiac and respiratory centres that control heart rate and breathing.

Note: medull/o also refers to bone marrow in the centre of long bones.

**medull**-ary, 1. pertaining to a medulla *e.g.* the medulla oblongata 2. pertaining to the spinal cord 3. pertaining to bone marrow

**medull**-ated, 1. containing or surrounded by a medulla such as a nerve fibre surrounded by a myelin sheath 2. myelinated

**medull/o**-blast, an immature cell or embryonic cell (of the neural tube in the embryo) that forms a neuroblast or spongioblast

**medull/o**-blast-oma, malignant tumour of medulloblasts (neuroblasts or spongioblasts), it often forms in the cerebellum most frequently in children aged 5–9 years

**medull/o**-epitheli-oma, a tumour formed from neuro-epithelial cells lining the tubular spaces

---

**Mening/i/o**, meninges

From a Greek word **meningx**, meaning membrane. Here, mening/i means the meninges, the three membranes that surround the brain and spinal cord. Beginning with the outermost membrane they are named dura mater, arachnid and pia mater.

hydro-**mening/o**-cele, a protrusion or hernia of the meninges (through the cranium or spine) containing a watery fluid

lepto-**mening**-eal, pertaining to the lepto-meninges

lepto-**meninges**, the thin meninges, the piamater and pia-arachnid together

lepto-**mening**-itis, inflammation of the thin meninges (leptomeninges)

lepto-**mening/o**-pathy, disease of the leptomeninges

**mening**-eal, pertaining to the meninges

**meningi**-oma, a tumour of the meninges

**mening**-ism, process of (forming symptoms of) meningitis without actual infection of the meninges

**mening**-ismus, process of (forming symptoms of) meningitis without actual infection of the meninges

**mening**-itic, pertaining to having meningitis

**mening**-itis, inflammation of the meninges (usually due to infection)

**mening/o**-blast-oma, a tumour of immature cells or embryonic cells of the meninges, a meningioma

**mening/o**-cele, a protrusion or hernia of the meninges (through the cranium or spine)

**mening/o**-cocc-aem-ia, condition of the blood infected with meningococci

**mening/o**-cocc-al, pertaining to meningococci

**mening/o**-cocc-ic, pertaining to meningococci

**mening/o**-cocc-us, a berry-like bacterium that infects the meninges, *Neisseria meningitidis.* Plural meningococci

**mening/o**-cortic-al, pertaining to the cerebral cortex and meninges

**mening/o**-cyte, a cell of the meninges, a type of histiocyte

**mening/o**-encephal-itis, inflammation of the brain and meninges Syn. encephalomeningitis

**mening/o**-encephal/o-cele, a protrusion or hernia of the brain and meninges (through the cranium) Syn. encephalomeningocele

**mening/o**-encephal/o-myel-itis, inflammation of the spinal cord, brain and meninges

**mening/o**-encephal/o-pathy, disease of the brain and meninges

**mening/o**-gen-ic, 1. pertaining to forming the meninges 2. pertaining to originating in the meninges

**mening/o**-malac-ia, condition of softening of the meninges

**mening/o**-myel-itis, inflammation of the spinal cord and meninges

**mening/o**-myel/o-cele, a protrusion or hernia of the spinal cord and meninges (through the spine)

**mening/o**-myel/o-radicul-itis, inflammation of spinal nerve roots, spinal cord and the meninges

**mening/o**-myelo-rrhaphy, stitching or suturing of the spinal cord and meninges (repair of a meningomyelocele)

**mening/o**-pathy, disease of the meninges

**mening/o**-rachid-ian, pertaining to or characteristic of the spine (spinal cord) and meninges

**mening/o**-radicul-ar, pertaining to spinal or cranial nerve roots and the meninges

**mening/o**-rrhag-ia, condition of bursting forth of blood from the meninges

**mening/o**-vascul-ar, pertaining to the (blood) vessels of the meninges

**pachy-mening**-itis, inflammation of the thick meninx (the dura mater)

**pachy-mening/o**-pathy, disease of the thick meninx (the dura mater), a non-inflammatory condition

**pachy-meninx**, the thick meninx, the dura mater

**pachy-lepto-mening**-itis, inflammation of the thin meninges (pia mater) and thick meninx (the dura mater)

**peri-mening**-itis, inflammation around the meninges (the dura mater) Syn. pachymeningitis

**meninx**, a membrane especially one of the meninges. Singular of meninges

---

**Myelin/o**, myelin, myelin sheath
From a Greek word **myelos** meaning marrow. Here myelin/o means myelin, the lipid substance that forms the myelin sheath of an axon.

**de-myelin-**ation, action of losing or destroying myelin Syn. myelinolysis

**myelin-**ated, having or covered with myelin or a myelin sheath

**myelin-**ic, pertaining to myelin

**myelin-**iz-ation, action of making myelin or a myelin sheath

**myelin/o**-genesis, formation of myelin or a myelin sheath

**myelin/o**-lysis, breakdown or disintegration of myelin Syn. demyelination

**myelin-**oma, a tumour of myelin producing cells

**myelin/o**-pathy, disease of myelin or a myelin sheath (degenerative change)

**myelin-**osis, abnormal condition of myelin (a fatty degeneration as myelin forms)

**myelin/o**-tox-ic, pertaining to poisonous to myelin (causing demyelination)

**Myel/o**, spinal cord

From a Greek word **myelos**, meaning marrow. Here myel/o means the spinal cord, the soft marrow contained within the spine.

Note: myel/o also refers to the bone marrow and to the myelocytes, the precursors of the polymorphonuclear series of granulocytes. Words containing mye/lo are also listed in Section 5 on Blood and Section 14 on the Skeletal system.

micro-**myel**-ia, condition of a small spinal cord

**myel**-atel-ia, condition of imperfect or incomplete development of the spinal cord

**myel**-a-trophy, without nourishment (wasting away) of the spinal cord

**myel**-encephal-ic, 1. pertaining to the brain and spinal cord 2. pertaining to the myelencephalon

**myel**-encephal-itis, inflammation of the brain and spinal cord

**myel**-encephalon, the posterior part of the hind brain (medulla oblongata continuous with the spinal cord)

**myel**-in, a lipid substance found in the myelin sheath covering the axons of myelinated nerve fibres

**myel**-itic, pertaining to having myelitis

**myel**-itis, inflammation of the spinal cord

**myel/o**-cele, a protrusion or hernia of the spinal cord (through the spine)

**myel/o**-cerebell-ar, pertaining to the cerebellum and spinal cord

**myel/o**-cyst, a cyst developing from the spinal cord (from its medullary cavity)

**myel/o**-cyst-ic, pertaining to a cyst developing from the spinal cord (from its medullary cavity)

**myel/o**-cyst/o-cele, a protrusion or hernia of a cyst containing spinal cord through a defect in the vertebral column

**myel/o**-cyst/o-meningi/o-cele, a protrusion or hernia of the meninges and spinal cord associated with a myelo-cystocele

**myel/o**-dys-plas-ia, condition of poor growth or development of the spinal cord

**myel/o**-encephal-ic, pertaining to the brain and spinal cord

**myel/o**-encephal-itis, inflammation of the brain and spinal cord

**myel/o**-genesis, 1. formation of the spinal cord, it refers to formation of the nervous system, particularly the spinal cord and brain 2. formation of the myelin sheath around a nerve fibre

**myel/o**-gram, a recording or X-ray picture of the spinal cord

**myel/o**-graphy, technique of making a recording or X-ray picture of the spinal cord

**myel**-oid, resembling the spinal cord

**myel/o**-malac-ia, condition of softening of the spinal cord

**myel/o**-mening/o-cele, a protrusion or hernia of the meninges and spinal cord (through the spine)

**myel/o**-mening-itis, inflammation of the meninges and spinal cord

**myel/o**-pathy, disease of the spinal cord

**myel/o**-pet-al, pertaining to moving towards the spinal cord

**myel/o**-phthisis, wasting away of the spinal cord

**myel/o**-radicul-itis, inflammation of the (posterior) spinal nerve roots and spinal cord

**myel/o**-scler-osis, abnormal condition of hardening of the spinal cord

**myel/o**-osis, abnormal condition of the spinal cord (tumour formation)

polio-**myel**-itis, inflammation of the grey matter of the spinal cord (a disease caused by infection with poliovirus)

---

**Narc/o**, narcosis, stupor

From a Greek word **narke**, meaning stupor. Here narc/o means a narcosis, an abnormally deep sleep induced by a drug (narcotic). Narcosis is a different level of consciousness from anaesthesia; patients are not oblivious to pain and can be woken up.

**narc/o**-analysis, type of psychotherapy in which patients are encouraged to talk under the influence of narcotics

**narc/o**-hypn-osis, hypnotism in which a narcotic drug is used

**narc/o**-lepsy, condition of sudden fit of sleep or desire to sleep

**narc**-osis, abnormal stupor (produced by narcotic drugs)

**narc/o**-t-ic, a drug that induces stupor or sleep

**narc/o**-t-ize, make subject to narcotic drugs

---

**Neur/i/o**, nerve

From a Greek word **neuron**, meaning nerve. Here neur/o means a nerve, nervous tissue or the nervous system.

endo-**neur/i**-al, pertaining to the endoneurium

endo-**neur/i**-um, the structure within a nerve, it refers to the delicate connective tissue within a nerve surrounding each nerve fibre

epi-**neur/i**-al, pertaining to the epineurium

epi-**neur/i**-um, the structure upon a nerve, it refers to the fibrous connective tissue that surrounds and encloses a number of bundles of nerve fibres

mono-**neur**-itis, inflammation of one nerve

**neur**-al, pertaining to a nerve or nerves

**neur**-alg-ia, condition of pain in a nerve

**neur**-ana-genesis, regeneration or reformation of nerves or nervous tissue

**neur/a**-prax-ia, condition of temporary paralysis or conduction failure of a nerve, due to compression injury or ischaemia

**neur**-asthen-ia, condition of weakness of nerves (characterized by fatigue, both physical and mental)

**neur**-a-troph-ic, 1. pertaining to without nourishment or wasting away of nerves 2. pertaining to atrophy of nerves

**neur**-ectas-ia, condition of dilation or stretching of a nerve (by surgical means)

**neur**-ectomy, removal of part of a nerve

**neur**-ec-top-ia, condition of displacement of a nerve or condition of a nerve in an abnormal position

**neur/i**-lemma, 1. the plasma membrane of a Schwann cell 2. the sheath of Schwann that overlies the myelin sheath of a nerve fibre

**neur/i**-lemm-itis, inflammation of a neurilemma

**neur**-itis, inflammation of a nerve

**neur/o**-anastom-osis, condition of anastomosis of nerves (joining one nerve to another by surgery)

**neur/o**-anatomy, the anatomy or structure of the nervous system

**neur/o**-arthr/o-pathy, disease of joints associated with disease of nerves

**neur/o**-astr/o-cyt-oma, a tumour of nervous tissue, composed mainly of astrocytes, a glioma

**neur/o**-blast, an immature cell or embryonic cell that forms a nerve cell

**neur/o**-blast-oma, a tumour of neuroblasts (a malignant sarcoma)

**neur/o**-cardi-ac, pertaining to the heart and nervous system

**neur/o**-chori/o-retin-itis, inflammation of the retina, choroid and optic nerve

**neur/o**-choroid-itis, inflammation of the choroid and optic nerve

**neur/o**-clon-ic, pertaining to a violent action of nerves (a sudden nervous spasm)

**neur/o**-crani-al, pertaining to the neurocranium

**neur/o**-crani-um, the structure, part of the cranium (skull) enclosing the nervous tissue (brain)

**neur/o**-cutane-ous, 1. pertaining to the skin and nerves 2. pertaining to the cutaneous nerves

**neur/o**-cyte, a nerve cell (of any type)

**neur/o**-cyt-oma, a tumour of nerve cells, it refers to a type of glioma with undifferentiated nerve cells

**neur/o**-dermat-itis, inflammation of the skin due to nerves (itching of psychological origin)

**neur/o**-dyn-ia, condition of pain in a nerve Syn. neuralgia

**neur/o**-encephal/o-myel/o-pathy, disease of the spinal cord, brain and nerves

**neur/o**-endocrin/o-logy, the study of the endocrine and nervous systems (in particular the interaction between nerves and the endocrine system)

**neur/o**-epitheli-oma, a tumour of a nerve cell epithelium, a type of glioma with undifferentiated nerve cells Syn. neurocytoma

**neur/o**-epitheli-um, 1. a layer of nerve cells specialized as sensory cells 2. cells from the lining of the neural tube in the embryo that give rise to nerve cells

**neur/o**-fibril, a small fibre (found within the cytoplasm of a nerve cell)

**neur/o**-fibrill-ar, pertaining to neurofibrils, small fibres found within the cytoplasm of a nerve cell

**neur/o**-fibr-oma, a nerve fibre tumour arising from connective tissue around nerves

**neur/o**-fibr-omat-osis, abnormal condition of neurofibromas found over the entire body (Von Recklinghausen's disease)

**neur/o**-genesis, formation of nerves or nervous tissue

**neur/o**-gen-ic, 1. pertaining to formation of nerves 2. pertaining to originating in nerves

**neur/o**-glia, the supporting cells of the nervous tissue (astrocytes, microglia and oligodendrocytes in the CNS)

**neur/o**-glia-cyte, a nerve glue cell, one of the cells that forms the neuroglial tissue Syn. neurogliocyte

**neur/o**-glia-cyt-oma, a tumour of neuroglial cells

**neur/o**-gli-al, pertaining to the neuroglia

**neur/o**-gli/o-cyte, a nerve glue cell, one of the cells that form the neuroglial tissue Syn. neurogliacyte

**neur/o**-gli-oma, a tumour composed of neuroglial tissue

**neur/o**-gli-osis, abnormal condition of multiple neurogliomas

**neur/o**-hist/o-logy, the study of nervous tissue

**neur/o**-hypophysis, the hypophysis (pituitary gland) connected to nerves,

it refers to the posterior lobe of the pituitary gland

**neur/o**-lept-ic, a chemical agent used as an antipsychotic

**neur/o**-log-ic, 1. pertaining to the study of nerves 2. pertaining to neurology

**neur/o**-log-ical, 1. pertaining to the study of nerves 2. pertaining to neurology

**neur/o**-log-ist, a medical specialist who studies neurology

**neur/o**-logy, the study of nerves or the nervous system (anatomy, diseases and treatment of)

**neur/o**-lysis, 1. breakdown or disintegration of nervous tissue 2. separation or stretching of a nerve sheath by surgery to prevent perineural adhesions

**neur**-oma, a tumour of nerve cells and nerve fibres

**neur/o**-malac-ia, condition of softening of nerves

**neur/o**-muscul-ar, pertaining to muscles and nerves

**neur/o**-myel-itis, inflammation of the spinal cord with inflammation of nerves

**neur/o**-my/o-path-ic, pertaining to disease of muscle and nerves

**neur/o**-neuron-itis, inflammation of neurons and nerves, it refers to the cells and roots of spinal nerves Syn. neuronitis

**neur/o**-ophthalm/o-logy, the study of the eye and neurological aspects relating to the eye

**neur/o**-papill-itis, inflammation of the optic disc and (optic) nerve Syn. optic neuritis

**neur/o**-paralysis, paralysis caused by disease of a nerve

**neur/o**-path/o-genic-ity, the ability to produce disease in nervous tissue

**neur/o**-path/o-logy, the study of diseases of the nervous system

**neur/o**-pathy, disease of nerves or the nervous system, also refers to noninflammatory lesions

**neur/o**-pharmac/o-logy, the study of effect of drugs on nerves or the nervous system

**neur/o**-phthisis, wasting or decay of nerves

**neur/o**-physi/o-logy, the study of the physiology (functioning) of the nervous system

**neur/o**-plastic-ity, state or condition of regeneration of nerves

**neur/o**-plasty, surgical repair or reconstruction of a nerve or nerves

**neur/o**-psych-iatr-ic, pertaining to psychiatry and neurology

**neur/o**-radi/o-logy, the study of radiology in relation to the nervous system, it refers to using X-rays and other forms of radiation to diagnose and treat disease of the nervous system

**neur/o**-retin-itis, inflammation of the retina and optic nerve

**neur/o**-retin/o-pathy, disease of the retina and optic nerve

**neur/o**-rrhaphy, stitching or suturing of a nerve (joining two ends of a cut nerve with a suture)

**neur/o**-sarc-oma, a sarcoma (a malignant tumour) containing nerve cells

**neur/o**-scler-osis, abnormal condition of hardening of nerves

**neur**-osis, abnormal condition of nerves (an illness of personality with functional derangement of mind or body giving rise to anxiety, obsessions or phobias, a complex meaning in psychiatry)

**neur/o**-spasm, sudden contraction (twitching) of a muscle caused by a nervous disorder

**neur/o**-splanchn-ic, pertaining to the sympathetic nervous system and cerebrospinal nervous system

**neur/o**-suture, stitching or suturing of a nerve (joining two ends of a cut nerve with a suture) Syn. neurorrhaphy

**neur/o**-syphilis, involvement of the central nervous system with syphilis

**neur/o**-tic, 1. pertaining to nerves 2. pertaining to affected by a neurosis 3. one suffering from a neurosis

**neur/o**-tome, a needle-like instrument for cutting nerves (micro dissection of)

**neur/o**-tom/o-graphy, technique of making a recording or X-ray picture of a slice or section of the nervous system

**neur/o**-tomy, incision into or cutting of a nerve

**neur/o**-tox-ic, pertaining to poisonous to nerves or nervous tissue

**neur/o**-toxic-ity, quality of being poisonous to nerves or nervous tissue

**neur/o**-tox-in, an agent poisonous to nerves or nervous tissue

**neur/o**-trauma, injury to nerves

**neur/o**-tripsy, crushing of a nerve (by surgery)

**neur/o**-troph-ic, pertaining to nourishing the nervous system

**neur/o**-trop-ic, pertaining to affinity for or stimulating nerves or the nervous system

**neur/o**-trop-ism, process of having an affinity for or stimulating nerves or the nervous system

**neur/o**-vascul-ar, 1. pertaining to (blood) vessels and nerves 2. pertaining to nerves that control (blood) vessels

**neur/o**-viscer-al, 1. pertaining to the viscera and nerves 2. pertaining to the sympathetic nervous system and cerebrospinal nervous system

**pan**-**neur**-osis, abnormal condition of all nerves (an illness of personality with functional derangement of mind or body giving rise to anxiety, obsessions, phobias and other symptoms at the same time)

**peri**-**neur**-al, 1. pertaining to around nerves 2. pertaining to the perineurium

**peri**-**neuri**-um, the structure around a nerve, it refers to the connective tissue around a bundle of nerve fibres

**poly**-**neur**-itis, inflammation of many nerves

**sub**-**neur**-al, pertaining to under or below a nerve

---

**Neuron-**, neuron

From a Greek word **neuron**, meaning nerve. Here neuron- means a neuron, a specialized cell that forms the basic structural and functional unit of the nervous system. Each neuron consists

139

of a cell 'body' plus long extensions known as dendrons or dendrites and axons that conduct nerve impulses. There are three basic types grouped according to their function: motor neurons, inter neurons and sensory neurons.

**neuron**-al, pertaining to neurons Syn. neuronic

**neuron**-a-trophy, without nourishment of neurons (degeneration of neurons)

**neuron**-ic, pertaining to neurons Syn. neuronal

**neuron**-itis, inflammation of neurons (cells and roots of spinal nerves) Syn. neuroneuronitis

---

**Parasympath/o**, parasympathetic nerves, parasympathetic nervous system

From the Greek words **sympathein** meaning to feel with and **para-** meaning beside. Here, parasympathetic/o means the parasympathetic nervous system or parasympathetic nerves. The parasympathetic nervous system is a branch of the autonomic nervous system that controls the functions of the body carried out automatically. Parasympathetic activity tends to slow down body processes except digestion and absorption of food and the functions of the genito-urinary system. Normally the parasympathetic and sympathetic systems work in an opposing manner to maintain a regular heartbeat, body temperature and constant internal environment.

**parasympath**-et-ic, pertaining to the parasympathetic nervous system

**parasympath/o**-lyt-ic, 1. an agent that breaks down or opposes parasympathetic activity 2. pertaining to the break down of parasympathetic nerve fibres

**parasympath/o**-mimet-ic, 1. an agent that produces effects that mimic or resemble those of the parasympathetic nervous system 2. pertaining to producing effects that mimic those

of stimulation of parasympathetic nerves

---

**Phob-**, aversion, irrational fear

From a Greek word **phobos**, meaning fear. Here, phob- means a condition of irrational fear or an aversion to something.

acro-**phob**-ia, condition of irrational fear of heights

agora-**phob**-ia, condition of irrational fear of open spaces

aqua-**phob**-ia, condition of irrational fear of water

arachn/o-**phob**-ia, condition of irrational fear of spiders

cancer/o-**phob**-ia, condition of irrational fear of cancer (developing a cancer)

claustr/o-**phob**-ia, condition of irrational fear of confined spaces

copr/o-**phob**-ia, condition of aversion to faeces or defaecation

necro-**phob**-ia, condition of irrational fear of dying or dead bodies

nyct/o-**phob**-ia, condition of irrational fear of being in the dark

pan-**phob**-ia, 1. condition of morbid apprehension of all things 2. irrational fear of an unknown harmful thing

**phob**-ia, condition of irrational fear or aversion to something

**phob**-ic, pertaining to having an irrational fear or aversion to something

photo-**phob**-ia, condition of irrational fear or intolerance of light

photo-**phob**-ic, 1. pertaining to having photophobia 2. pertaining to an irrational fear or intolerance of light

---

**phren/o**, mind

From a Greek word **phren** meaning mind. Here phren/o means mind.

Note: These terms have complex meanings in psychiatry.

**phren**-etic, 1. maniacal 2. a maniac

**phren/o**-trop-ic, pertaining to affecting the mind

schiz/o-**phren**-ia, condition of a split mind, the psychiatric meaning of this word is different and more complex, it refers to a group of severe psychotic disorders in which the personality is fragmented with loss of emotional stability, judgment and reality and is accompanied by disturbances of thought, hallucinations and delusions

schiz/o-**phren**-ic, 1. pertaining to schizophrenia 2. a person suffering from schizophrenia

schiz/o-**phren**/o-gen-ic, pertaining to forming schizophrenia

---

-**pleg**-ic, paralysis, stroke

From a Greek word **plege**, meaning a blow. Here, pleg- means a paralysis. Strokes or cerebrovascular accidents are often the cause of a paralysis; these occur when a blockage or haemorrhage in the brain leads to destruction of cells that control motor activities.

di-**pleg**-ia, condition of paralysis of similar parts on either side of the body

di-**pleg**-ic, pertaining to paralysis of similar parts on either side of the body

hemi-**pleg**-ia, condition of half paralysis (on one side of the body)

hemi-**pleg**-ic, pertaining to having half paralysis (on one side of the body)

mono-**pleg**-ia, condition of paralysis of one part

para-**pleg**-ia, condition of paralysis of lower limbs and trunk

para-**pleg**-ic, pertaining to having paralysis of lower limbs and trunk

poly-**pleg**-ia, condition of paralysis of many (muscles)

pre-hemi-**pleg**-ic, pertaining to before hemiplegia

pseudo-para-**pleg**-ia, condition of false paraplegia, a hysterical feigned paraplegia

pseudo-**pleg**-ia, condition of false paralysis, a hysterical feigned paralysis

quadri-**pleg**-ia, condition of paralysis of all four limbs Syn. tetraplegia

quadri-**pleg**-ic, pertaining to having paralysis of all four limbs Syn. tetraplegic

tetra-**pleg**-ia, condition of paralysis of all four limbs Syn. quadriplegia

tetra-**pleg**-ic, pertaining to having paralysis of all four limbs Syn. quadriplegic

tri-**pleg**-ia, condition of paralysis of three limbs

---

**Plex/i/o**, nerve plexus

From a Latin word **plexus**, meaning plaited. Here plex/o means a nerve plexus, a network of nerves.

**plex**-al, pertaining to a plexus or nerve plexus

**plex**-ectomy, removal of a nerve plexus

**plex**/i-form, having the form of a plexus

**plex**-itis, inflammation of a nerve plexus

**plex**/o-gen-ic, 1. pertaining to forming a nerve plexus 2. pertaining to originating in a nerve plexus

**plex**/o-pathy, disease of a nerve plexus

---

**Polio-**, grey matter, poliomyelitis

From a Greek word **polios** meaning grey. Here, polio- means the grey matter of the spinal cord or polio. Polio is a common name for poliomyelitis, a viral infection of the grey matter of the spinal cord and brain stem. Poliomyelitis may or may not lead to a paralysis of the lower motor neuron type with loss of muscular power and flaccidity.

**polio**-clast-ic, pertaining to the breakdown of grey matter of the nervous system (due to viral infection)

**polio**-dys-trophy, condition of poor nourishment or growth of the grey matter (of the cerebrum)

**polio**-encephal-itis, inflammation of the grey matter of the brain

**polio**-encephal/o-mening/o-myel-itis, inflammation of the meninges, and grey matter of the spinal cord and brain

**polio**-encephal/o-myel-itis, inflammation of the grey matter of the spinal cord and brain

**polio**-encephal/o-pathy, disease of the grey matter of the brain

**polio**-encephal/o-trop-ic, pertaining to having an affinity for the grey matter of the brain

**polio**-myel-itis, inflammation of the grey matter of the spinal cord and brain stem caused by infection with poliovirus

**polio**-myel/o-encephal-itis, inflammation of the grey matter of the brain and spinal cord

**polio**-myel/o-pathy, disease of the grey matter of the spinal cord

**polio**-virus, an infectious enterovirus that causes poliomyelitis, an inflammation of the grey matter of the spinal cord and brain stem

---

**Pont/o**, pons

From a Latin word **pons** meaning bridge. Here pont/o means the pons, part of the brain stem joining the midbrain and medulla. It contains fibres that form a bridge between the cerebellar hemispheres and of fibres passing between the higher levels of the brain and the spinal cord. There are groups of cells within the pons that act as relay stations and some of these are associated with cranial nerves. The pons is situated in front of the cerebellum, below the midbrain and above the medulla oblongata.

**pont**-ic, pertaining to the pons

**pont**-ine, pertaining to the pons

**pont/o**-bulb-ar, pertaining to the medulla oblongata and pons

**pont/o**-cerebell-ar, pertaining to the cerebellum and pons

**pont/o**-mes-encephal-ic, pertaining to the middle brain (mesencephalon) and pons

---

**Psych/o**, mind

From a Greek word **psyche**, meaning soul or mind. Here psych/o means the mind.

Note: Many psychiatric terms such as psychopathy have a simple literal meaning but have very complex medical meanings. Readers wanting details of these conditions should consult psychiatric textbooks.

anti-**psych/o**-tic, 1. pertaining to having an effect on a psychosis 2. an agent that acts against a psychosis (reduces the symptoms of)

ger/o-**psych**-iatry, speciality of medicine dealing with the mind (the study and treatment of mental illness) in the elderly

intra-**psych**-ic, pertaining to inside the mind

**psych**-alg-ia, condition of pain of the mind, it refers to pain of mental or hysterical origin

**psych**-alg-ic, pertaining to pain of the mind, it refers to pain of mental or hysterical origin

**psych**-a-tax-ia, condition of without ordered movement caused by the mind, a disordered mental state

**psych**-iatr-ic, pertaining to psychiatry

**psych**-iatr-ist, doctor who specializes in the study of the mind (the study and treatment of mental illness)

**psych**-iatry, speciality of medicine dealing with the mind (the study and treatment of mental illness)

**psych**-ic, pertaining to the mind

**psych/o**-act-ive, 1. an agent drug that affects the mind 2. affecting the mind

**psych/o**-analysis, procedure to diagnose and treat mental disorders by analysing a patient's emotional history (after Sigmund Freud)

**psych/o**-analytic-al, pertaining to diagnosing and treating mental disorders by analysing a patient's emotional history (after Sigmund Freud)

**psych/o**-bio-logy, the study of biology and the mind, it refers to the interactions of the body and mind in forming the personality

**psych/o**-chem/o-therapy, treatment of the mind using drugs

**psych**-drama, form of psychotherapy whereby patients act out their personal problems

**psych/o**-dynam-ic, pertaining to the power of the mind (mental powers, processes, behaviour and motivation)

**psych/o**-dynam-ics, the science of studying the power of the mind (mental powers, processes, behaviour and motivation)

**psych/o**-genesis, 1. forming the mind (mental development) 2. formation in the mind of a symptom or illness

**psych/o**-gen-ic, pertaining to originating in the mind

**psych/o**-ger-iatr-ics, the science of studying the mind (psychology) of the elderly (an old term)

**psych/o**-graph, a recording (chart) of the mind (personality traits and mental functions)

**psych/o**-lepsy, a sudden mild seizure (characterized by sudden mood change)

**psych/o**-log-ical, pertaining to the study of the mind, especially behaviour and mental processes

**psych/o**-log-ist, person who specializes in the study of the mind, especially behaviour and mental processes

**psych/o**-logy, pertaining to the study of the mind, especially behaviour and mental processes

**psych/o**-metr-ic, pertaining to the measurement of the mind (mental ability and intelligence)

**psych/o**-metr-ics, the science dealing with the measurement of the mind (mental ability and intelligence)

**psych/o**-metry, technique of measuring the mind (mental ability and intelligence)

**psych/o**-motor, pertaining to the motor effects of the mind (motor meaning muscular movements or response caused by the mind)

**psych/o**-neur-al, pertaining to the nervous system and mind

**psych/o**-neur/o-immun/o-logy, the study of the immune response in relation to the state of the nervous system and the mind

**psych/o**-neur-osis, abnormal condition of the nerves and mind, it refers to a neurosis characterized by a faulty emotional response to the stresses of life

**psych/o**-neur/o-tic, pertaining to having a psychoneurosis

**psych/o**-path, one with a diseased mind, it refers to a person who lacks empathy and may be aggressive and socially irresponsible. This term has a complex meaning in psychiatry

**psych/o**-path-ic, 1. pertaining to behaving like a psychopath 2.pertaining to psychopathy

**psych/o**-path/o-logy, the study of diseases of the mind (abnormal mental processes)

**psych/o**-pathy, disease of the mind (insanity)

**psych/o**-physic-al, 1. pertaining to the relationship between the body and mind 2. pertaining to physical conditions in the body in relation to the mind

**psych/o**-phys-ics, the science of studying physical stimuli and the mental responses induced by them

**psych/o**-physi/o-logy, the study of physiology in relation to the mind (interactions)

**psych/o**-pleg-ic, 1. pertaining to paralysis of the mind, it refers to a sudden unexpected attack of mental illness 2. an agent paralysing the mind (diminishing mental activity)

**psych/o**-prophylat-ic, pertaining to preventing emotional maladjustment of the mind

**psych/o**-sens-ory, pertaining to sensation in the mind (perception of sensory stimuli)

**psych/o**-sexu-al, pertaining to sex and the mind (the mental aspects of sex)

**psych**-osis, abnormal condition of the mind (due to organic disease of mind or brain) Psychoses are serious mental disorders commonly associated with madness

**psych/o**-soci-al, pertaining to social behaviour and the mind

**psych/o**-somat-ic, pertaining to the body and mind relationship

**psych/os/o**-mimet-ic, pertaining to mimicking a psychosis (producing similar symptoms to)

**psych/o**-stimul-ant, drug that stimulates the mind (increases psychomotor activity)

**psych/o**-surgery, surgery of the mind (treatment of disorders of the mind with brain surgery)

**psych/o**-therapy, treatment of the mind (using psychological methods rather than physical intervention)

**psychot**-ic, 1. pertaining to a psychosis 2. one who suffers from a psychosis

**psychot**/o-gen-ic, pertaining to forming a psychosis

**psychot**/o-mimet-ic, pertaining to mimicking a psychosis (producing similar symptoms to)

**psych/o**-trop-ic, pertaining to stimulating or affecting the mind

---

**Rachi/o**, spine

From a Greek word **rhachis**, meaning spine. Here rachi/o means the spine, the popular term for the bony vertebral column or spinal column.

hemi-**rachi**-schisis, cleaving of the half of the spine, it refers to rachischisis without prolapse of the spinal cord

**rachi**-alg-ia, condition of pain of the spine

**rachi**-an-aesthes-ia, 1. condition of without sensation in the spine 2. anaesthesia of the spine

**rachi**-cele, a protrusion or hernia of the spine (as in spina bifida)

**rachi**-centesis, puncture of the spine to remove fluid Syn. lumbar puncture

**rachi**-graph, an instrument that records the spine (outline)

**rachi**-lysis, loosening or breakdown of the spine (by medical intervention to correct curvatures by pressure and traction)

**rachi/o**-centesis, puncture of the spine to remove fluid Syn. lumbar puncture

**rachi/o**-dyn-ia, condition of pain of the spine

**rachi/o**-kyph-osis, abnormal condition of forward curvature of the spine (hump back)

**rachi/o**-meter, an instrument to measure the spine (degree of curvature)

**rachi/o**-paralysis, paralysis affecting the spine (muscles of)

**rachi/o**-phyma, a tumour of the spine

**rachi/o**-pleg-ia, condition of paralysis of the spine (muscles of)

**rachi/o**-scoli-osis, abnormal condition of lateral curvature of the spine

**rachi/o**-tome, an instrument for cutting the spine (dividing vertebral laminae)

**rachi/o**-tomy, incision into the spine (to divide vertebral laminae)

**rachi**-schisis, cleaving of the spine, it refers to a fissure of the vertebral column (spina bifida)

---

**Radic/ul/o**, spinal nerve root

From a Latin word **radicula**, meaning root. Here, radicul/o means the anterior and/or posterior root of a spinal nerve that emerges from the spinal cord. The anterior nerve root consists of motor fibres transmitting impulses away from the CNS; the posterior nerve root sensory nerve fibres transmitting impulses towards the CNS. Two roots join to form each spinal nerve.

poly-**radicul**-itis, inflammation of many spinal nerve roots

poly-**radicul/o**-neur-itis, inflammation of many nerves and spinal nerve roots

poly-**radicul/o**-neur/o-pathy, disease of many nerves and spinal nerve roots

**radic/o**-tomy, incision into a spinal nerve root

**radicul**-alg-ia, condition of pain in a spinal nerve root

**radicul**-ar, pertaining to or having characteristics of a spinal nerve root

**radicul**-ectomy, removal of a spinal nerve root

**radicul**-itis, inflammation of a spinal nerve root

**radicul/o**-ganglion-itis, inflammation of ganglia spinal and their nerve roots

**radicul/o**-gram, a recording or X-ray picture of spinal nerve roots

**radicul/o**-graphy, technique of making a recording or X-ray picture of spinal nerve roots

**radicul/o**-medull-ary, pertaining to the spinal cord and spinal nerve roots

**radicul/o**-mening/o-myel-itis, inflammation of the spinal cord, meninges and spinal nerve roots

**radicul/o**-myel/o-pathy, disease of the spinal cord and spinal nerve roots

**radicul/o**-neur-itis, inflammation of nerves and nerve roots Syn. polyneuritis

**radicul/o**-neur/o-pathy, disease of (spinal) nerves and spinal nerve roots

**radicul/o**-pathy, disease of spinal nerve roots

---

**Rhiz/o**, spinal nerve root

From a Greek word **rhiza** meaning root. Here, rhiz/o means the anterior and/or posterior root of a spinal nerve that emerges from the spinal cord. The anterior nerve root consists of motor fibres transmitting impulses away from the CNS; the posterior nerve root sensory nerve fibres transmitting impulses towards the CNS. Two roots join to form each spinal nerve.

**rhiz**-oid, resembling a root

**rhiz/o**-lysis, breakdown of a spinal nerve root (by medical intervention)

**rhiz/o**-mening/o-myel-itis, inflammation of the spinal cord, meninges and spinal nerve roots

**rhiz/o**-tomy, incision into a spinal nerve root

---

**Sympath/ic/o**, sympathetic nerves, sympathetic nervous system

From a Greek word **sympathein** meaning to feel with. Here, sympath/o means the sympathetic nervous system or sympathetic nerves. The sympathetic nervous system is a branch of the autonomic nervous system that controls the functions of the body carried out automatically. Sympathetic activity prepares the body to deal with stressful

situations. The adrenal glands are stimulated to release adrenaline and noradrenaline that prepares the body to fight. Normally the sympathetic and parasympathetic systems work in an opposing manner to maintain a regular heartbeat, body temperature and constant internal environment.

**sympath**-ectomy, removal of a section of a sympathetic nerve

**sympath**-etic, pertaining to the sympathetic nervous system

**sympathic/o**-blast, an immature cell or embryonic cell that develops into a sympathetic nerve cell

**sympathic/o**-blast-oma, a tumour containing sympatheticoblasts

**sympathic/o**-neur-itis, inflammation of the nerves of the sympathetic nervous system

**sympathic/o**-pathy, disease resulting from disturbance of the sympathetic nervous system

**sympathic/o**-ton-ia, condition of tone of the sympathetic nervous system, it refers to a state produced by stimulation of the sympathetic nervous system (high BP, vascular spasm, erection of hairs etc.)

**sympathic/o**-tripsy, surgical crushing of a sympathetic nerve or other part of the sympathetic nervous system

**sympathic/o**-trop-ic, 1. pertaining to having an affinity for the sympathetic nervous system 2. an agent that has an affinity for the sympathetic nervous system

**sympath/o**-adren-al, pertaining to the adrenal (medulla) and sympathetic nervous system (especially increased sympathetic activity)

**sympath/o**-lyt-ic, 1. an agent that breaks down or opposes sympathetic activity 2. pertaining to blocking transmission of nerve impulses from postganglionic fibres to effector organs

**sympath/o**-mimet-ic, 1. an agent that produces effects similar to those of stimulation of sympathetic nerves 2. pertaining to producing an effect that mimics the stimulation of organs and structures by the sympathetic nervous system *e.g.* by increasing the release of noradrenaline at post-ganglionic nerve endings

## Synapt-, synapse

From a Greek word **synaptein** meaning to join. Here synapt- means a synapse, a microscopic junction between two neurons. A nerve impulse passes from one neuron to another at this point when a neurotransmitter is released into the synaptic gap between the two cells.

mono-**synapt**-ic, pertaining to one synapse

oligo-**synapt**-ic, pertaining to few synapses (in a series)

pauci-**synapt**-ic, pertaining to few synapses (in a series)

poly-**synapt**-ic, pertaining to many synapses (more than two in a series)

post-**synapt**-ic, pertaining to after or distal to a synapse

pre-**synapt**-ic, pertaining to before or proximal to a synapse

**synapt**-ic, pertaining to a synapse

## Syring/o, fistula, pipe-like cavity

From a Greek word **syrigx** meaning pipe. Here syring/o means a cavity or fistula and refers to long pipe-like cavities that form in the spinal cord and brain stem.

**syring/o**-bulb-ia, condition of cavities in the bulb (medulla oblongata in the brain)

**syring/o**-cele, a protrusion or hernia (of the spinal cord) containing a cavity, it protrudes through the spine as in spina bifida

**syring/o**-coele, the cavity (central canal) of the spinal cord

**syring/o**-meningi/o-cele, a protrusion or hernia of the meninges with a cavity (it connects to the central canal of the spinal cord)

**syring/o**-myel-ia, condition of formation of cavities in the spinal cord (a pro-

gressive disease with neurological deficits)

**syring/o**-myel-itis, inflammation of the spinal cord marked by formation of cavities

**syring/o**-myel/o-cele, a protrusion or hernia of the spinal cord containing a cavity, it protrudes through the spine as in spina bifida

## Thalam/o, thalamus

From a Greek word **thalamos** meaning chamber. Here thalam/o means the thalamus, a collection of grey matter at the base of the cerebrum in the lateral wall of the 3rd ventricle of the brain. Sensory impulses pass through the thalamus on their way from the body to the cerebral cortex.

hypo-**thalam**-us, the structure below the thalamus, it refers to the highest centre of the autonomic nervous system that controls many physiological functions such as emotion, hunger, thirst and circadian rhythms

**thalam**-ic, pertaining to the thalamus

**thalam/o**-cortic-al, pertaining to the cerebral cortex and thalamus

**thalam/o**-lenticul-ar, pertaining to the lenticular nucleus and thalamus

**thalam/o**-tomy, incision into the thalamus, it refers to a stereotaxic operation to destroy groups of cells within the thalamus for relief of pain, tremor or rigidity

## Ventricul/o, ventricle

From a Latin word **ventriculum**, meaning ventricle or chamber. Here ventricul/o means a ventricle, a cavity in the brain filled with cerebrospinal fluid, a cerebral ventricle.

Note: Ventricul/o is also used to refer to one of the lower chambers of the heart, a heart ventricle.

**ventricul**-ar, pertaining to a ventricle

**ventricul**-itis, inflammation of the cerebral ventricles

**ventricul/o**-cistern/o-stomy, formation of an opening between (3rd) cerebral ventricle and the cisterna magna (cisterna meaning a closed space, here it refers to the sub-arachnoid space for drainage of CSF in hydrocephalus) or the name of the opening so created

**ventricul/o**-gram, a recording or X-ray picture of a cerebral ventricle

**ventricul/o**-graphy, technique of making a recording or X-ray picture of the cerebral ventricles (now rarely performed)

**ventricul/o**-metry, technique of measuring the cerebral ventricles (intracranial pressure)

**ventricul/o**-peritone-al, pertaining to the peritoneum (peritoneal cavity) and cerebral ventricles (as in a ventriculo-

peritoneal shunt used to treat hydrocephalus)

**ventricul/o**-puncture, surgical puncture of a cerebral ventricle

**ventricul/o**-scope, an instrument to view or examine the cerebral ventricles (with an endoscope)

**ventricul/o**-scopy, technique of viewing or examining cerebral ventricles

**ventricul/o**-stomy, formation of an opening into a cerebral ventricle or the name of the opening so created

**ventricul/o**-sub-arachnoid, pertaining to the subarachnoid space and cerebral ventricles

**ventricul/o**-tomy, incision into cerebral ventricles

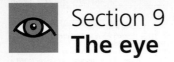

# Section 9
# The eye

The eye is the organ for the sense of sight and is positioned by extraocular muscles in the orbital cavity. It is almost spherical in shape and approximately 2.5 cm in diameter. Light enters the eye through the pupil and transparent cornea, it passes through the lens and is focused onto the light-sensitive retina. In the retina light stimulates receptors (rods and cones) to generate nerve impulses in sensory neurons; these impulses travel via neurons in the optic nerve (cranial nerve II) to areas of the brain concerned with vision. In the visual cortex of the brain the impulses are interpreted as an image.

Structurally the two eyes are separate, but their activities are coordinated so that they function as a pair. Using two eyes enables us to see a three dimensional image and judge distances.

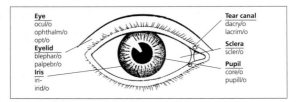

Figure 13  Anterior view of the eye

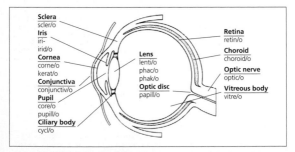

Figure 14  Sagittal section through the eye

The eye consists of:

- an outer fibrous layer – sclera and cornea
- a middle layer or uveal tract – choroid, ciliary body and iris
- an inner nervous tissue layer – retina
- structures within the eyeball – lens, aqueous humour and the vitreous body (vitreous humour)

Figures 13 and 14 show the anatomy of the eye and combining forms of roots associated with its components.

## Roots and combining forms, meanings

### Blephar/o, eyelid

From a Greek word **blepharon**, meaning eyelid. Here blephar/o means the eyelids, the moveable folds in front of the eyeball closing during sleep or to protect from injury. The upper fold is called the palpebra superior and the lower palpebra inferior. The palpebral fissure forms the longitudinal opening between the eyelids.,

See the combining form palpebr/o also meaning eyelid.

**blephar**-aden-itis, inflammation of the eyelid glands, the meibomian glands

**blephar**-al, pertaining to the eyelids

**blephar**-ectomy, surgical removal of part of an eyelid

**blephar**-ism, process of having a spasm of the eyelids

**blephar**-itis, inflammation of the eyelids

**blephar/o**-aden-oma, a tumour (adenoma) of the glandular epithelium of the eyelid

**blephar/o**-ather-oma, porridge-like tumour of the eye-lid, a sebaceous cyst

**blephar/o**-blenn/o-rrhoea, excessive flow or discharge of mucus from the eye-lid

**blephar/o**-chalasis, slack or loose eyelids, it refers to drooping of the eyelids

**blephar/o**-cleisis, abnormal closure of the eyelids. From a Greek word *kleiein* meaning to shut up

**blephar/o**-conjuctiv-itis, inflammation of the conjunctiva and eyelid

**blephar/o**-oedema, swelling of fluid in the eyelid

**blephar**on, the eyelid

**blephar**-onc-us, a tumour (neoplasm) on the eyelid

**blephar**-ophthalm-ia, condition of the eye and eyelid, it refers to inflammation

**blephar/o**-phim-osis, abnormal condition of closure or narrowing of the eyelids, it refers to narrowing of the palpebral fissure Syn. blepharo-stenosis

**blephar/o**-plasty, surgical repair or reconstruction of the eyelid

**blephar/o**-pleg-ia, condition of paralysis of the eyelid

**blephar/o**-ptosis, falling or drooping of the eyelid

**blephar/o**-py/o-rrhoea, flow or discharge of pus from the eyelid

**blephar/o**-rrhaphy, stitching or suturing of the eyelid

**blephar/o**-rrhoea, excessive flow or discharge from the eyelid

**blephar/o**-spasm, involuntary contraction of the eyelid

**blephar/o**-sten-osis, abnormal condition of narrowing of the eyelids, it refers to narrowing of the palpebral fissure Syn. blepharophimosis

**blephar/o**-synech-ia, condition of sticking together of eyelids

**blephar/o**-tomy, incision into an eyelid

macro-**blephar**-ia, condition of an abnormally large eyelid

micro-**blephar**-ia, condition of an abnormally small eyelid

pachy-**blephar**on, thickening of an eyelid

sym-**blephar**on, adhesion of an eyelid to the eyeball

### Chori/o, choroid/e/o, choroid

From a Greek word **choroeides**, meaning like a skin. Here choroid/o means the choroid, the middle, pigmented vascular coat of the posterior five-sixths of the eyeball. The choroid absorbs light and stops reflections within the eye.

**chori/o**-retin-al, pertaining to the retina and choroid Syn. choroidoretinal

**chori/o**-retin-itis, inflammation of the retina and choroid Syn. choroido-retinitis

**chori/o**-retin/o-pathy, disease of the retina and choroid (non-inflammatory)

**choroid**-al, pertaining to the choroid

**choroid**-itis, inflammation of the choroid

**choroid/o**-cycl-itis, inflammation of the ciliary body and choroid

**choroid/o**-ir-itis, inflammation of the iris and choroid

**choroid/o**-retin-al, pertaining to the retina and choroid Syn. chorioretinal

**choroid/o**-retin-itis, inflammation of the retina and choroid Syn. chorio-retinitis

ento-**choroide**-a, the inside layer of the choroid

peri-**choroid**-al, pertaining to around the choroid

supra-**choroid**, above the choroid

---

## Conjunctiv/o, conjunctiva

From a Latin word **conjunctivus** meaning connecting. Here conjunctiv/o means the conjunctiva, the delicate, transparent membrane that lines the inner surface of the eyelids (palpebral conjunctiva) and reflects over the front of the eyeball (ocular conjunctiva).

**conjunctiv**-al, pertaining to or belonging to the conjunctiva

**conjunctiv**-itis, inflammation of the conjunctiva

**conjunctiv/o**-dacryocyst/o-stomy, formation of an opening between the lacrimal sac and conjunctiva or the name of the opening so created

**conjunctiv**-oma, a tumour (on the eyelid) derived from the conjunctiva

**conjunctiv/o**-plasty, surgical repair or reconstruction of the conjunctiva

sub-**conjunctiv**-al, pertaining to beneath the conjunctiva

---

## Cor/e/o, pupil

From a Greek word **kore**, meaning pupil of eye. Here core/o means the pupil, the opening in the centre of the iris that allows the passage of light into the eye.

an-iso-**cor**-ia, condition of unequal pupils

**cor**-ectasis, dilation of a pupil

**cor**-ectop-ia, condition of displacement of the pupil from its normal position

**core**-dialysis, separation of the pupil (actually the separation of the iris from the ciliary body)

**core**-lysis, surgical destruction of the pupil, it refers to the cutting of adhesions between the lens and iris

**core**-morph-osis, condition of forming or shaping a pupil, it refers to forming an artificial pupil

**core/o**-pexy, surgical fixation of pupils into a new position

**core/o**-plasty, surgical repair or reconstruction of a pupil

**cor/o**-tomy, incision into the pupil, actually into the iris Syn. iridotomy

dys-**cor**-ia, condition of poor pupil, it refers to abnormality of shape or reaction of a pupil

iso-**cor**-ia, condition of equal pupils

---

## Corne/o, cornea

From a Latin word **corneus** meaning horny. Here, corne/o means the cornea, the transparent, avascular membrane covering the anterior outer coat of the eyeball. The cornea is situated in front of the iris and pupil and merges backwards into the sclera. The cornea provides strength and refractive power as well as transmitting light into the eye.

**corne**-al, pertaining to or belonging to the cornea

**corne**-itis, inflammation of the cornea

**corne/o**-blepharon, (adhesion between) the eyelid and cornea

**corne/o**-ir-itis, inflammation of the iris and cornea

**corne/o**-sclera, the sclera and cornea considered together

**corne/o**-scler-al, pertaining to or belonging to the sclera and cornea

**corne/o**-scler-ectomy, removal of the sclera and cornea

**corne/o**-plasty, surgical repair or reconstruction of the cornea (a corneal graft)

ento-**corne**-a, within or inside the cornea, it refers to Descemet's membrane, the inner posterior membrane of the cornea

---

## Cycl/o, ciliary body

From a Greek word **kyklos** meaning circle. Here, cycl/o means the circular ciliary body of the eye and or the ciliary muscle. The ciliary body connects the anterior part of the choroid to the circumference of the iris; it is composed of ciliary muscles and processes. When the ciliary muscles contract and relax, the thickness of the lens changes, this action refracts light rays entering the eye and focuses them on the retina. The ability of the lens to change shape in this way is known as accommodation.

cycl-ectomy, removal of part of the ciliary body or ciliary muscle

cycl-itis, inflammation of the ciliary body

cycl/o-choroid-itis, inflammation of the choroid and ciliary body

cycl/o-cryo-therapy, treatment by freezing the ciliary body, a treatment for glaucoma

cycl/o-dialysis, separation of the ciliary body, it refers to the formation of a communication between the anterior chamber of the eye and the perichoroidal space to reduce tension in glaucoma

cycl/o-dia-thermy, heating through the ciliary body (to destroy tissue)

cycl/o-kerat-itis, inflammation of the cornea and ciliary body

cycl/o-paresis, slight weakness or paralysis of a ciliary muscle

cycl/o-pleg-ia, condition of paralysis of a ciliary body, it leads to loss of accommodation

cycl/o-pleg-ic, 1. pertaining to paralysis of a ciliary body 2. an agent that causes paralysis of a ciliary body

cycl/o-spasm, sudden contraction of a ciliary body, causing a change in accommodation

cycl/o-tome, an instrument used to cut a ciliary body or ciliary muscle

cycl/o-tomy, incision into the ciliary body or ciliary muscle

---

**Dacry/o**, lacrimal apparatus (duct, gland or sac), tear

From a Greek word **dakryon**, meaning tear. Here, dacry/o refers to parts of the lacrimal apparatus and/or tears. The eye is cleansed and lubricated by fluid from the lacrimal apparatus which

consists of a gland, sac and ducts. The gland produces lacrimal (tear) fluid that washes over the eyeball and drains into the lacrimal sac through the lacrimal duct. The lacrimal sac in turn drains the fluid into the nose via the nasolacrimal duct.

dacry-aden-itis, inflammation of a lacrimal gland

dacry-agog-ic, pertaining to the stimulating or inducing the flow of tears

dacry-agogue, an agent that induces the flow of tears

dacry/o-aden-alg-ia, condition of pain in a lacrimal gland

dacry/o-aden-ectomy, removal of a lacrimal gland

dacry/o-blenn/o-rrhoea, excessive discharge of mucus from the duct of the lacrimal gland

dacry/o-cyst, a tear bladder (lacrimal sac). See the next combining form dacryocyst/o

dacry/o-haem/o-rrhoea, excessive flow or discharge of tears containing blood

dacry-oid, resembling tears

dacry/o-lith, a tear stone or calculus

dacry/o-lith-iasis, condition or presence of stones or calculi in the lacrimal apparatus

dacry-oma, swelling (tear-filled cyst) caused by obstruction of a lacrimal duct

dacry-ops, 1. condition of the eye with tears, it refers to excess of tears in the eye 2. distension of a lacrimal duct with tear fluid

dacry/o-py/o-rrhoea, excessive flow or discharge of pus in tears

dacry/o-py-osis, condition of pus in the lacrimal apparatus

dacry/o-rrhoea, excessive flow or discharge of tears

dacry/o-scint/i-graphy, technique of making a scintigram or scintiscan (radioisotope scan) of the lacrimal ducts

dacry/o-sinus-itis, inflammation of the ethmoidal sinus and lacrimal ducts

dacry/o-sten-osis, abnormal condition of narrowing of the lacrimal duct

**dacry/o**-syrinx, 1. the lacrimal duct 2. a fistula or abnormal passage in the lacrimal apparatus 3. an instrument for syringing the lacrimal ducts

---

**Dacryocyst/o,** lacrimal sac

From the Greek words **dakryon** meaning tear and **kystis** meaning bladder. Here, dacryocyst/o means the lacrimal sac, a structure that collects lacrimal (tear) fluid drained from the surface of the eye and passes it into the naso-lacrimal duct.

**dacryocyst**-ectomy, removal of the lacrimal sac (the wall of)

**dacryocyst**-itis, inflammation of the lacrimal sac (the wall of)

**dacryocyst/o**-blenn/o-rrhoea, flow or discharge of mucus from the lacrimal sac (with inflammation)

**dacryocyst/o**-cele, a dilation or hernia of the lacrimal sac (filled with mucus)

**dacryocyst/o**-gram, a recording or X-ray picture of the lacrimal sac

**dacryocyst/o**-graphy, technique of making a recording or X-ray picture of the lacrimal sac

**dacryocyst/o**-py-osis, abnormal condition of pus in the lacrimal sac

**dacryocyst/o**-rhin/o-sten-osis, narrowing of the duct between the nasal cavity and the lacrimal sac

**dacryocyst/o**-rhin/o-stomy, formation of an opening between the nose and lacrimal sac or the name of the opening so created

**dacryocyst/o**-sten-osis, abnormal condition of narrowing of the lacrimal sac

**dacryocyst/o**-stomy, formation of an opening into the lacrimal sac or the name of the opening so created

---

**Goni/o,** angle of the anterior chamber

From a Greek word **gonia,** meaning angle. Here goni/o means the peripheral angle of the anterior chamber of the eye. This angle is observed when evaluating types of glaucoma.

**goni/o**-meter, an instrument to measure the peripheral angle of the anterior chamber

**goni/o**-scope, an instrument used to view or examine the peripheral angle of the anterior chamber

**goni/o**-scopy, technique of viewing or examining the peripheral angle of the anterior chamber

**goni/o**-tomy, incision into the peripheral angle of the anterior chamber

**goni**-puncture, technique of puncturing the cornea across the angle of the anterior chamber (a treatment for glaucoma)

---

**Iri-,** irid/o, iris

From a Greek word **iris,** meaning rainbow. Here, irid/o means the iris, the circular, coloured membrane surrounding the pupil of the eye. Contraction of its muscle fibres regulates the size of the aperture (pupil) within the iris, thereby regulating the light entering the eye.

**irid**-aem-ia, condition of blood in the iris (haemorrhage)

**irid**-al, pertaining or belonging to the iris

**irid**-aux-esis, abnormal condition of increase in the iris, it becomes thick and swollen

**irid**-avulsion, action of tearing away the iris. From a Latin word *avellere* meaning to tear away

**irid**-ectome, an instrument used to cut the iris

**irid**-ecto-meso-dialysis, 1. surgical separation and cutting out of the middle of the iris to make an artificial pupil 2. separation and cutting out of adhesions around the inner edge of the iris

**irid**-ectomy, removal of the iris

**irid**-ec-tropi-um, an iris that is turned outwards

**irid**-en-tropi-um, an iris that is turned inward

**irides,** plural of iris

**iri**-desis, surgical fixation of the iris, a method of making an artificial pupil

**irid**-ic, pertaining to belonging to the iris

**irid/o**-avulsion, action of tearing away the iris. From a Latin word *avellere* meaning to tear away

**irid/o**-capsul-itis, inflammation of the lens capsule and iris

**irid/o**-cele, a protrusion or hernia of the iris

**irid/o**-choroid-itis, inflammation of the choroid and iris

**irid/o**-coloboma, a congenital fissure in the iris. From a Greek word *koloboma* meaning a defect

**irid/o**-constrict-or, 1. a muscle that constricts (reduces the diameter) of the iris 2. an agent that constricts (reduces the diameter) of the iris

**irid/o**-corne/o-scler-ectomy, removal of (part of) the sclera, cornea and iris

**irid/o**-cycl-ectomy, removal of the ciliary body and iris

**irid/o**-cycl-itis, inflammation of the ciliary body and the iris

**irid/o**-cycl/o-choroid-itis, inflammation of the choroid, ciliary body and iris

**irid/o**-cyst-ectomy, removal of a cyst on the iris

**irid/o**-desis, surgical fixation of the iris, a method of making an artificial pupil

**irid/o**-dialysis, separation of the iris (from its ciliary attachment)

**irid/o**-dilat-or, 1. a muscle that dilates (increases the diameter) of the iris 2. an agent that dilates (increases the diameter) of the iris

**irid/o**-donesis, abnormal condition of tremor in the iris. From a Greek word *donesis* meaning a tremor

**irid/o**-kerat-itis, inflammation of the cornea and iris

**irid/o**-kines-ia, condition of movement of the iris, it refers to its expansion and contraction

**irid/o**-kinesis, motion or movement of the iris, it refers to its expansion and contraction

**irid/o**-kinet-ic, pertaining to movement of the iris, it refers to its expansion and contraction

**irid/o**-leptynis, thinning or wasting of the iris. From a Greek word *leptynein* meaning to thin

**irid/o**-logy, the study of the iris, a branch of ophthalmology that studies the anatomy, diseases and treatment of the iris

**irid/o**-malac-ia, condition of softening of the iris

**irid/o**-meso-dialysis, surgical separation of adhesions around the inner edge (pupillary border) of the iris

**irid/o**-motor, pertaining to the action or movement of the iris

**irid**-onc-osis, abnormal condition of a swelling or tumour of the iris (causing thickening of the iris)

**irid**-onc-us, a swelling or tumour of the iris (causing thickening of the iris)

**irid/o**-paralysis, paralysis of muscles that move the iris Syn. iridoplegia

**irid/o**-paresis, slight paralysis of muscles that move the iris

**irid/o**-pathy, disease of the iris

**irid/o**-peri-phac-itis, inflammation around the lens capsule (its anterior portion) and iris

**irid/o**-peri-phak-itis, inflammation around the lens capsule (its anterior portion) and iris

**irid/o**-ptosis, falling or displacement of the iris

**irid/o**-pupill-ary, pertaining to the pupil and iris

**irid/o**-rrhexis, rupture or tearing of the iris

**irid/o**-schisis, splitting of the iris, the iris stroma separates into two layers

**irid/o**-scler/o-tomy, incision into the sclera and iris (a treatment for glaucoma)

**irid/o**-scope, an instrument used to view the iris (a type of ophthalmoscope)

**irid/o**-ster-esis, removal of a portion or whole of the iris. From a Greek word *steresis* meaning being in want of

**irid/o**-tasis, surgical stretching of the iris. From a Greek word *tasis* meaning a stretching, a treatment for glaucoma

**irid/o**-tome, an instrument for cutting the iris

**irid/o**-tomy, incision into the iris

**ir**-itic, pertaining to having iritis

**ir**-itis, inflammation of the iris

## Kerat/o, cornea

From a Greek word **keras**, meaning horn. Here, kerat/o means the cornea, the transparent, avascular membrane covering the anterior outer coat of the eyeball. The cornea is situated in front of the iris and pupil and merges backwards into the sclera. The cornea provides strength and refractive power as well as transmitting light into the eye.

Note: kerat/o is also used to mean the epidermis, see Section 11 The skin.

auto-**kerat**/o-plasty, surgical repair or reconstruction of the cornea (a corneal graft) from oneself, from one eye to the other

**kerat**-ectas-ia, condition of dilation of the cornea, it refers to a protrusion of the cornea

**kerat**-ectomy, removal of the cornea

**kerat**-ic, pertaining to the cornea

**kerat**-itis, inflammation of the cornea

**kerat**/o-cele, a protrusion or hernia of the cornea (of Descemet's membrane)

**kerat**/o-centesis, puncture of the cornea

**kerat**/o-chromat-osis, abnormal condition of colour or pigment in the cornea

**kerat**/o-conjunctiv-itis, inflammation of the conjunctiva and cornea

**kerat**/o-con/o-meter, an instrument to measure the conicity of the cornea

**kerat**/o-con-us, a cone-like protrusion of the cornea

**kerat**/o-glob-us, a ball-like cornea (a globe-shaped protrusion)

**kerat**/o-haem-ia, condition of blood in the cornea

**kerat**/o-helc-osis, abnormal condition of ulceration of the cornea

**kerat**/o-irid/o-cycl-itis, inflammation of the ciliary body, iris and cornea

**kerat**/o-ir-itis, inflammation of the iris and cornea

**kerat**/o-leptynis, removal of the anterior part of the cornea and replacement with conjunctiva. From a Greek word *leptynein* meaning to thin

**kerat**/o-leuc-oma, a white tumour of the cornea, it refers to a white opacity

**kerat**/o-leuk-oma, a white tumour of the cornea, it refers to a white opacity

**kerat**/o-malac-ia, condition of softening of the cornea

**kera**-tome, an instrument used to cut the cornea

**kerat**/o-meter, an instrument used to measure the cornea, it measures the curvature of the cornea

**kerat**/o-metry, technique of measuring the cornea (the curvature of the cornea)

**kerat**/o-mileusis, carving of the cornea, a form of keratoplasty

**kerat**/o-myc-osis, abnormal condition of fungi in the cornea

**kerat**/o-nyxis, puncture or pricking of the cornea

**kerat**/o-pathy, disease of the cornea (non inflammatory)

**kerat**/o-phak-ia, condition of the lens and cornea, it refers to a type of corneal grafting between a donor and recipient to change the curvature of the cornea

**kerat**/o-plast-ic, pertaining to plastic surgery of the cornea

**kerat**/o-plasty, surgical repair or reconstruction of the cornea (a corneal graft)

**kerat**/o-rrhexis, rupture of the cornea

**kerat**/o-scler-itis, inflammation of the sclera and cornea

**kerat**/o-scope, an instrument used to view or examine the cornea

**kerat**/o-scopy, technique of viewing or examining the cornea

**kerat**/o-tome, an instrument used to cut the cornea

**kerat**/o-tomy, incision into the cornea

**kerat**/o-tor-us, a swollen cornea, it refers to an arched protrusion of the cornea. From a Latin word *torus* meaning swelling

---

**Lacrim**/o, lacrimal apparatus (duct, gland or sac), tear

From a Latin word **lacrima**, meaning tear. Here, lacrim/o refers to parts of the lacrimal apparatus and/or tears.

The eye is cleansed and lubricated by fluid from the lacrimal apparatus which consists of a gland, sac and ducts. The gland produces lacrimal (tear) fluid that washes over the eyeball and drains into the lacrimal sac through the lacrimal duct. The lacrimal sac in turn drains the fluid into the nose via the nasolacrimal duct.

**lacrim**-al, pertaining to tears

**lacrim**-ation, action of secreting tears

**lacrim/o**-nas-al, pertaining to the nose and lacrimal apparatus

**lacrim/o**-tome, an instrument used to cut the lacrimal sac and lacrimal duct

**lacrim/o**-tomy, incision into the lacrimal apparatus (duct, gland or sac)

---

**Lent/i**, lenticul-, lens

From a Latin word **lens** meaning a lentil. Here lent/i means the crystalline lens of the eye, a small biconvex crystalline body supported by suspensory ligaments immediately behind the iris. The suspensory ligaments connect the lens capsule to the ciliary body that surrounds the lens.

Although the lens is elastic and tends to assume a spherical shape, tension in the suspensory ligaments can alter its shape and focus. Changes of tension in the suspensory ligaments are brought about by the action of ciliary muscles in the ciliary body. When the muscles are relaxed the ligaments are tensed by their attachments and the lens flattens, when contracted tension is reduced, and the lens assumes a more convex shape for near vision. The ability of the lens to change shape is known as accommodation and it enables light rays to focus precisely on the retina.

**lent**-ate, 1. having a lens 2. resembling a lens

**lenti**-con-us, a cone-shaped abnormal bulging of the lens

**lenticul**-ar, 1. pertaining to a lens 2. resembling a lens

**lenti**-form, having the form of a lens

**Ocul/o**, eye

From a Latin word **oculus**, meaning the eye. Here ocul/o means the eye.

bin-**ocul**-ar, pertaining to two eyes

electro-**ocul/o**-gram, a recording or picture of the electrical activity of the eye

extra-**ocul**-ar, pertaining to outside the eye

mon-**ocul**-ar, pertaining to one eye

**ocul**-ar, pertaining to the eye

**ocul**-ist, an eye specialist, medically qualified in ophthalmology

**ocul/o**-cephal/o-gyr-ic, pertaining to movements of the head in association with the eye (vision)

**ocul/o**-cutane-ous, pertaining to the skin and eyes

**ocul/o**-fac/i-al, pertaining to the face and eyes

**ocul/o**-front-al, pertaining to the forehead and eyes

**ocul/o**-gyr-ation, action of circular movement of the eye, around the anteroposterior axis

**ocul/o**-gyr-ic, pertaining to a circular movement of the eye

**ocul/o**-metr/o-scope, an instrument used for viewing and measuring the eye, it refers to a device for rotating trial lenses before the eyes

**ocul/o**-motor, eye action or movement caused by stimulation of the oculomotor nerve (cranial nerve III)

**ocul/o**-myc-osis, abnormal condition of fungi in the eyes

**ocul/o**-nas-al, pertaining to the nose and eye

**ocul/o**-pathy, disease of the eye

**ocul/o**-pupill-ary, pertaining to the pupil of the eye

**ocul/o**-spin-al, pertaining to the spinal cord and eye

**ocul/o**-zygomat-ic, pertaining to the zygomatic bone or process and the eye

**ocul**-us, the eye

uni-**ocul**-ar, pertaining to one eye

---

**Ophthalm/o**, eye

From a Greek word **ophthalmos**, meaning eye. Here ophthalm/o means the eye.

blenn-**ophthalm**-ia, condition of inflammation of the eye with mucus (discharge)

crypt-**ophthalm**-ia, condition of hidden eye, it refers to congenital adhesion or absence of the palpebral (eyelid) fissure so the eye cannot be seen

crypt-**ophthalmos**, hidden eye, it refers to congenital adhesion or absence of the palpebral (eyelid) fissure so the eye cannot be seen

end-**ophthalm**-itis, inflammation inside the eye, within its cavities and adjacent structures

en-**ophthalm**os, in eye, it refers to displacement of the eye into its socket

ex-**ophthalm**-ic, pertaining to exophthalmos

ex-**ophthalm/o**-metry, technique of measuring exophthalmos that is the extent of protrusion of the eye

ex-**ophthalm**os, out eye (bulging eye), an abnormal protrusion of the eye

heter-**ophthalm**-ia, condition of different eyes, it refers to a difference in the direction of the visual axes or colour of the eyes

hydr-**ophthalm**os, abnormal amount of water (fluid) in the eye, seen in infantile glaucoma

macr-**ophthalm**-ia, condition of an abnormal enlargement of the eye

megal-**ophthalm**os, abnormal enlargement of the eyes

meg-**ophthalm**os, abnormal enlargement of the eyes

micr-**ophthalm**-ia, condition of a small eye (small in all dimensions, unilateral or bilateral)

micr-**ophthalm**os, small eye (small in all dimensions, unilateral or bilateral)

nan-**ophthalm**-ia, condition of a small eye (congenitally small but no other abnormality)

nan-**ophthalm**os, a small eye (congenitally small but no other abnormality)

**ophthalm**-agra, sudden pain in the eye

**ophthalm**-alg-ia, condition of pain in the eye

**ophthalm**-a-trophy, without nutrition of the eye, it refers to wasting away or atrophy of the eye

**ophthalm**-ectomy, removal of the eye (enucleation of the eyeball)

**ophthalm**-ia, condition of the eye, it refers to inflammation of the whole eye

**ophthalm**-ic, pertaining to the eye

**ophthalm**-itic, pertaining to having ophthalmitis

**ophthalm**-itis, inflammation of the eye

**ophthalm/o**-blenn/o-rrhoea, excessive flow or discharge of mucus from the eye (due to gonorrhoea)

**ophthalm/o**-carcin/oma, a malignant tumour or carcinoma of the eye

**ophthalm/o**-cele, a protrusion or hernia of the eye Syn. exophthalmos

**ophthalm/o**-centesis, surgical puncture of the eye

**ophthalm/o**-donesis, abnormal condition of tremor in the eye. From a Greek word *donesis* meaning tremor

**ophthalm/o**-dynam/o-metry, technique of measuring force (blood pressure) in the eye (in the ophthalmic artery)

**ophthalm/o**-dyn-ia, condition of pain in the eye

**ophthalm/o**-eikon/o-meter, an instrument for measuring the image of the eyes (it determines refraction and the size and shape of the images in both eyes)

**ophthalm/o**-fund/o-scope, an instrument used to view or examine the fundus of the eye

**ophthalm/o**-gyr-ic, pertaining to a circular movement of the eye

**ophthalm/o**-lith, a stone or calculus in the eye (in the lacrimal apparatus)

**ophthalm/o**-log-ical, pertaining to ophthalmology

**ophthalm/o**-log-ist, a specialist who studies the eye, medically qualified

**ophthalm/o**-logy, the study of the eye (anatomy, diseases and treatment of)

**ophthalm/o**-malac-ia, condition of softening of the eye

**ophthalm/o**-melan-oma, a malignant pigmented tumour or melanoma of the eye

**ophthalm/o**-melan-osis, abnormal condition of melanoma (formation) in the eye

**ophthalm/o**-meter, an instrument used to measure the eye (the degree of curvature of the corneal surface

**ophthalm/o**-metr/o-scope, an instrument used to view and measure the eye (a type of ophthalmoscope that enables powers of refraction of the eye to be determined)

**ophthalm/o**-metry, technique of measuring the eye (refractive errors, powers and defects)

**ophthalm/o**-myc-osis, abnormal condition of fungi in the eye (fungal infection)

**ophthalm/o**-my-itis, inflammation of the (extrinsic) muscles of the eye

**ophthalm/o**-my/o-tomy, incision into the (extrinsic) muscles of the eye

**ophthalm/o**-neur-itis, inflammation of the optic nerve

**ophthalm/o**-neur/o-myel-itis, inflammation of the spinal cord associated with inflammation of the optic nerve

**ophthalm**-onc-us, a swelling or tumour of the eye

**ophthalm/o**-pathy, disease of the eye

**ophthalm/o**-phleb/o-tomy, incision into the veins of the eye

**ophthalm/o**-phyma, swelling or hypertrophy of the eye

**ophthalm/o**-plast-ic, pertaining to surgical repair or reconstruction of the eye

**ophthalm/o**-plasty, surgical repair or reconstruction of the eye

**ophthalm/o**-pleg-ia, condition of paralysis of the eye, it refers to paralysis of its extra-ocular muscles

**ophthalm/o**-pleg-ic, pertaining to paralysis of the eye

**ophthalm/o**-ptosis, drooping or falling of the eye (exophthalmos)

**ophthalm/o**-rrhag-ia, condition of bursting forth of blood from the eye (haemorrhage)

**ophthalm/o**-rrhexis, rupture of the eye

**ophthalm/o**-rrhoea, excessive flow or discharge from the eye (of mucus, pus or blood)

**ophthalm/o**-scope, an instrument to view or examine the eye

**ophthalm/o**-scop-ic, pertaining to viewing or examining the eye

**ophthalm/o**-spasm, sudden contraction of the eye

**ophthalm/o**-stas-ia, condition of fixation of the eye (in position with an ophthalmostat)

**ophthalm/o**-stasis, fixation of the eye (in position with an ophthalmostat)

**ophthalm/o**-stat, a device to hold the eyeball in a fixed position during an operation

**ophthalm/o**-tomy, incision into an eye

**ophthalm/o**-ton/o-meter, an instrument used to measure tension or pressure within the eye

**ophthalm/o**-trope, mechanical model eye used to demonstrate movements of the extrinsic eye muscles

**ophthalm/o**-trop/o-meter, an instrument used to measure a deviation of the eye, it measures the imbalance in ocular muscles

**ophthalm/o**-trop/o-metry, technique of measuring deviations of the eye, it refers to measuring imbalances in ocular muscles

**ophthalm/o**-vascul-ar, pertaining to (blood) vessels of the eye

**ophthalm/o**-xer-osis, abnormal condition of dry eyes

pan-**ophthalm**-itis, inflammation of all of the eye

par-**ophthalm**-ia, condition beside or near the eye, it refers to inflammation of connective tissues beside the eye

peri-**ophthalm**-ic, pertaining to inflammation around the eye

phot-**ophthalm**-ia, condition of the eye due to light, it refers to ophthalmia caused by exposure to intense light such as that reflected from snow or welding torches

xer-**ophthalm**-ia, condition of inflammation due to dryness

---

**-opia, opsia**, condition of vision
From a Greek word **ops** also meaning eye. Here the suffixes -opia and -opsia mean a condition of defective vision. Many focusing defects of vision can be

corrected by prescribing appropriate spectacles.

ambly-**op**-ia, condition of dim vision

anti-metr-**op**-ia, condition of defect in vision where the refractive error (measurement) in one eye is of a different kind from the refractive error in the other eye *e.g.* myopia in one eye, hypermetropia in the other

an-iso-metr-**op**-ia, condition of defect in vision where the refractive error measurement is without equality in the two eyes

asthen-**op**-ia, condition of weakness of vision, typically due to eyestrain

brachy-**metr**-op-ia, condition in which light is focused in front of the retina, it refers to short sightedness in which vision is better for near objects than for those further away

deuter-an-**op**-ia, condition of defect in vision where two of the three primary colours red and blue are perceived but green is not appreciated, it results in a form of colour blindness in which reds and greens are confused

deuter-an-**op**-ic, pertaining to having deuteranopia

dipl-**op**-ia, condition of double vision

dys-chromat-**ops**-ia, condition of poor colour vision, a disorder of colour vision

dys-**op**-ia, condition of painful or difficult vision

em-metr-**op**-ia, condition of sight in measure, here light is focused in correct position on retina (normal or ideal vision)

hemi-a-chromat-**ops**-ia, condition of half colour vision, it refers to faulty colour vision in half the field of view

hemi-an-**op**-ia, condition of without half vision, it refers to blindness in one half of the visual field in one or both eyes

hetero-metr-op-ia, condition of a defect in vision where refraction measured in the two eyes is different

heter-**ops**-ia, condition of a defect in vision where there is different or unequal vision in the two eyes

hyper-metr-**op**-ia, condition in which light is focused beyond the retina, it refers to long sightedness in which vision is better for far objects than for near

hyper-**op**-ia, condition in which light is focused beyond the retina, it refers to long sightedness in which vision is better for far objects than for near

macr-**op**-ia, condition of defect in vision where objects appear to be larger than their actual size

megal-**op**-ia, condition of defect in vision where objects appear to be larger than their actual size

megal-**ops**-ia, condition of defect in vision where objects appear to be larger than their actual size

micr-**ops**-ia, condition of defect in vision where objects appear to be smaller than their actual size

my-**op**-ia, condition in which light is focused in front of the retina, it refers to short sightedness in which vision is better for near objects than for those further away

my-**op**-ic, pertaining to having myopia

phot-**op**-ia, condition of light vision, day vision

phot-**op**-ic, pertaining to having photopia

phot-**ops**-ia, condition of defect in vision where flashes of light appear, caused by retinopathy

poly-**op**-ia, condition of defect in vision in which many images of the same object are seen

presby-**op**-ia, condition of old man's vision

prot-an-**op**-ia, condition of a defect in vision without the first primary colour (red), it refers to an inability to perceive red light and the confusion of red with green. From a Greek word *protos* meaning first

prot-an-**op**-ic, pertaining to having protanopia

quadrant-an-**op**-ia, condition of without vision in one quadrant of the field of vision

tetr-an-**ops**-ia, condition of without vision in one quadrant of the field of vision tripl-**op**-ia, condition of defect in vision in which three images of the same object are seen. From a Greek word *triplos* meaning triple

---

**Optic/o**, optic nerve

From **optikos**, a Greek word meaning sight. Here optic/o means the optic nerve, a nerve containing sensory neurons that originate in the retinae of the eyes. The nerve is directed backwards and medially through the posterior part of the orbital cavity. Nerve impulses travelling in the sensory neurons of the optic nerve pass to the cerebrum where they are perceived as sight.

**optic/o**-chiasmat-ic, pertaining to the chiasma and optic nerve

**optic/o**-chiasm-ic, pertaining to the chiasma and optic nerve

**optic/o**-cili-ary, pertaining to the ciliary nerve and optic nerve

**optic/o**-pupill-ary, pertaining to the pupil and optic nerve

---

**Opt/o**, eye, sight, vision

From **optikos**, a Greek word meaning sight. Here opt/o means sight or eye.

ent-**opt**-ic, pertaining to or originating within the eye

ent-**opt**/o-scopy, technique of viewing or examining the inside of the eye

**opt**-aesthes-ia, condition of sensation of sight (ability to perceive visual stimuli)

**opt**-ic, pertaining to or belonging to the eye

**opt**-ical, pertaining to the eye or vision

**opt**-ician, person who specializes in vision, it refers to a person who makes and sells spectacles in accordance with an ophthalmic prescription

**opt**-ics, the science of studying vision and light

**opt**/o-gram, a picture or recording of vision (of the image formed on the retina)

**opt**/o-kinet-ic, pertaining to movement of the eyes as in nystagmus

**opt**/o-meter, an instrument that measures sight

**opt**/o-metr-ist, a specialist who measures sight (and provides corrective measures for eye defects)

**opt**/o-metry, 1. technique of measuring sight 2. the profession of an optometrist in providing primary eye and vision care

**opt**/o-my/o-meter, an instrument for measuring the muscles of sight, it measures the power of the ocular muscles

orth-**opt**-ic, pertaining to straight or correct sight, it refers to the study and treatment of muscle imbalances of the eye known as squints

orth-**opt**-ics, the science dealing with straightening vision, it refers to correcting squints using ocular exercises

orth-**opt**-ist, a specialist dealing with straightening vision, it refers to a specialist who corrects squints using ocular exercises

orth-**opt**/o-scope, an instrument that enables eyes to view straight, it refers to an optical device that induces a patient with a squint to achieve binocular vision

peri-**opt**/o-metry, technique of measuring sight around the visual field, it refers to measuring visual acuity to the edge of peripheral vision

phot-**opt**/o-meter, an instrument used to measure light, it refers to an instrument that measures the smallest amount of light that allows an object to be seen

---

**Orbit/o**, orbit

From a Latin word **orbita** meaning wheel track. Here, orbit/o means the orbit of the eye, the large, bony cavity containing the eyeball and its associated vessels, nerves and muscles.

infra-**orbit**-al, pertaining to beneath the orbit

**orbit**-a, orbit

**orbit**-ae, plural of orbita

**orbit**-al, pertaining to the orbit of the eye

**orbit/o**-meter, an instrument for measuring the orbit, it refers to an instrument to measure the backward movement of the eyeball when pressure is applied to its anterior surface

**orbit/o**-metry, technique of measuring the orbit, it refers to measuring the compressibility of its contents

**orbit/o**-nas-al, pertaining to the nose and orbit of the eye

**orbit/o**-tempor-al, pertaining to the temporal and orbital regions

**orbit/o**-tomy, incision into an orbit

sub-**orbit**-al, pertaining to beneath an orbit

supra-**orbit**-al, pertaining to above an orbit

---

**Palpebr/o**, eyelid

From a Latin word **palpebra** meaning eyelid. Here palpebr/o means the eyelids, the movable folds in front of the eyeball closing during sleep or to protect from injury. The upper fold is called the palpebra superior and the lower palpebra inferior. The palpebral fissure forms the longitudinal opening between the eyelids.

See the combining form blephar/o also meaning eyelid.

**palpebr**-al, pertaining to the eyelids

**palpebr**-ate, having eyelids

**palpebr**-ation, action of the eyelids, winking

**palpebr**-itis, inflammation of the eyelids Syn. blepharitis

**palpebr/o**-front-al, pertaining to the forehead and eyelids

---

**Papill/o**, optic disc, optic papilla

From a Latin word **papilla**, meaning nipple-shaped. Here papill/o means the optic disc or optic papilla, a nipple-shaped point where the sensory neurons collect and form the optic nerve in the retina. Sensory neurons leave the retina and travel through the

optic nerve at the back of the eye towards the visual cortex in the brain. The optic disc is visible through the pupil using an ophthalmoscope.

**papill**-ary, pertaining to a papilla

**papill**-itis, inflammation of the optic disc or optic papilla

**papill**-oedema, swelling of fluid in the optic disc or optic papilla

**papill/o**-retin-itis, inflammation of the retina and optic disc or optic papilla

---

**Phac/o, phak/o**, lens

From a Greek word **phakos**, meaning lentil. Here, phac/o means the lentil-shaped lens of the eye, a small biconvex crystalline body supported by suspensory ligaments immediately behind the iris. The suspensory ligaments connect the lens capsule to the ciliary body that surrounds the lens.

Although the lens is elastic and tends to assume a spherical shape, tension in the suspensory ligaments can alter its shape and focus. Changes of tension in the suspensory ligaments are brought about by the action of ciliary muscles in the ciliary body. When the muscles are relaxed the ligaments are tensed by their attachments and the lens flattens, when contracted tension is reduced, and the lens assumes a more convex shape for near vision. The ability of the lens to change shape is known as accommodation and it enables light rays to focus precisely on the retina.

a-**phak**-ia, condition of without a lens

**phac/o**-ana-phylaxis, an allergic reaction to lens protein, that escapes from a lens

**phac/o**-cele, a protrusion or hernia of a lens

**phac/o**-cyst, the capsule of the lens

**phac/o**-cyst-ectomy, removal of a phacocyst or lens capsule

**phac/o**-cyst-itis, inflammation of a lens capsule

**phac/o**-emulsific-ation, action of emulsifying a lens, the lens is fragmented and removed using an ultrasonic probe

**phac/o**-erysis, sucking out of a lens

**phac**-oid, resembling a lens (shape)

**phacoid**-itis, inflammation of a lens Syn. phacitis

**phacoid/o**-scope, an instrument used to view or examine a lens (its variations occurring during accommodation)

**phac/o**-lysis, breakdown or disintegration of a lens (by surgical means)

**phac/o**-lyt-ic, pertaining to breakdown or disintegration of a lens (by surgical means)

**phac**-oma, a tumour of a lens

**phac/o**-malac-ia, condition of softening of a lens (a soft cataract)

**phac/o**-metachoresis, condition of displacement of the lens. From a Greek word *metachoresis* meaning a change of place

**phac/o**-meter, an instrument used to measure a lens (its refractive power)

**phac/o**-scler-osis, abnormal condition of hardening of the lens (a hard cataract)

**phac/o**-scope, an instrument used to view the lens (to view changes in its shape)

**phac/o**-scopy, technique of viewing or examining a lens

**phac/o**-tox-ic, pertaining to poisoning of a lens

**phak**-itis, inflammation of a lens Syn. phacoiditis

**phak/o**-emulsific-ation, action of emulsifying a lens, the lens is fragmented and removed using as ultrasonic probe

---

**-phoria**, phoria

From a Greek word **phora** meaning orbit. Here -phoria is used as a suffix to mean a latent (hidden) deviation of the visual axis of one or both eyes. The visual axis of the eye is an imaginary line passing from the object of regard (the object being looked at) to the fovea centralis in the retina. The deviation becomes apparent or manifest when one eye is covered or when they view

dissimilar objects. The suffix -phoria is used synonymously with heterophoria to mean a condition in which there is a tendency for the eyes to move out of alignment *i.e.* have different visual axes when one eye is covered or when they view dissimilar objects.

ana-**phor-ia**, a condition in which the visual axes tend to turn upwards when one eye is covered (a type of heterophoria)

an-iso-**phor-ia**, a condition in which the visual axes are without equality, it refers to an unequal heterophoria in the two eyes

cata-**phor-ia**, 1. a condition in which the visual axis of either eye tends to turn downwards when covered 2. a condition in which the visual axes of both eyes turn downwards in the absence of a fixation stimulus Syn. kataphoria

cycl/o-**phor-ia**, a condition in which the visual axes tend to rotate around the anteroposterior axis when one eye is covered (a type of heterophoria)

eso-**phor-ia**, a condition in which the visual axes tend to turn inwards when one eye is covered (a type of heterophoria)

exo-**phor-ia**, a condition in which the visual axes tend to turn outwards when one eye is covered (a type of heterophoria)

ex-cycl/o-**phor-ia**, a condition in which the top pole of the eye tends to rotate outwards around the anteroposterior axis (towards the temple) when one eye is covered (a type of heterophoria)

hetero-**phor-ia**, a condition of different visual axes, it refers to a failure of the axes to remain parallel when one eye is covered or when they view dissimilar objects

hyper-exo-**phor-ia**, condition of deviation of the visual axes outward and upward when one eye is covered (a type of heterophoria)

hyper-**phor-ia**, condition of deviation of the visual axis of one eye upwards relative to the other when one eye is covered (a type of heterophoria)

in-cycl/o-**phor-ia**, condition of deviation of the visual axes in which the top pole of the eye rotates inwards on its anteroposterior axis when one eye is covered (a type of heterophoria)

kata-**phor-ia**, 1. a condition in which the visual axis of either eye tends to turn downwards when covered 2. a condition in which the visual axes of both eyes turn downwards in the absence of a fixation stimulus (a type of heterophoria)

ortho-**phor-ia**, condition of straight (perfect) visual axes, muscle balance in which no deviations of the axes occur when one eye is covered (no heterophoria or heterotropia present)

ortho-**phor-ic**, pertaining to having orthophoria

---

**Pupill/o**, pupil

From a Latin word **pupilla**, meaning little girl. Here, pupill/o means the pupil, the opening in the centre of the iris that allows the passage of light into the eye.

**pupill**-ary, pertaining to a pupil

**pupill**-a-ton-ia, condition of without tone of the pupil, the pupil does not respond to light

**pupill/o**-metry, technique of measuring pupils

**pupill/o**-motor, pertaining to the action (movement) of the pupil

**pupill/o**-pleg-ia, condition of paralysis of the pupils

**pupill/o**-scope, an instrument used for viewing or examining the pupils, it measures reactions of the pupils and refractive errors

**pupill/o**-scopy, technique of viewing or examining the pupils, in this procedure, the reactions and refractive errors of the pupils are measured

**pupill/o**-stat/o-meter, an instrument used to measure fixed distance between the pupils

**pupill/o**-ton-ia, condition of a tonic pupil, it refers to a pupil with an abnormal action

---

**Retin/o**, retina

From a mediaeval Latin word **retina**, probably derived from rete, meaning net. It refers to the retina, the light-sensitive internal coat of the eyeball consisting of eight superimposed layers, seven of which are nervous and one pigmented. The retina contains specialized nerve cells called rods and cones, rods are sensitive to light of low intensity while cones are sensitive to colour and bright light. Light is focused onto the retina by the lens.

electro-**retin/o**-gram, a picture or recording of the electrical activity of the retina

electro-**retin/o**-graph, an instrument that records the electrical activity of the retina in response to light

ento-**retin/a**, within or inside the retina, it refers to the inner nervous layer of the retina

photo-**retin**-itis, inflammation of the retina caused by exposure to intense light

**retin**-al, 1. pertaining to the retina 2. an aldehyde of retinol, it combines with opsins in the retina to form visual pigments

**retin**-itis, inflammation of the retina

**retin/o**-blast-oma, a tumour of immature cells or embryonic cells of the retina (it arises from the neuroglial elements of the retina in children)

**retin/o**-choroid, pertaining to or belonging to the choroid and retina

**retin/o**-choroid-itis, inflammation of the choroid and retina Syn. choroido-retinitis, chorioretinitis

**retin/o**-dialysis, separation of the retina, it refers to a tear in the anterior part of the retina

**retin/o**-graph, a recording or photograph of the retina

**retin**-oid, 1. resembling the retina 2. a derivative of retinal

**retin**-ol, a chemical with vitamin A activity essential for the formation of rhodopsin (visual pigment) in the retina

**retin/o**-malac-ia, condition of softening of the retina

**retin/o**-mening/o-encephal-itis, inflammation of the brain, meninges and retina

**retin/o**-papill-itis, inflammation of the optic papilla and retina

**retin/o**-path-ia, condition of disease of the retina

**retin/o**-pathy, disease of the retina

**retin/o**-schisis, splitting (separation) of the retina

**retin/o**-scope, an instrument used to view or examine the retina

**retin/o**-scopy, technique of viewing or examining the retina to determine refractive errors

**retin**-osis, abnormal condition of the retina (degeneration, not inflammation)

**retin/o**-top-ic, pertaining to the place of the retina, its visual pathways and relation to the visual cortex of the brain

**retin/o**-tox-ic, pertaining to poisonous to the retina

sub-**retin**-al, pertaining to beneath the retina

---

**Scler/o**, sclerotic/o, sclera

From a Greek word **skleros**, meaning hard. Here scler/o means the sclera, the tough outer coat of the eye. The opaque, white part of the sclera forms five-sixths of the outer coat of the eyeball and merges with the transparent cornea at the front of the eye.

**scler**-al, pertaining to or belonging to the sclera

**scler**-ectas-ia, condition of dilation or bulging of the sclera

**scler**-ectasis, dilation or bulging of the sclera

**scler**-ecto-irid-ectomy, removal of the iris (iridectomy) and part of the sclera (sclerectomy)

**scler**-ecto-irid/o-dialysis, separation of the iris (from its ciliary attachment) and removal of part of the sclera

(sclerectomy), an operation for glaucoma

**scler**-ectomy, removal of the sclera (part of)

**scler**-ir/i-tomy, incision into the iris and sclera

**scler**-itis, inflammation of the sclera

**scler/o**-cataract, a hard cataract (an opacity of the lens or lens capsule)

**scler/o**-choroid-itis, inflammation of the choroid and sclera

**scler/o**-conjunctiv-al, pertaining to or belonging to the conjunctiva and sclera

**scler/o**-conjunctiv-itis, inflammation of the conjunctiva and sclera

**scler/o**-cornea, the cornea and sclera considered together

**scler/o**-corne-al, pertaining to the cornea and sclera

**scler/o**-cycl/o-tomy, incision into the ciliary muscle through the sclera

**scler/o**-irid/o-dialysis, separation of the iris and sclera

**scler/o**-irid/o-tomy, incision into the iris and sclera

**scler/o**-ir-itis, inflammation of the iris and sclera

**scler/o**-kerat-itis, inflammation of the cornea and sclera

**scler/o**-kerat/o-ir-itis, inflammation of the iris, cornea and sclera

**scler/o**-kerat-osis, abnormal condition of the cornea and sclera

**scler/o**-malac-ia, condition of softening of the sclera (degeneration)

**scler/o**-nyxis, puncture of the sclera

**scler/o**-ophthalm-ia, condition of the eye and sclera (a developmental defect in which only the central part of the cornea is clear, due to a failure of differentiation from the sclera)

**scler/o**-opt-ic, pertaining to the optic nerve and sclera

**scler/o**-plasty, surgical repair or reconstruction of the sclera

**scler/o**-stomy, formation of an opening into the sclera or the name of the opening so created

**scler/o**-tic, pertaining to or belonging to the sclera

**sclerotic**-a, the sclera

**sclerotic**-ectomy, removal of the sclera (part of)

**sclerotic/o**-choroid-itis, inflammation of the choroid and sclera Syn. sclero-choroiditis

**sclerotic/o**-nyxis, puncture of the sclera Syn. scleronyxis

**sclerotic/o**-puncture, puncture of the sclera Syn. scleronyxis

**sclerotic/o**-tomy, incision into the sclera

**scler/o**-tome, an instrument used to cut the sclera

**scler/o**-tomy, incision into the sclera

---

**Scot/o**, **scotoma/t-**, dark, scotoma

From a Greek word **skotos**, meaning darkness. Here scot/o means dark or scotoma, a normal or abnormal blind spot in the visual field where vision is poor.

**scotoma**-graph, an instrument used to record scotomas in the visual field

**scotoma**-meter, an instrument used to measure scotomas in the visual field

**scot**-omat-a, pleural of scotoma

**scotomat**-ous, pertaining to or having scotomas in the visual field

**scot/o**-meter, an instrument used to measure scotomas in the visual field

**scot/o**-metry, the technique of measuring scotomas in the visual field

**scot**-opia, condition of dark vision (the ability to adapt to seeing in the dark)

**scotop**-ic, pertaining to having scotopia (condition of dark vision or the ability to adapt to seeing in the dark)

---

**Strabism/o**, **strab/o**, strabismus, a squint

From a Greek word **strabismos** meaning squinting. Here strabism/o means a strabismus or squint, a manifest (visible) condition in which the visual axes of the eyes are misaligned and one eye deviates from the point of fixation when uncovered. The visual axis of the

eye is an imaginary line passing from the object of regard (the object being looked at) to the fovea centralis in the retina. The word strabismus is used synonymously with heterotropia, see the suffix -tropia.

**strab**-ism, condition of strabismus, a squint

**strabism**-al, pertaining to or affected by strabismus or squint

**strabism**-ic, pertaining to or affected by strabismus or squint

**strabism/o**-meter, an instrument used to measure the angle of a strabismus or squint

**strabism/o**-metry, technique of measuring the angle of a strabismus or squint

**strab/o**-tomy, incision to correct a strabismus (by cutting an ocular tendon)

---

**Synech/i/o**, synechia

From a Greek word **synechia** meaning a continuity. Here, synechi/o means an adhesion between the iris and the posterior surface of the cornea or iris and the anterior surface of the lens.

**synechi/o**-tomy, incision into a synechia

**synech/o**-tome, an instrument to cut a synechia

**synech/o**-tomy, incision into a synechia

---

**-tropia**, strabismus, a squint

From a Greek word **trope** meaning to turn. Here -tropia is used as a suffix, it means a condition of turning but is used to denote the presence of a stabismus or squint. A strabismus is a manifest (visible) condition in which the visual axes are misaligned and one eye deviates from the point of fixation when uncovered. The visual axis of the eye is an imaginary line passing from the object of regard (the object being looked at) to the fovea centralis in the retina. Strabismus is used synonymously with heterotropia, see the combining form strabism/o.

an-iso-**trop-ia**, a condition of an unequal strabismus in the two eyes

cyclo-**trop-ia**, a condition of a strabismus in which there is a permanent rotation of one eye around an anteroposterior axis relative to the other (a type of heterotropia)

eso-**trop-ia**, a condition of a strabismus in which there is a permanent deviation of the visual axis of one eye inwards, towards the other giving a cross-eyed appearance (a type of heterotropia)

exo-**trop-ia**, a condition of a strabismus in which there is a permanent deviation of the visual axis of one eye outwards, away from the other (a type of heterotropia)

hetero-**trop-ia**, a condition of having different visual axes, it refers to having a strabismus

hyper-**trop-ia**, a condition of a strabismus in which there is a permanent upward deviation of the visual axis of one eye relative to the other (a type of heterotropia)

hypo-**trop-ia**, a condition of a strabismus in which there is a permanent downward deviation of the visual axis of one eye relative to the other (a type of heterotropia)

in-cyclo-**trop-ia**, a condition of a strabismus in which the upper pole of the visual axis of one eye rotates inwards on its anteroposterior axis towards the nose (a type of heterotropia)

micro-**trop-ia**, a condition of a small strabismus in which the heterotropia is difficult to detect by cover testing

**Uve/o**, uvea

From a Latin word **uva** meaning grape. Here, uve/o means the uvea, the middle, pigmented coat of the eyeball. It includes the iris, ciliary body and choroid together.

**uve**-al, pertaining to or belonging to the uvea

**uve**-itic, pertaining to having uveitis

**uve**-itis, inflammation of the uvea (all or part of)

**uve/o**-parotid, involving the parotid gland and uvea

**uve/o**-parotid-itis, inflammation of the parotid glands and uvea

**uve/o**-plasty, surgical repair or reconstruction of the uvea

**uve/o**-scler-itis, inflammation of the sclera and uvea

**Vitre/o**, the vitreous body of the eye

From a Latin word **vitreus** meaning glass-like. Here vitre/o means the glass-like vitreous body lying behind the lens and filling the posterior cavity. The vitreous body consists of a soft, colourless, transparent, jelly-like substance composed of 99% water, some salts and mucoprotein. It maintains sufficient intraocular pressure to support the retina against the choroid and prevent the walls of the eyeball from collapsing.

**vitr**-ectomy, removal of the vitreous body of the eye

**vitre/o**-retin-al, pertaining to the retina and vitreous body

**vitre/o**-us, 1. pertaining to glass-like 2. the vitreous body

# Section 10
# The ear

The ear is a major sense organ concerned with two important functions: hearing and balance. It is divided into three distinct parts:

- the outer or external ear
- the middle ear or tympanic cavity
- the inner ear.

Sound waves collected by the auricle enter the external auditory meatus and vibrate the ear drum. The vibrations are amplified and transmitted to the oval window of the cochlea by the ear ossicles in the middle ear. The cochlea is the organ of hearing and contains special receptor cells that generate nerve impulses in response to sound. Nerve impulses from the cochlea are relayed via sensory neurons in cranial nerve VIII to auditory areas in the brain where they are interpreted as sounds. Having two ears enables us to sense the direction of sound.

The vestibule and semi-circular canals of the inner ear contain receptors

**Quick Reference**
Combining forms relating to the ear:

| | | Page |
|---|---|---|
| Acous- | hearing | 168 |
| -acusis | hearing | 168 |
| Audi/o | hearing | 168 |
| Aur/i | ear | 169 |
| Auricul/o | auricle, pinna | 169 |
| Cochle/o | cochlea | 169 |
| Incud/o | incus (an ear ossicle) | 169 |
| Labyrinth/o | labyrinth of the inner ear | 170 |
| Malle/o | malleus (an ear ossicle) | 170 |
| Mastoid/o | mastoid process, mastoid air cells | 170 |
| Myring/o | ear drum, tympanic membrane | 170 |
| Ossicul/o | ossicle | 171 |
| Ot/o | ear | 171 |
| Saccul/o | saccule of inner ear | 172 |
| Salping/o | auditory tube, Eustachian tube, pharyngotympanic tube | 172 |
| Stapedi/o | stapes (an ear ossicle) | 172 |
| Tympan/o | ear drum, middle ear | 173 |
| Utricul/o | utricle of inner ear | 173 |
| Vestibul/o | vestibule, vestibular apparatus (of inner ear) | 173 |

**Quick Reference**
Common words and combining forms relating to the ear:

| | | Page |
|---|---|---|
| Auditory tube | salping/o | 172 |
| Auricle | auricul/o | 169 |
| Cochlea | cochle/o | 169 |
| Ear | aur/i, ot/o | 169/171 |
| Ear drum | myring/o, tympan/o | 170/173 |
| Eustachian tube | salping/o | 172 |
| Hearing | acous-, -acusis, audi/o | 168 |
| Incus | incud/o | 169 |
| Labyrinth | labyrinth/o | 170 |
| Malleus | malle/o | 170 |
| Mastoid air cells | mastoid/o | 170 |
| Mastoid process | mastoid/o | 170 |
| Middle ear | tympan/o | 173 |
| Ossicle | ossicul/o | 171 |
| Pharyngotympanic tube | salping/o | 172 |
| Pinna | auricul/o | 169 |
| Saccule of inner ear | saccul/o | 172 |
| Stapes | stapedi/o | 172 |
| Tympanic membrane | myring/o, tympan/o | 170/173 |
| Utricle of inner ear | utricul/o | 173 |
| Vestibular apparatus | vestibul/o | 173 |
| Vestibule | vestibul/o | 173 |

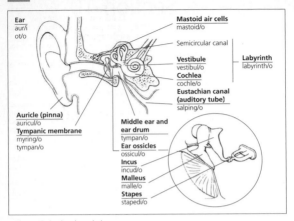

Ear
aur/i
ot/o

Mastoid air cells
mastoid/o

Semicircular canal

Vestibule
vestibul/o

Cochlea
cochle/o

Labyrinth
labyrinth/o

Eustachian canal
(auditory tube)
salping/o

Auricle (pinna)
auricul/o

Tympanic membrane
myring/o
tympan/o

Middle ear and
ear drum
tympan/o

Ear ossicles
ossicul/o

Incus
incud/o

Malleus
malle/o

Stapes
stapedi/o

Figure 15  Section through the ear

that detect changes in velocity and position of the body. Sensory impulses from the inner ear are relayed via sensory neurons to centres in the cerebellum and other regions of the brain. There they are used in the neural processes that allow us to maintain our balance and upright posture.

Figure 15 shows a section through the ear and the combining forms associated with its components.

**Roots and combining forms**, meanings

**Acous-, acusis-,** hearing
From a Greek word **akouein** meaning to hear. Here acous- means a sense of hearing.

**acous**-ia, condition of ability to hear
**acous**-tic, pertaining to hearing or sound
hyper-**acous**-ia, condition of above normal sense of hearing (acute hearing)

hyper-**acusis**, condition of above normal sense of hearing (acute hearing)
hypo-**acous**-ia, condition of below normal sense of hearing
hypo-**acusis**, below normal sense of hearing
par-**acous**-ia, condition of wrong hearing, it refers to any abnormal condition of hearing sense
par-**acusis**, condition of wrong hearing, it refers to any abnormal condition of hearing sense
presby-**acusis**, condition of old man's hearing, it refers to progressive loss of hearing in both ears with increasing age

**Audi/o**, hearing
From a Latin word **audire**, meaning to hear. Here audi/o means the sense of hearing.

**audi**-mut-ism, process of being mute with hearing

**audi/o**-gen-ic, 1. pertaining to formed by sound 2. having origin in sound

**audi/o**-gram, a tracing or recording made by an audiometer

**audi/o**-logy, the study of hearing

**audi/o**-meter, an instrument that measures hearing

**audi/o**-metry, technique of measuring hearing using an audiometer

**audi**-tion, process of hearing or sense of hearing

**audit**-ory, 1. pertaining to audition 2. pertaining to having the sense of hearing

---

**Aur/i**, ear

From a Latin word **auris**, meaning ear. Here aur/i means the ear.

**aur**-al, pertaining to the ear

**aur/i**-cle, small ear, it refers to the ear flap or pinna of the external ear. Syn. auricula. See the combining form auricul/o

**aur/i**-cula, small ear, it refers to the ear flap or pinna of the external ear Syn. auricle. See the combining form auricul/o

**aur/i**-scope, an instrument used to view or examine the ear

bin-**aur**-al, pertaining to two ears

dextro-**aur**-al, pertaining to the ear, right ear (superior hearing in the right ear)

end-**aur**-al, pertaining to within the ear

sinistr-**aur**-al, pertaining to the ear, left ear (superior hearing in the left ear)

sub-**aur**-al, pertaining to below the ear

---

**Auricul/o**, auricle, pinna

From a Latin word **auricula**, meaning little ear. Here, auricul/o means the auricle or pinna of the external ear. The auricle is the expanded, visible portion of the ear projecting from the side of the head.

**auricula**, auricle

**auric**ulae, plural of auricula

**auricul**-ar, pertaining to an auricle

**auricul/o**-crani-al, pertaining to the cranium and auricle of the ear

**auricul/o**-tempor-al, pertaining to the temple and auricle of the ear

post-**auricul**-ar, pertaining to behind the auricle of the ear

pre-**auricul**-ar, pertaining to in front of the auricle of the ear

supra-**auricul**-ar, pertaining to above the auricle of the ear

---

**Cochle/o**, cochlea

From a Latin word **cochlea**, meaning snail. Here cochle/o means the cochlea, the snail-shaped anterior bony labyrinth of the inner ear.

**cochle**-ar, pertaining to the cochlea

**cochle**-itis, inflammation of the cochlea

**cochle/o**-top-ic, pertaining to the position or place of the cochlea (in relation to the auditory pathways and auditory area of the brain)

**cochle/o**-stomy, formation of an opening into the cochlea or the name of the opening so created

**cochle/o**-vestibul-ar, pertaining to the vestibule and cochlea

electro-**cochle/o**-graphy, technique of recording electrical potentials of the cochlea (in the eighth cranial nerve) in response to acoustic stimuli

retro-**cochle**-ar, pertaining to behind the cochlea

---

**Incud/i/o**, incus (an ear ossicle)

From a Latin word **incus**, meaning anvil. Here incud/o means the incus, the middle anvil-shaped ear ossicle that connects the malleus to the stapes. The ear ossicles amplify vibrations from the ear drum and transmit them to the oval window of the cochlea.

**incud**-al, pertaining to the incus

**incud**-ectomy, removal of the incus

**incud/i**-form, having the form or shape of an incus or anvil

**incud/o**-malle-al, pertaining to the malleus and incus

**incud/o**-stapedi-al, pertaining to the stapes and incus

**Labyrinth/o**, labyrinth of the inner ear
From a Greek word **labyrinthos**, meaning maze. Here labyrinth/o means the labyrinth, a group of maze-like passageways that form the inner ear. The bony labyrinth is a cavity within the temporal bone enclosing the membranous labyrinth. Within the membranous labyrinth lie the cochlea, the vestibule and three semi-circular canals, these enable us to hear and balance.

**labyrinth**-ectomy, removal of the labyrinth (of the inner ear)

**labyrinth**-ine, pertaining to or belonging to a labyrinth

**labyrinth**-itis, inflammation of the labyrinth (of the inner ear)

**labyrinth/o**-tomy, incision into the labyrinth (of the inner ear)

**labyrinth**-us, a labyrinth

peri-**labyrinth**-itis, inflammation of the tissues around the labyrinth

---

**Malle/o**, malleus (an ear ossicle)
From a Latin word **malleus**, meaning hammer. Here malle/o means the malleus, the lateral hammer-shaped ear ossicle that connects the tympanic membrane to the incus. The ear ossicles amplify vibrations from the ear drum and transmit them to the oval window of the cochlea.

**malle**-al, pertaining to the malleus

**malle/o**-incud-al, pertaining to the incus and malleus

**malle/o**-tomy, incision into the malleus

---

**Mastoid/e/o**, mastoid air cells, mastoid process
From a Greek word **mastos**, meaning breast. Here, mastoid/o means the nipple-shaped air cells found in the mastoid process that forms part of the temporal bone behind the external ear. The air cells are small air spaces, or air sinuses that communicate with the middle ear, they are lined with squamous epithelium.

Note: words using mast/o meaning breast are listed in Section 16 The female reproductive system.

**mastoid**, 1. pertaining to the mastoid process (part of temporal bone) 2. resembling a nipple

**mastoid**-al, pertaining to the mastoid process (part of temporal bone)

**mastoid**-alg-ia, condition of pain in the mastoid region

**mastoid**-ectomy, removal of the mastoid air cells, it refers to removal of tissue from the mastoid process

**mastoide/o**-centesis, surgical puncture of the mastoid air cells

**mastoid**-itis, inflammation of the mastoid air cells of the mastoid process

**mastoid/o**-tomy, incision into the mastoid air cells of the mastoid process

**mastoid/o**-tympan-ectomy, removal of the tympanic (antrum) and mastoid air cells of the mastoid process

---

**Myring/o**, ear drum, tympanic membrane
A New Latin word **myringa**, meaning membrane. Here myring/o means the tympanic membrane or ear drum. The tympanic membrane vibrates when sound is produced, and the vibrations are transmitted via the ear ossicles from the tympanic membrane to the oval window of the inner ear.

**myring**-ectomy, removal of the ear drum (tympanic membrane)

**myring**-itis, inflammation of the ear drum (tympanic membrane)

**myring/o**-dermat-itis, inflammation of the skin (of external ear) and the ear drum (tympanic membrane)

**myring/o**-myc-osis, abnormal condition of fungi in the ear drum (tympanic membrane)

**myring/o**-plast-ic, 1. pertaining to myringoplasty 2. pertaining to surgical repair or reconstruction of the ear drum

**myring/o**-plasty, surgical repair or reconstruction of the ear drum (tympanic membrane)

**myring/o**-scope, an instrument to view or examine the ear drum (tympanic membrane)

**myring/o**-tome, an instrument used to cut the ear drum (tympanic membrane)

**myring/o**-tomy, incision into the ear drum (tympanic membrane)

---

**Ossicul/o**, ossicle

From the Latin words **os** meaning bone and **-cle** meaning small. Here, ossicul/o means the ossicles, the smallest bones in the body found in the middle ear. There are three bones named malleus, incus and stapes. The function of the ossicles is to transmit vibrations from the tympanic membrane to the oval window of the inner ear.

**ossicul**-ectomy, removal of the ear ossicles

**ossicul/o**-plasty, surgical repair reconstruction of the ear ossicles

**ossicul/o**-tomy, incision of an ear ossicle

**ossicul**-um, an ear ossicle

---

**Ot/o**, ear

From a Greek word **ous**, meaning ear. Here ot/o means the ear, the organ of hearing and balance.

macr-**ot**-ia, condition of large ears

micr-**ot**-ia, condition of small ears

**ot**-acous-tic, pertaining to a sense of hearing

**ot**-alg-ia, condition of pain in the ear (ear ache)

**ot**-alg-ic, pertaining to pain in the ear (ear ache)

**ot**-antr-itis, inflammation of the mastoid antrum and ear (in the attic of the tympanum)

**ot**-haem/o-rrhag-ia, condition of bursting forth of blood from the ear

**ot**-haem/o-rrhoea, excessive discharge of blood from the ear

**ot**-ic, pertaining to the ear or hearing

**ot**-itis, inflammation of the ear

**ot/o**-antr-itis, inflammation of the (mastoid) antrum and ear (in the attic of the tympanum)

**ot/o**-crani-al, pertaining to the oto-cranium

**ot/o**-crani-um, 1. structure or part of the skull containing the (inner) ear 2. the auditory part of the cranium

**ot/o**-encephal-itis, inflammation of the brain from the (middle) ear

**ot/o**-gen-ic, pertaining to forming or originating in the ear

**ot/o**-gen-ous, pertaining to forming or originating in the ear

**ot/o**-laryng/o-logy, the study of the larynx and ear (laryngology and otology considered together)

**ot/o**-lith, an ear stone or calculus

**ot/o**-log-ical, 1. pertaining to otology 2. pertaining to the study of the ear

**ot/o**-log-ist, a (medical) specialist who studies ears (anatomy, diseases and treatment of)

**ot/o**-logy, the study of the ear (anatomy, diseases and treatment of)

**ot/o**-mastoid-itis, inflammation of the mastoid air cells and ear

**ot/o**-micro-scope, a microscope used to view or examine the ear

**ot/o**-myc-osis, abnormal condition of fungi in the ear

**ot/o**-neur/o-log-ic, 1. pertaining to the study of the parts of the nervous system relating to the ear 2. pertaining to otoneurology

**ot/o**-neur/o-logy, the study of the parts of the nervous system relating to the ear

**ot/o**-pathy, disease of the ear

**ot/o**-pharyng-eal, pertaining to the pharynx and (middle) ear

**ot/o**-plasty, surgical repair or reconstruction of the ear

**ot/o**-polyp-us, a polyp in the ear

**ot/o**-py/o-rrhoea, excessive flow of pus from the ear

**ot/o**-py-osis, abnormal condition of pus in the ear

**ot/o**-ophthalm-ic, pertaining to the eye and ear

**ot/o**-rhin/o-laryng/o-logy, the study of the larynx, nose and ear (laryngology, rhinology and otology considered together)

**ot/o**-rhin/o-logy, the study of the nose and ear (rhinology and otology considered together)

**ot/o**-rrhag-ia, condition of bursting forth of blood (haemorrhage) from the ear

**ot/o**-rrhoea, excessive discharge from the ear

**ot/o**-salpinx, the auditory tube, also known as the Eustachian tube or pharyngotympanic tube

**ot/o**-scler-osis, abnormal condition of hardening of the ear, it refers to new bone formation in the middle ear

**ot/o**-scler/o-tic, pertaining to hardening of the ear, it refers to new bone formation in the middle ear

**ot/o**-scope, an instrument to view or examine the ear

**ot/o**-scop-ic, 1. pertaining to otoscopy 2. pertaining to viewing or examining the ear

**ot/o**-scopy, technique of viewing or examining the ear

**ot/o**-spongi-osis, abnormal condition of spongy (bone) in the ear (in the bony labyrinth)

**ot/**-ost-eal, pertaining to the bones of the ear, it refers to the ossicles

**ot/o**-tox-ic, pertaining to poisonous to the ear, it refers to an agent affecting the auditory nerve, hearing and or balance

pan-**ot**-itis, inflammation of all of the ear

par-**ot**-ic, pertaining to beside the ear *e.g.* the parotid gland

peri-**ot**-ic, pertaining to around the ear

pro-**ot**-ic, pertaining to in front of the ear

---

**Saccul/o**, saccule

From a Latin word **sacculus** meaning a small sac. Here saccul/o means the saccule, the smaller of the two divisions of the membranous labyrinth. The saccule contains specialized epithelial cells (hair cells) that detect changes in position of the head, it is concerned with maintaining balance.

**saccul**-ar, 1. pertaining to a saccule 2. sac-shaped

**saccul/o**-cochle-ar, pertaining to the cochlea and saccule

**saccul**-us, a saccule

---

**Salping/o**, auditory tube, Eustachian tube, pharyngotympanic tube

From a Greek word **salpigx**, meaning trumpet tube. Here salping/o means the Eustachian tube, a trumpet-shaped tube that connects the middle ear to the nasopharynx. The Eustachian tube is also called the auditory tube or pharyngotympanic tube, it was first named by Bartolomeo Eustachio (b 1520)

Note: Salping/o is also used to mean the oviduct, Fallopian tube or uterine tube that transports eggs from the ovary to the uterus. See Section 11 The female reproductive system.

**salping**-emphraxis, blocking up of the auditory tube

**salping**-ian, pertaining to auditory tube

**salping**-itic, pertaining to having salpingitis

**salping**-itis, inflammation of the auditory tube

**salping/o**-palat-al, pertaining to the palate and the auditory tube

**salping/o**-palat-ine, pertaining to the palate and auditory tube

**salping/o**-pharyng-eal, pertaining to the pharynx and auditory tube

**salping/o**-scope, an instrument to view or examine the auditory tube

**salping/o**-scopy, technique of viewing or examining the auditory tube

**salping/o**-staphyl-ine, pertaining to the uvula and the auditory tube

**salpinx**, the auditory tube, also known as the Eustachian tube or pharyngo-tympanic tube

---

**Staped/i/o**, stapes

From a Latin word **stapes**, meaning stirrup. Here stapedi/o means the stapes, the stirrup-shaped ear ossicle that connects the incus to the oval window of the cochlea. The ear ossicles amplify vibrations from the ear drum and transmit them to the oval window of the cochlea.

**staped**-ectomy, removal of the stapes

**stapedi**-al, pertaining to the stapes

**stapedi/o**-lysis, breakdown of the stapes (surgical freeing of a fixed stapes)

**stapedi/o**-ten/o-tomy, incision into the tendon of the stapes

**stapedi/o**-vestibul-ar, pertaining to the vestibule and stapes

---

**Tympan/o**, middle ear, tympanum, tympanic membrane (ear drum)

From a Greek word **tympanon**, meaning a drum. Here tympan/o means the cavity of the middle ear or the tympanic membrane (ear drum).

epi-**tympan**-um, part upon or above the tympanic cavity, it refers to the upper part of the tympanic cavity

intra-**tympan**-ic, pertaining to within the cavity of the middle ear

meso-**tympan**-um, middle part of the tympanic cavity, it refers to the part of the middle ear medial to the ear drum

**tympan/o**-gen-ic, pertaining to originating in the tympanic cavity or middle ear

**tympan/o**-gram, a recording of the compliance (mobility) and impedance of the tympanic membrane

**tympan/o**-metry, technique of measuring the compliance (mobility) and impedance of the tympanic membrane

**tympan/o**-plast-ic, pertaining to tympanoplasty

**tympan/o**-plasty, surgical repair or reconstruction of the ear drum or middle ear

**tympan/o**-centesis, puncture of the ear drum

**tympan/o**-scler-osis, abnormal condition of hardening of the middle ear, it refers to deposition of dense connective tissue around the ear ossicles

**tympan**-itis, inflammation of the ear drum or middle ear

**tympan/o**-tomy, incision into the ear drum or middle ear

**tympan/o**-mastoid-itis, inflammation of the mastoid air cells and tympanic cavity (middle ear)

**tympan**-um, 1. the tympanic membrane 2. the cavity of the middle ear

---

**Utricul/o**, utricle

From a Latin word **utriculus** meaning a small bag or sac. Here utricul/o means the utricle, a membranous sac in the bony labyrinth of the inner ear into which the semi-circular canals open. The utricle is the larger of the two divisions of the membranous labyrinth; it contains specialized epithelial cells (hair cells) that detect changes in position of the head, it is concerned with maintaining balance.

**utricul**-ar, 1. pertaining to the utricle of the inner ear 2. shaped like a utricle (small sac)

**utricul**-itis, inflammation of the utricle of the inner ear

**utricul/o**-ampull-ar, pertaining to the ampullae (expanded ends of the semi-circular canals) and utricle of the inner ear

**utricul/o**-saccul-ar, pertaining to the saccule and utricle of the inner ear

**utricul**-us, the utricle

---

**Vestibul/o**, vestibule

From the Latin word **vestibulum**, meaning entrance. Here vestibul/o means the vestibule, the oval cavity in the middle of the bony labyrinth between the semi-circular canals and the cochlea. The vestibule contains the utricle and saccule, structures concerned with detecting the position of the head and maintaining balance.

**vestibul**-ar, pertaining to the vestibule

**vestibul/o**-cochle-ar, pertaining to the cochlea and vestibule

**vestibul/o**-gen-ic, pertaining to or originating in a vestibule

**vestibul/o**-ocul-ar, 1. pertaining to visual stability during movement of the head (vestibule) 2. pertaining to occulomotor nerves and vestibular nerves

**vestibul/o**-tomy, incision into a vestibule

# Section 11
## The skin

The skin completely covers the body and is continuous with membranes lining the body orifices. It can be regarded as the largest organ in the body. The skin consists of two layers:

- the outer **epidermis**
- the inner **dermis**.

The skin protects us from the environment, plays a major role in thermoregulation and contains sensory nerve endings that detect pain, temperature and touch. In its protective role, the skin prevents the body dehydrating, resists the invasion of micro-organisms and provides protection from the harmful effects of ultraviolet light. Cells in the lower stratum germinativum of the epidermis divide continuously, enabling worn cells at the surface to be replaced. Complete replacement of the epidermis takes approximately 40 days. The underlying dermis contains elastic fibres and collagen fibres that make the skin tough and elastic. Between the skin and underlying structures there is a layer of subcutaneous fat.

Figure 16 shows a section through the skin and combining forms associated with its components.

**Roots and combining forms**, meanings

**Acanth/o**, prickle-cell, spiny
From a Greek word **akantha** meaning thorn. Here, acanth/o means prickle-cell or the prickle-cell layer in the stratum spinosum of the epidermis. These cells are named because of the spines that project from their surface connecting them to neighbouring cells.

**acanth**-oid, resembling a spine

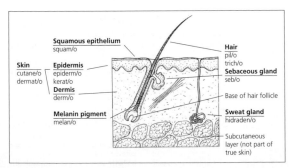

Figure 16 Section through the skin

acanth/o-lysis, separation of the prickle-cell layer of the epidermis, due to breakdown of intercellular bridges (desmosomes)

acanth/o-lyt-ic, pertaining to separation of the prickle-cell layer of the epidermis, due to breakdown of intercellular bridges (desmosomes)

acanth-oma, a tumour of the prickle-cells of the epidermis, it results in hypertrophy of the epidermis

acanth/o-rrhexis, rupture of the prickle-cell layer of the epidermis, due to rupture of intercellular bridges (desmosomes)

acanth-osis, abnormal condition of the prickle-cell layer of the epidermis (hyperplasia and thickening)

acanth/o-tic, pertaining to having acanthosis

pseudo-acanth-osis, false acanthosis, it refers to a condition clinically resembling acanthosis

---

**Quick Reference**

Combining forms of roots relating to the skin:

| | | Page |
|---|---|---|
| Acanth/o | prickle-cell, spiny | 174 |
| Cutane/o | skin | 175 |
| Cut/i | skin | 175 |
| Derm/at/o | skin | 175 |
| Epiderm/o | epidermis | 177 |
| Hidraden/o | sweat gland | 178 |
| Hidr/o | sweat | 178 |
| Ichthy/o | fish-like | 178 |
| Keratin/o | keratin | 179 |
| Kerat/o | epidermis, horny | 179 |
| Melan/o | black, melanin | 180 |
| Onych/o | nail | 180 |
| Pil/o | hair | 181 |
| Rhytid/o | wrinkle | 182 |
| Seb/o | sebum, sebaceous gland | 182 |
| Squam- | scaly | 182 |
| Trich/o | hair | 182 |

---

**Quick Reference**

Common words and combining forms relating to the skin:

| | | Page |
|---|---|---|
| Black | melan/o | 180 |
| Epidermis | epiderm/o, kerat/o | 177/179 |
| Fish-like | ichthy/o | 178 |
| Hair | pil/o, trich/o | 181/182 |
| Horny | kerat/o | 179 |
| Keratin | keratin/o | 179 |
| Melanin | melan/o | 180 |
| Nail | onych/o | 180 |
| Prickle-cell | acanth/o | 174 |
| Scaly | squam- | 182 |
| Sebaceous gland | seb/o | 182 |
| Sebum | seb/o | 182 |
| Skin | cutane/o, cut/i, derma/t/o | 175 |
| Spiny | acanth/o | 174 |
| Sweat | hidr/o | 178 |
| Sweat gland | hidraden/o | 178 |
| Wrinkle | rhytid/o | 182 |

---

**Cutane/o, cut/i/cul-**, skin

From a Latin word **cutis** meaning skin. Here cutane/o means the skin.

cutane-ous, pertaining to the skin

cut/i-cle, 1. small skin, it refers to the epidermis 2. the epidermis that spreads over the base of the nail from the surrounding skin

cuticul-ar, pertaining to a cuticle

cuticul-ar-iz-ation, process or action of making skin (over a wound)

cut/i-reaction, inflammation or other reaction of the skin, for example to an irritant produced by an infective agent

cut-is, the skin

cut/i-sect-or, device that cuts small sections of skin for examination

sub-cutane-ous, pertaining to under the skin

sub-cuticul-ar, 1. pertaining to under the epidermis 2. pertaining to under a cuticle

---

**Derm/a/t/o**, skin

From a Greek word **derma**, meaning skin. Here dermat/o is used to mean the skin.

ecto-**derm**, outer skin, it refers to the primary germ layer in the early embryo that gives rise to epithelia and nervous tissue

electro-**derm**-al, pertaining to the electrical activity or property of the skin (its electrical resistance)

endo-**derm**, inner skin, it refers to the primary germ layer in the early embryo that gives rise to the epithelium of the pharynx, digestive tract, bladder and urethra

epi-**dermis**, the structure upon the dermis (the stratified, squamous, keratinized epithelium that forms the outer part of the skin). See the combining form epiderm/o

**derm**-abras-ion, action of abrasion on the skin (skin planing of superficial lesions)

**derm**-al, pertaining to or belonging to the skin or dermis

**dermat**-alg-ia, condition of pain of the skin (a local sensation, that may be due to nervous disease)

**dermat**-itis, inflammation of the skin

**dermat/o**-auto-plasty, surgical repair or reconstruction of the skin from one's self (a graft from one part of the body to another)

**dermat/o**-chalasis, slackening or loosening of the skin

**dermat/o**-conjunctiv-itis, inflammation of the conjunctiva and skin (around the conjunctiva)

**dermat/o**-cyst, a bladder-like tumour of the skin (a closed epithelium-lined cavity)

**dermat/o**-cyst-oma, a bladder-like tumour of the skin (a closed epithelium-lined cavity)

**dermat/o**-dyn-ia, condition of pain of the skin (a local sensation, that may be due to nervous disease)

**dermat/o**-fibr-oma, a fibrous tumour of the skin

**dermat/o**-fibr/o-sarc-oma, a malignant fibrous tumour (sarcoma) of the skin

**dermat/o**-gen-ic, pertaining to producing or forming skin or a skin disease

**dermat/o**-glyph-ics, the science of studying carvings of the skin (the line and ridge patterns of the fingers, palms and soles as genetic indicators and to

discover developmental anomalies). From a Greek word *glyphos* meaning carved

**dermat/o**-graph-ia, condition of writing on the skin (a condition in which a red weal develops when the skin is scratched with a blunt instrument) Syn. dermographia

**dermat/o**-graph-ic, pertaining to dermatographia

**dermat/o**-graph-ism, process of writing on the skin (a condition in which a red weal develops when the skin is scratched with a blunt instrument)

**dermat/o**-heter/o-plasty, surgical repair or reconstruction of the skin taken from a different species (a skin graft taken from another species, only human autografts and allografts are used in man)

**dermat/o**-log-ist, a medical specialist who studies the skin (anatomy, diseases and treatment of)

**dermat/o**-logy, the study of the skin (anatomy, diseases and treatment of)

**dermat/o**-lysis, loosening of the skin (the skin hangs loosely in folds, an inherited condition called cutis laxa)

**dermat**-oma, a tumour of the skin

**dermat/o**-malac-ia, condition of softening of the skin

**derma**-tome, an instrument for cutting skin (thin slices for grafting)

**dermat/o**-myc-osis, abnormal condition of fungi in the skin (fungal infection) Syn. dermomycosis

**dermat/o**-myi-asis, presence of disease of the skin caused by flies or maggots. From a Greek word *myia* meaning fly

**dermat/o**-my-oma, a tumour of (smooth) muscle of the skin

**dermat/o**-myos-itis, inflammation of muscles and skin

**dermat/o**-ophthalm-itis, inflammation of the eye and skin

**dermat/o**-path-ic, pertaining to disease of the skin

**dermat/o**-pathy, disease of the skin

**dermat/o**-pharmac/o-logy, the study of pharmacology in relation to skin diseases and disorders

**dermatophil**-osis, abnormal condition or disease caused by the fungus *Dermatophilus*

**Dermatophilus**, a genus of pathogenic fungi (actinomycetes) infecting the skin of animals and sometimes man

**dermat/o**-phyte, a skin plant (a fungus parasitic on the skin)

**dermat/o**-phyt-osis, abnormal condition or disease of skin plants (fungi infecting the skin, hair and nails such as *Tinea pedis* or Athlete's foot)

**dermat/o**-plas-ia, condition of forming skin or skin cells

**dermat/o**-plast-ic, pertaining to surgical reconstruction or repair of the skin (plastic surgery or skin grafting)

**dermat/o**-plasty, surgical reconstruction or repair of the skin (plastic surgery, skin grafting)

**dermat/o**-scler-osis, abnormal condition or disease of hardening of the skin

**dermat/o**-scopy, technique of viewing or examining the skin (*e.g.* with a microscope to see superficial capillaries)

**dermat**-osis, abnormal condition or disease of the skin

**dermat/o**-zoon, a skin animal (an animal parasite of the skin *e.g.* an ectoparasite such as Scabies)

**derm**-ic, 1. pertaining to or belonging to the skin 2. pertaining to or belonging to the dermis of the skin

**derm/o**-actinomyc-osis, abnormal condition or skin disease caused by fungi belonging to the genus Actinomyces

**derm/o**-blast, a layer of immature cells or embryonic cells in the mesoderm that develop into the dermis

**derm/o**-graph-ia, condition of writing on the skin (a condition in which a red weal develops when the skin is scratched with a blunt instrument) Syn. dermatographia

**derm**-oid, 1. resembling skin 2. a dermoid cyst (a teratoma often found in the ovary that contains keratinous material)

**dermoid**-ectomy, removal of a dermoid cyst

**derm/o**-labi-al, pertaining to the lips and skin

**derm/o**-myc-osis, abnormal condition of fungi in the skin (fungal infection) Syn. dermatomycosis

**derm/o**-necr/o-tic, 1. pertaining to dead tissue in the skin 2. pertaining to necrosis of the skin

**derm/o**-phleb-itis, inflammation of (superficial) veins and surrounding skin

**derm/o**-synov-itis, inflammation of a synovial membrane (tendon sheath or bursa) and (overlying) skin

**derm/o**-vascul-ar, pertaining to blood vessels of the skin

hetero-**derm**-ic, pertaining to skin from a different species (for use as a skin graft)

hypo-**derm**-ic, pertaining to under the skin

hypo-**dermis**, tissue below the skin, the subcutaneous tissue

intra-**derm**-al, pertaining to within the skin

meso-**derm**, middle skin, it refers to the primary germ layer in the early embryo that gives rise to muscle, connective tissue and some epithelial tissue

pachy-**derma**, thickening of the skin

tri-**derm**-ic, pertaining to three skins, it refers to originating from the three germ layers of the embryo ectoderm, mesoderm and endoderm

xanth/o-**derma**, yellowing of the skin

xero-**derm**-ia, condition of dry skin

---

**Epiderm/o**, epidermis

From the Greek words **derma** meaning skin and **epi-** meaning upon. Here epiderm/o means the epidermis, the upper layer of the skin also known as the cuticle. There are several layers (strata) of cells in the epidermis which extend from dividing cells in the stratum germinativum to the surface stratum corneum. The cells on the surface are dead, flat, non-nucleated and their cytoplasm has been replaced by keratin. As cells wear off at the surface, they are replaced by cells originating in the germinative layer.

The epidermis is waterproof and protects the body against abrasion, invasion by micro-organisms and damage from ultraviolet light.

**epiderm**-al, pertaining to the epidermis

**epiderm**-ic, pertaining to the epidermis

**epiderm**-itis, inflammation of the epidermis

**epiderm**/o-dys-plas-ia, condition of poor growth of cells of the epidermis

**epiderm**-oid, 1. resembling epidermis 2. a tumour containing epidermal elements found at sites away from the skin

**epiderm**/o-lysis, breakdown or loosening of the epidermis usually with the formation of blisters

**epiderm**/o-myc-osis, abnormal condition of fungal infection of the epidermis

**epiderm**/o-phyt-osis, abnormal condition of plants (fungi) in the epidermis *e.g.* ringworm

**epiderm**/o-trop-ic, pertaining to having an affinity for the epidermis

sub-**epiderm**-al, pertaining to under the epidermis

---

**Hidraden**/o, sweat gland

From the Greek words **hidros**, meaning sweat and **aden** meaning gland. Here, hidraden/o means the sudoriferous gland or sweat gland found in the dermis of the skin. The sweat gland passes its secretion to a pore on the surface via a sweat duct that runs through the epidermis. The evaporation of sweat from the skin cools the body and plays a major role in the homeostatic regulation of body temperature.

**hidraden**-itis, inflammation of the sweat glands

**hidraden**/o-carcin-oma, a malignant tumour derived from a sweat gland

**hidraden**-oid, resembling a sweat gland

**hidraden**-oma, a tumour of a sweat gland (used as a general term for skin tumours containing epithelial cells similar to those found in sweat glands)

---

**Hidr**/o, sweat

From a Greek word **hidros**, meaning sweat. Here, hidr/o means sweat or sweating (perspiration).

an-**hidr**-osis, abnormal condition of without sweat (diminished or absent secretion)

an-**hidr**/o-tic, 1. pertaining to having anhidrosis 2. pertaining to without sweat 3. an agent that inhibits sweating

dys-**hidr**-osis, 1. abnormal condition of poor or bad sweating (any disturbance of the sweat mechanism) 2. pompholyx, an itchy, vesicular skin eruption occurring on the hands and feet

hemi-**hidr**-osis, abnormal condition of sweating on half (one side) of the body

**hidr**/o-cyst-oma, a cystic, bladder-like tumour originating in a sweat gland

**hidr**/o-poiesis, the formation or production of sweat

**hidr**/o-poie-tic, pertaining to the formation or production of sweat

**hidr**/o-schesis, 1. retention of sweat 2. suppression of sweating. From a Greek word *schesis* meaning a checking

**hidr**-osis, abnormal condition of sweating

**hidr**/o-tic, 1. pertaining to having hidrosis 2. an agent that stimulates sweating

hyper-**hidr**-osis, condition of above normal or excessive sweating

hyper-**hidr**/o-tic, 1. pertaining to above normal or excessive sweating 2. pertaining to having hyperhidrosis

hypo-**hidr**-osis, condition of below normal or diminished sweating

hypo-**hidr**/o-tic, 1. pertaining to below normal or diminished sweating 2. pertaining to having hypohidrosis

poly-**hidr**-osis, condition of much or excessive sweating

---

**Ichthy**/o, fish, fish-like

From a Greek word **ichthys** meaning fish. Here ichty/o means fish or fish-like particularly when referring to a scaly skin.

**ichthy**-oid, resembling fish, fish-like

**ichthy**-osis, abnormal condition of fish (skin), It refers to a congenital condition in which the skin is dry and scaly

**ichthy/o**-tic, pertaining to or having the characteristics of ichthyosis

---

**Keratin/o,** keratin

From a Greek word **keras**, meaning horn, horny tissue. Here, keratin/o means keratin, the waterproof scleroprotein found in the outer layers of the epidermis, nails and hair.

hyper-**keratin**-iz-ation, process of producing above normal amounts of keratin in the epidermis

**kerat**-ic, pertaining to keratin

**keratin**-ase, an enzyme that digests keratin

**keratin**-iz-ation, process of forming keratin or horny tissue

**keratin**-ize, to form or become keratin or horny tissue

**keratin/o**-cyte, a keratin cell, a type of epidermal cell that synthesizes keratin

**keratin**-oid, resembling keratin

**keratin**-ous, pertaining to keratin or horny tissue

---

**Kerat/o,** epidermis

From a Greek word **keras**, meaning horn, horny tissue. Here kerat/o means the epidermis, or the outer or horny layer of the epidermis (stratum corneum) that contains keratin, a waterproof protein.

Note: kerat/o is also used to mean the cornea of the eye, see Section 9 The eye.

dys-**kerat**-osis, abnormal condition or disease of the horny tissue of the epidermis, it refers to poor keratinization of cells in the epidermis

hyper-**kerat**-osis, abnormal condition above normal growth or thickening of the horny tissue of the epidermis

hyper-**kerat/o**-tic, pertaining to above normal growth (hypertrophy) of the horny tissue of the epidermis

**kerat**-ic, pertaining to keratin or horny tissue

**kerat/o**-acanth-oma, a tumour of the epidermis derived from prickle cells

**kerat/o**-angi-oma, a tumour or swelling of the epidermis made up of (blood) vessels

**kerat/o**-derma, a growth (hypertrophy) of the horny layer of the skin

**kerat/o**-dermat-itis, inflammation of the horny layer of the skin

**kerat/o**-dermat-osis, abnormal condition or disease of the horny layer of the skin

**kerat/o**-genesis, formation of horn-like tissue

**kerat/o**-genet-ic, pertaining to the formation of horny tissue

**kerat/o**-gen-ous, pertaining to the formation of horny tissue

**kerat/o**-hyal-in, a glass-like chemical (eleidin) found in the epidermis (in the granular layer )

**kerat/o**-hyal-ine, pertaining to glass-like (transparent) and horny

**kerat/o**-lysis, breakdown or separation of the epidermis

**kerat/o**-lyt-ic, 1. pertaining to breakdown or separation of the epidermis 2. an agent that breaks down the epidermis (used for removing warts)

**kerat**-oma, a tumour or swelling of the epidermis, it refers to any wart-like growth or hypertrophy of the epidermis

**kerat/o**-malac-ia, condition of softening of the horny layer of the skin

**kerat**-onc-us, a tumour or swelling of the epidermis Syn. keratoma, keratosis

**kerat/o**-plas-ia, condition of formation of horny layer of the epidermis, due to an increase in cells of the epidermis

**kerat**-ose, horny or presence of horny tissue

**kerat**-osis, abnormal condition or disease of the horny tissue of the epidermis, it refers to any wart-like growth or hypertrophy of the epidermis

179

**Melan/o**, melanin, black, dark

From a Greek word **melas** meaning black. Here melan/o means melanin, the black pigment found in hair, skin and the choroid of the eye.

**melan**-ism, process of darkening of skin and other tissues

**melan/o**-blast, an immature cell or embryonic cell that develops into a melanocyte

**melan/o**-blast-oma, a tumour of embryonic or undifferentiated cells that produce melanin

**melan/o**-carcin-oma, a carcinoma containing melanin (malignant)

**melan/o**-cyte, a cell containing or forming melanin

**melan/o**-cyt-oma, a tumour composed of melanocytes

**melan/o**-derma, skin containing melanin, an abnormal increase causing a discoloration of the skin

**melan/o**-dermat-itis, inflammation of the skin with deposition of melanin

**melan/o**-derm-ic, pertaining to dark or pigmented skin

**melan/o**-gen, an agent (colourless chromogen) found in the body that can be converted into melanin

**melan/o**-genesis, the formation of melanin

**melan/o**-hidr-osis, abnormal condition of pigmented sweat

**melan**-oid, resembling melanin

**melan**-oma, a tumour of dark melanin containing cells (melanocytes)

**melan**-omat-osis, abnormal condition of having (malignant) melanomas

**melan**-onych-ia, condition of nails pigmented with melanin

**melan/o**-path-ia, any condition of disease accompanied by pigmentation of the skin or other tissue

**melan/o**-pathy, any disease accompanied by pigmentation of the skin or other tissue

**melan/o**-phage, a cell that engulfs melanin (a histiocyte containing melanin)

**melan/o**-phore, a pigment cell containing melanin

**melan/o**-sarc-oma, a malignant fleshy tumour containing melanin

**melan/o**-sarc-omat-osis, abnormal condition of having multiple malignant melanosarcomas

**melan**-osis, abnormal condition of pigment deposition in the skin or other tissues

**melan/o**-some, an intracellular body containing melanin

**melan/o**-tic, pertaining to melanosis

**melan/o**-troph, nourishing melanin, it refers to a cell in the pituitary gland that produces MSH melanocyte stimulating hormone

**melan/o**-trop-ic, pertaining to having an affinity for melanin

**melan**-ur-ia, condition of dark pigment in the urine

**melan**-ur-ic, 1. pertaining to dark pigment in the urine 2. pertaining to melanuria

---

**Onych/o**, nail

From a Greek word **onychos,** meaning nail. Here, onych/o means the nail, a structure that protects the tip of a finger or toe.

an-**onych**-ia, condition of absence of nails (congenital)

ep-**onych**-ium, band of epidermal cells that extends onto the proximal lunula of the nail

hyp-**onych**-ial, pertaining to the hyponychium

hyp-**onych**-ium, structure below the nail, it refers to thickened epidermis under the free edge of the nail

leuc-**onych**-ia, condition of white nails (patchy discoloration)

macr-**onych**-ia, condition of large nails (abnormally long)

**onych**-alg-ia, condition of pain in the nails Syn. onychodynia

**onych**-a-troph-ia, 1. condition of without nourishment or wasting away of the nails 2. atrophy of the nails

**onych**-a-trophy, 1. without nourishment or wasting away of the nails 2. atrophy of the nails

**onych**-auxis, overgrowth of the nails (hypertrophy)

**onych**-ectomy, removal of a nail

**onych**-ia, condition of the nails (abnormality due to inflammation of the nail bed with loss of the nail)

**onych**-itis, inflammation of the nail (bed or matrix) Syn. onychia

**onych/o**-crypt-osis, abnormal condition of a hidden nail (an ingrowing nail)

**onych/o**-dyn-ia, condition of pain in the nails Syn. onychalgia

**onych/o**-dys-trophy, poor growth or poor nutrition of nails (malformation from impaired nutrition)

**onych/o**-gen-ic, pertaining to formation of nails or nail tissue

**onych/o**-graph, an instrument that records the nail, it records the nail pulse and blood pressure under the nail

**onych/o**-gryph-osis, abnormal condition of curved or claw-like nails. From a Greek word *gryphein* meaning to curve

**onych/o**-gryp-osis, abnormal condition of curved or claw-like nails. From a Greek word *gryphein* meaning to curve

**onych/o**-helc-osis, abnormal condition of ulcers affecting the nails

**onych/o**-heter/o-top-ia, condition of nails in a different place, it refers to abnormally placed nails

**onych**-oid, resembling a nail

**onych/o**-lysis, separation of a nail from its bed

**onych**-oma, a tumour arising from cells in the nail matrix

**onych/o**-madesis, total loss of the nail. From a Greek word *madein* meaning to fall off

**onych/o**-malac-ia, condition of softening of the nails

**onych/o**-myc-osis, abnormal condition or disease of fungi in the nails

**onych/o**-nos-us, a disease of the nails Syn. onychopathy

**onych**-opac-ity, condition or state of shaded nails, it refers to white patches in a nail Syn. leuconychia. From a Latin word *opacus* meaning shaded

**onych/o**-path-ic, pertaining to disease of the nails

**onych/o**-path/o-logy, the study of disease of the nails

**onych/o**-pathy, disease of the nails

**onych/o**-phag-ia, condition of eating nails (biting)

**onych/o**-phagy, condition of eating nails (biting)

**onych/o**-phyma, swelling of the nails (thickening or hypertrophy)

**onych/o**-ptosis, falling or displacement of the nails (results in loss of the nail)

**onych/o**-rrhex-ia, condition of breaking or rupturing of the nails

**onych/o**-rrhexis, breaking or rupturing of the nails

**onych/o**-schiz-ia, condition of split nails Syn. onycholysis

**onych**-osis, abnormal condition or disease of nails (deformity of)

**onych/o**-till/o-man-ia, manic condition in which nails are torn out or picked. From a Greek word *tillein* meaning to pull

**onych/o**-tomy, incision into a nail

**onych/o**-trophy, nourishment or development of the nails

pachy-**onych**-ia, condition of thickening of the nails

par-**onych**-ia, a condition beside a nail (inflammation in tissue around a nail)

par-**onych**-ial, 1. pertaining to paronychia 2. a condition beside a nail (inflammation in tissue around a nail)

schiz/o-**onych**-ia, condition of split nails

## Pil/o, hair

From a Latin word **pilus**, meaning hair. Here pil/o means hair, the epidermal structure that grows from a hair follicle. Hairs are present on all parts of human skin except palms, sole, lips, glans penis and that surrounding the terminal phalanges.

**pil/o**-cyst-ic, pertaining to a (dermoid) cyst containing hair

**pil/o**-gen-ic, 1. pertaining to forming hair 2. pertaining to originating in hair

**pil/o**-logy, the study of hair (anatomy, diseases and treatment of)

**pil/o**-matrix-oma, a tumour derived from cells of the hair matrix (mitotic cells from which a hair develops, at the base of a follicle)

**pil/o**-motor, pertaining to action or movement of a hair (piloerection by arrector pili muscles)

**pil/o**-nid-al, pertaining to (growth) of hair in a cyst, nidus or other internal part

**pil**-ose, full of hair (covered with hair)

**pil/o**-sebace-ous, pertaining to sebaceous glands and hair (follicles)

**pil**-osis, abnormal condition or disease of hair, it refers to excessive growth of hair or hair in an unusual place

**pilos**-ity, state or condition of hair, it refers to excessive growth of hair or hair in an unusual place

**pil**-ous, pertaining to hair (covered with hair) Syn. pilose

**pil**-us, a hair

---

**Rhytid/o**, wrinkle

From a Greek word **rhytis** meaning wrinkle. Here, rhytid/o means a wrinkle of the skin.

**rhytid**-ectomy, surgical elimination of wrinkles (by removal of the skin)

**rhytid/o**-plasty, surgical repair or reconstruction to remove wrinkles from the skin

**rhytid**-osis, abnormal condition of wrinkling

---

**Seb/o**, sebace/o, sebum,
sebaceous gland

From a Latin word **sebum**, meaning fat or grease. Here seb/o and sebace/o mean sebum or sebaceous gland. Sebum is the oily secretion of the sebaceous glands, it contains fatty acids, cholesterol and dead cells. Sebum keeps hair soft and shiny, is waterproof and acts as a bactericidal and fungicidal agent preventing the growth of microbes on the skin.

**sebace/o**-follicul-ar, pertaining to hair follicles and sebaceous glands

**seb/o**-cyst-oma, a sebaceous cyst (a bladder-like tumour of a sebaceous gland)

**seb/o**-lith, a stone or calculus in a sebaceous gland

**seb/o**-rrhoea, excessive flow or discharge of sebum (also used to mean seborrhoeic dermatitis)

**seb/o**-rrhoe-al, pertaining to excessive flow or discharge of sebum

**seb/o**-rrhoe-ic, pertaining to excessive flow or discharge of sebum

**seb/o**-troph-ic, pertaining to nourishment of the sebaceous glands (producing excessive secretion)

**seb/o**-trop-ic, pertaining to stimulating the sebaceous glands (producing excessive secretion)

**seb**-um, the fatty secretion of the sebaceous gland

---

**Squam-**, scale, scaly

From a Latin word **squama** meaning scale. Here squam- means scaly. The epidermis is composed of a squamous, stratified, keratinized epithelium that is scaly in appearance when viewed through a microscope.

**squam**-ate, pertaining to scales, scale-like or covered with scales

**squam**-ous, pertaining to scales, scale-like or covered with scales

---

**Trich/o**, hair

From a Greek word **trichos**, meaning hair. Here trich/o means hair, the epidermal structure that grows from a hair follicle. Hairs are present on all parts of human skin except palms, sole, lips, glans penis and that surrounding the terminal phalanges.

hyper-**trich**-iasis, abnormal condition of having more than the normal amount of hair

hyper-**trich**-osis, abnormal condition of having more than the normal amount of hair

hypo-**trich**-osis, abnormal condition of having less than the normal amount of hair

**182**

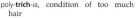

poly-**trich**-ia, condition of too much hair

schiz/o-**trich**-ia, condition of splitting of hairs at their ends

**trich**-itis, inflammation of hair, it refers to inflammation of the bulb at the base of each hair follicle

**trich/o**-aesthes-ia, condition of hair sensitivity (when touched)

**trich/o**-an-aesthes-ia, condition of without hair sensitivity (when touched)

**trich/o**-clas-ia, condition of breaking of hair (due to brittleness)

**trich/o**-epitheli-oma, a tumour formed from epithelial cells of hair follicles

**trich/o**-gen, an agent that produces or promotes hair (growth)

**trich/o**-gen-ous, pertaining to the formation of hair

**trich**-oid, resembling hair

**trich/o**-logy, the study of hair (anatomy, diseases and treatment of)

**trich/o**-megaly, having large hairs (excessive growth of eyebrows and eyelashes)

**trich/o**-myc-osis, abnormal condition or disease of fungi in the hair (follicles)

**trich/o**-nod-osis, abnormal condition or disease of nodes (knots) in the hairs

**trich/o**-pathy, disease of hair

**trich/o**-phag-ia, condition of eating (biting) hair (a neurotic habit)

**trich/o**-phagy, process of eating (biting) hair (a neurotic habit)

**trich/o**-phyt-osis, abnormal condition or disease of plants in the hair (fungal infection)

**trich/o**-poli-osis, abnormal condition of greying of the hair

**trich/o**-ptil-osis, abnormal condition of splitting of hairs (at the end). From a Greek word *ptilosis* meaning plumage. Here, it refers to the feathery end of the hairs

**trich/o**-rrhexis, rupture or breaking of hairs

**trich/o**-schisis, splitting of hairs (at the end) Syn. trichoptilosis, schizotrichia

**trich**-osis, abnormal condition or disease of hair

**trich/o**-till/o-man-ia, manic condition in which hair is plucked out or pulled. From a Greek word *tillein* meaning to pull

**trich/o**-trophy, the nourishment or development of hair

# Section 12
# The nose and mouth

## The nose

Air enters the nose through two nostrils or anterior nares into a large irregular nasal cavity that is separated into two equal passages by a septum. The roof of the nasal cavity is formed by the cribriform plate of the ethmoid bone, sphenoid bone, frontal bone and nasal bone. The floor is formed by the palate, the medial walls by the nasal septum and the lateral walls by the maxilla, ethmoid bone and inferior conchae. The posterior wall is formed by the posterior wall of the pharynx and on its surface lies the pharyngeal tonsil or adenoids, a structure prominent in children that atrophies in adults. The nasal cavity is lined with a very

**Quick Reference**
Combining forms relating to the nose and mouth:

| | | Page |
|---|---|---|
| **Adenoid-** | adenoids | 187 |
| **Antr/o** | Antrum of Highmore (maxillary sinus) | 187 |
| **Bucc/o** | cheek, buccal cavity | 187 |
| **Cement/o** | cementum of a tooth | 188 |
| **Cheil/o** | lip | 188 |
| **Dentin/o** | dentine | 188 |
| **Dent/o** | teeth | 189 |
| **Ethm/o** | ethmoid bone | 189 |
| **Ethmoid/o** | ethmoid bone | 189 |
| **Faci/o** | face | 190 |
| **Gingiv/o** | gum | 190 |
| **Gloss/o** | tongue | 190 |
| **Gnath/o** | jaw | 191 |
| **Labi/o** | lip | 192 |
| **Lal/o** | speech | 192 |
| **Lingu/o** | tongue | 193 |
| **Log/o** | speech, words | 193 |
| **Mandibul/o** | mandible (lower jaw bone) | 193 |
| **Maxill/o** | maxilla (upper jaw bone) | 194 |
| **Ment/o** | chin | 194 |
| **Nas/o** | nose | 194 |
| **Nasopharyng/o** | nasopharynx | 195 |
| **Odont/o** | teeth | 195 |
| **Or/o** | mouth | 196 |
| **Osm/o** | smell, odour, olfaction | 197 |
| **Osphresi/o** | smell, odour, olfaction | 197 |
| **Palat/o** | palate | 197 |
| **Parotid/o** | parotid gland | 198 |
| **Parot/o** | parotid gland | 198 |
| **Pharyng/o** | pharynx | 198 |
| **-phas-** | speech | 199 |
| **Phasi/o** | speech | 199 |
| **Phon/o** | sound, speech, voice | 199 |
| **Prosop/o** | face | 200 |
| **Ptyal/o** | saliva | 200 |
| **Rhin/o** | nose | 200 |
| **Sept/o** | nasal septum, septum | 202 |
| **Sial/o** | saliva, salivary gland or duct | 202 |
| **Sin/o** | sinus | 203 |
| **Sinus/o** | sinus | 203 |
| **Staphyl/o** | uvula | 203 |
| **Stomat/o** | mouth | 203 |
| **Tonsill/o** | tonsil | 204 |
| **Turbin/o** | nasal conchae, turbinate bones | 205 |
| **Uran/o** | palate | 205 |
| **Uvul/o** | uvula | 205 |

vascular ciliated epithelium containing
mucus-secreting cells.

The function of the nose is to begin
the process by which inspired air is
warmed, moistened and filtered. In
addition, the nose is the organ of the
sense of smell or olfaction; its receptors
are located in the olfactory epithelium
in the roof of the nasal cavity. The
receptors for olfaction lie in the region
of the cribriform plate, ethmoid bones
and superior conchae. In order for us to
smell a substance it must be volatile,
so it can be carried into the nose and
dissolve in the mucus covering the
receptors. Humans can distinguish
between 2000 and 4000 different
odours.

The paranasal sinuses are cavities in
the bones of the face and cranium that
open into the nasal cavity through
tiny passageways. The sinuses play an
important role in giving resonance to
the voice and serve to lighten the skull.

Inspired air enters the nose through
the nostrils (anterior nares), passes
through the nasal cavity and leaves
via the posterior nares into the nasopharynx.

## The mouth

The mouth or oral cavity is bounded by
the closed lips and facial muscles, the
palate and lower jaw. The palate forms
the roof of the mouth and is divided
into the anterior hard palate and the
posterior soft palate. The uvula, a soft
fold of muscle covered with mucous
membrane, hangs down from the
middle of the free border of the soft
palate. In the folds formed by the soft
palate and oropharynx lie the palatine
tonsils, patches of lymphoid tissue
containing cells that form antibodies
and lymphocytes to defend against
infection. Another pair of tonsils, the
lingual tonsils lie near the base of the
tongue.

The mouth contains the upper and
lower teeth embedded in the alveoli or
sockets of the alveolar ridges on the
mandible and maxilla. By their cutting

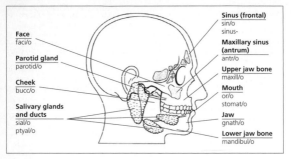

Figure 17 Sagittal section through the head

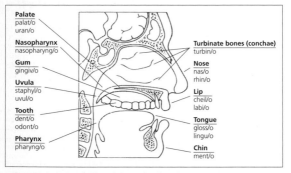

Figure 18 Sagittal section through the nasal and buccal cavity

and grinding action teeth increase the surface area of food and make it easy to swallow. The tongue occupies the floor of the mouth, it plays an important role in speech, mastication (chewing), deglutition (swallowing), and gustation (the sense of taste). When a substance is eaten, four types of receptor can be stimulated on the tongue, producing sensations for sweet, bitter, salty, and sour.

Three pairs of salivary glands (parotid, submaxillary and sublingual) secrete saliva into the mouth to lubricate the food and begin the digestion of starch. Once food has been mixed with saliva and masticated, it is rolled into a bolus by the tongue and muscles of the cheek and is swallowed into the stomach via the pharynx and oesophagus.

Figures 17 and 18 show sagittal sections through the nose and mouth and combining forms associated with their components.

## Roots and combining forms, meanings

### Adenoid-, adenoids

From the Greek words **aden** meaning gland and **eidos** meaning form. Here adenoid- means the adenoids, an enlarged pharyngeal tonsil that extends into the nasopharynx of children. Sometimes it obstructs the passage of air or interferes with hearing when it blocks the entrance to the auditory tube.

Note: although ending with an 's', **adenoids** is used to mean the single enlarged pharyngeal tonsil.

**aden**-oid, 1. resembling a gland 2. hypertrophy of adenoid tissue of a pharyngeal tonsil

**adenoid**-ectomy, removal of the adenoids (the pharyngeal tonsil)

**adenoid**-ism, process of describing the presence of enlarged adenoids (giving characteristic adenoid face, facial pallor and breathing through the mouth)

**adenoid**-itis, inflammation of the adenoids (the pharyngeal tonsil)

**adenoids**, the condition of having an enlarged pharyngeal tonsil (formed by hypertrophy of lymphoid tissue into the nasopharynx)

### Antr/o, antrum

From a Greek word **antron**, meaning cave. Here antr/o means the superior maxillary sinus, the Antrum of Highmore.

**antr**-al, pertaining to an antrum

**antr**-ectomy, removal of an antrum (the walls of)

**antr**-itis, 1. inflammation of an antrum 2. inflammation of the Antrum of Highmore (maxillary sinus)

**antr/o**-bucc-al, pertaining to a cheek or buccal cavity and Antrum of Highmore (maxillary sinus)

**antr/o**-cele, 1. a protrusion or hernia of an antrum 2. a protrusion or hernia of the Antrum of Highmore (maxillary sinus)

**antr/o**-dyn-ia, 1. condition of pain in an antrum 2. condition of pain in the Antrum of Highmore (maxillary sinus)

**antr/o**-nas-al, pertaining to the nose and Antrum of Highmore (maxillary sinus)

**antr/o**-or-al, pertaining to the mouth and Antrum of Highmore (maxillary sinus)

**antr/o**-scope, 1. an instrument to view the Antrum of Highmore (maxillary sinus)

**antr/o**-scopy, technique of viewing or examining an antrum especially the Antrum of Highmore (maxillary sinus)

**antr/o**-stomy, formation of an opening into the Antrum of Highmore (maxillary sinus) or the name of the opening so created

**antr/o**-tome, an instrument for cutting into an antrum

**antr/o**-tomy, incision into an antrum

### Bucc/o, buccal cavity, cheek

From a Latin word **bucca** meaning cheek. Here, bucc/o means cheek or buccal cavity (the cavity of the mouth).

**bucc**-al, pertaining to or belonging to a cheek or buccal cavity

**bucc/o**-cervic-al, pertaining to the cervical margin (neck of a tooth) and the cheek surface

**bucc/o**-dist-al, pertaining to the distal surface (of a tooth) and the cheek surface

**bucc/o**-gingiv-al, pertaining to the gums and cheeks

**bucc/o**-lingu-al, pertaining to the tongue and cheek

**bucc/o**-mesi-al, pertaining to the mesial surface (of a tooth) and the cheek surface

**bucc/o**-nas-al, pertaining to the nose (nasal cavity) and the buccal cavity (mouth)

**bucc/o**-nas/o-pharyng-eal, pertaining to the pharynx, nose (nasal cavity) and buccal cavity (mouth)

**bucc/o**-pharyng-eal, pertaining to the pharynx and buccal cavity (mouth)

**bucc/o**-pulp-al, pertaining to the pulp (in the cavity of a tooth) and the buccal surface

**bucc/o**-vers-ion, process of turning (of a tooth) towards the cheek surface

mesi-**bucc**-al, pertaining to the buccal surface and mesial surface (of a tooth)

---

**Cement/i/o**, cementum of a tooth

From a Latin word **caementum** meaning unhewn stone. Here cement/o means cementum, the supporting layer of calcified tissue covering the surface of the root of a tooth.

**cement/i**-cle, small body of cementum in the periodontal membrane of a tooth root

**cement/o**-blast, an immature cell or embryonic cell that forms cementum

**cement/o**-blast-oma, a tumour formed from cementoblasts (an odontogenic fibroma containing a little calcified tissue)

**cement/o**-clas-ia, condition of breakdown and resorption of cementum on a tooth root

**cement/o**-cyte, a cementum cell

**cement/o**-genesis, formation of cementum on a tooth root

**cement**-oma, a tumour or swelling of cementum (may be a reaction to a damaged tooth)

peri-**cement**-itis, inflammation around the cementum, it refers to inflammation around the supporting tissue of the teeth in the periodontium

---

**Cheil/o**, lip

From a Greek word **cheilos**, meaning lip. Here cheil/o means a lip, and refers to either of the two fleshy folds, upper and lower, bordering the external entrance to the mouth.

**cheil**-alg-ia, condition of pain in the lips

**cheil**-ecto-trop-ion, lip that is turned outwards (everted)

**cheil**-itis, inflammation of the lip

**cheil/o**-carcin-oma, a malignant tumour of the lip

**cheil/o**-gnath/o-palat-osis, abnormal condition of palate, jaw and lip, it refers to a cleft palate and cleft lip involving the jaw

**cheil/o**-gnath/o-prosopo-schisis, a facial cleft continuing into the face, jaw and (upper) lip

**cheil/o**-gnath/o-schisis, a cleft lip (harelip) involving the jaw

**cheil/o**-gnath-us, a cleft lip (hare-lip) involving the jaw

**cheil**-onc-us, a tumour of a lip

**cheil/o**-phag-ia, pertaining to eating the lip, it refers to the habit of biting the lip

**cheil/o**-plast-ic, 1. pertaining to cheiloplasty 2. surgical repair or reconstruction of a lip

**cheil/o**-plasty, surgical repair or reconstruction of a lip

**cheil/o**-rrhaphy, stitching or suturing of a lip

**cheil/o**-schisis, a split or cleft lip

**cheil/o**-scopy, technique of viewing or examining the lips (to identify patterns)

**cheil**-osis, abnormal condition of the lips (drying with fissures, seen in riboflavin deficiency)

**cheil/o**-stomat/o-plasty, surgical repair or reconstruction of the mouth and lips

**cheil/o**-tomy, incision into a lip

macro-**cheil**-ia, condition of abnormally large lips

micro-**cheil**-ia, condition of abnormally small lips

pachy-**cheil**-ia, condition of thickening of the lips

syn-**cheil**-ia, condition of fusion of the lips (a congenital condition)

---

**Dentin/o**, dentine

From a Latin word **dens** meaning tooth. Here, dentin/o means dentine, the

188

calcified tissue forming the body of a tooth beneath the enamel and cementum enclosing the pulp chamber and root canals.

**dentin/o**-genesis, formation of dentine

**dentin/o**-gen-ic, pertaining to forming dentine

**dentin**-oma, a tumour originating in teeth composed of dentine

**dentin**-um, dentine

**Dent/i/o**, teeth

From a Latin word **dens** meaning tooth. Here dent/o means a tooth or teeth. The teeth are used for mastication, the chewing of food. The first teeth are known as deciduous teeth, milk teeth or the primary set. There are twenty deciduous teeth that are usually shed by the age of seven, they are replaced by the permanent teeth or secondary set. The permanent set, thirty-two in number, is usually complete by the late teens.

**dens**, a tooth

**dent**-al, pertaining to the teeth

**dent**-alg-ia, condition of pain in the teeth or toothache

**dent**-ate, 1. tooth-shaped 2. having one's own teeth

**dent**-ia, condition of teeth, it refers to the development and eruption of teeth or teething

**dent/i**-cle, 1. a small, projecting tooth-like process 2. a deposition of calcium or a pulp stone within the pulp chamber of a tooth

**dent/i**-form, having the form of teeth or tooth-shaped

**dent/i**-frice, an agent used for rubbing the teeth, it refers to any liquid, powder or paste used for cleaning the teeth. From a Latin word *fricare* meaning to rub.

**dent/i**-lab/i-al, pertaining to the lips and teeth

**dent**-ine, the hard, calcified tissue forming the body of a tooth beneath the enamel and cementum, enclosing the pulp chamber and root canals

**dent**-ist, a specialist in teeth *i.e.* a practitioner of dentistry

**dent**-istr-y, 1. branch of medicine that deals with the oral cavity, the teeth, the bone of the jaws and overlying soft tissue together with diagnosis and treatment of disease in these structures 2. the work performed by a dentist

**dent/i**-tion, the natural state of one's teeth in position in their alveoli

**dent/o**-alveol-ar, pertaining to the alveoli of teeth, alveoli are the sockets or cavities into which the roots of teeth are embedded

**dent/o**-cement-al, pertaining to the the cementum and (dentine) of a tooth

**dent/o**-faci-al, pertaining to the face and teeth in their dental arch

**dent/o**-lingu-al, pertaining to the tongue or lingual nerve and the teeth

**dent/o**-logy, 1. the scientific study of teeth (anatomy, physiology and diseases of) 2. dentistry Syn. odontology

**dent/o**-ment-al, pertaining to the chin and teeth

**dent/o**-nas-al, pertaining to the nose and teeth

**dent/o**-trop-ic, 1. pertaining to turning towards the tissues composing the teeth 2. pertaining to having an affinity for the tissues composing the teeth

**dent**-ure, a set of teeth, natural or artificial

inter-**dent**-al, pertaining to between the teeth, it refers to between the proximal surfaces of teeth in the same arch

**Ethm/o**, ethmoid/o, ethmoid bone, sieve-like

From a Greek word **ethmos** meaning a sieve. Here, ethm/o means the ethmoid bone, a spongy bone with a sieve-like plate (cribriform plate) forming the lateral walls of the nose and the upper portion of the bony nasal septum.

**ethm**-oid, 1. the ethmoid bone 2. resembling a sieve (cribriform)

189

**ethmoid**-ectomy, removal of part of the ethmoid bone or ethmoidal cells

**ethmoid**-itis, inflammation of the ethmoid bone or ethmoidal sinuses

**ethmoid/o**-front-al, pertaining to the frontal bone and ethmoid bone

**ethmoid/o**-lacrim-al, pertaining to the lacrimal bone and ethmoid bone

**ethmoid/o**-nas-al, pertaining to the nasal bone and ethmoid bone

**ethmoid/o**-palat-al, pertaining to the bones of the palate and ethmoid bone

**ethmoid/o**-palat-ine, pertaining to the palatine bone and ethmoid bone

**ethmoid/o**-sphenoid, pertaining to the sphenoid bone and ethmoid bone

**ethmoid/o**-tomy, incision into the ethmoid sinus

**ethm/o**-maxill-ary, pertaining to the maxilla and ethmoid bone

**ethm/o**-nas-al, pertaining to the nasal bone and ethmoid bone

**ethm/o**-palat-al, pertaining to the bones of the palate and ethmoid bone

**ethm/o**-palat-ine, pertaining to the palatine bone and ethmoid bone

**ethm/o**-sphenoid, pertaining to the sphenoid bone and ethmoid bone

**ethm/o**-turbin-al, pertaining to the ethmoid turbinate bones (superior and middle nasal conchae)

---

**Faci/o**, face

From a Latin word **facies**, meaning face. Here faci/o means the face.

**faci**-al, pertaining to the face

**faci**-es, 1. the face 2. facial expression

**faci/o**-brachi-al, pertaining to the arms and face

**faci/o**-ceph-alg-ia, condition of pain in the head and face

**faci/o**-cervic-al, pertaining to the neck and face

**faci/o**-lingu-al, pertaining to the tongue and face

**faci/o**-maxill-ary, pertaining to the jaws and face

**faci/o**-plasty, surgical repair or reconstruction of the face

**faci/o**-pleg-ia, condition of paralysis of the face

**faci/o**-pleg-ic, 1. pertaining to paralysis of the face 2. pertaining to having facioplegia

**faci/o**-scapul/o-humer-al, pertaining to the humerus, scapula and face

---

**Gingiv/o**, gum

From a Latin word **gingiva**, meaning gum. Here, gingiv/o means the gums or gingivae consisting of the vascular tissue surrounding the necks of erupted teeth.

**gingiv**-al, pertaining to the gingivae (gums)

**gingiv**-ectomy, removal of gum

**gingiv**-itis, inflammation of the gingivae (gums)

**gingiv/o**-gloss-itis, inflammation of the tongue and gingivae (gums)

**gingiv/o**-labi-al, pertaining to the lips and gingivae (gums)

**gingiv/o**-plasty, surgical repair or reconstruction of the gingivae (gums)

**gingiv**-osis, abnormal condition of the gingivae (gums), it refers to inflammation

**gingiv/o**-stomat-itis, inflammation of the mouth and gingivae (gums)

---

**Gloss/o**, tongue

From a Greek word **glossa**, meaning tongue. Here gloss/o means the tongue, the mobile muscular organ in the mouth. The tongue plays a vital role in speech, mastication (chewing of food) and swallowing. Papillae on the surface of the tongue contain nerve endings (chemoreceptors) that produce the sense of taste and are sometimes called the taste buds. The chemoreceptors detect chemicals in our food that we describe as sweet, sour, bitter or salty.

**gloss**-al, pertaining to the tongue

**gloss**-alg-ia, condition of pain in the tongue

**gloss**-aux-esis, condition of increase in size of the tongue

**gloss**-ectomy, removal of the tongue

**gloss**-itic, pertaining to having glossitis

**gloss**-itis, inflammation of the tongue

**gloss/o**-cele, a protrusion or swelling of the tongue

**gloss/o**-dynam/o-meter, an instrument used to measure the force or power of the tongue

**gloss/o**-dyn-ia, condition of pain in the tongue

**gloss/o**-epi-glott-ic, pertaining to the epiglottis and tongue

**gloss/o**-graph, an instrument that records the tongue (movements during speech)

**gloss/o**-hy-al, pertaining to the hyoid bone and tongue

**gloss**-oid, resembling a tongue

**gloss/o**-labi-al, pertaining to the lips and tongue

**gloss/o**-logy, the study of the tongue (anatomy, diseases and treatment of)

**gloss**-onc-us, a swelling of the tongue

**gloss/o**-palat-ine, pertaining to or belonging to the palate and tongue

**gloss/o**-pathy, disease of the tongue

**gloss/o**-pharyng-eal, 1. pertaining to the pharynx and tongue 2. pertaining to the glossopharyngeal nerve IX

**gloss/o**-phob-ia, condition of fear of using the tongue (speaking)

**gloss/o**-plasty, surgical repair or reconstruction of the tongue

**gloss/o**-pleg-ia, condition of paralysis of the tongue

**gloss/o**-ptosis, falling or downward displacement of the tongue

**gloss/o**-rrhaphy, stitching or suturing of the tongue

**gloss/o**-scopy, technique of viewing or examining the tongue

**gloss/o**-spasm, sudden contraction of the muscles of the tongue

**gloss/o**-trich-ia, condition of hairy tongue

**gloss/o**-tomy, incision into the tongue

hemi-**gloss**-ectomy, removal of one-half of the tongue

hemi-**gloss**-itis, inflammation of one-half of the tongue

idi/o-**gloss**-ia, condition of one's own tongue, it refers to defective, meaningless vocal sounds always used to express the same idea

macro-**gloss**-ia, condition of having a large tongue

micro-**gloss**-ia, condition of having a small tongue

pachy-**gloss**-ia, condition of having an abnormally thick tongue

sub-**gloss**-al, pertaining to below the tongue

---

**Gnath/o**, jaw

From a Greek word **gnathos**, meaning jaw. Here gnath/o means jaw a common term used to describe the bones of the face supporting the teeth and concerned with mastication. The inferior maxilla forms the lower jaw or mandible and two superior maxillae the upper jaw or maxilla.

brachy-**gnath**-ia, condition of an abnormally short jaw

dys-**gnath**-ia, condition of a poor jaw, it refers to any abnormality outside the teeth and extending to the maxilla or mandible

**gnath**-alg-ia, condition of pain in the jaw

**gnath**-ic, pertaining to the jaw

**gnath**-itis, inflammation of the jaw

**gnath/o**-dynam-ics, the science of studying the force or power of the jaws (in mastication)

**gnath/o**-dynam/o-meter, an instrument that measures the force of the jaw (closing force)

**gnath/o**-dyn-ia, condition of pain in the jaws

**gnath/o**-graphy, technique of recording the jaws (strength of a patient's bite)

**gnath/o**-logy, the study of the jaws (anatomy, diseases and treatment of)

**gnath/o**-plasty, surgical repair or reconstruction of the jaw

**gnath/o**-rrhag-ia, condition of bursting forth of blood or haemorrhage from the jaws

**gnath/o**-schisis, split or cleft jaw

**gnath/o**-stomat-ics, the science of studying the mouth and jaws

macro-**gnath**-ia, condition of having a large jaw

macro-**gnath**-ic, 1. pertaining to having a large jaw 2. pertaining to having macrognathia

micro-**gnath**-ia, condition of having a small jaw

micro-**gnath**-ic, 1. pertaining to having a small jaw 2. pertaining to having micrognathia

pro-**gnath**-ic, pertaining to having a jaw in front, it refers to an abnormal protrusion of one or both jaws

retro-**gnath**-ia, condition of having a backward jaw, it refers to poor development of the mandible and maxilla

retro-**gnath**-ic, 1. pertaining to a backward jaw 2. pertaining to having retrognathia

---

**Labi/o**, lip

From a Latin word **labium**, meaning lip. Here labi/o means a lip, and refers to either of the two fleshy folds, upper and lower, bordering the external entrance to the mouth.

labi-al, pertaining to the lips

labi/o-alveol-ar, 1. pertaining to the dental alveoli and lips 2. pertaining to the labial side of a dental alveolus

labi/o-cervic-al, pertaining to the neck (of a tooth) and its labial surface

labi/o-chorea, rapid, jerky, involuntary spasm of the lips (causes stammering)

labi/o-clina-tion, action or process of leaning of a tooth (from its normal position) towards the lips or labial surface

labi/o-dent-al, 1. pertaining to the teeth and lips 2. pertaining to the labial surface of a tooth

labi/o-gingiv-al, pertaining to the gingivae (gums) and lips

labi/o-gloss/o-laryng-eal, pertaining to the larynx, tongue and lips

labi/o-gloss/o-pharyng-eal, pertaining to the pharynx, tongue and lips

labi/o-graph, an instrument that records the lips (movement during speech)

labi/o-lingu-al, pertaining to the tongue and lips

labi/o-logy, the study of the lips (movement in speech)

labi/o-mandibul-ar, pertaining to the mandible and lip

labi/o-ment-al, pertaining to the chin and lips

labi/o-myc-osis, abnormal condition of fungi in the lips

labi/o-nas-al, pertaining to the nose and lips

labi/o-palat-ine, pertaining to the palate and lips (as one structure)

labi/o-plasty, surgical repair or reconstruction of the lips

labi/o-tenacul-um, an instrument that holds a lip in position during an operation. From a Latin word **tenaculum** meaning a holder

labi/o-vers-ion, process of turning (of a tooth) towards the lip (from its line of occlusion)

labi-um, a lip

mesi/o-**labi**-al, pertaining to the lip surface and mesial surface (of a tooth)

---

**Lal/o**, speaking, speech

From a Greek word **lalia** meaning speech. Here lal/o means speaking or speech.

copr/o-**lal**-ia, condition of speaking words relating to faeces, it refers to the use of obscene language as in Tourette's Syndrome

dys-**lal**-ia, condition of difficult or poor speech, it refers to difficulty in speaking because of an abnormality of the tongue or other organs of speech

lal/o-pathy, disease of speech, it refers to any disorder giving rise to a speech defect

lal/o-phob-ia, condition of aversion to speaking

lal/o-pleg-ia, condition of paralysis of the organs of speech

lal/o-rrhoea, excessive flow of speech, an abnormal talkativeness

para-**lal**-ia, condition of wrong speech, particularly the substitution of one letter for another or the utterance

of a sound other than the one intended

---

**Lingu/o**, tongue

From a Latin word **lingua** meaning tongue. Here lingu/o means the tongue, the mobile muscular organ in the mouth. The tongue plays a vital role in speech, mastication (chewing of food) and swallowing. Papillae on the surface of the tongue contain nerve endings (chemoreceptors) that produce the sense of taste and are sometimes called the taste buds. The chemoreceptors detect chemicals in our food that we describe as sweet, sour, bitter or salty.

**lingu**-al, pertaining to the tongue

**lingu**-ally, in the direction of the tongue

**lingu/o**-clina-tion, condition or process of deviation bending (of a tooth from its normal position) towards the lingual side

**lingu/o**-dent-al, pertaining to the teeth and tongue

**lingu/o**-dist-al, pertaining to the distal and lingual surfaces (of a tooth)

**lingu/o**-gingiv-al, pertaining to the gums and tongue

**lingu/o**-papill-itis, inflammation of the papillae (small nipple-like projections) at the edge of the tongue

**lingu/o**-trite, an instrument to crush the tongue (actually to grasp and pull it forward)

**lingu/o**-vers-ion, process of turning towards the tongue (*e.g.* the turning of a tooth)

mesi/o-**lingu**-al, pertaining to the lingual (tongue) surface and mesial surface (of a tooth)

sub-**lingu**-al, pertaining to below the tongue

sub-**lingu**-itis, inflammation below the tongue, it refers to inflammation of the sublingual glands

---

**Log/o**, speech, words

From a Greek word **logos** meaning word. Here log/o means speech or words.

**log**-amnes-ia, 1. condition of inability to understand written and spoken words. From a Greek word *amnesia* meaning forgetfulness 2. receptive aphasia

**log**-a-phas-ia, 1. condition of without word speech 2. expressive aphasia in which a patient understands words but cannot say them

**log/o**-graph-ic, pertaining to written words

**log/o**-koph-osis, abnormal condition of word deafness or loss of power of understanding what is said. From a Greek word *kophos* meaning deaf

**log/o**-man-ia, condition of excessive talkativeness to the point of mania

**log/o**-paed-ics, a branch of medical science dealing with the physiology and pathology of speech and the correction of speech defects (originally meaning science of studying speech in children)

**log/o**-pathy, disease of speech, it refers to any speech disorder caused by a lesion in the CNS

**log/o**-rrhoea, excessive flow of words or excessive talkativeness

**log/o**-spasm, condition in which words are produced in sudden spasms, stuttering in character

---

**Mandibul/o**, mandible, the lower jaw bone

From a Latin word **mandere** meaning to chew. Here mandibul/o means the mandible, the lower jaw or inferior maxilla.

**mandibula**, the mandible or lower jaw, plural mandibulae

**mandibul**-ar, pertaining to the mandible

**mandibul**-ectomy, removal of part of the mandible

**mandibul/o**-faci-al, pertaining to the facial bones and mandible

**mandibul/o**-pharyng-eal, pertaining to the pharynx and mandible

sub-**mandibul**-ar, pertaining to beneath the mandible

**Maxill/o**, maxilla, upper jaw

From a Latin word **maxilla**, meaning jaw. Here maxill/o means the maxilla, a common name for the upper jaw or superior maxillae composed of two bones that fuse before birth.

**maxilla**, the maxilla or upper jaw bone, plural maxillae

**maxill**-ary, pertaining to the maxilla

**maxill**-itis, inflammation of the maxilla

**maxill/o**-dent-al, pertaining to the teeth and maxillae

**maxill/o**-ethmoid-ectomy, removal of ethmoid cells and part of the maxilla (around the maxillary sinus)

**maxill/o**-faci-al, pertaining to the face and maxilla

**maxill/o**-labi-al, pertaining to the lips and maxilla

**maxill/o**-mandibul-ar, pertaining to the mandible (lower jaw bone) and maxilla (upper jaw bone)

**maxill/o**-palat-ine, pertaining to the palatine bone and the maxilla

**maxill/o**-pharyng-eal, pertaining to the pharynx and maxilla

**maxill/o**-tomy, incision into a maxilla

**maxill/o**-turbin-al, pertaining to a turbinate bone (the inferior nasal concha) and maxilla

pre-**maxilla**, in front of the maxilla, it refers to the incisive bone of the maxilla. The premaxilla is incorporated into the anterior part of the maxilla

pre-**maxill**-ary, 1. pertaining to in front of the maxilla 2.pertaining to the premaxilla

sub-**maxilla**, the mandible

sub-**maxillar**-itis, inflammation of a submaxillary gland, it refers to a submandibular salivary gland

sub-**maxill**-ary, pertaining to beneath the maxilla

supra-**maxilla**, the maxilla

supra-**maxill**-ary, 1. pertaining to above the maxilla 2. pertaining to the upper jaw or maxilla

**Ment/o**, chin

From a Latin word **mentum** meaning the chin. Here ment/o means the chin.

Note: mental is also used to mean pertaining to the mind.

**ment**-al, pertaining to the chin

**ment/o**-anterior, pertaining to an anterior view of the chin

**ment/o**-hyoid, pertaining to the hyoid bone and chin

**ment/o**-labi-al, pertaining to the lips and chin

**ment/o**-plasty, surgical repair or reconstruction of the chin

**ment**-um, the chin

sub-**ment**-al, pertaining to beneath the chin

**Nas/o**, nose

From a Latin word **nasus** meaning nose. Here nas/o means the nose, the organ that acts to warm, filter and moisten air entering the respiratory system. The nose is the the organ of the sense of smell (olfaction). Nerve endings that detect odours are located in the roof of the nose in the area of the cribriform plate of the ethmoid bone and nasal conchae.

**nas**-al, pertaining to the nose

**nas**-endo-scope, an instrument used to view or examine inside the nose (its nasal passages, post nasal space and larynx)

**nas**-endo-scopy, technique of viewing or examining inside the nose (its nasal passages, post nasal space and larynx) using a fibre-optic endoscope

**nas**-itis, inflammation of the nose

**nas/o**-antr-al, pertaining to the Antrum of Highmore (maxillary sinus) and nose

**nas/o**-antr-itis, inflammation of the Antrum of Highmore (maxillary sinus) and nose

**nas/o**-antr/o-stomy, formation of an opening between the Antrum of Highmore (maxillary sinus) and the nose or the name of the opening so created

**nas/o**-aur-al, pertaining to the ears and nose

**nas/o**-bucc-al, pertaining to the buccal cavity and nose

**nas/o**-bucc/o-pharyng-eal, pertaining to the pharynx, buccal cavity and nose

**nas/o**-cili-ary, pertaining to the eyelids and nose

**nas**-ocul-ar, pertaining to the eyes and nose

**nas/o**-duoden-al, pertaining to the duodenum and nose

**nas/o**-endo-scope, an instrument used to view or examine inside the nose (its nasal passages, post-nasal space and larynx) Syn. nasendoscope

**nas/o**-endo-scopy, technique of viewing or examining inside the nose (its nasal passages, post-nasal space and larynx) using a fibre-optic endoscope Syn. nasendoscopy

**nas/o**-front-al, pertaining to the frontal bones and nose

**nas/o**-gastr-ic, pertaining to the stomach and nose

**nas/o**-graph, an instrument that records the nose (it determines the patency of the nasal passages)

**nas/o**-jejun-al, pertaining to the jejunum and nose

**nas/o**-labi-al, pertaining to the lips and nose

**nas/o**-lacrim-al, pertaining to the lacrimal apparatus and the nose

**nas/o**-logy, the study of the nose (anatomy, diseases and treatment of)

**nas/o**-man/o-meter, an instrument used to measure pressure in the nose (during breathing)

**nas/o**-occipt-al, pertaining to the occiput and nose

**nas/o**-oesophag-eal, pertaining to the oesophagus and nose

**nas/o**-palat-ine, pertaining to the palate and nose

**nas/o**-palpebr-al, pertaining to the eyelids and nose

**nas/o**-pharyng-eal, 1. pertaining to the pharynx and nose 2. pertaining to the nasopharynx

**nas/o**-pharyng-itis, inflammation of the nasopharynx. See the combining form nasopharyng/o

**nas/o**-pharynx, part of the pharynx above the soft palate near the nose. See the combining form nasopharyng/o

**nas/o**-rostr-al, pertaining to the rostrum (of the sphenoid bone) and the nose

**nas/o**-scope, an instrument used to view or examine the nose

**nas/o**-sept-al, pertaining to the septum of the nose (it divides the nasal cavity)

**nas/o**-sinus-itis, inflammation of the (paranasal) sinuses and the nose

**nas**-us, the nose

---

**Nasopharyng/o**, nasopharynx

From the Latin word **nasus**, meaning nose and the Greek word **pharynx** meaning throat. Here nasopharyng/o means the nasopharynx, the portion of the pharynx above the soft palate.

**nasopharyng**-eal, pertaining to the nasopharynx

**nasopharyng**-itis, inflammation of the nasopharynx

**nasopharyng/o**-laryng/o-scope, an instrument used for viewing or examining the larynx, and the nasopharynx (a fibre-optic endoscope)

**nasopharyng/o**-scope, an instrument used for viewing or examining the nasopharynx (a fibre-optic endoscope)

**nasopharynx**, part of the pharynx above the soft palate near the nose

---

**Odont/o**, teeth

From a Greek word **odontos**, meaning tooth. Here odont/o means tooth or teeth. The teeth are used for mastication, the chewing of food. The first teeth are known as deciduous teeth, milk teeth or the primary set. There are twenty deciduous teeth that are usually shed by the age of seven, they are replaced by the permanent teeth or secondary set. The permanent set, thirty-two in number, is usually complete by the late teens.

end-**odont**-ic, pertaining to inside teeth (the pulp, roots, dentine *etc.*)

end-**odont**-ics, the branch of dentistry dealing with inside teeth (the pulp, roots, dentine *etc.*)

end-**odont**-ology, the study of the inside of teeth (the pulp, roots, dentine *etc.*)

ger-**odont**-ics, branch of dentistry dealing with the aged

heter-**odont**, having different teeth, premolars, molars *etc.*

**odont**-alg-ia, condition of pain in a tooth or toothache

**odont**-alg-ic, pertaining to pain in a tooth or toothache

**odont**-ectomy, removal of a tooth

**odont**-ic, pertaining to teeth

**odont**/o-blast, an immature cell or embryonic cell that forms teeth (forms the dentine and outer surface of the dental pulp)

**odont**/o-blast-oma, a tumour formed by immature cells or embryonic cells (odontoblasts) that form teeth

**odont**/o-ceram-ic, 1. pertaining to porcelain teeth 2. pertaining to the porcelain filling in a tooth

**odont**/o-clasis, a break or fracture of a tooth

**odont**/o-clast, a cell that breaks down teeth (it removes roots of deciduous teeth)

**odont**/o-genesis, the formation of teeth

**odont**/o-gen-ic, 1. pertaining to forming teeth 2. pertaining to originating in teeth

**odont**-oid, resembling a tooth

**odont**/o-lith, a stone or calculus on a tooth

**odont**/o-log-ist, 1. a specialist who studies teeth (anatomy, diseases and treatment of) 2. a dentist

**odont**/o-logy, 1. the study of teeth (anatomy, diseases and treatment of) 2. dentistry

**odont**/o-lysis, the breakdown or disintegration of teeth (resorption)

**odont**-oma, a tumour of a tooth (derived from cells concerned with tooth development)

**odont**/o-pathy, disease of teeth

**odont**/o-prisis, grinding of teeth. From a Greek word *prisis* meaning a sawing

**odont**/o-therapy, treatment of the teeth (for routine hygiene and dental disease)

**odont**/o-tomy, incision into a tooth

orth-**odont**-ic, pertaining to straight or correct teeth

ortho-**odont**-ics, a branch of dentistry dealing with straightening or correcting teeth

ortho-**odont**-ist, a specialist who straightens or corrects teeth

peri-**odont**-ic, pertaining to around teeth

peri-**odont**-ics, branch of dentistry dealing with supporting tissues around teeth

peri-**odont**-itis, inflammation of the periodontium

peri-**odont**-ium, the structure around the teeth, it refers to the tissues that support the teeth including the alveolar bone, gum, cementum and periodontal ligament

prostho-**odont**-ic, pertaining to adding teeth, it refers to fitting artificial teeth or other oral prostheses

prosth-**odont**-ics, the branch of dentistry dealing with adding teeth, it refers to fitting artificial teeth or other oral prostheses

prosth-**odont**-ist, a specialist who adds teeth, it refers to a specialist who fits artificial teeth or other oral prostheses

---

**Or/o**, mouth

From a Latin word **oris**, meaning mouth. Here or/o means the mouth, a cavity bounded by the closed lips and facial muscles, the hard and soft palate and lower jaw. It contains upper and lower teeth and the tongue. Three pairs of salivary glands (parotid, submaxillary and sublingual) secrete saliva into the mouth.

circum-**or**-al, pertaining to around the mouth

intra-**or**-al, pertaining to inside the mouth

**or**-al, pertaining to the mouth

**or**-al-ity, state pertaining to the mouth (a stage of psychosexual development involving an interest in sucking)

**or/o**-antr-al, pertaining to the Antrum of Highmore (maxillary sinus) and the mouth

**or/o**-genit-al, pertaining to the external genitalia and mouth

**or/o**-lingu-al, pertaining to the tongue and mouth

**or/o**-maxill-ary, pertaining to the maxilla and mouth

**or/o**-nas-al, pertaining to the nose and mouth

**or/o**-pharyng-eal, pertaining to the pharynx and mouth

**or/o**-pharynx, the part of the pharynx behind the mouth (and below the soft palate)

peri-**or**-al, pertaining to around the mouth

---

**Osm/a/o**, odour, olfaction (sense of smell), smell

From a Greek word **osme** meaning odour. Here osm/o means an odour or sense of smell (olfaction).

Note: osm/o is also used to mean osmosis, the movement of water molecules across cell membranes.

an-**osm**-ia, condition of without a sense of smell or olfaction

cac-**osm**-ia, condition of having a bad odour, for example from a nasal infection

dys-**osm**-ia, bad or poor sense of smell, it refers to a distortion in odour perception

hyper-**osm**-ia, condition of above normal acuteness of the sense of smell or olfaction

hyp-**osm**-ia, condition of below normal sense of smell, refers to partial loss of the sense of smell

**osm**-aesthes-ia, condition of having a sense of smell or olfaction

**osm/a**-tic, pertaining to the sense of smell or olfaction

**osm**-ics, the branch of medical science dealing with the sense of smell or olfaction

**osm/o**-meter, an instrument used to measure the sense of smell or olfaction

**osm/o**-receptor, a specialized sensory nerve ending sensitive to odours

par-**osm**-ia, condition of wrong sense of smell, it refers to a distortion of perception of the external stimulus

phant-**osm**-ia, condition of phantom (imaginary) smell, it refers to smell perception without an external stimulus

---

**Osphresi/o**, odour, olfaction (sense of smell), smell

From a Greek word **osphresis** meaning smell. Here osphresi/o means an odour or sense of smell (olfaction).

**osphresi/o**-logy, the study of the sense of smell and the production of odours

**osphresi/o**-meter, an instrument that measures a patient's sense of smell or olfaction

**osphresi/o**-phil-ia, condition of liking smells, it refers to a morbid interest in odours

**osphresi/o**-phob-ia, condition of aversion or dislike of odours

**osphr**-esis, condition of a sense of smell or olfaction

---

**Palat/o**, palate

From a Latin word **palatum** meaning palate. Here palat/o means the palate, the roof of the mouth. The hard palate at the front of the mouth is formed by two palatal bones; the posterior soft palate consists of muscle covered by mucous membrane.

**palat**-al, pertaining to or belonging to the palate

**palat**-ic, pertaining to or belonging to the palate

**palat**-ine, pertaining to or belonging to the palate

**palat**-itis, inflammation of the palate

**palat/o**-gloss-al, pertaining to the tongue and palate

**palat/o**-gnath-ic, pertaining to the jaws and palate

197

**palat/o**-gnath-ous, pertaining to the jaw and palate, it refers to having a cleft palate

**palat/o**-gnath-us, the jaw and palate, it refers to a cleft palate

**palat/o**-graphy, technique of recording the palate (movements while speaking)

**palat/o**-my/o-graph, an instrument that records the muscles of the palate (movements while speaking)

**palat/o**-nas-al, pertaining to the nose and palate

**palat/o**-pharyng-eal, pertaining to the pharynx and palate

**palat/o**-plasty, surgical repair or reconstruction of the palate

**palat/o**-pleg-ia, condition of paralysis of the palate

**palat/o**-pterygoid, pertaining to the pterygoid process (of the sphenoid bone) and palate

**palat/o**-rrhaphy, stitching or suturing of the palate (usually a cleft palate)

**palat/o**-schisis, a split or cleft palate

**palat**-um, the palate

post-**palat**-al, pertaining to after or behind the palate

---

**Parotid/o, parot/o,** parotid gland
From the Greek words **para** meaning beside and **ous** meaning ear. Here, parotid/o means the parotid gland, the gland beside the ear that secretes saliva into the mouth. The parotid glands are situated one on each side of the face just below the external acoustic meatus. Each has a parotid duct opening to the mouth near the second upper molar tooth.

**parotid**-ectomy, removal of a parotid gland

**parotid**-itis, inflammation of a parotid gland, for example mumps

**parotid/o**-scler-osis, abnormal condition of hardening of a parotid gland

**parot**-itis, inflammation of a parotid gland, for example mumps

**parot/o**-megaly, enlargement of a parotid gland

---

**Pharyng/o,** pharynx
From a Greek word **pharynx** meaning throat. Here pharyng/o means the pharynx, the cone-shaped cavity at the back of the mouth lined with mucous membrane. The pharynx varies in length (average 75 mm) and has three parts, the nasopharynx, oropharynx and laryngopharynx. At its lower end the pharynx opens into the oesophagus.

**pharyng**-alg-ia, condition of pain in the pharynx

**pharyng**-eal, pertaining to the pharynx

**pharyng**-ectas-ia, condition of widening or dilation of the pharynx

**pharyng**-ectomy, removal of the pharynx

**pharyng**-emphraxis, stopping up or obstruction of the pharynx

**pharyng**-ismus, process or state of the pharynx (a sudden spasm)

**pharyng**-itic, pertaining to having pharyngitis

**pharyng**-itis, inflammation of the pharynx

**pharyng/o**-cele, a protrusion or hernia of the pharynx

**pharyng/o**-dyn-ia, condition of pain in the pharynx

**pharyng/o**-epiglott-ic, pertaining to the epiglottis and pharynx

**pharyng/o**-gloss-al, pertaining to the tongue and pharynx

**pharyng/o**-laryng-eal, pertaining to the larynx and pharynx

**pharyng/o**-laryng-itis, inflammation of the larynx and pharynx

**pharyng/o**-lith, a calculus or stone in the pharynx

**pharyng/o**-logy, the study of the pharynx (anatomy, diseases and treatment of)

**pharyng/o**-maxill-ary, pertaining to the maxilla (jaw) and pharynx

**pharyng/o**-myc-osis, abnormal condition of fungi in the pharynx

**pharyng/o**-nas-al, pertaining to the nose and pharynx

**pharyng/o**-oesophag-eal, pertaining to the oesophagus and pharynx

**pharyng/o**-or-al, pertaining to the mouth and pharynx

**pharyng/o**-palat-ine, pertaining to the palate and pharynx

**pharyng/o**-paralysis, paralysis (of muscles) of the pharynx

**pharyng/o**-plasty, surgical repair or reconstruction of the pharynx

**pharyng/o**-pleg-ia, condition of paralysis of the pharynx

**pharyng/o**-rhin-itis, 1. inflammation of the nose and pharynx 2. inflammation of the nasopharynx

**pharyng/o**-rhin/o-scopy, technique of viewing or examining the nose and pharynx (with a rhinoscope)

**pharyng/o**-rrhag-ia, condition of bursting forth of blood from the pharynx (haemorrhage)

**pharyng/o**-rrhoea, excessive flow or discharge from the pharynx

**pharyng/o**-salping-itis, inflammation of the Eustachian tube (auditory tube) and pharynx

**pharyng/o**-scope, an instrument used to view or examine the pharynx

**pharyng/o**-scopy, technique of viewing or examining the pharynx

**pharyng/o**-spasm, involuntary contraction (of muscles) in the pharynx

**pharyng/o**-sten-osis, abnormal condition of narrowing of the pharynx

**pharyng/o**-tomy, incision into the pharynx

**pharyng/o**-tonsill-itis, inflammation of the tonsils and the pharynx

**pharyng/o**-tympan-ic, pertaining to the middle ear and pharynx

**pharyng/o**-xer-osis, abnormal condition of dry pharynx (due to lack of secretions)

---

**phas/i/o, -phas-ia**, speech
From a Greek word **phasis**, meaning speech. Here phas/i/o means speech.

a-**phas**-ia, condition of without speech (inability to speak), note there are many types of aphasia

a-**phas**-iac, person suffering from aphasia (inability to speak)

a-**phas**-ic, 1. pertaining to aphasia (inability to speak) 2. pertaining to without speech

a-**phasi/o**-log-ist, a specialist who studies aphasia

a-**phasi/o**-logy, the study of aphasia (inability to speak)

cata-**phas**-ia, condition of wrong speech, it refers to a speech disorder in which the same word or phrase is repeated involuntarily

dys-**phas**-ia, condition of difficult or disordered speech

dys-**phas**-iac, person suffering from dysphasia (difficulty in speaking)

dys-**phas**-ic, pertaining to dysphasia (difficulty in speaking)

mono-**phas**-ia, condition of one speech, it refers to a type of aphasia in which one word or phrase is spoken

mono-**phas**-ic, pertaining to having monophasia

para-**phas**-ia, condition of near speech, it refers to using wrong words or using words in meaningless phrases

---

**Phon/o**, sound, speech, voice
From a Greek word **phone** meaning voice. Here phon/o means speech or voice.

dys-**phon**-ia, condition of difficulty in speaking

dys-**phon**-ic, pertaining to having dysphonia

**phon**-al, pertaining to the voice

**phon**-asthen-ia, condition of having a weak voice, it refers to difficulty in producing sound

**phon**-iatr-ics, 1. branch of medical science dealing with the treatment of disorders and defects of speech 2. speech therapy

**phon**-ic, 1. pertaining to the voice 2. pertaining to speech sounds

**phon/o**-meter, an instrument used to measure sound intensity (loudness)

**phon/o**-pathy, disease of speech, it refers to any disease of the vocal cords or organs of speech

**phon/o**-receptor, a receptor sensitive to sound

trach-y-**phon**-ia, condition of a rough sounding voice

**Prosop/o**, face

From a Greek word **prosopon** meaning face. Here prosop/o means face.

micro-**prosop**-us, a thing (fetus) with a small or underdeveloped face

**prosop**-a-gnos-ia, condition of being unable to know (recognize) a face, due to brain damage in the occipital lobes

**prosop**-alg-ia, 1. condition of pain in the face 2. trigeminal neuralgia

**prosop**-ectas-ia, condition of dilation of the face, it refers to an abnormally large face

**prosop**-ic, pertaining to the face or facial

**prosop/o**-di-pleg-ia, condition of paralysis in the two lower limbs and face

**prosop/o**-neur-alg-ia, condition of pain in the nerves of the face (facial neuralgia)

**prosop/o**-pleg-ia, condition of paralysis of the face

**prosop/o**-pleg-ic, 1. pertaining to paralysis of the face 2. pertaining to having prosopoplegia

**prosop/o**-schisis, splitting or fissure of the face, a congenital abnormality

**prosop/o**-spasm, a sudden involuntary contraction of facial muscles

---

**Ptyal/o**, saliva

From a Greek word **ptyalon**, meaning saliva. Here ptyal/o means saliva, a secretion produced by the three pairs of salivary glands (parotid, submaxillary and sublingual) in the mouth. Saliva contains water, mucin and the enzyme amylase (ptyalin) that can digest starch into maltose sugar.

**ptyal**-agogue, an agent that stimulates the flow of saliva

**ptyal**-ectasis, dilation of a salivary duct

**ptyal**-in, a chemical in the saliva (the enzyme amylase)

**ptyal**-ism, process of salivation (excessive secretion of saliva)

**ptyal/o**-cele, a protrusion containing saliva, it refers to a salivary cyst

**ptyal/o**-gen-ic, 1. pertaining to formation of saliva 2. pertaining to originating in saliva

**ptyal/o**-lith, a stone or calculus in the saliva

**ptyal/o**-lith-iasis, abnormal condition of stones or calculi in the saliva

**ptyal/o**-lith/o-tomy, incision to remove a salivary stone or calculus (from a salivary duct)

**ptyal**-osis, abnormal condition of saliva (excessive secretion) Syn. ptyalism

**ptyal/o**-react-ion, 1. a chemical reaction occurring in the saliva 1. a chemical reaction resulting from a test performed on the saliva

**ptyal/o**-rrhoea, excessive flow of saliva

---

**Rhin/o**, nose

From a Greek word **rhinos**, meaning nose. Here rhin/o means the nose, the organ that acts to warm, filter and moisten air entering the respiratory system. The nose is the organ of the sense of smell (olfaction). Nerve endings that detect odours are located in the roof of the nose in the area of the cribriform plate of the ethmoid bone and nasal conchae.

**rhin**-aesthes-ia, condition of the sense of the nose, it refers to the sense of smell or olfaction

**rhin**-al, pertaining to the nose

**rhin**-alg-ia, condition of pain in the nose

**rhin**-eurynter, a device to distend or widen the nose, it widens the nostrils

**rhin**-iatry, 1. treatment of the nose by a doctor 2. the medical speciality of treatment of the nose

**rhin**-ic, pertaining to the nose

**rhin**-itis, inflammation of the nose

**rhin/o**-anem/o-meter, an instrument for measuring air in the nose (during respiration)

**rhin/o**-antr-itis, inflammation of the Antrum of Highmore (maxillary sinus) and nose (nasal cavity)

**rhin/o**-blen/o-rrhoea, excessive discharge of mucus from the nose

**rhin/o**-canth-ectomy, removal of the inner canthus of the eye (nearest to the nose)

**rhin/o**-cheil/o-plasty, surgical repair or reconstruction of the lips and nose

**rhin/o**-cleisis, obstruction of the nose (its nasal passages)

**rhin/o**-dacry-lith, a stone or calculus in the nasal duct of the lacrimal (tear) apparatus

**rhin/o**-dyn-ia, condition of pain in the nose

**rhin/o**-gen-ous, pertaining to forming or arising in the nose

**rhin/o**-kyph-ectomy, removal of a hump on the nose (by cosmetic surgery)

**rhin/o**-kyph-osis, abnormal condition of hump (ridge) on the nose

**rhin/o**-lal-ia, condition of speaking with a nasal voice

**rhin/o**-laryng-itis, inflammation of the larynx and nose

**rhin/o**-laryng/o-logy, the study of the larynx and nose (anatomy, diseases and treatment of)

**rhin/o**-lith, a stone or calculus in the nose

**rhin/o**-lith-iasis, presence of stones or calculi in the nose

**rhin/o**-log-ical, 1. pertaining to the study of the nose 2. pertaining to rhinology

**rhin/o**-log-ist, a specialist who studies the nose (anatomy, diseases and treatment of)

**rhin/o**-logy, the study of the nose (anatomy, diseases and treatment of)

**rhin/o**-man/o-metry, technique of measuring pressure in the nose (air flow)

**rhin/o**-melosis, shortening or reduction in the size of the nose (by surgery)

**rhin/o**-miosis, shortening or reduction in the size of the nose (by surgery)

**rhin/o**-myc-osis, abnormal condition of fungi in the nose

**rhin/o**-necr-osis, abnormal condition of dead tissue in the nose (due to destruction of nasal bones)

**rhin/o**-neur-osis, 1. abnormal nervous condition or neurosis characterized by nasal symptoms 2. abnormal condition of the nerves in the nose, it refers to any functional nervous disease of the nose

**rhin/o**-ops-ia, condition of nasal sight, it refers to eyes converging towards the nose, a convergent squint

**rhin/o**-path-ia, condition of disease of the nose (any morbid condition)

**rhin/o**-pathy, disease of the nose

**rhin/o**-pharyng-eal, pertaining to the pharynx and nose (nasal part of the pharynx)

**rhin/o**-pharyng-itis, inflammation of the pharynx and nose

**rhin/o**-pharyng/o-cele, a protrusion or swelling (an air-filled cyst) arising from the nasal part of the pharynx (rhinopharynx)

**rhin/o**-pharyng/o-lith, a stone or calculus in the nasal part of the pharynx (rhinopharynx)

**rhin/o**-pharynx, the nasal part of the pharynx

**rhin/o**-phon-ia, condition of having a nasal sound to the voice (speech through the nose)

**rhin/o**-phyma, swelling of the nose (nodular enlargement of the skin)

**rhin/o**-plast-ic, 1. pertaining to reconstructive surgery of the nose 2. pertaining to rhinoplasty

**rhin/o**-plasty, surgical repair or reconstruction of the nose

**rhin/o**-polyp-us, a nasal polyp

**rhin/o**-rrhag-ia, condition of excessive flow of blood from the nose, it refers to a nosebleed or epistaxis

**rhin/o**-rrhaphy, 1. stitching or suturing of the nose 2. an operation to remove an epicanthus, a vertical fold of skin on either side of the nose

**rhin/o**-rrhoea, excessive flow or discharge from the nose

**rhin/o**-salping-itis, inflammation of the Eustachian tube (auditory tube) and nose

**rhin/o**-scler-oma, a hard tissue or swelling in the nose, due to infection with *Klebsiella*

**rhin/o**-scope, an instrument used to view or examine the nose

**rhin/o**-scop-ic, 1. pertaining to viewing or examining the nose 2. pertaining to rhinoscopy

**rhin/o**-scopy, technique of viewing or examining the nose

**rhin/o**-sinus-itis, inflammation of the sinuses and nose

**rhin/o**-sinus/o-path-ia, condition of disease of the sinuses and nose

**rhin/o**-sten-osis, abnormal condition of narrowing of the nose (the nasal passage)

rhin/o-tomy, incision into the nose

**rhin/o**-virus, a virus that affects the nose (*e.g.* picornavirus that causes a cold)

---

**Sept/o**, septum

From a Latin word **saeptum** meaning fence. Here, sept/o means the nasal septum; a partition dividing the nasal cavity. The posterior bony part of the septum is formed by the perpendicular plate of the ethmoid bone and the vomer. Anteriorly it consists of hyaline cartilage.

**sept**-al, pertaining to a septum

**sept**-ate, having a septum

**sept**-ectomy, removal of part of the nasal septum

**sept/o**-margin-al, pertaining to the margin or edge of a septum

**sept/o**-nas-al, pertaining to the septum of the nose

**sept/o**-tome, an instrument to cut the nasal septum

**sept/o**-tomy, incision into a nasal septum

---

**Sial/o**, saliva, salivary duct, salivary gland

From a Greek word **sialon**, meaning saliva. Here sial/o means saliva, salivary glands or salivary ducts. Three pairs of salivary glands, the parotid, submaxillary and sublingual secrete saliva into the mouth via ducts. Amylase, an enzyme present in saliva, begins the digestion of starch in food to maltose sugar.

anti-**sial**-agog-ic, pertaining to acting against the secretion of saliva

anti-**sial**-agogue, an agent that acts against the secretion of saliva

anti-**sial**-ic, 1. pertaining to acting against the secretion of saliva 2. an agent that acts against the secretion of saliva

poly-**sial**-ia, condition of too much saliva

**sial**-aden-ectomy, removal of a salivary gland

**sial**-aden-itis, inflammation of a salivary gland

**sial**-aden-osis, abnormal condition of a salivary gland (linflammation) Syn. sialadenitis

**sial**-agogue, an agent that stimulates secretion of saliva

**sial**-angi/o-graphy, technique of making a recording or X-ray picture of salivary vessels

**sial**-ectas-ia, condition of dilation of a salivary duct

**sial**-ectasis, dilation of a salivary duct

**sial**-ine, pertaining to saliva

**sial**-ism, process of secreting saliva or salivation

**sial**-ismus, process of secreting saliva or salivation

**sial**-itis, inflammation of a salivary duct or gland

**sial/o**-aden-ectomy, removal of a salivary gland

**sial/o**-aden-itis, inflammation of a salivary gland Syn. sialadenitis

**sial/o**-aden/o-tomy, incision into a salivary gland

**sial/o**-aer/o-phag-ia, condition of eating (swallowing) air and saliva

**sial/o**-aer/o-phagy, process of eating (swallowing) air and saliva

**sial/o**-angi-ectasis, abnormal condition of dilation of a salivary vessel (duct) Syn. sialectasia

**sial/o**-angi-itis, inflammation of a salivary vessel (duct)

**sial/o**-angi/o-graphy, technique of making a recording or X-ray picture of the salivary vessels (ducts and glands)

**sial/o**-cele, a swelling or protrusion of saliva, it refers to a salivary cyst

**sial/o**-doch-itis, inflammation of a salivary duct Syn. sialangiitis

**sial/o**-doch-ium, a duct of a salivary gland

**sial/o**-doch/o-gram, a recording or X-ray picture of the salivary ducts (and glands)

**sial/o**-doch/o-plasty, surgical repair or reconstruction of a salivary duct

**sial/o**-duct-itis, inflammation of a salivary duct Syn. sialangiitis, sialodochitis

**sial/o**-gen-ous, pertaining to producing saliva

**sial/o**-gram, a recording or X-ray picture of salivary glands and ducts

**sial/o**-graphy, technique of making a recording or X-ray picture of the salivary ducts (and glands) Syn. sialangiography

**sial**-oid, resembling saliva

**sial**-oma, a tumour of a salivary gland or duct

**sial**-onc-us, a tumour or swelling caused by saliva (obstruction in its flow)

**sial/o**-lith, a stone or calculus in the saliva (duct or gland)

**sial/o**-lith-iasis, condition of stones or calculi in the saliva

**sial/o**-lith/o-tomy, incision to remove a stone or calculus from a salivary duct or gland

**sial/o**-meta-plas-ia, condition of growth of cells of the salivary glands that are changed in form

**sial/o**-phag-ia, condition of eating (swallowing) saliva (in abnormal amounts)

**sial/o**-rrhoea, excessive flow or secretion of saliva Syn. ptyalism

**sial/o**-schesis, reduction or suppression in the secretion of saliva

**sial**-osis, abnormal condition of saliva (excessive flow) Syn. ptyalism

**sial/o**-sten-osis, abnormal condition of narrowing of a salivary duct

**sial/o**-syrinx, 1. a salivary fistula (abnormal passage) 2. a tube used to drain the salivary ducts 3. a syringe for washing out the salivary ducts

**sial/o**-tic, pertaining to having an excessive flow of saliva

---

**Sin/o, sinus-,** sinus

From a Latin word **sinus** meaning a curve or hollow. Here, sin/o means a nasal sinus, a hollow or cavity within a bone of the skull. The paranasal sinuses give resonance to the voice and lighten the skull, they are lined with mucous membrane continuous with that of the nasal cavity.

peri-**sinus**-itis, inflammation of tissue around a sinus

**sin/o**-bronch-itis, inflammation of bronchi and sinuses

**sin/o**-gram, a recording or X-ray picture of a sinus

**sin**-us, a hollow or cavity in bone, an anatomical part

**sinus**-al, pertaining to a sinus hollow or cavity in bone

**sinus**-itis, inflammation of a sinus

**sinus**-oid, resembling a sinus

**sinus/o**-tomy, incision into a sinus

---

**Staphyl/o,** soft palate, uvula

From a Latin word **staphyle**, meaning bunch of grapes. Here staphyl/o means the uvula, the central tag-like structure extending downwards from the soft palate. It can also be used to mean the soft palate.

**staphyl/o**-dialysis, loosening or relaxation of the uvula resulting in its elongation

**staphyl/o**-haemat-oma, swelling or effusion of blood in the uvula

**staphyl**-onc-us, a tumour of the uvula

**staphyl/o**-pharyng/o-rrhaphy, stitching or suturing of the pharynx and uvula (as in a procedure to repair a cleft palate or modify the length of the soft palate)

**staphyl/o**-plasty, surgical repair or reconstruction of the uvula or soft palate

**staphyl/o**-ptosis, falling or drooping of the uvula, due to relaxation bringing about its elongation

**staphyl/o**-rrhaphy, stitching or suturing of the uvula or soft palate (as in a procedure to repair a cleft palate)

**staphyl/o**-schisis, a fissure in the uvula or a fissure in the uvula and soft palate

**staphyl/o**-tomy, incision into the uvula

---

**Stomat/o,** mouth

From a Greek word **stomatos**, meaning mouth. Here stomat/o means the

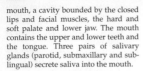 

mouth, a cavity bounded by the closed lips and facial muscles, the hard and soft palate and lower jaw. The mouth contains the upper and lower teeth and the tongue. Three pairs of salivary glands (parotid, submaxillary and sublingual) secrete saliva into the mouth.

macro-**stom**-ia, condition of having a large mouth (abnormally wide)

**stomat**-alg-ia, condition of pain in the mouth Syn. stomatodynia

**stomat**-ic, pertaining to or belonging to the mouth

**stomat**-itis, inflammation of the mouth

**stomat**-o-dyn-ia, condition of pain in the mouth Syn. stomatalgia

**stomat**/o-dysod-ia, condition of a bad odour from the mouth. From a Greek word *dysodes* meaning ill-smelling

**stomat**/o-gastr-ic, pertaining to the stomach and mouth

**stomat**/o-gnath-ic, pertaining to the jaw and mouth

**stomat**/o-lal-ia, condition of speaking through the mouth (due to blocked or obstructed nares)

**stomat**/o-log-ic, 1. pertaining to the study of the mouth 2. pertaining to stomatology

**stomat**/o-log-ical, 1. pertaining to the study of the mouth 2. pertaining to stomatology

**stomat**/o-log-ist, a specialist who studies the mouth (anatomy, diseases and treatment of)

**stomat**/o-logy, the study of the mouth

**stomat**/o-malac-ia, condition of softening of the mouth

**stomat**/o-men-ia, condition of bleeding from the mouth (at the time of menstruation)

**stomat**/o-myc-osis, abnormal condition of fungi in the mouth

**stomat**/o-necr-osis, abnormal condition of dead tissue in the mouth (gangrenous stomatitis)

**stomat**/o-pathy, disease of the mouth

**stomat**/o-plast-ic, pertaining to surgical repair or reconstruction of the mouth

**stomat**/o-plasty, surgical repair or reconstruction of the mouth

**stomat**/o-rrhag-ia, condition of excessive flow of blood from the mouth

**stomat**/o-scope, an instrument for viewing or examining the mouth (oral cavity)

**stomat**-osis, abnormal condition or disease of the mouth

xero-**stom**-ia, condition of a dry mouth, due to lack of secretion of saliva

---

**Tonsil/l/o**, tonsil

From a Latin word **tonsillae**, meaning tonsils. Here, tonsill/o means a tonsil; a patch of lymphoid tissue located in the mouth or nasopharynx. The pharyngeal tonsil (or adenoids) is found in the posterior wall of the nasopharynx, and the palatine tonsils in the folds formed by the soft palate and oropharynx. The palatine tonsils are known more commonly as the 'tonsils'. The lingual tonsils are found at the base of the tongue. Tonsils are important in the formation of antibodies and lymphocytes that defend against infection.

peri-**tonsill**-ar, pertaining to around a tonsil

**tonsill**-ar, pertaining to a tonsil

**tonsill**-ectomy, removal of the tonsils

**tonsill**-itic, pertaining to having tonsillitis

**tonsill**-itis, inflammation of the tonsils

**tonsill**/o-lith, a stone or calculus in a tonsil

**tonsill**/o-monil-iasis, abnormal condition or disease of the fungus Monilia (now known as Candida) in the tonsils

**tonsill**/o-myc-osis, abnormal condition or disease of fungi in the mouth

**tonsill**/o-pathy, disease of the tonsils

**tonsill**/o-pharyng-eal, pertaining to the pharynx and tonsils

**tonsill**/o-scope, an instrument used to view or examine the tonsils

**tonsill**/o-scopy, technique of viewing or examining the tonsils

**tonsill**/o-tome, an instrument used to cut a tonsil

**tonsill**/o-tomy, technique of cutting a tonsil

**tonsil**-sect-or, an instrument used to cut a tonsil

---

**Turbin/o**, turbinate bones, nasal conchae

From a Latin word **turbinatus**, meaning like a top. Here turbin/o means the turbinate bones or nasal conchae, three on either side forming the lateral walls of the nose. The turbinates increase mucosal surface area within the nose and cause air turbulence.

**turbin**-al, 1. top-shaped 2. pertaining to being turbinate

**turbin**-ate, 1. top-shaped 2. a turbinate bone (nasal concha)

**turbin**-ectomy, removal of a turbinate bone

**turbin/o**-tomy, incision into a turbinate bone

---

**Uran/o**, the palate

From a Greek word **ouranos** meaning palate. Here uran/o means the palate, the roof of the mouth. The hard palate at the front of the mouth is formed by two palatal bones; the posterior soft palate consists of muscle covered by mucous membrane.

**uran/o**-plasty, surgical repair or reconstruction of the palate, an operation for a cleft palate

**uran/o**-pleg-ia, condition of paralysis of the soft palate

**uran/o**-rrhaphy, stitching or suturing of the palate *e.g.* of a cleft palate

**uran/o**-schisis, a cleft palate

**uran/o**-staphyl/o-plasty, surgical repair or reconstruction of the uvula and palate *e.g.* of a cleft palate

**uran/o**-staphyl/o-schisis, fissure of the uvula (soft palate) and hard palate

---

**Uvul/o**, uvula

From a Latin word **uva** meaning grape. Here uvul/o means the uvula, the central tag-like structure extending downwards from the soft palate.

**uvul**-ar, pertaining to or belonging to the uvula

**uvul**-ectomy, removal of the uvula

**uvul**-itis, inflammation of the uvula

**uvul/o**-ptosis, falling or displacement of the uvula, it refers to the uvula in a relaxed state

**uvul/o**-tome, an instrument to cut the uvula

**uvul/o**-tomy, incision into the uvula

Muscles compose 40–50 per cent of the body's weight. The function of muscle is to effect the movement of the body as a whole and to move internal organs involved in the vital processes required to keep the body alive. There are three types of muscles tissue:

- Skeletal muscle moves the vocal chords, diaphragm and limbs. This type of muscle may also be described as striated, striped or voluntary muscle. It is called

voluntary because its contraction is under conscious control.
- Cardiac muscle moves the heart; it is not under conscious control.
- Smooth muscle moves the internal organs, bringing about movement of food through the intestines and urine through the urinary tract. It is also found in the walls of blood vessels where it acts to maintain blood pressure.

**Quick Reference**
Combining forms relating to the muscular system:

| | | Page |
|---|---|---|
| **Aponeur/o** | aponeurosis | 207 |
| **Chore/o** | chorea | 207 |
| **Cinema-** | motion, movement | 207 |
| **Cinesi/o** | motion, movement | 207 |
| **Fasci/a** | fascia | 208 |
| **Fascicul-** | fascicle | 208 |
| **Fibr/o** | fibre, fibrous tissue | 208 |
| **Kinesi/o** | movement | 209 |
| **Kinet/o** | movement | 209 |
| **Leiomy/o** | smooth muscle | 210 |
| **Muscul/o** | muscle | 210 |
| **My/o** | muscle | 210 |
| **Ortho-** | correct, right, straight | 212 |
| **Rhabdomy/o** | striated muscle | 213 |
| **Spasm/o** | spasm | 213 |
| **-tax-** | ordered movement | 213 |
| **Tendin/o** | tendon | 214 |
| **Tend/o** | tendon | 214 |
| **Ten/o** | tendon | 214 |
| **Tenont/o** | tendon | 214 |
| **Thec/o** | theca, tendon sheath | 214 |
| **Ton/o** | tension, tone | 214 |

**Quick Reference**
Common words and combining forms relating to the muscular system:

| | | Page |
|---|---|---|
| Aponeurosis | **aponeur/o** | 207 |
| Chorea | **chore/o** | 207 |
| Correct | **ortho-** | 212 |
| Fascia | **fasci/o** | 208 |
| Fascicle | **fascicul-** | 208 |
| Fibre | **fibr/o** | 208 |
| Fibrous tissue | **fibr/o** | 208 |
| Motion | **cinema-, cinesi/o,** | 207 |
| | **kinesi/o, kinet/o** | 209 |
| Movement | **cinema-, cinesi/o,** | 207 |
| | **kinesi/o, kinet/o** | 209 |
| Muscle | **muscul/o, my/o** | 210 |
| Ordered movement | **-tax-** | 213 |
| Right | **ortho-** | 212 |
| Smooth muscle | **leiomy/o** | 210 |
| Spasm | **spasm/o** | 213 |
| Straight | **ortho-** | 212 |
| Striated muscle | **rhabdomy/o** | 213 |
| Tendon | **tendin/o tend/o,** | 214 |
| | **ten/o, tenont/o** | 214 |
| Tendon sheath | **thec/o** | 214 |
| Tension | **ton/o** | 214 |
| Theca | **thec/o** | 214 |
| Tone | **ton/o** | 214 |

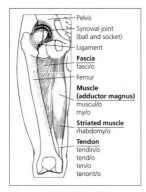

- Pelvis
- Synovial joint (ball and socket)
- Ligament
- **Fascia**
  fasci/o
- Femur
- **Muscle (adductor magnus)**
  muscul/o
  my/o
- **Striated muscle**
  rhabdomy/o
- **Tendon**
  tendin/o
  tend/o
  ten/o
  tenont/o

Figure 19 A muscle arrangement in the thigh

This type of muscle may also be described as non-striated or involuntary. It is not under conscious control.

A typical skeletal muscle consists of a large number of muscle fibres also called striated muscle cells. Each muscle fibre is enclosed in and attached to fine fibrous connective tissue called endomysium. Small bundles of fibres are enclosed in perimysium, and the whole muscle in epimysium. The fibrous tissue enclosing the fibres, the bundles and the whole muscle extends beyond the muscle fibres to become the tendon, that attaches muscle to bone. Figure 19 shows the arrangement of a skeletal muscle in the thigh.

**Roots and combining forms**, meanings

**Aponeur/o**, aponeurosis (a flat, wide tendon)
From the Greek words **apo** meaning detached, neuron meaning tendon and **osis** condition of, note neuron is also

the origin of neur/o mean nerve. Here aponeur/o means an aponeurosis, a broad tendon-like tissue that serves to invest and attach muscles to each other and to the parts which they move.

**aponeur**-ectomy, removal of an aponeurosis
**aponeur**-itis, inflammation of an aponeurosis
**aponeur/o**-rrhaphy, stitching or suturing of an aponeurosis
**aponeur/o**-tic, pertaining to an aponeurosis

---

**Chore/i/o**, chorea
From a Greek word **choreia** meaning to dance. Here chore/o means chorea; a disease manifested by irregular and spasmodic movements beyond a patient's control. Voluntary movements are also affected being jerky and ungainly, for example Huntington's Chorea.

**chore**-al, 1. pertaining to or of the nature of chorea 2. caused by chorea
**chore**-ic, 1. pertaining to or of the nature of chorea 2. caused by chorea
**chore/i**-form, having the form of or resembling chorea
**chore/o**-athet-oid, resembling choreoathetosis
**chore/o**-athet-osis, abnormal condition of athetosis and chorea (athetosis is a condition marked by repetitive, involuntary, purposeless movements, especially of the hands)
**chore**-oid, resembling chorea
ortho-**chorea**, straight chorea, it refers to a type of chorea in which the jerky movements occur when the patient is standing up straight or walking in the erect position

---

**Cinema-, cinesi/o, cin/et/o**, motion, movement
From a Greek word **kinema**, meaning motion. Here cinesi/o means movement or motion of the body.

**cinema**-tics, the science of studying movement particularly, movement of the body Syn. kinematics

**cine**-plast-ic, pertaining to surgical repair or reconstruction for movement, it refers to using the stump of an amputated limb to move a prosthesis

**cine**-plasty, surgical repair or reconstruction for movement, it refers to using the stump of an amputated limb to move a prosthesis

**cines**-alg-ia, condition of pain caused by movement of muscles Syn. kinesalgia

**cines**-ia, abnormal condition due to motion *e.g.* sea-sickness Syn. kinetosis

**cines**-iatr-ics, the science of medical treatment using active and passive movements Syn. kinesiotherapy

**cinesi/o**-logy, the study of movement of the body musculature (including movement disorders and their treatment)

**cinesi/o**-therapy, treatment using active and passive movements as a primary form of rehabilitation *e.g.* for amputees Syn. kinesiotherapy

**cin**-esis, condition of movement or motion Syn. kinesis

**cinesi**-therapy, treatment using active and passive movements as a primary form of rehabilitation *e.g.* for amputees Syn. kinesiotherapy

**cinet/o**-graph-ic, pertaining to recording movements

dys-**cines**-ia, condition of difficult or painful movement

---

**Fasci/a/o**, fascia of a muscle
From a Latin word **fascia** meaning band. Here fasci/o means a fascia, a layer, sheet or band of fibrous connective tissue separating or enclosing groups of muscles or other organs.

**fasciae**, plural of fascia

**fasci**-al, pertaining to or having the property of a fascia

**fasci/a**-plasty, surgical repair or reconstruction of a fascia

**fasci**-ectomy, removal of a fascia

**fasci**-gram, a recording or X-ray picture of a fascia

**fasci**-itis, inflammation of a fascia

**fasci/o**-desis, surgical fixation of a fascia *e.g.* to bone or other fascia

**fasci/o**-rrhaphy, stitching or suturing of a fascia

sub-**fasci**-al, pertaining to beneath a fascia

---

**Fascicul-**, fascicle, fasciculus
From the Latin word **fasciculus** meaning a little bundle. Here, fascicul- means a little bundle or collection of fibres with the same orientation; it refers to muscle or nerve fibres.

**fascicul**-ar, pertaining to a fasciculus

**fascicul**-ate, arranged into little bundles or fasciculi

**fascicul**-ation, 1. process of formation of fasciculi 2. process of arranging into little bundles 3. involuntary twitching of small bundles of muscle fibres

**fascicul**-i, plural of fasciculus

**fascicul**-us, a little bundle of fibres (muscle or nerve). Singular of fasciculi

---

**Fibr/o**, fibre, fibrous tissue
From a Latin word **fibra**. Here, fibr/o means fibrous tissue particularly that associated with muscle and the musculoskeletal system.

**fibr/o**-aden-oma, a glandular tumour in which there is formation of fibrous tissue

**fibr/o**-blast, 1. an immature cell that forms (collagen) fibres or fibrous connective tissue 2. an immature cell that forms precursor cells that produce connective tissue

**fibr/o**-blast-oma, a tumour developing from fibroblasts Syn. fibroma, fibrosarcoma

**fibr/o**-calcif-ic, 1. pertaining to calcium salts in fibrous tissue 2. pertaining to calcification of fibrous tissue

**fibr/o**-cartilage, cartilage containing bundles of white fibrous (collagenous) tissue

**fibr/o**-chondr-itis, inflammation of fibrocartilage

**fibr/o**-collagen-ous, pertaining to collagen fibres

**fibr/o**-cyst, a cyst or bladder-like tumour composed of fibrous or fully developed connective tissue

**fibr/o**-cyst-ic, pertaining to having fibrocysts

**fibr/o**-cyte, a fibre cell, it refers to 1. an immature cell that forms (collagen) fibres or fibrous connective tissue 2. an immature cell that forms precursor cells that produce connective tissue Syn. fibroblast

**fibr/o**-elast-ic, pertaining to being elastic and fibrous

**fibr/o**-elast-osis, abnormal condition of elastic and fibrous tissue (proliferation of)

**fibr**-oid, 1. resembling fibrous tissue 2. the name for a fibroma especially in the uterus

**fibroid**-ectomy, removal of a fibroma especially from the uterus

**fibr**-oma, a tumour composed of fibrous or fully developed connective tissue

**fibr/o**-muscul-ar, pertaining to or composed of muscular and fibrous tissue

**fibr/o**-my-alg-ia, condition of pain in muscles and surrounding fibrous tissues

**fibr/o**-my-itis, inflammation of a muscle resulting in fibrous degeneration

**fibr/o**-my-oma, a tumour of muscle and fibrous tissue

**fibr/o**-plas-ia, condition of formation or growth of fibrous tissue

**fibr/o**-sarc-oma, a malignant fleshy tumour formed from (collagen-producing) fibroblasts

**fibr/o**-osis, abnormal condition of (formation) of fibrous tissue (in an organ)

**fibros**-itis, inflammation of fibrous tissue (especially of muscle sheaths and fascia)

**fibr/o**-tic, 1. pertaining to or of the nature of fibrosis, 2. pertaining to having fibrosis

**fibr**-ous, pertaining to or of the nature of fibres

**fibr/o**-vascul-ar, pertaining to (blood) vessels and fibrous tissue

**Kinesi/o, kin/et/o,** movement
From a Greek word **kinein,** meaning movement. Here kinesi/o means movement or motion.

brady-**kines**-ia, condition of abnormally slow movement

brady-**kines**-ic, 1. pertaining to bradykinesia 2. pertaining to having slow movement

centro-**kines**-ia, condition of movement resulting from central stimulation (by the CNS)

dys-**kines**-ia, condition of difficult or painful movement

hyper-**kines**-ia, condition of above normal power of movement

hypo-**kines**-ia, condition of below normal power of movement

**kin**-aesthes-ia, condition of sensation of movement (the overall sensations by which weight, position and muscular movement are perceived)

**kin**-aesth-esis, condition of sensation of movement (the overall sensations by which weight, position and muscular movement are perceived)

**kin**-aesthe-tic, pertaining to having the sensation of movement (the overall sensations by which weight, position and muscular movement are perceived)

**kin**-an-aesthes-ia, condition of loss of sensation of movement

**kine**-plasty, surgical repair or reconstruction for movement, it refers to using stump of an amputated limb to move a prosthesis

**kines**-alg-ia, condition of pain caused by movement of muscles Syn. cinesalgia

**kines**-ia, condition due to motion *e.g.* sea-sickness

**kines**-iatr-ics, the science of medical treatment using active and passive movements Syn. kinesiotherapy

**kines**-ics, the science of studying body movement

**kinesi/o**-logy, the study of movement of the body musculature, including movement disorders and their treatment

**kinesi/o**-meter, 1. an instrument that measures degree of movement 2. a device that moves across the body to measure skin sensibility

**kinesi/o**-neur-osis, abnormal nervous condition that results in movement (a motor disturbance *e.g.* a nervous tic or spasm)

**kinesi/o**-therap-ist, a specialist in kinesio-therapy

**kinesi/o**-therapy, treatment using active and passive movements as a primary form of rehabilitation *e.g.* for amputees

**kin**-esis, condition of movement or motion

**kinet/o**-cardi/o-graphy, technique of recording heart movements (low frequency vibrations through the chest wall)

**kinet/o**-gen-ic, pertaining to forming movements

**kinet**-osis, abnormal condition due to motion *e.g.* sea-sickness Syn. cinesia

my/o-**kines/i**-meter, an instrument that measures movement of muscle

syn-**kin**-esis, condition of moving together, it refers to an involuntary movement occurring in one part of the body at the same time as a deliberate movement in another part

---

**Leiomy/o**, smooth muscle

From the Greek words **leios** meaning smooth and **mys** meaning muscle. Here leiomy/o means smooth muscle, a type of involuntary muscle found in the walls of hollow organs. Smooth muscle is also known as non-striated and involuntary muscle.

**leiomy/o**-fibr-oma, a tumour of fibrous tissue (fibroma) and smooth muscle cells (leiomyoma)

**leiomy**-oma, a tumour formed from smooth muscle (often of the uterus)

**leiomy/o**-sarc-oma, a malignant, fleshy tumour containing smooth muscle cells

---

**Muscul/o**, muscle

From a Latin word **musculus**, meaning muscle. Here muscul/o means a muscle or muscle tissue.

intra-**muscul**-ar, pertaining to within a muscle

**muscul**-ar, pertaining to muscle

**muscul**-ar dys-trophy, poor nourishment of muscle, it refers to poor growth and development

**muscul/o**-aponeur-o-tic, pertaining to an aponeurosis and its muscle

**muscul/o**-cutane-ous, pertaining to the skin and muscle

**muscul/o**-derm-ic, pertaining to the skin and muscle Syn. musculocutaneous

**muscul/o**-phren-ic, pertaining to the muscles of the diaphragm

**muscul/o**-skelet-al, pertaining to the skeleton (bones) and muscle

**muscul/o**-tendin-ous, pertaining to tendon and muscle

**muscul/o**-ton-ic, 1. pertaining to tone of muscle 2. pertaining to contractility of muscle

**muscul/o**-trop-ic, 1. pertaining to an affinity for muscle 2. pertaining to stimulating muscle

---

**My/o/s**, **mys/i**, muscle

From a Greek word **mys**, meaning muscle. Here my/o means a muscle or muscle tissue.

electro-**my/o**-graphy, technique of recording the electrical activity of muscle

endo-**mys/i**-um, a structure within a muscle, refers to the thin connective tissue around individual muscle fibres

epi-**mys/i**-um, a structure upon a muscle, it refers to the fibrous connective tissue that encloses an entire muscle

**my/o**-a-trophy, 1. without nourishment or wasting away of muscle 2. muscular atrophy

**my/o**-blast, an immature cell or embryonic cell that forms into a muscle fibre

**my/o**-blast-oma, a tumour of myoblasts (its histiogenesis is now in doubt,

**my/o**-cardi-al, pertaining to heart muscle or myocardium

**my/o**-cardi/o-graph, an instrument that records heart muscle or myocardium (heart movements)

**my/o**-cardi/o-pathy, disease of heart muscle

**my/o**-card-itis, inflammation of the heart muscle or myocardium

**my/o**-card-um, the heart muscle (the thick, middle layer of muscle in the heart)

**my/o**-card-osis, abnormal condition of the heart muscle or myocardium (a degenerative condition) Syn. myo-cardiopathy

**my/o**-cele, a protrusion or hernia of a muscle through its sheath

**my/o**-cer-osis, abnormal condition of wax in muscle (waxy degeneration)

**my/o**-clon-us, a violent action (sudden shock-like contractions) of muscles

**my/o**-cyte, a muscle cell

**my/o**-dynam-ic, pertaining to the force or power of muscle

**my/o**-dys-ton-ia, condition of poor tone of muscle

**my/o**-dys-trophy, poor nourishment (growth and development) of muscle Syn. muscular dystrophy

**my/o**-electr-ical, pertaining to the electrical properties of muscle

**my/o**-fasc-itis, inflammation of a fascia and its muscle

**my/o**-fibr-il, a small muscle fibre, found in the cytoplasm of muscle cells

**my/o**-fibr/o-blast, an immature cell or embryonic cell that produces fibres with features of a smooth muscle cell (an atypical cell)

**my/o**-fibr-oma, a tumour composed of fibrous and muscle tissue (a myoma with fibrous tissue)

**my/o**-fibr-osis, abnormal condition of fibres in muscle

**my/o**-fibros-itis, inflammation of fibrous tissue around muscle fibres (in the perimysium)

**my/o**-filament, a thread-like muscle filament found within the myofibrils

of muscle cells, composed of actin or myosin

**my/o**-genesis, the formation or development of muscle tissue

**my/o**-gen-ic, 1. pertaining to forming from muscle tissue 2. pertaining to originating in muscle tissue

**my/o**-gen-ous, 1. pertaining to forming from muscle tissue 2. pertaining to originating in muscle tissue

**my/o**-globin, a muscle protein, it is similar to haemoglobin and functions as an oxygen carrier in muscle cells

**my/o**-globin-ur-ia, condition of myoglobin (muscle protein) in the urine

**my/o**-gram, a tracing or recording of a muscle (made by a myograph)

**my/o**-graph, an instrument that records muscle (contraction)

**my/o**-graphy, 1. technique of recording muscles (contracting) 2. technique of making a recording or X-ray picture of muscle

**my**-oid, resembling muscle

**my/o**-kinesi/o-meter, an instrument that measures movement of muscle (its contraction following artificial stimulation)

**myo**-kin-esis, condition of movement of muscle

**my/o**-kinet-ic, 1. pertaining to the movement of muscle 2. pertaining to myokinesis

**my/o**-kym-ia, condition of involuntary twitching of a muscle

**my/o**-logy, the study of muscles and associated structures (anatomy, diseases and treatment of)

**my/o**-lysis, breakdown or disintegration of muscle tissue

**my**-oma, a tumour of a muscle

**my/o**-malac-ia, condition of softening of a muscle

**my**-omat-osis, abnormal condition of having multiple myomas

**my**-om-ectomy, removal of a muscle tumour or myoma

**my/o**-melan-osis, abnormal condition of pigmented or dark muscle

**my/o**-meter, an instrument that measures muscle (contraction)

**my/o**-metri-al, pertaining to the muscle of the uterus ( the myometrium)

**my/o**-metr-itis, inflammation of the muscle of the uterus (the myometrium)

**my/o**-metri-um, the muscle of the uterus (the tunica muscularis)

**my/o**-neur-al, pertaining to nerve and muscle

**my/o**-palm-us, muscle twitching or clonic spasm of muscle. From a Greek word *palmus* meaning a quivering

**my/o**-paralysis, paralysis of a muscle

**my/o**-paresis, slight paralysis of a muscle

**my/o**-path-ic, pertaining to disease of muscle

**my/o**-pathy, disease of muscle

**my/o**-peri-card-itis, inflammation of the pericardium and heart muscle (myocardium)

**my/o**-plast-ic, pertaining to surgical repair or reconstruction of muscle

**my/o**-plasty, surgical repair or reconstruction of muscle

**my/o**-rrhexis, rupture of a muscle

**my/o**-sarc-oma, a malignant fleshy tumour derived from muscle cells

**my/o**-scler-osis, abnormal condition of hardening of a muscle

**myos**-in, a chemical (protein) found in myofibrils of muscle cells (it participates in the contraction of the cell)

**myos**-itis, inflammation of muscle

**my/o**-spasm, involuntary contraction of muscle

**my/o**-tact-ic, pertaining to the tactile (touch) sense of muscles

**my/o**-tasis, stretching (tension) of muscle. From a Greek word *tasis* meaning a straining

**my/o**-tenos-itis, inflammation of a tendon and its muscle

**my/o**-tomy, incision into a muscle

**my/o**-ton-ia, condition of muscle tone, it refers to any disorder involving a prolonged contraction of muscle (a tonic spasm)

**my/o**-ton-ic, pertaining to having myotonia

**my/o**-ton-us, muscle tone (a slight continuous contraction or tension always present in healthy muscle)

**my/o**-troph-ic, 1. pertaining to nourishing muscle (increasing its mass) 2. pertaining to myotrophy

**my/o**-trophy, nourishment of muscle

peri-**myos**-itis, inflammation around a muscle ( its connective tissue)

peri-**mys/i**-itis, inflammation of the perimysium Syn. myofibrositis

peri-**mys/i**-um, the structure around a muscle, it refers to the fibrous connective tissue that encloses bundles of muscle fibres

---

**Ortho-**, correct, right, straight

From a Greek word **orthos** meaning right or straight. Here, ortho- is used as a prefix meaning correct, right or straight.

**ortho**-chorea, jerky movements that occur when standing straight (erect)

**ortho**-dactyl-ous, pertaining to straight fingers or toes

**ortho**-grade, walking with the body in the straight (erect) position

**ortho**-paed-ic, 1. pertaining to a straight child, now a branch of surgery that deals with the restoration of function of the musculoskeletal system in children or adults 2. pertaining to orthopaedics

**ortho**-paed-ics, literally meaning the art or science of making a child straight, it now means the branch of surgery that deals with the restoration of function of the musculoskeletal system in children or adults

**ortho**-paed-ist, a specialist in orthopaedics, the branch of surgery that deals with the restoration of function of the musculoskeletal system

**ortho**-prax-ia, condition of normal, purposeful movement, it refers to the process of surgical correction of deformities to make straight, purposeful movements

**ortho**-prax-is, process of normal, purposeful movement, it refers to the process of surgical correction of deformities to make straight, purposeful movements

**ortho**-praxy, process of normal, purposeful movement, it refers to the process of surgical correction of deformities to make straight, purposeful movements

**orth**-oses, structures or appliances used to straighten deformities. Plural of orthosis

**orth**-osis, a structure or appliance used to straighten a deformity. Singular of orthoses

**ortho**-stat-ic, pertaining to standing straight (erect)

**ortho**-stat-ism, process of standing in a straight position (erect)

**ortho**-therapy, treatment by standing straight (right or correct posture)

**ortho**-tics, a branch of medical science dealing with the design, manufacture and fitting of orthoses

**orth**-ot-ist, a specialist in orthotics or the use of orthoses (structures and appliances to correct deformities)

**ortho**-ton-us, a muscular spasm that fixes the head, body and limbs in a rigid, straight line

**ortho**-top-ic, pertaining to the correct or normal place

**Rhabdomy/o**, striated muscle
From a Greek word **rhabdos**, meaning stripe. Here, rhabdomy/o means striped muscle, a type of muscle under voluntary control that moves the limbs. Striped muscle is also known as striated or voluntary muscle.

**rhabdomy/o**-blast-oma, a malignant tumour of immature cells or embryonic cells that form striated muscle cells Syn. rhabdomyosarcoma

**rhabdomy/o**-chondr-oma, a tumour containing cartilage cells and striated muscle cells

**rhabdomy/o**-lysis, breakdown of striated muscle

**rhabdomy**-oma, a tumour containing striated muscle

**rhabdomy/o**-sarcoma, a malignant tumour derived from immature cells or embryonic cells that form striated muscle cells

**rhabd/o**-sarc-oma, a malignant tumour derived from immature cells or embryonic cells that form striated muscle cells Syn. rhabdomyosarcoma

**Spas/m/o, spasmod-**, spasm
From a Greek word **spasmos** meaning spasm. Here spasm/o means a sudden, powerful, involuntary contraction of a muscle.

**spasmod**-ic, 1. pertaining to or having the form of a spasm 2. pertaining to occurring in spasms

**spasm/o**-lysis, breaking down (stopping) a spasm

**spasm/o**-lyt-ic, 1. pertaining to breaking down (stopping) a spasm 2. an agent that acts against a spasm (an antispasmodic)

**spasm/o**-phil-ia, condition of tendency to have spasms. From a Greek word *philein* meaning to love

**spasm**-us, a spasm

**spas**-tic, 1. produced by a spasm 2. pertaining to or of the nature of a spasm 3. state of rigid (hypertonic) muscles 4. a person exhibiting spasticity

**spas**-tic-ity, 1. condition or state of being spastic 2. condition of rigid (hypertonic) muscles

**-tax-**, ordered movement
From a Greek word **taxis** meaning order. Here -tax- means an ordered movement.

a-**tax**-ia, condition of without ordered movement or disordered movement (irregular jerky movements)

a-**tax**-ic, pertaining to without ordered movement or disordered movement (irregular jerky movements)

a-**tax**-y, condition of without ordered movements, it refers to irregular jerky movements

di-a-**tax**-ia, condition of ataxia affecting two (both) sides of the body

dys-**tax**-ia, condition of difficulty in controlling ordered (voluntary) movement

213

**Ten/o, tend/o, tendin/o, tenont/o, tendon**

From a Greek word **tenon**, meaning to stretch. Here, ten/o means a tendon, a firm, white, fibrous inelastic cord that attaches muscle to bone.

poly-**tendin**-itis, inflammation of many tendons at the same time

poly-**tendin/o**-burs-itis, inflammation of many bursae and tendon sheaths at the same time

poly-**ten/o**-synov-itis, inflammation of many synovia of tendon sheaths

**ten**-alg-ia, condition of pain in a tendon Syn. tenontodynia, tenodynia

**ten**-ectomy, removal of a tendon or tendon sheath

**tendin**-itis, inflammation of tendons Syn. tendinitis, tenontitis, tenonitis

**tendin/o**-plasty, surgical repair or reconstruction of a tendon

**tendin/o**-suture, stitching or suturing of a tendon Syn. tenorrhaphy

**tendin**-ous, pertaining to or of the nature of a tendon

**tendon**-itis, inflammation of a tendon Syn. tendinitis, tenontitis, tenonitis

**ten/o**-desis, surgical fixation of a tendon (the end of a tendon to a new point)

**ten/o**-dyn-ia, condition of pain in a tendon Syn. tenalgia, tenontodynia

**ten/o**-lysis, surgical loosening of a tendon (from adhesions)

**ten/o**-my/o-plasty, surgical repair or reconstruction of muscle and tendons

**ten/o**-my/o-tomy, incision into muscle and a tendon

**tenon**-ectomy, removal of a tendon or part of a tendon

**tenon**-itis, inflammation of a tendon Syn. tendonitis, tendinitis, tenontitis

**tenont/o**-dyn-ia, condition of pain in a tendon Syn. tenalgia, tenodynia

**tenont/o**-logy, the study of tendons (anatomy, diseases and treatment of)

**ten/o**-phyte, a plant-like growth of a tendon

**ten/o**-plast-ic, 1. pertaining to surgical repair or reconstruction of a tendon 2. pertaining to tenoplasty

**ten/o**-plasty, surgical repair or reconstruction of a tendon

**ten/o**-recept-or, a sensory nerve ending in a tendon that gives information about movement and position (a proprioceptor)

**ten**-ost-osis, abnormal condition of ossification (bone formation) in a tendon

**ten/o**-suture, stitching or suturing of a tendon Syn. tenorrhaphy

**ten/o**-synov-ectomy, removal of a tendon sheath

**ten/o**-synov-itis, inflammation of a tendon sheath

**ten/o**-rrhaphy, stitching or suturing of a tendon

**ten/o**-tomy, incision into a tendon

**Thec/o, theca**

From a Greek word **theke** meaning sheath. Here thec/o means a theca, an enveloping sheath particularly of a tendon.

**thec**-al, pertaining to a theca

**thec**-ate, having a theca or sheath

**thec**-itis, inflammation of a theca, here it refers to a tendon sheath Syn. tenosynovitis

**thec/o**-stegn-osis, abnormal narrowing of a tendon sheath. From a Greek word *stegnosis* meaning a narrowing

**Ton/o, tension, tone**

From a Greek word **tonos** meaning tension. Here ton/o means muscle tone, a slight tension present in muscles when they are not undergoing active contraction.

a-**ton**-ia, condition of without muscle tone or strength

a-**ton**-ic, 1. pertaining to without muscle tone or strength 2. pertaining to having atonia

a-**ton**-ic-ity, state or quality of muscles being atonic Syn. atony

a-**ton**-y, condition of without muscle tone

dys-**ton**-ia, condition of bad or impaired muscle tone

dys-**ton**-ic, 1. pertaining to bad or impaired muscle tone 2. pertaining to having dystonia

hetero-**ton**-ia, condition of different (variable) muscular tension or tone

hyper-**ton**-ia, condition of increased or above normal muscle tone

hyper-**ton**-ic, 1. pertaining to increased or above normal muscle tone 2. pertaining to having hypertonia

hyper-**ton**-ic-ity, state or quality of muscles being hypertonic

hypo-**ton**-ia, condition of decreased or below normal muscle tone

hypo-**ton**-ic, 1. pertaining to decreased or below normal muscle tone 2. pertaining to having hypotonia

hypo-**ton**-ic-ity, state or quality of muscles being hypotonic

**ton**-ic, 1. pertaining to producing normal muscle tone 2. pertaining to having continuous tone or tension in muscle

**ton**-ic-ity, state or quality of muscle tension

# The skeletal system

The supporting structure of the body consisting of 206 bones is known as the skeletal system. Bones have a variety of functions including:

- supporting all tissues by providing a framework for the body
- enabling movement of the body by forming joints and points of attachment for the muscles
- protecting vital organs and soft tissues
- forming red bone marrow, the substance in which blood cells develop by haemopoiesis
- storing minerals, especially calcium phosphate, that can be released into the blood.

The point at which any two bones or more meet is called a joint. Some joints have no movement (fibrous), some only slight movement (cartilaginous) and some are freely movable (synovial).

Synovial joints have features that enable a wide range of movements. The parts of the bone in contact within a synovial joint are always covered with hyaline cartilage; this provides a smooth articular surface and is strong enough to withstand compression and bear the weight of the body. The cavity of a synovial joint contains a thick sticky fluid of egg-white consistency called synovia or synovial fluid secreted by membranes surrounding the synovial cavity. Synovial fluid has a variety of functions: it provides nutrients for structures within the

## Quick Reference

Common words and combining forms relating to the skeletal system:

joint cavity, acts as a lubricant, helps maintain joint stability, prevents the ends of bone becoming separated and contains phagocytes that remove cell debris. Little sacs of synovial fluid called bursae are present in some joints, for example the knee. These act as cushions to help prevent friction between a bone and a ligament or tendon.

Tough bands of fibrous connective tissue called ligaments prevent synovial joints from separating and give them additional stability. Ligaments connect bone to bone around a joint.

Figure 20 shows the combining forms associated with the skeleton. Figures 21 and 22 show combining forms associated with a synovial joint and the vertebral column.

Tables 1–4 at the end of this section list words associated with specific bones, components of the skeleton and movements at synovial joints.

### Roots and combining forms, meanings

**Ankyl/o,** fusion, stiffness
From a Greek word **agkylosis** meaning stiffness of a joint. Here ankyl/o means a joint that becomes fixed or fused in position.

**ankyl**-ose, 1. pertaining to fixed by ankylosis 2. pertaining to becoming fused

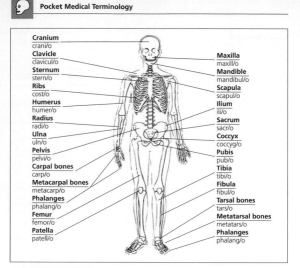

Figure 20  The skeleton

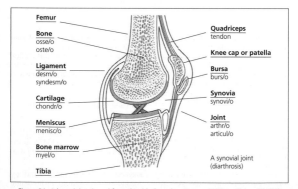

Figure 21  A knee joint viewed from the side (based on Ross and Wilson, Figure 17.12B)

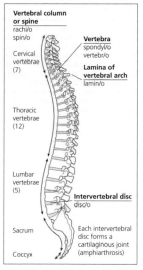

**Vertebral column or spine**
rachi/o
spin/o

Cervical vertebrae (7)

**Vertebra**
spondyl/o
vertebr/o

**Lamina of vertebral arch**
lamin/o

Thoracic vertebrae (12)

Lumbar vertebrae (5)

**Intervertebral disc**
disc/o

Sacrum

Each intervertebral disc forms a cartilaginous joint (amphiarthrosis)

Coccyx

Figure 22 The vertebral column, lateral view (based on Ross and Wilson, Figure 16.16)

ankylos-ing, process of becoming fused

ankyl-osis, abnormal condition of fusion of a joint (results in immobility of the joint)

ankyl/o-tic, 1. pertaining to ankylosis 2. pertaining to suffering from ankylosis

**Arthr/o**, joint

From a Greek word **arthron**, meaning joint. Here arthr/o means a joint, the point where two or more bones or cartilages meet. There are three main classes 1. Fibrous, immovable joints (synarthroses) 2. Cartilaginous, slightly movable joints (amphiarthroses) sub-divided into synchondroses and symphyses 3. Freely movable synovial joints (diarthroses).

amphi-**arthr**-osis, a cartilaginous, slightly movable joint with both surfaces connected by a fibrocartilaginous disc or by synovial membranes

**arthr**-agra, sudden pain in a joint (due to gout)

**arthr**-al, pertaining to or belonging to a joint

**arthr**-alg-ia, condition of pain in a joint Syn. arthrodynia

**arthr**-ectomy, removal of a joint

**arthr**-itic, pertaining to having arthritis

**arthr**-itis, inflammation of a joint

**arthr/o**-centesis, puncture of a joint (for aspiration of fluid)

**arthr/o**-chondr-itis, inflammation of the cartilage of a joint

**arthr/o**-clas-ia, condition of breaking of a joint, it refers to breaking adhesions within a joint by surgical means to improve mobility

**arthr/o**-clasis, breaking of a joint, it refers to breaking adhesions within a joint by surgical means to improve mobility

**arthr/o**-desis, surgical fixation of a joint

**arthr/o**-dys-plas-ia, condition of poor formation of joints (an inherited deformity of joints)

**arthr/o**-em-py-esis, condition of pus within a joint

**arthr/o**-endo-scope, an instrument used to view or examine the inside of a joint

**arthr/o**-desis, surgical fixation of joints

**arthr/o**-dyn-ia, condition of pain in a joint Syn. arthralgia

**arthr/o**-gram, a recording or X-ray picture of a joint

**arthr/o**-graphy, technique of making a recording or X-ray picture of a joint

**arthr/o**-gryp-osis, abnormal retention of a joint in a flexed (bent) position. From a Greek word *grypsis* meaning curve

**arthr/o**-lith, a stone or calculus in a joint

**arthr/o**-logy, the study of joints (anatomy, diseases and treatment of)

**arthr/o**-neur-alg-ia, condition of pain in nerves in or around a joint

**arthr/o**-ophthalm/o-pathy, disease of the eyes associated with (degenerative) disease of joints

**arthr/o**-path-ic, 1. pertaining to disease of joints 2. pertaining to having arthropathy

**arthr/o**-pathy, disease of a joint

**arthr/o**-plast-ic, 1. pertaining to surgical repair or reconstruction of a joint 2. pertaining to arthroplasty

**arthr/o**-plasty, surgical repair or reconstruction of a joint

**arthr/o**-py-osis, abnormal condition of pus in a joint

**arthr/o**-scinti-gram, a scintiscan recording of a joint, it refers to a recording of a radioisotope scan

**arthr/o**-scler-osis, abnormal condition of hardening of a joint (inflexibility)

**arthr/o**-scope, an instrument used to view or examine a joint (a type of endoscope)

**arthr/o**-scopy, technique of viewing or examining a joint

**arthr/o**-osis, 1. a joint or articulation 2. abnormal condition of a joint

**arthr/o**-stomy, formation of an opening into a joint (for drainage) or the name of the opening so created

**arthr/o**-synov-itis, inflammation of a synovial joint

**arthr/o**-tomy, incision into a joint

di-**arthr/o**-ic, pertaining to two joints or affecting two different joints

di-**arthr/o**-osis, a freely movable synovial joint. From the Latin words *di* meaning opposite and *articulare* meaning to divide into joints

en-**arthr/o**-osis, condition of a joint, it refers to a ball and socket joint where the head of one bone fits into the socket of another

mon-**arthr/o**-itis, inflammation of one joint

poly-**arthr/o**-itis, inflammation of many joints

pseudo-**arthr/o**-osis, condition of a false joint, it refers to an ununited fracture

syn-**arthr/o**-osis, condition of a joint fixed or fused together, it refers to a fibrous immovable joint

**Articul**-, articulation, joint

From a Latin word **articulare** meaning to divide into joints. Here articul-means a joint or articulation, the point where two or more bones or cartilages meet. There are three main classes 1. Fibrous, immovable joints (synarthroses) 2. Cartilaginous, slightly movable joints (amphiarthroses) subdivided into synchondroses and symphyses 3. Freely movable synovial joints (diarthroses).

**articul**-ar, 1. pertaining to a joint 2. pertaining to an articulation

**articul**-ate, 1. arranged into joints 2. to unite in a joint or divide to form a joint 3. united so as to form a joint

**articul**-ation, a junction between two bones or cartilages

bi-**articul**-ar, pertaining to two joints

bi-**articul**-ate, having two joints

di-**articul**-ar, pertaining to two joints or affecting two different joints

ex-**articul**-ation, 1. process of removing part of a joint 2. amputation of a limb through a joint 3. a dislocation

mon-**articul**-ar, pertaining to one joint

peri-**articul**-ar, pertaining to around a joint

**Burs/o**, bursa

From a Latin word **bursa** meaning purse. Here burs/o means a bursa, a small sac lined with a synovial membrane secreting synovial fluid. Bursae are found between joints, muscles and tendons where they act to reduce friction.

**burs**-al, pertaining to a bursa

**burs**-ectomy, removal of a bursa

**burs**-itis, inflammation of a bursa

**burs/o**-lith, a stone or calculus in a bursa

**burs/o**-pathy, disease of a bursa

**burs/o**-tomy, incision into a bursa

**Chondr/o**, cartilage

From a Greek word **chondros**, meaning cartilage. Here chondr/o means cartilage, the plastic-like connective tissue found at the ends of bones, for example in joints where it forms a smooth surface for movement at a joint.

**chondr**-al, pertaining to cartilage

**chondr**-alg-ia, condition of pain in a cartilage

**chondr**-ectomy, removal of a cartilage

**chondr**-ic, pertaining to cartilage

**chondr**-itis, inflammation of cartilage

**chondr/o**-aden-oma, a tumour of glandular epithelium containing cartilage elements

**chondr/o**-angi-oma, a tumour of blood vessels (angioma) with cartilage elements

**chondr/o**-blast, an immature cell or embryonic cell that forms cartilage

**chondr/o**-blast-oma, a tumour formed from chondroblasts (embryonic cells that form cartilage)

**chondr/o**-calcin-osis, abnormal condition of calcified cartilage

**chondr/o**-carcin-oma, a carcinoma (malignant tumour) containing cartilage elements

**chondr/o**-clast, a cell that breaks down cartilage

**chondr/o**-cost-al, pertaining to a rib cartilage

**chondr/o**-crani-um, the cartilage cranium (present in the embryo before ossification)

**chondr/o**-cyte, a cartilage cell (mature)

**chondr/o**-dermat-itis, inflammation of the skin and cartilage

**chondr/o**-dyn-ia, condition of pain in a cartilage

**chondr/o**-dys-plas-ia, condition of poor growth or development of cartilage, it refers to a benign growth of cartilage arising in the metaphysis of a bone

**chondr/o**-dys-troph-ia, condition of poor or bad nourishment of cartilage, it leads to poor formation of cartilage Syn. chondrodystrophy

**chondr/o**-dys-trophy, poor or bad nourishment of cartilage, it leads to poor formation of cartilage

**chondr/o**-epiphys-eal, pertaining to the epiphyseal cartilages (at the ends of long bones)

**chondr/o**-epiphys-itis, inflammation of epiphyseal cartilages

**chondr/o**-fibr-oma, a tumour composed of fibrous connective (fibroma) tissue and cartilage elements

**chondr/o**-genesis, formation of cartilage

**chondr/o**-gen-ic, pertaining to forming cartilage

**chondr**-oid, resembling cartilage

**chondr/o**-lip-oma, a tumour in which there are elements of fatty tissue and cartilaginous tissue

**chondr/o**-lysis, breakdown of cartilage

**chondr**-oma, a tumour of cartilage cells or cartilaginous tissue

**chondr/o**-malac-ia, condition of softening of cartilage

**chondr**-omat-osis, abnormal condition of multiple chondromas

**chondr/o**-meta-plas-ia, condition of change in form or change in growth of cartilage (cells)

**chondr/o**-my-oma, a tumour of muscle tissue (myoma) and cartilaginous tissue (chondroma)

**chondr/o**-myx-oma, a tumour of mucoid tissue (myxoma) and cartilaginous tissue (chondroma)

**chondr/o**-myx/o-sarc-oma, a tumour in which there are elements of sarcoma, myxoma and chondroma

**chondr/o**-osse-ous, 1. pertaining to bone and cartilage 2. made up of bone and cartilage

**chondr/o**-oste/o-dys-trophy, poor or bad nourishment of bone and cartilage, it results in deformities of the epiphyses leading to dwarfism and kyphosis

**chondr/o**-pathy, disease of cartilage

**chondr/o**-plas-ia, condition of formation or development of cartilage (cells)

**chondr/o**-plast-ic, 1. pertaining to surgical repair or reconstruction of cartilage 2. pertaining to chondroplasty

**chondr/o**-plasty, surgical repair or reconstruction of cartilage

**chondr/o**-phyte, a cartilage plant, it refers to a plant-like growth of cartilage

**chondr/o**-por-osis, abnormal condition of pores in cartilage

**chondr/o**-sarc-oma, a malignant fleshy tumour derived from cartilage cells

**chondr**-osis, abnormal condition of cartilage, it refers to an abnormal increase in the formation of cartilage

**chondr/o**-oste-oma, a tumour of bone covered with cartilage Syn. osteochondroma

**chondr/o**-stern-al, pertaining to the sternum and (costal) cartilage

**chondr/o**-stern/o-plasty, surgical repair or reconstruction of the sternum and (costal) cartilage to correct funnel chest

**chondr/o**-tome, an instrument used to cut cartilage

**chondr/o**-tomy, incision into cartilage

**chondr/o**-xiph-oid, pertaining to the cartilage of the xiphoid process

dys-**chondr/o**-plas-ia, condition of poor growth of cartilage (cells), it refers to poor endochondral ossification of long bones

endo-**chondr**-al, pertaining to within cartilage

hypo-**chondr**-ial, pertaining to the hypochondrium

hypo-**chondr**-ium, the upper abdominal region on either side of the body below the cartilages of the lower ribs

syn-**chondr**-osis, a joint formed when two bones are connected by cartilage, this is usually temporary as between a epiphysis and diaphysis of a long bone

---

**Condyl/o**, condyle

From a Greek word **condylos** meaning knuckle. Here condyl/o means a condyle, a rounded, articular projection found at the ends of some bones.

**condyl**-ar, pertaining to a condyle

**condyl**-arthr-osis, 1. condition of a joint with condyles 2. a condyloid articulation

**condyl**-ectomy, removal of a condyle

**condyl**-oid, 1. resembling or shaped like a condyle 2. knuckle-shaped

**condyl/o**-tomy, incision into a condyle

epi-**condyl**-alg-ia, condition of pain in an epicondyle (of the humerus) it refers to muscular pain around the elbow as a result of over strain of the arm

epi-**condyl**-ar, pertaining to an epicondyle

epi-**condyle**, structure upon a condyle, it refers to an eminence (projection) upon a bone above its condyle

epi-**condyl**-itis, inflammation of an epicondyle (of the humerus) and surrounding tissues

---

**Crani/o**, cranium, skull

From a Greek word **kranion** meaning skull. Here crani/o means the cranium, the part of the skull enclosing the brain. It consists of eight bones: the occipital, two parietals, frontal, two temporals, sphenoid and ethmoid.

**crani**-ad, in the direction of the cranium

**crani**-al, pertaining to the cranium

**crani/o**-acromi-al, pertaining to the acromion and the cranium

**crani/o**-caud-al, pertaining to the tail and cranium (head and tail as of an axis in embryology)

**crani/o**-cele, a protrusion or hernia (of the brain) through the cranium

**crani/o**-cervic-al, pertaining to the neck and cranium

**crani/o**-clasis, 1. breaking of the cranium or skull e.g. to deliver a dead fetus 2. craniotomy

**crani/o**-clasty, 1. process of breaking of the cranium e.g. to deliver a dead fetus 2. craniotomy

**crani/o**-cleid/o-dys-oste-osis, condition of defective formation of bones of the clavicle and cranium (head), due to defective ossification in the fetus

**crani/o**-faci-al, pertaining to the face and cranium

**crani/o**-fenestr-ia, condition of windows in the cranium, it refers to areas in which no bone has formed

**crani/o**-lacun-ia, condition of lacunae (hollows) in the cranium, it refers to poor development of the fetal skull

**crani/o**-malac-ia, condition of softening of the cranium

**crani/o**-mening/o-cele, a protrusion or hernia of the meninges through a defect in the cranium

**crani/o**-meter, an instrument used to measure the cranium (diameters)

**crani/o**-metry, technique of measuring the cranium

**crani/o**-plasty, surgical repair or reconstruction of the cranium

**crani/o**-rachi-schisis, splitting (congenital fissure) of the spinal column and cranium

**crani/o**-sacr-al, pertaining to the sacrum and cranium

**crani/o**-schisis, splitting (congenital fissure) of the cranium

**crani/o**-scler-osis, abnormal condition of hardening (thickening) of the cranium

**crani/o**-sten-osis, abnormal condition of narrowing of the cranium, it refers to premature closure of sutures (fixed, fibrous joints) in the cranium

**crani**-ost-osis, abnormal, congenital condition of ossification of cranial sutures

**crani/o**-syn-ost-osis, abnormal condition of (premature) fusion of cranial sutures

**crani/o**-tabes, wasting of the cranium or skull, it refers to thinning of the infant skull

**crani/o**-tome, an instrument used to cut the cranium

**crani/o**-tomy, incision into the cranium

**crani/o**-tympan-ic, pertaining to the tympanum (middle ear) and cranium

epi-**crani**-um, structure upon the cranium, it refers to the structures that cover the cranium forming the scalp

---

**-dactyl-**, a digit, finger or toe
From a Greek word **daktylos** meaning finger. Here, -dactyl- means a finger or toe.

brachy-**dactyl**-y, condition of abnormally short fingers and toes

hexa-**dactyl**-y, condition of six fingers or toes on a limb

iso-**dactyl**-ism, condition of having the same length of fingers or toes on a limb

mega-syn-**dactyl**-y, condition of abnormally large fused (webbed) fingers and toes

pachy-**dactyl**-y, condition of thick (enlarged) fingers and toes

poly-**dactyl**-ism, condition of more than the normal number of fingers or toes on a limb

poly-**dactyl**-y, condition of more than the normal number of fingers or toes on a limb

poly-syn-**dactyl**-y, condition of syndactyly and polydactyly in association

syn-**dactyl**-ous, pertaining to syndactyly

syn-**dactyl**-y, condition of fused fingers or toes, the fusion may be complete or partial giving a webbed appearance

zygo-**dactyl**-y, condition of joined fingers and joined toes (by soft tissues, not bones)

---

**Desm/o**, ligament
From a Greek word **desmos** meaning band. Here, desm/o means a ligament, a band of tough, fibrous connective tissue. Ligaments join bones or other structures together.

**desm**-alg-ia, condition of pain from a ligament

**desm**-ectasis, dilation or stretching of a ligament

**desm**-itis, inflammation of a ligament

**desm/o**-gen-ous, pertaining to originating in ligaments

**desm/o**-graphy, description or study of ligaments

**desm**-oid, 1. resembling a ligament 2. a fibrous tumour arising in a muscle sheath resembling a fibrosarcoma

**desm/o**-pathy, disease of ligaments

**desm/o**-pex-ia, surgical fixation of ligaments *e.g.* the round ligaments to the wall of the uterus

**desm/o**-tomy, incision into a ligament

**Disc/o, disk/o,** intervertebral disc

From a Latin word **diskus,** meaning disc. Here, disc/o means an intervertebral disc, a pad of connective tissue that acts as a shock absorber between vertebrae.

**disc**-ectomy, removal of an intervertebral disc

**disc**-itis, inflammation of an intervertebral disc

**disc/o**-gen-ic, 1. pertaining to forming in a disc 2. pertaining to originating in a disc

**disc/o**-graphy, technique of making a recording or X-ray picture of an intervertebral disc

**disc**-oid, resembling a disc

**disc/o**-pathy, disease of an an intervertebral disc

**disk**-ectomy, removal of an intervertebral disc

**disk**-itis, inflammation of an intervertebral disc

**disk/o**-graphy, technique of making a recording or X-ray picture of an intervertebral disc

**Gon-, gony-,** knee

From a Greek word **gony** meaning knee. Here, gon- means the knee; the hinge joint formed by the lower end of the femur and the head of the tibia. The triangular sesamoid bone called the patella forms the knee cap in front of the knee joint.

Note: the root gon- derived from the Greek word *gone* means semen and goni- derived from the Greek word **gonia** means the angle of the anterior chamber of the eye. See Section 15 The male reproductive system and Section 9 The eye.

**gon**-agra, pain in a knee due to gout

**gon**-alg-ia, condition of pain in a knee

**gon**-arthr-itis, inflammation of a knee joint

**gon**-arthr/o-tomy, incision into a knee joint

**gon**-itis, inflammation of a knee

**gony**-campsis, deformity of the knee caused by abnormal curvature. From a Greek word *kampe* meaning a bending

**gony**-cele, a protrusion or hernia of the knee

**gony**-onc-us, a tumour of the knee

**Kyph/o,** crooked, forward curvature of the thoracic spine, hunch-backed

From a Greek word **kyphos** meaning hunch-backed. Here, kyph/o means a kyphosis, an excessive forward curvature of the thoracic spine.

**kyph/o**-lord-osis, abnormal condition of lordosis (forward curvature of the lumbar spine) with kyphosis (anteroposterior deformity of the thoracic spine with the formation of a hump)

**kyphos,** the hump of the spine present in kyphosis

**kyph/o**-scoli-osis, abnormal condition of scoliosis (lateral curvature of the spine) with kyphosis (anteroposterior deformity of the thoracic spine with the formation of a hump)

**kyph/o**-scoli/o-tic, 1. pertaining to or affected by kyphoscoliosis 2. pertaining to scoliosis and kyphosis

**kyph**-osis, abnormal condition of crooked hunched spine (anteroposterior deformity of the thoracic spine with the formation of a hump)

**kyph/o**-tic, pertaining to or affected by kyphosis

**Lamin/o,** lamina of a vertebral arch

From a Latin word **lamina** meaning thin plate. Here, lamin/o means a vertebral lamina, a thin plate of bone lying on the posterolateral part of a vertebral arch on each side.

hemi-**lamin**-ectomy, removal of the laminae of half a vertebral arch (on one side only)

**lamin**-ar, 1. pertaining to a lamina 2. composed of laminae

**lamin**-ectomy, removal of the laminae of a vertebral arch (to gain access to the spinal cord)

**lamin/o**-tomy, incision into the laminae of a vertebral arch

**Lord/o**, forward curvature of the lumbar spine
From a Greek word **lordos** meaning bent so as to be convex in front. Here, lord/o means a lordosis, a forward curvature of the lumbar spine.

**lord/o**-scoli-osis, abnormal condition of scoliosis (lateral curvature of the spine) with lordosis (forward curvature of the lumbar spine)
**lord**-osis, abnormal condition of forward curvature of the lumbar spine
**lord/o**-tic, pertaining to having lordosis (forward curvature of the lumbar spine)

**Menisc/o**, meniscus
From a Greek word **meniskos** meaning crescent. Here, menisc/o, a meniscus, a crescent-shaped (semi-lunar) fibro-cartilage found in a knee joint.

**menisc**-ectomy, removal of a meniscus (the semi-lunar cartilage of a knee joint)
**menisc**-itis, inflammation of a meniscus (the semi-lunar cartilage of a knee joint)
**menisc/o**-synovi-al, pertaining to a synovial membrane and meniscus (the semi-lunar cartilage of a knee joint)

**Myel/o**, bone marrow, marrow
From a Greek word **myelos**, meaning marrow. Here, myel/o means the marrow of bones.
Note: myel/o also refers to the spinal marrow *i.e.* the spinal cord and to myelocytes, the precursors of the poly-morphonuclear series of granulocytes. Words containing myel/o are also listed in Section 5 on Blood and Section 8 on the Nervous system.

**myel**-itic, pertaining to having myelitis
**myel**-itis, inflammation of bone marrow

**myel/o**-blast, an immature cell or embryonic cell of the bone marrow, a precursor of the polymorphonuclear series of granulocytes
**myel/o**-fibr/o-scler-osis, abnormal condition of hardening bone marrow with fibrous tissue Syn. myelofibrosis
**myel/o**-fibr-osis, abnormal condition of fibres in bone marrow, refers to replacement of bone marrow with fibrous tissue
**myel/o**-gen-ic, pertaining to forming or originating in bone marrow
**myel/o**-gen-ous, 1. pertaining to forming in bone marrow 2. pertaining to originating in bone marrow
**myel**-oid, 1. resembling bone marrow 2. originating in bone marrow
**myel/o**-path-ic, pertaining to disease of bone marrow
**myel/o**-pathy, disease of bone marrow
**myel/o**-phthisis, wasting away of bone marrow, it refers to a reduction in production of cells by bone marrow
**myel/o**-poiesis, formation of marrow or marrow cells
**myel/o**-poiet-ic, 1. pertaining to formation of marrow or marrow cells 2. pertaining to myelopoiesis
**myel/o**-sarc-oma, a malignant fleshy tumour made up of bone marrow cells
**myel/o**-scler-osis, abnormal condition of hardening of bone marrow
**myel**-osis, abnormal condition of bone marrow, it refers to an abnormal increase of bone marrow tissue leading to myelocytic leukaemia
**myel/o**-tox-ic, pertaining to poisonous to bone marrow
**myel/o**-toxic-osis, abnormal condition of the bone marrow due to poisoning
**myel/o**-tox-in, an agent that poisons bone marrow, it causes destruction of cells in the bone marrow

**Ortho-**, correct, right, straight
From a Greek word **orthos** meaning right or straight. Here, ortho- is used as a prefix meaning straight, correct or right.

**ortho**-chorea, jerky movements that occur when standing straight (erect)

**ortho**-dactyl-ous, pertaining to straight fingers or toes

**ortho**-grade, walking with the body in the straight (erect) position

**ortho**-paed-ic, 1. pertaining to a straight child, now a branch of surgery that deals with the restoration of function of the musculoskeletal system in children or adults 2. pertaining to orthopaedics

**ortho**-paed-ics, literally meaning the art or science of making a child straight, it now means the branch of surgery that deals with the restoration of function of the musculoskeletal system in children or adults.

**ortho**-paed-ist, a specialist in orthopaedics, the branch of surgery that deals with the restoration of function of the musculoskeletal system

**ortho**-prax-ia, condition of normal, purposeful movement, it refers to the process of surgical correction of deformities to make straight, purposeful movements

**ortho**-prax-is, process of normal, purposeful movement, it refers to the process of surgical correction of deformities to make straight, purposeful movements

**ortho**-praxy, process of normal, purposeful movement, it refers to the process of surgical correction of deformities to make straight, purposeful movements

**orth**-oses, structures or appliances used to straighten deformities. Plural of orthosis

**orth**-osis, 1. a structure or appliance used to straighten a deformity 2. a force system designed to correct a bone deformity

**ortho**-stat-ic, pertaining to standing straight (erect)

**ortho**-stat-ism, process of standing in a straight position (erect)

**ortho**-therapy, treatment by standing straight (in the right or correct posture)

**ortho**-tic, pertaining to an orthosis

**ortho**-tics, a branch of medical science dealing with the design, manufacture and fitting of orthoses

**orth**-ot-ist, a specialist in orthotics or the use of orthoses (structures and appliances to correct deformities)

**ortho**-ton-us, a muscular spasm that fixes the head, body and limbs in a rigid, straight line

**ortho**-top-ic, pertaining to the correct or normal place

---

**Osse/o, oss/i, bone**
From a Latin word **os** meaning bone. Here osse/o means bone, the connective tissue that forms the separate bones of the skeleton. Salts such as calcium carbonate and calcium phosphate are deposited in the matrix of bone making it hard and dense. Bone is strong in compression and tension enabling the skeleton to support all tissues and organs in the body.

**osse**-in, a chemical found in bone (collagen)

**osse/o**-aponeur/o-tic, pertaining to an aponeurosis and bone

**osse/o**-cartilagin-ous, 1. pertaining to cartilage and bone 2. composed of cartilage and bone

**osse/o**-fibr-ous, 1. pertaining to fibrous tissue and bone 2. composed of fibrous tissue and bone

**osse/o**-muc-in, a mucin-like chemical found in the matrix of bone that binds together its collagenous fibres

**osse**-ous, 1. pertaining to bone 2. having the property of bone

**oss/i**-cle, a small bone *e.g.* an ear ossicle

**oss/i**-fer-ous, pertaining to bearing bone (used to mean forming bone)

**oss/i**-fication, process of forming bone. From a Latin word *facere* meaning to make

**oss/i**-form, having the form of bone

**oss/i**-fy, to form or develop into bone. From a Latin word *facere* meaning to make

**Oste/o**, bone

From a Greek word *osteon*, meaning bone. Here, oste/o means bone, the connective tissue that forms the separate bones of the skeleton. Salts such as calcium carbonate and calcium phosphate are deposited in the matrix of bone making it hard and dense. Bone is strong in compression and tension enabling the skeleton to support all tissues and organs in the body.

dys-**ost**-osis, abnormal condition of poor bones, it refers to defective formation of bones or defective ossification of fetal cartilage

ect-**ost**-osis, condition on the outside of bone, it refers to ossification beginning under the periosteum of a bone

end-**oste**-al, 1. pertaining to the endosteum 2. pertaining to within a bone

end-**oste**-um, the structure on the inside of bone, it refers to the tissue lining the medullary cavity of bone

ex-**ost**-osis, condition away from bone, it refers to a benign growth protruding from a bone surface

oste-al, pertaining to bone

oste-alg-ia, condition of pain in bones

**oste**-alg-ic, 1. pertaining to pain in bones 2. pertaining to having ostealgia

**oste**-itic, pertaining to having osteitis

oste-itis, inflammation of bone

ost-em-py-esis, abnormal condition of pus in a bone

**oste/o**-ana-genesis, formation of bone again (bone regeneration)

**oste/o**-arthr-itis, inflammation of joints and bones, it refers to a degenerative joint disease accompanied by pain and stiffness, often associated with increasing age

**oste/o**-arthr/o-pathy, disease of joints and bones

**oste/o**-arthr-osis, abnormal condition of joints and bones (non-inflammatory bone disease)

**oste/o**-arthr/o-tomy, incision (to remove) the joint end of a bone

**oste/o**-blast, an immature or embryonic cell that forms bone, it synthesizes the collagen and glycoproteins that form the matrix of bone

**oste/o**-blast-ic, pertaining to osteoblasts

**oste/o**-blast-oma, a tumour of osteoblasts (the condition leads to formation of primitive bone or osteoid tissue)

**oste/o**-camps-ia, condition of curving of a bone. From a Greek word *campsis* meaning a curving

**oste/o**-chondr-al, pertaining to cartilage and bone

**oste/o**-chondr-itis, inflammation of cartilage and bone

**oste/o**-chondr/o-dys-plas-ia, condition of poor growth or poor development of cartilage and bone cells

**oste/o**-chondr/o-dys-trophy, poor nourishment and development of cartilage and bone (congenital Morquio's syndrome), a condition in which the cartilage of bone contains multiple ossification centres causing them to twist and deform

**oste/o**-chondr-oma, a (benign) tumour of bone covered with cartilage Syn. chondrosteoma

**oste/o**-chondr-omat-osis, abnormal condition of multiple osteochondromas

**oste/o**-chondr-osis, abnormal condition of cartilage and bone, it refers to disease of ossification centres in which there is necrosis followed by repair and regeneration

**oste/o**-clas-ia, 1. condition of breaking down (and absorption) of bone by osteoclasts 2. the surgical breaking of a bone by surgery

**oste/o**-clasis, 1. breaking down (and absorption) of bone by osteoclasts 2. surgical breaking of a bone by surgery

**oste/o**-clast, 1. a cell that breaks down bone 2. a surgical instrument used for breaking bone

**oste/o**-clast-ic, 1. pertaining to osteoclasts, cells that break down bone 2. pertaining to osteoclasis

**oste/o-clast-oma,** a tumour formed from osteoclasts (cells that break down bone)

**oste/o-cope,** pain in bone. From a Greek word *kopos* meaning pain

**oste/o-cop-ic,** pertaining to pain in bone. From a Greek word *kopos* meaning pain

**oste/o-crani-um,** the bony cranium, it refers to the cranium of a fetus following ossification

**oste/o-cyst-oma,** a cyst-like tumour of a bone

**oste/o-cyte,** a bone cell

**oste/o-diastasis,** an abnormal separation of (adjacent) bones. From a Greek word *diastasis* meaning separation

**oste/o-dyn-ia,** condition of pain in bones

**oste/o-dys-trophy,** poor or bad nourishment of bone (poor growth)

**oste/o-epiphysis,** an epiphysis of a bone, it refers to the end of a long bone separated from the shaft by a cartilaginous plate

**oste/o-gen,** a substance that forms bone (found on the inner layer of the periosteum of bones)

**oste/o-genesis,** formation of bone

**oste/o-gen-ic,** 1. pertaining to forming bone 2. pertaining to originating in bone

**oste/o-hali-steresis,** condition of shortage or deficiency of salt in bone (a mineral deficiency resulting in the softening of bone). From a Greek word *hals* meaning salt and *steresis* meaning privation

**oste-oid,** 1. resembling bone 2. the basic tissue of bone before calcification

**oste/o-lip/o-chondr-oma,** a tumour of bone covered with cartilage (an osteochondroma) containing fatty elements

**oste/o-log-ist,** a specialist who studies osteology

**oste/o-logy,** the study of bones (anatomy, diseases and treatment of)

**oste/o-lysis,** 1. the breakdown or disintegration of bone 2. the breakdown and removal of calcium from bones (by osteoclasts)

**oste/o-lyt-ic,** 1. pertaining to osteolysis 2. pertaining to the breakdown of bone

**oste-oma,** a tumour of bone

**oste/o-malac-ia,** condition of softening of the bones

**oste/o-malac-ic,** 1. pertaining to the softening of bones 2. pertaining to having osteomalacia

**oste/o-metry,** technique of measuring bones

**oste/o-myel-itis,** inflammation of bone marrow

**oste/o-myel/o-dys-plas-ia,** condition of poor growth or development of bone marrow, it results in the reduction of bone tissue, increase in size of marrow cavities and leucopenia

**oste/o-myx/o-chondr-oma,** a tumour of cartilaginous tissue (chondroma) with primitive connective tissue and stroma (myxoma) and bone Syn. osteochondromyxoma

**oste-on,** a microscopic unit of compact bone centred on a Haversian canal and surrounded by concentric rings of bony lamellae

**oste/o-necr-osis,** abnormal condition of dead bone tissue

**oste/o-neur-alg-ia,** condition of pain in the nerves of a bone

**oste/o-path,** one who practises osteopathy

**oste/o-path-ia,** condition of disease of bone

**oste/o-path-ic,** 1. pertaining to disease of bone 2. pertaining to osteopathy

**oste/o-pathy,** 1. disease of bone 2. a system of treatment of disease by manipulation of bones

**oste/o-pen-ia,** condition of a reduction of bone mass

**oste/o-peri-oste-al,** pertaining to a periosteum and its underlying bone

**oste/o-peri-ost-itis,** inflammation of a periosteum and its underlying bone

**oste/o-petr-osis,** abnormal condition of stone-like bones, it refers to an increased density of bones that results in an increased tendency to fracture

**oste/o**-phleb-itis, inflammation of veins in a bone

**oste/o**-phony, process of conduction of sound through bone

**oste/o**-phyma, a swelling or tumour of bone (outgrowth)

**oste/o**-phyte, a bone plant, it refers to a plant-like growth of bone

**oste/o**-plast-ic, 1. pertaining to osteoplasty 2. pertaining to surgical repair or reconstruction of bones 3. pertaining to formation or development of bone

**oste/o**-plasty, surgical repair or reconstruction of bones

**oste/o**-poikil-osis, abnormal condition of irregular bone, it refers to a congenital condition in which bones appear mottled on radiographs, due to patches of hard, dense bone tissue

**oste/o**-por-osis, abnormal condition of pores in bone

**oste/o**-radi/o-necr-osis, abnormal condition of death of bone from exposure to radiation

**oste/o**-rrhag-ia, bursting forth of blood from bones (haemorrhage)

**oste/o**-rrhaphy, stitching or suturing of bone (with sutures or wire)

**oste/o**-sarc-oma, a malignant, fleshy tumour derived from bone

**oste/o**-sarc-omat-ous, 1. pertaining to or having multiple osteosarcomas 2. pertaining to or having the properties of an osteosarcoma

**oste/o**-scler-osis, abnormal condition of hardening of bone

**oste**-osis, abnormal condition of bone, it refers to an abnormal increase of bony tissue

**oste/o**-suture, stitching or suturing of bones Syn. osteorrhaphy

**oste/o**-synov-itis, inflammation of synovial membranes and surrounding bones

**oste/o**-synthesis, formation of bones, it refers to fixation of the ends of fractured bones by means of plates, wires or sutures

**oste/o**-tabes, condition of wasting away of bone (a condition seen mainly in children in which the bone marrow cells break down and the bone marrow disappears)

**oste/o**-thromb-osis, abnormal condition of clots (in the blood vessels) of a bone

**oste/o**-tome, an instrument that cuts bone

**oste/o**-tomy, incision of a bone

**ost**-itis, inflammation of bone Syn. osteitis

**pachy-peri-ost**-itis, inflammation of the periosteum producing abnormal thickening of long bones

**par-oste**-osis, abnormal condition beside a bone, it refers to ossification of tissues beside the periosteum

**peri-oste**-itis, inflammation of the periosteum

**peri-oste**-oma, a tumour around a bone, it refers to any bony growth surrounding a bone

**peri-oste/o**-myel-itis, inflammation of bone marrow and the periosteum (all of the bone)

**peri-oste/o**-phyte, a plant (bony growth) on the periosteum

**peri-oste/o**-tomy, incision into the periosteum

**peri-oste**-um, the structure around a bone, it refers to the connective tissue covering around a bone with osteogenic properties

**peri-ost**-itis, inflammation of the periosteum

**peri-ost**-osis, abnormal condition of the periosteum, it refers to deposition of bone forming periosteomas in the periosteum

---

**Pelvi/o**, pelvis

From a Latin word **pelvis** meaning basin. Here, pelvi/o means the pelvis; the basin-shaped bony ring at the lower end of the trunk formed by the two innominate bones, the sacrum and coccyx. It also refers to the basin-shaped cavity bounded by the bony pelvis. The bones of the pelvis protect the bladder, rectum and in the female the organs of reproduction.

Note: pelvi/o is also used to mean the basin-like renal pelvis.

endo-**pelv**-ic, pertaining to within the pelvis

**pelv**-ic, pertaining to the pelvis

**pelvi**-cephal/o-metry, technique of measuring the fetal head in proportion to the diameter of the maternal pelvis

**pelvi**-fix-ation, surgical fixation of a displaced or floating pelvic organ

**pelvi**-meter, an instrument used to measure the pelvic capacity and diameters for obstetric purposes

**pelvi**-metr-ic, pertaining to pelvimetry

**pelvi**-metry, technique of measuring the pelvic capacity and diameters for obstetric purposes

**pelvi/o**-periton-itis, inflammation of the peritoneum within the pelvis

**pelvi/o**-plasty, surgical repair or reconstruction of the pelvis *e.g.* to enlarge its outlet

**pelvi/o**-spondyl-itis, inflammation of the vertebrae and pelvis, it refers to inflammation of the pelvic portion of of the spinal column

**pelvi/o**-tomy, incision into the pelvic bones

**pelvi**-periton-itis, inflammation of the peritoneum within the pelvis

**pelvi**-rect-al, pertaining to the rectum and pelvis

supra-**pelv**-ic, pertaining to above the pelvis

---

**Phalang/o**, phalanges, phalanx

From a Greek word **phalagx** meaning a line of soldiers. Here phalang/o means the phalanges, the small bones of the fingers or toes arranged in a line.

hyper-**phalang**-ism, condition of having more than the normal number of phalanges in a finger or toe

**phalang**-eal, pertaining to a phalanx

**phalang**-ectomy, removal of a phalanx

**phalang**-itis, inflammation affecting a phalanx or phalanges

**phalang/o**-phalang-eal, pertaining to a phalanx and another phalanx (two adjacent phalanges)

**phalanx**, any bone of a finger or toe. Singular of phalanges

poly-**phalang**-ia, condition of many (excess) phalanges in a finger or toe

poly-**phalang**-ism, condition of many (excess) phalanges in a finger or toe

---

**Pod/o**, foot

From a Greek word **pous** meaning foot. Here pod/o means a foot or feet.

**pod**-agra, pain in a foot (gout in the big toe)

**pod**-alg-ia, condition of pain in the feet

**pod**-arthr-al, pertaining to joints of the feet (metatarsophalangeal joints)

**pod**-arthr-itis, inflammation of joints of the feet

**pod**-iatr-ic, pertaining to podiatry

**pod**-iatr-ist, a health care specialist who treats the feet, a chiropodist

**pod**-iatr-y, process of treating the feet, chiropody

**pod/o**-dyn-ia, condition of pain in the feet (of neuralgic origin)

**pod/o**-logy, 1. the study of the feet (anatomy, disorders and treatment of) 2. podiatry

---

**Rachi/o**, backbone, spine, vertebral column

From a Greek word **rhachis**, meaning spine. Here, rachi/o means the spine, a popular term for the vertebral column or backbone.

See the combining forms spin/o and vertebr/o.

hemi-**rachi**-schisis, cleaving of half of the spine, it refers to rachischisis without prolapse of the spinal cord

**rachi**-alg-ia, condition of pain of the spine

**rachi**-an-aesthes-ia, condition of without sensation of the spine, it refers to spinal anaesthesia

**rachi**-cele, a protrusion or hernia of the spine (as in spina bifida)

**rachi**-centesis, puncture of the spine to remove fluid Syn. lumbar puncture

**rachi**-graph, an instrument that records the spine (outline)

**rachi**-lysis, loosening or breakdown of the spine (to correct curvatures by pressure and traction)

**rachi/o**-centesis, puncture of the spine to remove fluid Syn. lumbar puncture

**rachi/o**-dyn-ia, condition of pain of the spine

**rachi/o**-kyph-osis, abnormal condition of forward curvature of the spine (a hunched back)

**rachi/o**-meter, an instrument used to measure the spine (degree of curvature)

**rachi/o**-myel-itis, inflammation of the spinal cord and spine

**rachi/o**-paralysis, paralysis affecting the spine (muscles of)

**rachi/o**-phyma, a tumour of the spine

**rachi/o**-pleg-ia, condition of paralysis of the spine (muscles of)

**rachi/o**-scoli-osis, abnormal condition of lateral curvature of the spine

**rachi/o**-tome, an instrument used for cutting the spine (dividing vertebral laminae)

**rachi/o**-tomy, incision into the spine (to divide vertebral laminae)

**rachi**-schisis, cleaving of the spine (congenital fissure of the vertebral column, spina bifida)

---

**Scoli/o, scolios/i/o,** lateral curvature of the spine

From a Greek word **skolios** meaning crooked or twisted. Here, scoli/o means a scoliosis, a lateral curvature of the spine.

**scoli/o**-kyph-osis, abnormal condition of kyphosis (anteroposterior deformity of the thoracic spine with the formation of a hump) with scoliosis (lateral curvature of the spine)

**scoli/o**-lord-osis, abnormal condition of lordosis (forward curvature of the lumbar spine) with scoliosis (lateral curvature of the spine)

**scoli**-osis, abnormal condition of lateral curvature of the spine

**scolios/o**-meter, an instrument used to measure the lateral curvature of the spine

**scolios/o**-metry, technique of measuring the lateral curvature of the spine

**scoli/o**-tic, 1. pertaining to scoliosis 2. pertaining to having scoliosis

---

**Spin/i/o,** spine

From a Latin word **spina** meaning the backbone. Here, spin/o means the spine, spinal cord or any sharp bony projection. Spine is a popular term for the vertebral column or backbone.

See the combining forms rachi/o and vertebr/o.

infra-**spin**-ous, 1. pertaining to below a spine of a vertebra 2. pertaining to below the spine of the scapula

**spin**-al, 1. pertaining to the spine or vertebral column 2. pertaining to a spine or any spinous process

**spin**-ate, 1. having spines 2. thorn-like

**spin/i**-fug-al, pertaining to conducting or moving away from the spinal cord

**spin/i**-pet-al, pertaining to conducting or moving towards the spinal cord

**spin/o**-bulb-ar, pertaining to the medulla oblongata and spinal cord

**spin/o**-cerebell-ar, pertaining to the cerebellum and spinal cord

**spin/o**-cortic-al, pertaining to the cerebral cortex and spinal cord

**spin/o**-thalam-ic, pertaining to the thalamus and spinal cord

**spin**-ous, 1. pertaining to being spine-like 2. pertaining to having spines or a thorny process 3. belonging to the spine or vertebral column

supra-**spin**-al, pertaining to above the spine

---

**Spondyl/o,** vertebra

From a Greek word **spondylos**, meaning vertebra. Here spondyl/o means a vertebra, one of the thirty-three or thirty-four irregular bones making up the spinal column or backbone. There are twenty-four individual bones comprising seven cervical, twelve thoracic and five lumbar vertebrae plus nine or ten fused bones. The latter consist of five sacral and four or five coccygeal bones.

**spondyl**-alg-ia, condition of pain in vertebrae

**spondyl**-arthr-itis, inflammation of vertebral joints (arthritis of the spine)

**spondyl**-itic, pertaining to having spondylitis

**spondyl**-itis, inflammation of vertebrae

**spondyl/o**-cace, bad vertebrae (destruction of vertebrae due to TB)

**spondyl/o**-dyn-ia, condition of pain in vertebrae

**spondyl/o**-graphy, technique of recording the vertebrae (the degree of kyphosis)

**spondyl**-olisthesis, slipping or dislocation of vertebrae

**spondyl/o**-olisthe-tic, pertaining to slipping or dislocation of vertebrae

**spondyl/o**-lysis, 1. breakdown or disintegration of vertebrae 2. breakdown of the normally stable attachment between one vertebra and the next

**spondyl/o**-malac-ia, condition of softening of the vertebrae

**spondyl/o**-meter, an instrument used to measure vertebrae (the degree of spinal movement)

**spondyl/o**-myel-itis, inflammation of the spinal cord and vertebrae

**spondyl/o**-pathy, disease of vertebrae

**spondyl/o**-ptosis, falling or dislocation of vertebrae Syn. spondylolisthesis

**spondyl/o**-py-osis, abnormal condition of pus in vertebrae

**spondyl/o**-schisis, splitting of a vertebra, it refers to a congenital fissure in a vertebral arch (spina bifida)

**spondyl**-osis, 1. abnormal condition of the vertebrae (any non-inflammatory, degenerative disease) 2. vertebral ankylosis

**spondyl/o**-syn-desis, surgical fixation or fusion of vertebrae (arthrodesis of the spine)

**spondyl/o**-therapy, treatment of disease of the vertebrae

**spondyl/o**-tomy, incision into a vertebra (to expose the spinal cord)

---

**Symphys/i/o**, symphysis

From a Greek word **symphysis** meaning a growing together. Here symphysi/o means a symphysis, a type of slightly movable, cartilaginous joint where a pad of fibrocartilage separates two bones *e.g.* the symphysis pubis, the joint formed between the two pubic bones.

**symphys**-eal, pertaining to a symphysis

**symphys**es, plural of symphysis

**symphys/i**-al, pertaining to a symphysis

**symphysi**-ectomy, removal of part of a symphysis, particularly the sympysis pubis to facilitate a future delivery

**symphysi/o**-lysis, breakdown or parting of a symphysis, particularly the symphysis pubis

**symphysi/o**-tomy, incision into the symphysis pubis (to facilitate delivery)

**symphysi/o**-rrhaphy, stitching or suturing of a symphysis

---

**Syndesm/o**, ligament

From a Greek word **syndesmos** meaning ligament. Here, syndesm/o means a ligament, a band of tough, fibrous connective tissue. Ligaments join bones or other structures together.

**syndesm**-ectomy, removal of a ligament

**syndesm**-ec-top-ia, condition of a displaced ligament

**syndesm**-itis, inflammation of a ligament

**syndesm/o**-graphy, a description or study of ligaments

**syndesm/o**-pexy, surgical fixation of ligaments (to fix a joint in position)

**syndesm/o**-plasty, surgical repair or reconstruction of ligaments

**syndesm/o**-rrhaphy, stitching or suturing of a ligament

**syndesm/o**-tomy, incision into a ligament

---

**Synov/i, synovia**, synovial fluid, synovial joint

From a New Latin word **synovia**, possibly from **syn-** meaning together and **ov** meaning egg. Here synov/i means synovia, the fluid (similar to egg-white) secreted by a synovial membrane. Synovial fluid is found in tendon sheaths, bursae and the cavities of joints. Here the combining form means synovial fluid, synovial membrane or a synovial joint that secretes synovial fluid.

arthr/o-**synov**-itis, inflammation of a synovial joint

poly-**synov**-itis, inflammation of many synovial membranes

**synov**-ectomy, removal of a synovial membrane

**synov/i**-al, 1. pertaining to synovia or synovial fluid 2. consisting of synovia or synovial fluid

**synov/i**-oma, a tumour or swelling of a synovial membrane

**synov/i**-par-ous, pertaining to bearing (producing) synovia or synovial fluid

**synov**-itis, inflammation of a synovial membrane

**synov/i**·um, a synovial membrane

---

**Vertebr/o**, vertebra

From a Latin word **vertebra** meaning joint. Here, vertebr/o means a vertebra, one of the thirty-three or thirty-four irregular bones making up the spinal column or backbone. There are twenty-four individual bones comprising seven cervical, twelve thoracic and five lumbar vertebrae plus nine or ten fused bones. The latter consist of five sacral and four or five coccygeal bones.

**vertebra**e, plural of vertebra

**vertebr**-al, 1. pertaining to a vertebra 2. possessing vertebrae

**vertebr**-ate, 1. having vertebrae, a vertebral column or spine 2. an animal with a backbone belonging to the sub-phylum Vertebrata

**vertebr**-ectomy, removal of a vertebra

**vertebr/o**-basil-ar, pertaining to the basilar and vertebral arteries

**vertebr/o**-chondr-al, pertaining to a (rib) cartilage and a vertebra

**vertebr/o**-cost-al, 1. pertaining to a rib and a vertebra 2. pertaining to a rib cartilage and vertebra

**vertebr/o**-femor-al, pertaining to the femur and vertebral column

**vertebr/o**-gen-ic, pertaining to originating in a vertebra or vertebral column

**vertebr/o**-stern-al, pertaining to the sternum and a vertebra

Table 1

## Bones and their combining forms

Use this list to find the names of major bones, their combining forms and locations within the body. The combining forms can be used with prefixes and suffixes to make many medical terms:

| Bone | Combining form | Location |
|---|---|---|
| calcaneus | **calcane/o** | leg (heel) |
| carpal | **carp/o** | lower arm |
| clavicle | **clavicul/o, cleid/o** | shoulder |
| coccyx | **coccyg/o** | lower back |
| cuboid | **cub/o, cuboide/o** | leg |
| cuneiform | **cune/o** | ankle |
| ethmoid | **ethmoid/o** | skull |
| femur | **femor/o** | thigh |
| fibula | **fibul/o** | leg |
| frontal | **front/o** | skull |
| humerus | **humer/o** | upper arm |
| hyoid | **hy/o** | neck |
| ilium | **ili/o** | pelvis |
| incus | **incud/o** | ear |
| ischium | **ischi/o** | pelvis |
| lacrimal | **lacrim/o** | skull |
| malleus | **malle/o** | ear |
| mandible | **mandibul/o** | lower jaw |
| maxilla | **maxill/o** | upper jaw |
| metacarpal | **metacarp/o** | hand |
| metatarsal | **metatars/o** | foot |
| nasal | **nas/o** | skull |
| navicular | **navicul/o** | foot |
| occipital | **occipit/o** | skull |
| palatine | **palat/o** | skull |
| parietal | **pariet/o** | skull |
| patella | **patell/o** | knee |
| phalanges | **phalang/o** | fingers and toes |
| pubis | **pub/o** | pelvis |
| radius | **radi/o** | forearm |
| rib | **cost/o** | chest |
| sacrum | **sacr/o** | lower back |
| scaphoid | **scaph/o** | wrist |
| scapula | **scapul/o** | shoulder |
| sphenoid | **sphen/o, sphenoid/o** | skull |
| stapes | **stapedi/o** | ear |
| sternum | **stern/o** | chest |
| talus | **tal/o** | ankle |
| tarsal | **tars/o** | ankle and foot |
| temporal | **tempor/o** | skull |
| tibia | **tibi/o** | leg |
| trapezium | **trapezi/o** | wrist |
| turbinate (nasal concha) | **turbin/o** | skull |
| ulnar | **uln/o** | forearm |
| vertebra | **spondyl/o, vertebr/o** | back (spine) |
| vomer | **vomer/o** | skull |
| zygomatic | **zygomatic/o** | skull |

Table 2

## Combining forms relating to bones

Use this table to find the meaning of combining forms relating to the major bones and their location within the body:

| Combining form | Bone | Location |
|---|---|---|
| calcane/o | calcaneus | leg (heel) |
| carp/o | carpal | lower arm |
| clavicul/o | clavicle | shoulder |
| cleid/o | clavicle | shoulder |
| coccyg/o | coccyx | lower back |
| cost/o | rib | chest |
| cub/o, cuboide/o | cuboid | leg |
| cune/o | cuneiform | ankle |
| ethmoid/o | ethmoid | skull |
| femor/o | femur | thigh |
| fibul/o | fibula | leg |
| front/o | frontal | skull |
| humer/o | humerus | upper arm |
| hy/o | hyoid | neck |
| ili/o | ilium | pelvis |
| incud/o | incus | ear |
| ischi/o | ischium | pelvis |
| lacrim/o | lacrimal | skull |
| malle/o | malleus | ear |
| mandibul/o | mandible | lower jaw |
| maxill/o | maxilla | upper jaw |
| metacarp/o | metacarpal | hand |
| metatars/o | metatarsal | foot |
| nas/o | nasal | skull |
| navicul/o | navicular | foot |
| occipit/o | occipital | skull |
| palat/o | palatine | skull |
| pariet/o | parietal | skull |
| patell/o | patella | knee |
| phalang/o | phalanges | fingers and toes |
| pub/o | pubis | pelvis |
| radi/o | radius | forearm |
| sacr/o | sacrum | lower back |
| scaph/o | scaphoid | wrist |
| scapul/o | scapula | shoulder |
| sphen/o, sphenoid/o | sphenoid | skull |
| spondyl/o | vertebra | back |
| stapedi/o | stapes | ear |
| stern/o | sternum | chest |
| tal/o | talus | ankle |
| tars/o | tarsal | ankle and foot |
| tempor/o | temporal | skull |
| tibi/o | tibia | leg |
| trapezi/o | trapezium | wrist |
| turbin/o | turbinate (nasal concha) | skull |
| uln/o | ulnar | forearm |
| vomer/o | vomer | skull |
| zygomatic/o | zygomatic | skull |

Table 3

**Terminology associated with movements at synovial joints**

Use this table to find words associated with the direction of movements at synovial joints:

| Movement | Definition |
| --- | --- |
| Flexion | Bending, usually forward but occasionally backward, *e.g.* knee joint |
| Extension | Straightening or bending backward |
| Abduction | Movement away from the midline of the body |
| Adduction | Movement towards the midline of the body |
| Circumduction | Combination of flexion, extension, abduction and adduction |
| Rotation | Movement around the long axis of a bone |
| Pronation | Turning the palm of the hand down |
| Supination | Turning the palm of the hand up |
| Inversion | Turning the sole of the foot inwards |
| Eversion | Turning the sole of the foot outwards |

Table 4

**Terminology related to components of the skeleton**

Use this table to find words associated with the anatomy of bones:

| Term | Definition |
| --- | --- |
| Articulating surface | The part of the bone that enters into the formation of a joint |
| Articulation | A joint between two or more bones |
| Bony sinus | A hollow cavity within a bone |
| Border | A ridge of bones separating two surfaces |
| Condyle | A smooth rounded projection of bone that forms part of a joint |
| Facet | A small generally rather flat articulating surface |
| Fissure or cleft | A narrow slit |
| Foramen (plural foramina) | A hole in a structure |
| Fossa (plural fossae) | A hollow or depression |
| Meatus | A tube-shaped cavity within a bone |
| Septum | A partition separating two cavities |
| Spine, spinous process or crest | A sharp ridge of bone |
| Styloid process | A sharp downward projection of bone that gives attachment to muscles and ligaments |
| Suture | An immovable joint, *e.g.* between bones of the skull |
| Trochanter, tuberosity or tubercle | Roughened bony projections, usually for attachment of muscles or ligaments. The different names are used according to the size of the projection. Trochanters are the largest and tubercles the smallest |

# Section 15
# The male reproductive system

The male reproductive system consists of the following organs:

- two testes
- two seminal vesicles
- two epididymes
- two ejaculatory ducts
- two deferent ducts (vas deferens)
- one prostate gland
- two spermatic cords
- one penis

The male possesses paired reproductive organs or gonads known as the testes (synonymous with testicles); they are held in position outside the main cavities of the body by a sac known as the scrotum. The testes are suspended in the scrotum by sheaths of smooth muscle and fibrous tissue called spermatic cords. Each cord contains a testicular artery and vein, lymphatics, a deferent duct, and testicular nerves. Each testis produces millions of sperm cells (spermatozoa) that carry the male's genetic information. The testes also act as endocrine glands releasing the male sex-hormone testosterone into the blood.

During intercourse, at the moment of orgasm, spermatozoa leave the epididymis and pass through the vas deferens, the ejaculatory duct and the urethra. The seminal vesicles and prostate gland add their secretion to the spermatozoa as they pass down the ejaculatory duct and urethra, forming the thin, milky fluid called semen. The semen is propelled by powerful rhythmical contraction of the smooth muscle in the walls of the vas deferens, seminal vesicles and prostate gland. The force generated by these contractions leads to ejaculation of semen through the external urethral sphincter at the end of the penis. A single ejaculate contains between 2 and 5 ml of semen and contains 40–100 million sperm per ml. If not ejaculated, sperm lose their fertility, die and are broken down and reabsorbed.

Figure 23 shows combining forms of roots associated with the anatomy of the male reproductive system:

**Roots and combining forms**, meanings

**Andr/o**, male, masculine
From a Greek word **aner** meaning man. Here andr/o means male or masculine.

**andr/o**-blast-oma, 1. a (benign) tumour of immature male cells, it refers to a virilizing ovarian tumour in women containing cells that mimic those of the testis by secreting testosterone 2. an arrhenoblastoma 3. a rare (benign) tumour of immature cells or embryonic cells of the testis seen in males

**andr/o**-gen, an agent that produces male or masculine characteristics *e.g.* testosterone

**andr/o**-gen-ic, pertaining to producing a male or masculine characteristics

**Quick Reference**

Combining forms relating to the male reproductive system:

|  |  | Page |
|---|---|---|
| **Andr/o** | male, masculine | 237 |
| **Arrhen/o** | male, masculine | 239 |
| **Balan/o** | glans penis | 239 |
| **Epididym/o** | epididymis | 239 |
| **Genit/o** | genitalia, reproductive organs | 240 |
| **Gonad/o** | gonad | 240 |
| **Gon/e/o** | sperm, spermatozoa | 240 |
| **Orchid/o** | testicle, testis | 240 |
| **Orchi/o** | testicle, testis | 240 |
| **Pen/o** | penis | 241 |
| **Phall/o** | penis, phallus | 242 |
| **Posth/o** | foreskin, prepuce | 242 |
| **Preputi/o** | foreskin, prepuce | 242 |
| **Prostat/o** | prostate gland | 242 |
| **Scrot/o** | scrotum | 243 |
| **Semin/i** | semen, testis | 243 |
| **-spad-** | cleft or rent of the male urethra | 243 |
| **Spermat/o** | sperm, spermatozoa | 244 |
| **Sperm/i** | sperm, spermatozoa | 244 |
| **Testicul-** | testicle | 245 |
| **Test/o** | testis | 245 |
| **Varic/o** | varicose vein, varix | 245 |
| **Vas/o** | sperm duct, vas deferens | 245 |
| **Vesicul/o** | seminal vesicle | 246 |

**Quick Reference**

Common words and combining forms relating to the male reproductive system:

|  |  | Page |
|---|---|---|
| Cleft of the male urethra | **-spad-** | 243 |
| Epididymis | **epididym/o** | 239 |
| Foreskin | **posth/o, preputi/o** | 242 |
| Glans penis | **balan/o** | 239 |
| Genitalia | **genit/o** | 240 |
| Gonad | **gonad/o** | 240 |
| Male | **andr/o, arrhen/o** | 237 239 |
| Masculine | **andr/o, arrhen/o** | 237/239 |
| Penis | **pen/o, phall/o** | 241/242 |
| Phallus | **phall/o** | 242 |
| Prepuce | **posth/o, preputi/o** | 242 |
| Prostate gland | **prostat/o** | 242 |
| Rent of the male urethra | **-spad-** | 243 |
| Reproductive organs | **genit/o** | 240 |
| Scrotum | **scrot/o** | 243 |
| Semen | **semin/i** | 243 |
| Seminal vesicle | **vesicul/o** | 246 |
| Sperm | **gone/o, spermat/o, sperm/i** | 240 242 244 |
| Spermatozoa | **gone/o, spermat/o, sperm/i** | 240 244 244 |
| Sperm duct | **vas/o** | 245 |
| Testicle | **orchid/o, orchi/o, semin/i, testicul-, test/o** | 240 245 245 |
| Testis | **orchid/o, orchi/o, semin/i, testicul-, test/o** | 240 243 245 |
| Varicose vein | **varic/o** | 245 |
| Varix | **varic/o** | 245 |
| Vas deferens | **vas/o** | 245 |

**andr/o**-gen-ous, pertaining to producing a male or masculine characteristics

**andr/o**-gloss-ia, condition of having a male tongue (masculine sound to a woman's voice)

**andr/o**-gyne, a male with secondary sexual organs like a woman (male pseudo-hermaphrodite)

**andr/o**-gyn-ism, condition of a female with male characteristics (female hermaphrodite)

**andr/o**-gyn-oid, a male resembling a female (male hermaphrodite)

**andr/o**-gyn-ous, pertaining to male and female (of doubtful sex, hermaphroditic)

**andr**-oid, resembling a male

**andr/o**-logy, the study of the male (particularly the anatomy, diseases of and treatment of the male reproductive system)

**andr/o**-pathy, disease of the male, it refers to any disease found only in a male

**andr/o**-phob-ia, condition of irrational fear or dislike of men

**andr/o**-sterone, a steroid hormone that produces male or masculine characteristics (a breakdown product of testosterone found in urine)

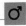

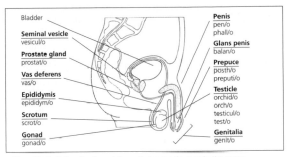

Figure 23 Sagittal section through the male showing the reproductive system

**Arrhen/o**, male, masculine

From a Greek word **arrhen** meaning male. Here arrhen/o means male or masculine.

**arrhen/o**-blast-oma, 1. a (benign) tumour of immature male cells, it refers to a virilizing ovarian tumour in women containing cells that mimic those of the testis by secreting testosterone

**arrhen/o**-gen-ic, pertaining to forming a male or masculine characteristics

**Balan/o**, glans penis

From a Greek word **balanos**, meaning acorn. Here balan/o means the sensitive, swollen end of the penis known as the glans penis. The glans is covered with the prepuce or foreskin.

**balan**-ic, pertaining to or belonging to the glans penis

**balan**-itis, inflammation of the glans penis

**balan/o**-blenn/o-rrhoea, excessive flow or discharge of mucus from the glans penis (of gonorrhoeal origin)

**balan/o**-cele, a protrusion or hernia of the glans penis (through a ruptured foreskin)

**balan/o**-plasty, surgical repair or reconstruction of the glans penis

**balan/o**-posth-itis, inflammation of the prepuce and glans penis

**balan/o**-posth/o-myc-osis, abnormal condition of fungi in the prepuce and glans penis

**balan/o**-preputi-al, pertaining to the prepuce and glans penis

**balan/o**-rrhag-ia, condition of bursting forth (of pus) from the glans penis (of gonorrhoeal origin)

**balan/o**-rrhoea, excessive flow or discharge (of pus) from the glans penis

**balan**-us, the glans penis

**Epididym/o**, epididymis

Derived from the Greek words **epi**-meaning on and **didymos**- meaning twins (the testicles). Here epididym/o means the epididymis, the coiled tube that forms the first part of the duct system of each testis; the epididymes store sperm.

**epididym**-al, pertaining to or belonging to an epididymis

**epididym**-ectomy, removal of the epididymis

**epididym**-itis, inflammation of the epididymis

**epididym/o**-orch-itis, inflammation of a testis and epididymis

239

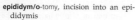

**epididym/o**-tomy, incision into an epididymis

**epididym/o-vas**-ectomy, removal of (part of) the vas deferens and epididymis

**epididym/o-vas/o**-stomy, formation of an opening between the vas deferens and epididymis or the name of the opening so created

---

**Genit/o**, genitalia, the organs of reproduction

From a Latin word **genitalis** meaning to beget. Here genit/o means the genitalia, the organs of reproduction especially the external organs.

**genit**-al, 1. pertaining to the genitalia or organs of reproduction 2. a reproductive organ

**genital**-ia, the reproductive organs

**genit/o-femor**-al, pertaining to the thigh and genitalia

**genit/o**-plasty, surgical repair or reconstruction of the genitalia

**genit/o-urin**-ary, pertaining to the urinary tract and genitalia

pre-**genit**-al, pertaining to before the genital stage (in psychosexual development)

---

**Gonad/o**, gonad

From a Greek word **gone** meaning seed or semen. Here, gonad/o means gonad *i.e.* a reproductive organ, it can refer to an ovary or a testis.

**gonad**-al, pertaining to the gonads

**gonad/o**-troph-ic, pertaining to nourishing or stimulating the gonads

**gonad/o**-troph-in, an agent or hormone that stimulates the gonads *e.g.* follicle-stimulating hormone and luteinizing hormone

**gonad/o**-trop-ic, pertaining to stimulating the gonads

---

**Gon/e/o**, sperm

From a Greek word **gone** meaning seed. Here gon/e means sperm, the male gametes. Combined with -cyst meaning bladder, gonecyst/o means a seminal

vesicle. These are small pouches lying near the base of the bladder secreting a nutrient fluid that becomes a component of semen. The seminal fluid forms 60% of the semen ejaculated at orgasm and contains nutrients to support the metabolic activities of the sperm.

Note: the root gon- derived from the Greek word **gony** means knee and goni- derived from the Greek word **gonia** means the angle of the anterior chamber of the eye. See Section 14 The skeletal system and Section 9 The eye, for words containing these roots.

**gon/e**-cyst, sperm bladder, it refers to a seminal vesicle

**gon/e**-cyst-itis, inflammation of the seminal vesicle

**gon/e-cyst/o**-lith, a stone or calculus in a seminal vesicle

**gon/e-cyst/o-py**-osis, abnormal condition of pus in a seminal vesicle (suppuration)

**gon/o**-cele, a swelling or protrusion containing sperm *e.g.* a swollen epididymis Syn. spermatocele

---

**Orchid/o**, **orch/i/o**, testicle, testis

From a Greek word **orchi**, meaning testis (or testicle). Here, orchi/o and orchid/o mean a testis or testicle. These male reproductive organs are present in pairs, and their function is to produce spermatozoa and male sex-hormones called androgens. The testes are enclosed in the scrotum that hangs behind the penis, in this position they maintain a temperature compatible with the viability of spermatozoa.

crypt-**orchid/o**-pexy, surgical fixation of hidden testes, it refers to fixing into their normal position in the scrotum

crypt-**orch**-ism, condition of having hidden testes, it refers to undescended testes that remain in the abdomen

mon-**orchid**-ism, condition of having one testis or one descended testis

mon-**orch**-ism, condition of having one testis or one descended testis

**orchi**-alg-ia, condition of pain in a testis

**orch**-ic, pertaining to a testis Syn. orchidic

**orchid**-alg-ia, condition of pain in a testis Syn. orchiodynia, orchiodynia

**orchid**-ectomy, removal of a testis

**orchid**-ic, pertaining to a testis Syn. orchic

**orchid**-itis, inflammation of a testis Syn. orchitis

**orchid/o**-cele, a protrusion or hernia of a testis, it refers to a scrotal hernia, tumour of a testis or hernia of a testis

**orchid/o**-dyn-ia, condition of pain in a testis

**orchid/o**-meter, an instrument used to measure a testicle (its volume)

**orchid**-onc-us, a swelling or tumour of the testis Syn. orchioncus

**orchid/o**-pathy, disease of the testes

**orchid/o**-pex-ia, surgical fixation of a testis, it refers to fixing of an undescended testicle into the scrotum

**orchid/o**-pexy, surgical fixation of the testis, it refers to fixing of an undescended testicle into the scrotum Syn. orchiopexy

**orchid/o**-plasty, surgical repair or reconstruction of a testis Syn. orchioplasty

**orchid/o**-ptosis, prolapse or displacement of a testis

**orchid/o**-rrhaphy, stitching or suturing of a testis *e.g.* suturing an undescended testis to the scrotum Syn. orchiorrhaphy

**orchid/o**-sche/o-cele, a protrusion or hernia of the scrotum and testis, it refers to a scrotal tumour with a scrotal hernia. From a Greek word *oscheon* meaning scrotum.

**orchid/o**-tomy, incision into a testis Syn. orchiotomy

**orch/i**-epididym-itis, inflammation of an epididymis and testis

**orch/i**-lyt-ic, pertaining to breakdown or disintegration of a testis

**orchi/o**-cele, a protrusion or hernia of the testes (through the scrotum)

**orchi/o**-dyn-ia, condition of pain in a testis Syn. orchidalgia, orchiodynia

**orchi/o**-myel-oma, a myeloma (a malignant tumour of plasma cells) in the testis

**orch/i**-onc-us, a swelling or tumour of the testis Syn. orchidoncus

**orchi/o**-neur-alg-ia, condition of pain in the nerves of the testis Syn. orchidalgia

**orchi/o**-pathy, disease of the testes

**orchi/o**-pexy, surgical fixation of a testis, it refers to fixing of an undescended testicle into the scrotum Syn. orchidopexy

**orchi/o**-plasty, surgical repair or reconstruction of a testis Syn. orchidoplasty

**orchi/o**-rrhaphy, stitching or suturing of a testis *e.g.* suturing an undescended testis to the scrotum Syn. orchidorrhaphy

**orchi/o**-sche/o-cele, a protrusion or hernia of the scrotum, it refers to a scrotal tumour with a scrotal hernia. From a Greek word *oscheon* meaning scrotum

**orchi/o**-schirr-us, a hard testis or hard (tumour) of the testis

**orchi/o**-tomy, incision into a testis Syn. orchidotomy

**orchis**, a testis

**orch**-itic, pertaining to having orchiditis

**orch**-itis, inflammation of a testis Syn. orchiditis

**peri-orch**-itis, inflammation of around a testis, it refers to inflammation of the tunica vaginalis that surrounds the testis

**syn-orch**-ism, condition of fusion or association of the testes into one

**tri-orchid**-ism, condition of having three testes

---

**Pen/o**, penis

From a Latin word **penis**, meaning the male copulatory organ. Here pen/o means the penis, the male organ that transfers urine from the bladder to the outside of the body via the urethra. The erect penis also transfers semen into the female during sexual intercourse.

**pen**-ial, pertaining to or belonging to the penis

**pen**-ile, pertaining to or belonging to the penis

**pen**-itis, inflammation of the penis

**pen/o**-plasty, surgical repair or reconstruction of the penis Syn. phalloplasty

**pen/o**-scrot-al, pertaining to the scrotum and penis

---

**Phall/o**, penis, phallus

From a Greek word **phallos**, meaning the penis. Here phall/o means the penis, the male organ that transfers urine from the bladder to the outside of the body via the urethra. The erect penis also transfers semen into the female during sexual intercourse.

megalo-**phall**-us, an abnormally large penis

**phall**-alg-ia, condition of pain in the penis

**phall**-ana-strophe, upward twisting of the penis. From a Greek word *anastrophe* meaning a turning back

**phall**-aneurysm, an aneurysm (dilation of a blood vessel) in the penis

**phall**-ectomy, removal of the penis

**phall**-ic, pertaining to the penis

**phall**-itis, inflammation of the penis

**phall/o**-campsis, condition of curving of the penis, a structural defect. From a Greek word *campsis* meaning a curving

**phall/o**-crypsis, condition of hidden (retracted) penis. From a Greek word *krypsis* meaning concealment

**phall/o**-dyn-ia, condition of pain in the penis

**phall**-oid, 1. resembling the penis 2. penis-shaped

**phall**-onc-us, a tumour or mass in the penis

**phall/o**-plasty, surgical repair or reconstruction of the penis Syn. penoplasty

**phall/o**-rrhag-ia, condition of bursting forth of blood from the penis (penile haemorrhage)

**phall/o**-rrhoea, excessive flow or discharge from the penis (of gonorrhoeal origin)

**phall/o**-tomy, incision into the penis

**phall**-us, the penis

---

**Posth/i/o**, foreskin, prepuce

From a Greek word **posthe** meaning foreskin. Here posth/o means the foreskin or prepuce, a thin fold of skin that covers and overhangs the glans penis.

**posthi/o**-plast-ic, pertaining to posthioplasty

**posthi/o**-plasty, surgical repair or reconstruction of the prepuce

**posth**-itis, inflammation of the prepuce

**posth/o**-lith, a stone or calculus in the prepuce

**posth**-onc-us, a tumour or swelling in the prepuce

---

**Preput/i/o**, foreskin, prepuce

From a Latin word **praeputium** meaning foreskin. Here preputi/o means the foreskin or prepuce, a thin fold of skin that covers and overhangs the glans penis.

**preputi**-al, pertaining to the prepuce or foreskin

**preputi/o**-tomy, incision into the prepuce or foreskin

**preput/i**-um, the foreskin or prepuce

---

**Prostat/o**, prostate gland

From a Greek word **prostates**, meaning one who stands before. Here, prostat/o means the prostate gland, a structure that surrounds the neck of the bladder and urethra in males. Secretions from the prostate gland are added to the semen during intercourse. The prostate gland secretion forms about 30% of the semen, it acts to protect sperm in the acidic environment of the vagina.

peri-**prostat**-itis, inflammation around the prostate gland

**prostat**-alg-ia, condition of pain in the prostate gland

**prostat**-ectomy, removal of the prostate gland

**prostat**-helc-osis, abnormal condition of ulceration of the prostate gland

**prostat**-ic, pertaining to or belonging to the prostate gland

**prostat**-ism, abnormal condition of the prostate gland (a symptom complex caused by an enlarged prostate gland such as benign prostatic hyperplasia). BPH results in increased frequency and hesitation of micturition and retention of urine

**prostat**-itic, pertaining to having prostatitis

**prostat**-itis, inflammation of the prostate gland

**prostat/o**-cyst-itis, inflammation of the bladder and prostate gland, it refers to inflammation of the neck of the bladder (the prostatic urethra)

**prostat/o**-cyst/o-tomy, incision into the bladder and prostate gland

**prostat/o**-dyn-ia, condition of pain in the prostate gland

**prostat/o**-graphy, technique of recording or making an X-ray picture of the prostate gland

**prostat/o**-lith, a stone or calculus in the prostate gland

**prostat/o**-lith/o-tomy, incision to remove a stone or calculus from the prostate gland

**prostat/o**-megaly, enlargement of the prostate gland

**prostat**-onc-us, a tumour or mass in the prostate gland

**prostat/o**-rrhoea, excessive flow or discharge from the prostate gland (as in a gonorrhoeal infection)

**prostat/o**-tomy, incision into the prostate gland

**prostat/o**-vesicul-ectomy, removal of the seminal vesicles and the prostate gland

**prostat/o**-vesicul-itis, inflammation of the seminal vesicles and the prostate gland

---

**Scrot/o**, scrotum

From a Latin word **scrotum**, a name for the pouch that contains the testicles. Here scrot/o means the scrotum, the pouch that hangs behind the penis containing the testicles. In this position

the testicles maintain a temperature compatible with the viability of spermatozoa.

**scrot**-al, pertaining to or belonging to the scrotum

**scrot**-ectomy, removal of the scrotum

**scrot**-itis, inflammation of the scrotum

**scrot/o**-cele, a protrusion or hernia of the scrotum (Syn. with orchiocele)

**scrot/o**-pexy, surgical fixation of the scrotum

**scrot/o**-plasty, surgical repair or reconstruction of the scrotum

**scrot**-um, the scrotum, it refers to the bag of pigmented skin and fascia containing the testicles

trans-**scrot**-al, pertaining to through or across the scrotum

---

**Semin/i**, semen

From a Latin word **seminis**, meaning seed. Here semin/i means semen; the sperm-containing liquid ejaculated from the male at orgasm. Semin/o is also used to mean testicle.

in-**semin**-ation, action of depositing semen in the vagina or uterus (by natural or artificial means)

**semin**-al, pertaining to semen or of the nature of semen

**semin**-ation, action of depositing semen in the vagina or uterus (by natural or artificial means)

**semin/i**-fer-ous, pertaining to carrying semen

**semin**-oma, a tumour or swelling of the testis

**semin**-ur-ia, condition of semen in the urine

---

**-spad-**, cleft or rent of the male urethra

From a Greek word **spadon** meaning rent. Here -spad- means a congenital, abnormal opening of the male urethra onto the wrong part of the penis.

epi-**spad**-ia, condition of a rent or abnormal opening above or upon the urethra, it refers to a congenital defect in which the urethra opens

onto the dorsal surface of the penis

epi-**spad**-iac, pertaining to epispadias

epi-**spad**-ial, pertaining to an epispadia or epispadias

epi-**spad**-ias, condition of a rent or abnormal opening above or upon the urethra, it refers to a congenital defect in which the urethra opens onto the dorsal surface of the penis

hypo-**spad**-ia, condition of a rent or abnormal opening below the urethra, it refers to a congenital defect in which the urethra opens onto the underside of the penis or onto the perineum

hypo-**spad**-iac, pertaining to a hypospadia or hypospadias

hypo-**spad**-ias, condition of a rent or abnormal opening below the urethra, it refers to a congenital defect in which the urethra opens onto the underside of the penis or onto the perineum

---

**Spermat/o, sperm/i/o**, sperm, spermatozoa

From a Greek word **sperma**, meaning seed. Here spermat/o means sperm cells or spermatozoa (sing. spermatozoon). Spermatozoa travel in the semen and are ejaculated from the male during the peak of sexual excitement known as orgasm. In a few words sperm/o means spermatic cord, spermatic duct or semen.

a-**sperm**-ia, condition of being without sperm

oligo-**sperm**-ia, condition of few sperm, it refers to a low sperm count

poly-**sperm**-ia, 1. condition of many sperm 2. condition of more than one sperm penetrating an egg 3. condition of excessive seminal secretion

poly-**sperm**-y, 1. condition of many sperm 2. condition of more than one sperm penetrating an egg 3. condition of excessive seminal secretion

**spermat**-emphraxis, blocking or stopping of sperm, it refers to the obstruction of the passage of sperm

**spermat**-ic, pertaining to sperm or semen

**spermat**-id, a cell formed from a secondary spermatocyte that develops into a spermatozoon

**spermat**-itis, inflammation of a spermatic cord

**spermat/o**-blast, an immature spermatozoon or spermatid

**spermat/o**-cele, a swelling or protrusion containing sperm *e.g.* a swollen epididymis

**spermat/o**-cel-ectomy, removal of a spermatocele

**spermat/o**-cid-al, pertaining to the killing or destruction of sperm

**spermat/o**-cyst, 1. a bladder containing sperm, it refers to a seminal vesicle 2. a spermatocele

**spermat/o**-cyst-ectomy, removal of a sperm bladder, here meaning removal of a seminal vesicle

**spermat/o**-cyst-itis, inflammation of a sperm bladder, here meaning inflammation of a seminal vesicle

**spermat/o**-cyst/o-tomy, incision into a sperm bladder, here meaning incision into a seminal vesicle

**spermat/o**-cyte, a sperm cell, it refers to an early stage of development of a spermatozoon

**spermat/o**-cyt/o-genesis, the formation of sperm cells, it refers to the first stage in the formation of spermatozoa from spermatogonia

**spermat/o**-blast, an immature sperm cell or spermatid

**spermat/o**-cide, an agent that kills or destroys spermatozoa

**spermat/o**-genesis, formation of sperm

**spermat/o**-gen-ic, pertaining to forming sperm or semen

**spermat/o**-goni-um, an immature germ cell that forms spermatocytes

**spermat**-oid, resembling sperm or semen

**spermat/o**-lysis, breakdown or disintegration of sperm

**spermat/o**-lyt-ic, pertaining to breakdown or disintegration of sperm

**spermat/o**-path-ia, condition of disease (abnormality) of the sperm

**spermat/o**-pathy, disease of sperm

**spermat/o**-rrhoea, excessive flow of sperm

**spermat/o**-schesis, suppression of sperm, it refers to suppression of semen secretion

**spermat/o**-zoa, animals of the semen, it refers to the mature male gametes or sperm

**spermat/o**-zo-al, pertaining to the spermatozoon or spermatozoa

**spermat/o**-zoon, a mature sperm cell, the mature male gamete

**spermat**-ur-ia, condition of sperm (semen) in the urine Syn. seminuria

**sperm**-ectomy, removal of sperm, it refers to removal of the spermatic cord

**sperm/i**-cid-al, pertaining to the killing or destruction of sperm

**sperm/i**-cide, an agent that kills sperm, used as a contraceptive

**sperm/i**-duct, the duct that carries sperm, it refers to the vas deferens and ejaculatory duct together

**sperm/o**-lith, a stone or calculus in the spermatic duct

**sperm/o**-neur-alg-ia, condition of pain in nerves of the spermatic cord

**sperm/o**-phleb-ectas-ia, condition of dilated spermatic veins (a varicosity of)

---

**Testicul-, test/o**, testicle, testis
From a Latin word **testiculus** meaning testicle. Here test/o means a testicle or testis, the male reproductive organ. The testicles are present in pairs, and their function is to produce spermatozoa and male sex-hormones called androgens. The testicles are enclosed in the scrotum that hangs behind the penis, in this position they maintain a temperature compatible with the viability of spermatozoa.

**test**-alg-ia, condition of pain in a testis
**test**-ectomy, removal of a testis
**testes**, the paired male gonads or male reproductive organs. Plural of testis
**testicle**, the male gonad or male reproductive organ

**testicul**-ar, pertaining to a testicle

**testicul**-oma, tumour of a testicle or testicular tissue

**test-is**, the male gonad or male reproductive organ. Singular of testes

**test**-itis, inflammation of a testis

**test**-oid, resembling a testis

**test/o**-pathy, disease of the testes

**test/o**-sterone, a steroid hormone produced by the testis, the principle androgenic hormone

---

**Varic/o, varicos-**, a varicose vein, varix
From a Latin word **varix** meaning a dilated vein. Here varic/o means a varix, a dilated, twisted vein. A varix can sometimes develop in the testicular vein producing a swelling in the scrotum.

**varic**-ation, action of forming a varix or varicosity

**varic**-eal, pertaining to a varix or of the nature of a varix

**varic**es, dilated twisted veins. Plural of varix

**varic/o**-cele, a swelling or protrusion of a dilated vein, it refers to swelling of a testicular vein that produces a swelling of the scrotum

**varic/o**-cel-ectomy, removal of a varicocele

**varic**-ose, having the nature of a varix or swollen vein

**varic**-osis, abnormal condition of varicosity of veins

**varicos**-ity, 1. a varicose vein or varix 2. state or condition of being varicose

**varix**, a dilated twisted vein. Singular of varices

---

**Vas/o**, sperm duct, vas deferens
From a Latin word **vas** meaning a vessel. Here, vas/o means vas deferens or ductus deferens, the main secretory duct of the testis along which mature sperms move towards the penis.

**vas**-al, 1. pertaining to the vas deferens 2. pertaining to a vessel

**vas**-ectomy, removal of the vas deferens

**vas**-itis, inflammation of the vas deferens

**vas/o**-epididym/o-graphy, technique of making a recording or X-ray picture of the epididymis and the vas deferens

**vas/o**-epididym/o-stomy, formation of an opening (anastomosis) between the epididymis and the vas deferens or the name of the opening so created

**vas/o**-ligation, process of tying off a vas deferens

**vas/o**-orchid/o-stomy, formation of an opening (anastomosis) between the testis and the vas deferens or the name of the opening so created

**vas/o**-puncture, puncture of the vas deferens

**vas/o**-resection, the cutting and removal of part of the vas deferens

**vas/o**-rrhaphy, stitching or suturing of the vas deferens

**vas/o**-sect-ion, cutting or excision of the vas deferens

**vas/o**-stomy, formation of an opening into the vas deferens or the name of the opening so created

**vas/o**-tomy, incision into the vas deferens

**vas/o**-vas/o-stomy, formation of an opening between the vas deferens and another remote part of the vas deferens or the name of the opening so created

**vas/o**-vesicul-ectomy, removal of the seminal vesicles and vas deferens

**vas/o**-vesicul-itis, inflammation of the seminal vesicles and vas deferens

---

**Vesicul/o**, seminal vesicle

From a Latin word **vesicula**, meaning vesicle or little bladder. Here, vesicul/o means the seminal vesicles, small pouches lying near the base of the bladder. The vesicles secrete seminal fluid that forms about 60% of the semen ejaculated at orgasm, it contains nutrients that support the metabolic activities of the sperm.

Note: vesicul/o is also used to refer to vesicles seen in various types of skin rash.

**vesicul**-ectomy, removal of the seminal vesicles

**vesicul**-itis, inflammation of a seminal vesicle

**vesicul/o**-gram, a recording or X-ray picture of the seminal vesicles

**vesicul/o**-graphy, technique of making a recording or X-ray picture of the seminal vesicles

**vesicul/o**-tomy, incision into the seminal vesicles

# Section 16
## The female reproductive system and obstetrics

The female reproductive system consists of:

**the internal genitalia**
- two ovaries
- two Fallopian tubes or uterine tubes
- one uterus
- one vagina

**the external genitalia**
- the vulva.

The female possesses paired reproductive organs known as ovaries; these are located in the upper pelvic cavity on either side of the uterus. The ovaries produce reproductive cells known as ova (or eggs) and secrete the female sex hormones oestrogen and progesterone; they pass through a regular ovarian cycle in which one egg is released (ovulation) every 28 days. The egg passes into the oviduct where it may be fertilized by sperms ejaculated into the female reproductive tract by the male. If the egg is not fertilized, it will disintegrate and may pass out of the body at menstruation. The branch of medicine dealing with diseases and treatment of the female reproductive system is known as gynaecology.

If an egg is fertilized, it may implant into the lining of the uterus beginning pregnancy. Pregnancy, also known as the period of gestation, lasts for approximately 40 weeks until birth. At term (the end of pregnancy), smooth muscle in the wall of the uterus forcefully expels the baby through powerful rhythmical contractions called labour. Following birth (parturition) the newborn baby is fed by milk secreted from the mammary glands (lactation). The medical specialism known as obstetrics deals with pregnancy, labour, and the period following birth known as the puerperium.

Figures 24 and 25 show combining forms of roots associated with the anatomy of the female reproductive system.

---

**Roots and combining forms**, meanings

---

**Amni/o, amnion-**, amnion
From a Greek word **amnia**, meaning a bowl in which blood was caught. Here amni/o means the amnion, the strong, translucent, fetal membrane that retains the amniotic fluid surrounding a developing fetus.

**amni/o**-cele, a protrusion or hernia of the amnion Syn. omphalocele, an umbilical hernia

**amni/o**-centesis, puncture of the amnion, by a needle to remove amniotic fluid

## Quick Reference

Combining forms relating to the female reproductive system and obstetrics:

| | | Page |
|---|---|---|
| **Amni/o** | amnion | 247 |
| **Bartholin/o** | Bartholin's glands of the vagina, the greater vestibular glands | 250 |
| **Cervic/o** | cervix | 250 |
| **Chori/o** | chorion | 250 |
| **Clitor/o** | clitoris | 251 |
| **Colp/o** | vagina | 251 |
| **Culd/o** | Douglas pouch, recto-uterine pouch | 252 |
| **Cyesi/o** | pregnancy | 253 |
| **Embry/o** | embryo | 253 |
| **Endometr/i** | endometrium | 253 |
| **Episi/o** | pudendum, vulva | 253 |
| **Fet/o** | fetus | 254 |
| **Galact/o** | milk | 254 |
| **Genit/o** | genitalia, reproductive organs | 255 |
| **-gravida** | pregnancy, a pregnant woman | 255 |
| **Gynaec/o** | gynaecology, woman | 255 |
| **Hyster/o** | uterus | 256 |
| **Lact/o** | milk | 258 |
| **Lochi/o** | lochia | 258 |
| **Mamill/o** | nipple | 259 |
| **Mamm/o** | breast, mammary gland | 259 |
| **Mast/o** | breast, mammary gland | 259 |
| **Men/o** | menses, menstruation | 260 |

| | | |
|---|---|---|
| **Metr/o** | uterus | 261 |
| **Nat/o** | birth | 262 |
| **Nymph/o** | labia minora, nymphae | 262 |
| **Obstetr/** | midwifery, obstetrics | 262 |
| **Omphal/o** | navel, umbilicus, umbilical cord | 262 |
| **Oo-** | egg | 263 |
| **Oophor/o** | ovary | 263 |
| **Ovari/o** | ovary | 264 |
| **-para** | to bear, bring forth offspring | 264 |
| **Parturi/o** | childbirth, labour, parturition | 265 |
| **Perine/o** | perineum | 265 |
| **Placent/o** | placenta | 265 |
| **Pub/o** | pubis, pubic region | 266 |
| **Pudend-** | pudendum, vulva | 266 |
| **Puerper-** | puerperium | 266 |
| **Salping/o** | Fallopian tube, oviduct, uterine tube | 266 |
| **Terat/o** | monster-like, monstrosity | 267 |
| **Thel/e** | nipple | 268 |
| **Toc/o** | childbirth, labour | 268 |
| **Tub/o** | Fallopian tube, oviduct, uterine tube | 268 |
| **Uter/o** | uterus | 269 |
| **Vagin/o** | vagina | 270 |
| **Vulv/o** | vulva | 270 |
| **Zygot-** | fertilized egg, zygote | 271 |

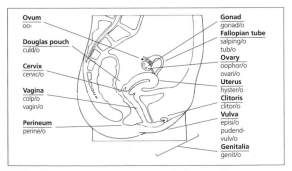

**Ovum**
oo-

**Douglas pouch**
culd/o

**Cervix**
cervic/o

**Vagina**
colp/o
vagin/o

**Perineum**
perine/o

**Gonad**
gonad/o

**Fallopian tube**
salping/o
tub/o

**Ovary**
oophor/o
ovari/o

**Uterus**
hyster/o

**Clitoris**
clitor/o

**Vulva**
episi/o
pudend-
vulv/o

**Genitalia**
genit/o

Figure 24  Sagittal section through the female showing the reproductive system

## Quick Reference

Common words and combining forms relating to the female reproductive system:

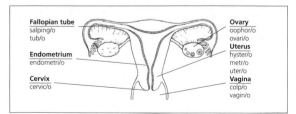

Figure 25  The female reproductive system

**amni/o**-clepsis, escape or loss of fluid from the amnion. From a Greek word *kleptein* meaning to steal

**amni/o**-genesis, formation or development of the amnion

**amni/o**-gram, a recording or X-ray picture of the amnion

**amni/o**-graphy, technique of making a recording or X-ray picture of the amnion

**amni**-oma, a tumour formed from the amnion

**amnion**, the amnion or fetal membrane

**amnion**-ic, pertaining to or belonging to the amnion

**amnion**-itis, inflammation of the amnion

**amni/o**-rrhex-ia, condition of rupture of the amnion

**amni/o**-rrhoea, excessive flow or discharge (of fluid) from the amnion

**amni/o**-scope, an instrument used to view or examine the amnion, a type of endoscope

**amni/o**-scopy, technique of viewing or examining the amnion, with an amnioscope

**amni/o**-tic, pertaining to or belonging to the amnion

**amni/o**-tome, an instrument to cut the amnion

**amni/o**-tomy, incision into the amnion

mono-**amni/o**-tic, pertaining to or having one amnion or one amniotic cavity

---

**Bartholin/o**, Bartholin's glands, the greater vestibular glands of the vagina
Named after Caspar Bartholin, the Copenhagen anatomist who described the structures now called the greater vestibular glands. There are two glands, one on each side of the vagina that secrete mucus into the vestibule through ducts. The mucus is produced during coitus to lubricate the vagina.

**bartholin**-itis, inflammation of the greater vestibular glands or Bartholin's glands

**Cervic/o**, cervix
From a Latin word **cervix**, meaning neck. Here cervic/o means the neck of the uterus, the cervix uteri.
Note: cervic/o also means neck as in cervical vertebrae of the neck.

**cervic**-al, pertaining to the cervix or cervix uteri

**cervic**-ectomy, removal of the cervix

**cervic**-itis, inflammation of the cervix

**cervic/o**-colp-itis, inflammation of the vagina and cervix uteri

**cervic/o**-vagin-al, pertaining to the vagina and cervix uteri

**cervic/o**-vagin-itis, inflammation of the vagina and cervix uteri

**cervic/o**-vesic-al, pertaining to the bladder and cervix uteri

intra-**cervic**-al, pertaining to within the cervix uteri

retro-**cervic**-al, pertaining to behind the cervix uteri

---

**Chori/o, chorion-**, chorion
From a Greek word **chorion** meaning a skin. Here, chori/o means the chorion, the outer membrane that surrounds a fetus. The chorion grows from a layer of cells called the trophoblast and develops extensions called villi that become part of the placenta.

**chori**-al, pertaining to the chorion Syn. chorionic

**chori/o**-aden-oma, an adenoma of the chorion (a sometimes malignant glandular tumour)

**chori/o**-allantois, a membrane formed by fusion of the allantois and chorion (the allantois is an extra-embryonic membrane that forms part of the umbilical cord in man)

**chori/o**-amnion-ic, pertaining to the amnion and chorion

**chorio**-amnion-itis, inflammation of the amnion and chorion

**chori/o**-angio-fibr-oma, an angioma (vascular tumour) containing fibrous connective tissue that develops from the chorion

**chori/o**-angi-oma, an angioma (vascular tumour) that develops from the chorion

**chori/o**-blast-oma, a tumour of (trophoblast) cells in the chorion

**chori/o**-carcin-oma, a malignant tumour of the chorion, formed from trophoblast cells Syn. chorioepithelioma

**chori/o**-cele, a protrusion or hernia of the chorion

**chori/o**-epitheli-oma, a malignant tumour of epithelial cells (trophoblasts) in the chorion Syn. choriocarcinoma

**chori/o**-genesis, formation or development of the chorion

**chori**-oma, a tumour of the chorion (formed from trophoblast cells, it can be benign or malignant)

**chorion**-ic, pertaining to the chorion

di-**chori**-al, pertaining to having two chorions

di-**chorion**-ic, pertaining to having two chorions

epi-**chori**-al, 1. pertaining to upon the chorion 2. pertaining to the epichorion

epi-**chori**-on, the part of the uterine mucosa upon and surrounding the developing conceptus

mono-**chorion**-ic, pertaining to one chorion

---

**Clito/r/i/d/o**, clitoris

From a Greek word **kleitoris** meaning clitoris. Here, clitor/o means the clitoris, a small erectile organ situated in the anterior part of the labia minora of the female, homologous to the penis in males; it contains abundant nervous tissue and is in involved in the female sexual response (orgasm).

**clitor**-al, pertaining to or belonging to the clitoris

**clitor**-alg-ia, condition of pain in the clitoris

**clitorid**-ectomy, removal of the clitoris

**clitorid**-itis, inflammation of the clitoris Syn. clitoritis

**clitorid/o**-tomy, incision into the clitoris (female circumcision) Syn. clitorotomy

**clitori**-megaly, enlargement of the clitoris, it refers to an abnormally large clitoris

**clitor**-ism, condition of the clitoris, it refers to enlargement or persistent erection of the clitoris

**clitor**-itis, inflammation of the clitoris Syn. clitoriditis

**clitor/o**-man-ia, condition of mania associated with the clitoris Syn. with nymphomania, an exaggerated sexual excitement in women

**clitor/o**-plasty, surgical repair or reconstruction of the clitoris

**clitor/o**-tomy, incision into the clitoris (female circumcision) Syn. clitoridotomy

**clito**-rrhag-ia, condition of bursting forth of blood (haemorrhage) from the clitoris

---

**Colp/o**, vagina

From a Greek word **colpos**, meaning hollow. Here, colp/o means vagina, the hollow chamber that receives the penis during copulation and through which the baby will pass at birth.

**colp**-alg-ia, condition of pain in the vagina

**colp**-atres-ia, condition of without an opening of the vagina, an imperforate vagina

**colp**-ectas-ia, condition of dilation of the vagina

**colp**-ectasis, dilation of the vagina

**colp**-ectomy, removal of the vagina

**colp**-eurynter, device (an inflatable bag) used to dilate the vagina

**colp**-eurysis, dilation of the vagina

**colp**-ismus, spasm of the vagina (muscles of) Syn. vaginismus

**colp**-itic, pertaining to having colpitis

**colp**-itis, inflammation of the vagina

**colp/o**-cele, a protrusion or hernia into the vagina (of rectum or bladder)

**colp/o**-cleisis, closure of the vagina. From a Greek word *kleisis* meaning closure

**colp/o**-cyst-ic, pertaining to the (urinary) bladder and vagina

**colp/o**-cyst-itis, inflammation of the (urinary) bladder and vagina

**colp/o**-cyst/o-cele, a protrusion or hernia of the (urinary) bladder into the vagina

**colp/o**-cyst/o-plasty, surgical repair of the (urinary) bladder and vagina (its vesicovaginal wall)

**colp/o**-cyst/o-tomy, incision into the bladder through the wall of the vagina

**colp/o**-cyt/o-gram, a recording or picture of cells of the vagina (from vaginal smears)

**colp/o**-cyt/o-logy, the study of cells of the vagina (from vaginal smears)

**colp/o**-desm/o-rrhaphy, stitching or suturing the bands of the vagina, it refers to the ruptured bands of bulbospongiosus muscle of the perineum

**colp/o**-dyn-ia, condition of pain in the vagina

**colp/o**-gram, a recording (a differential list) of vaginal cells

**colp/o**-hyper-plas-ia, condition of above normal growth or development (of cells) of the vagina

**colp/o**-hyster-ectomy, removal of the uterus through the vagina

**colp/o**-hyster/o-tomy, incision of the uterus through the vagina

**colp/o**-micro-scope, a microscope used to view or examine the lining of the vagina in situ

**colp/o**-perine/o-plasty, surgical repair or reconstruction of the perineum and vagina

**colp/o**-perine/o-rrhaphy, stitching or suturing of the perineum and vagina

**colp/o**-pexy, surgical fixation of the vagina

**colp/o**-photo-graphy, technique of recording by photography the lining of the vagina (and cervix) in women with abnormal smears

**colp/o**-myc-osis, abnormal condition of fungi in the vagina

**colp/o**-myom-ectomy, removal of a myoma (from the uterus) through the vagina

**colp/o**-pathy, disease of the vagina

**colp/o**-perine/o-plasty, surgical repair or reconstruction of the perineum and vagina

**colp/o**-pexy, surgical fixation of the vagina (to the abdominal wall to correct relaxation and prolapse)

**colp/o**-plasty, surgical repair or reconstruction of the vagina

**colp/o**-ptosis, displacement or prolapse of the vagina

**colp/o**-rect/o-pexy, surgical fixation of a (prolapsed) rectum to the walls of the vagina

**colp/o**-rrhag-ia, condition of bursting forth of blood (haemorrhage) from the vagina

**colp/o**-rrhaphy, 1. stitching or suturing of the vagina 2. a surgical procedure to narrow the lumen of the vagina

**colp/o**-rrhexis, rupture or laceration of the vaginal wall

**colp/o**-rrhoea, 1. excessive discharge (of mucus) from the vagina 2. leucor-rhoea

**colp/o**-scope, an instrument used to view or examine the vagina

**colp/o**-scopy, technique of viewing or examining the vagina

**colp/o**-spasm, spasm of the vagina, it refers to a sudden contraction of muscles of the vagina

**colp/o**-sten-osis, abnormal condition of narrowing or constriction of the vagina

**colp/o**-sten/o-tomy, incision into a narrowing (stricture) of the vagina

**colp/o**-tomy, incision into the vagina

**colp/o**-ureter/o-tomy, incision into a ureteral stricture through the vagina

**colp/o**-xer-osis, abnormal condition of a dry vagina

peri-**colp**-itis, inflammation of tissues around the vagina

---

**Culd/o**, Douglas pouch, recto-uterine pouch

From a French word **cul-de-sac**, meaning bottom of the bag or sack. Here, culd/o means the blindly ending Douglas pouch or recto-uterine pouch that lies above the posterior vaginal fornix.

**culd/o**-centesis, puncture of the recto-uterine pouch (Douglas pouch)

**culd/o-scope**, an instrument used to view or examine the recto-uterine pouch (Douglas pouch)

**culd/o-scopy**, technique of viewing or examining the recto-uterine pouch (Douglas pouch)

**culd/o-tomy**, incision into the recto-uterine pouch (Douglas pouch)

---

**Cye/si/o, -cyesis**, pregnancy

From a Greek word **kyesis** meaning pregnancy. Here -cyesis means pregnancy.

**cyesi/o-gnosis**, knowledge of pregnancy, it refers to diagnosis of pregnancy

**cye-tic**, pertaining to cyesis or pregnancy

en-**cyesis**, in pregnancy, it refers to a normally-sited pregnancy in the uterus

pseudo-**cyesis**, condition of a false pregnancy

---

**Embry/o**, embryo

From a Greek word **embruon** meaning embryo. Here, embry/o means an embryo, the early stage of development starting two weeks after fertilization of the oocyte until the end of week eight of gestation.

**embry-ectomy**, removal of an embryo, it refers to removal of an ectopic pregnancy from its extra-uterine position

**embry/o-gen-ic**, 1. pertaining to forming an embryo 2. pertaining to embryogeny

**embry/o-gen-y**, process of forming an embryo

**embry/o-log-ical**, pertaining to embryology

**embry/o-log-ist**, a specialist who studies embryology

**embry/o-logy**, 1. the study of the embryo or embryonic stage of development 2. the study of the development of an organism from fertilization to extra-uterine life

**embry-oma**, a tumour of embryonic origin e.g. a teratoma, a monster-like tumour of embryonic origin composed of different tissues in the wrong positions.

**embryon**, an embryo

**embryon-ic**, pertaining to an embryo

**embry/o-path-ic**, pertaining to disease of the embryo

**embry/o-path/o-logy**, the study of disease of the embryo

**embry/o-pathy**, disease of the embryo

**embry/o-plast-ic**, pertaining to the growth or formation of the embryo

**embry/o-tomy**, incision into an embryo, it refers to mutilation of the fetus to facilitate its removal from the uterus

**embry/o-trophy**, nourishment of the embryo

---

**Endometri/o**, endometrium (the lining of the uterus)

From the Greek words **metra**, meaning womb and **endo-** meaning inside. Here endometri/o means the endometrium, the mucous membrane lining the uterus.

**endometr-ectomy**, removal of the endometrium

**endometri-al**, pertaining to or belonging to the endometrium

**endometri-oid**, resembling the endometrium

**endometri-oma**, a tumour of the endometrium

**endometri-osis**, abnormal condition of the endometrium, it refers to endometrial tissue in abnormal locations in the pelvic cavity

**endometr-itis**, inflammation of the endometrium

**endometri-um**, the mucous membrane lining the uterus

**endometr/o-rrhag-ia**, condition of bursting forth of blood from the endometrium (irregular inter menstrual bleeding). Syn. metrorrhagia

---

**Episi/o**, pudendum, vulva

From a Greek word **episeion** meaning pudenda, the external genitalia of the female. Here, episi/o means the vulva or pudendum, comprising the mons pubis, labia majora and minora, the clitoris, the vaginal orifice, the vestibule, the hymen and the greater vestibular glands (Bartholin's glands).

**episi/o**-cele, a protrusion or hernia into the vulva

**episi/o**-perine/o-plasty, surgical repair or reconstruction of the perineum and vulva

**episi/o**-perine/o-rrhaphy, stitching or suturing of the perineum and vulva

**episi/o**-plasty, surgical repair or reconstruction of the vulva

**episi/o**-rrhag-ia, condition of bursting forth of blood (haemorrhage) from the vulva

**episi/o**-rrhaphy, 1. stitching or suturing of the vulva (labia majora) 2. stitching or suturing of the perineum

**episi/o**-sten-osis, abnormal condition of narrowing of the vulva (the vulval orifice)

**episi/o**-tomy, incision into the vulva or perineum to prevent tearing of the perineum during childbirth

**Fetal/o, fet/i/o,** fetus
From a Latin word **fetus**, meaning an unborn baby. Here, fet/o means a fetus, the stage of development following the embryonic period. A human embryo becomes a fetus eight weeks after fertilization when the organ systems have been laid down.

**fet**-al, 1. pertaining to or belonging to a fetus 2. at the stage of a fetus

**fetal**-ization, process of retaining fetal structures in an adult

**fetal/o**-metry, technique of measuring a fetus (particularly the head)

**fet**-ation, 1. process of forming or developing a fetus 2. pregnancy

**feti**-cide, the killing of a fetus

**fet/o**-amni-o-tic, pertaining to the amnion and fetus

**fet/o**-logy, the study of the fetus

**fet/o**-metry, technique of measuring a fetus

**fet/o**-placent-al, pertaining to a placenta and fetus

**fet/o**-scope, an instrument used for viewing or examining a fetus

**fet/o**-scopy, technique of viewing or examining a fetus

**fet/o**-tox-ic, pertaining to being toxic or poisonous to a fetus

**Galact/o,** milk
From a Greek word **gala**, meaning milk. Here, galact/o means milk, the secretion produced by the mammary gland during lactation.

**galacta**-cras-ia, condition of abnormal (composition) of milk. From a Greek word *krasis* meaning a mingling

**galact**-agogue, an agent that stimulates milk (production)

**galact**-ic, 1. pertaining to or belonging to milk 2. an agent that stimulates milk (a galactagogue)

**galact**-isch-ia, condition of holding back or stopping milk

**galact/o**-blast, a milk cell (colostrum corpuscle) found in the acini of the mammary gland

**galact/o**-cele, a swelling or protrusion of milk, it refers to a milk-filled cyst in a mammary gland due to obstruction of a duct

**galact**-oedema, a swelling (of the breast) caused by accumulation of milk

**galact/o**-graphy, technique of making a recording or X-ray picture of the milk ducts

**galact/o**-meter, an instrument used to measure milk (to estimate fat content)

**galact**-onc-us, a swelling or protrusion of milk, it refers to a milk-filled cyst in a mammary gland due to obstruction of a duct Syn. galactocele

**galact/o**-phag-ous, pertaining to feeding on milk

**galact/o**-phore, a duct that carries milk, it refers to a lactiferous duct

**galact/o**-phor-ous, 1. pertaining to carrying milk 2. lactiferous

**galact/o**-phyg-ous, pertaining to retarding or causing the cessation of milk production. From a Greek word *phyge* meaning banishment

**galact/o**-plan-ia, condition of secreting milk on an abnormal part of the body

**galact/o**-poiesis, formation of milk

**galact/o**-poie-tic, 1. pertaining to the formation of milk 2. an agent that stimulates the formation of milk (galactagogue)

**galact/o**-rrhoea, excessive flow of milk, spontaneous and/or persistent

**galactos**-aem-ia, condition of the presence of galactose (a component of milk sugar) in the blood, an inborn error of galactose metabolism

**galact**-ose, a monosaccharide found in the disaccharide lactose (milk sugar)

**galact**-osis, condition of milk, it refers in physiology to the secretion of milk by the mammary glands

**galact/o**-stas-ia, 1. condition of cessation or stopping of milk secretion 2. condition of abnormal amounts of milk in a mammary gland due to cessation of its flow

**galact/o**-stasis, 1. condition of cessation or stopping of milk secretion 2. condition of abnormal amounts of milk in a mammary gland due to cessation of its flow

**galactos**-ur-ia, condition of galactose (a component of milk sugar) in the urine

**galact/o**-tox-ism, process of poisoning by milk

**galact/o**-troph-ic, pertaining to stimulating the secretion of milk

**galact/o**-trophy, nourishing with milk only

hyper-**galact**-ia, condition of excessive secretion of milk

hyper-**galact**-osis, abnormal condition of excessive secretion of milk

hyper-**galact**-ous, pertaining to the excessive secretion of milk

hypo-**galact**-ia, condition of (producing) a small quantity of milk

---

**Genital-**, **genit/o**, genitalia
From a Latin word **genitalis** meaning to beget. Here genit/o means genitalia, the organs of reproduction especially the external organs.

**genit**-al, 1. pertaining to the genitalia or organs of reproduction 2. a reproductive organ

**genital**-ia, the reproductive organs

**genit/o**-femor-al, pertaining to the thigh and genitalia

**genit/o**-plasty, surgical repair or reconstruction of the genitalia

**genit/o**-urin-ary, pertaining to the urinary tract and genitalia

pre-**genit**-al, pertaining to before the genital stage in psychosexual development

---

**Gravid/o**, **-gravida**, pregnancy, pregnant woman
From a Latin word **gravidus** meaning heavy or pregnant. Here -gravida means a woman in relation to her pregnancies; for example, GI - gravida one, a woman pregnant for the first time, GII a woman pregnant for the second time *etc*.

**gravid**, pregnant

**gravida**, a pregnant woman

**gravid**-ic, pertaining to a pregnant woman or pertaining to during pregnancy

**gravid**-ity, state of pregnancy

**gravid/o**-cardi-ac, pertaining to heart (disease) during pregnancy

multi-**gravida**, a woman who is pregnant and has been pregnant at least twice before

primi-**gravida**, a woman pregnant for the first time (GI)

pro-**gravid**, before pregnancy, it refers to the phase of preparation of the lining of the uterus (endometrium) before implantation

secundi-**gravida**, a woman pregnant for the second time (GII)

terti-**gravida**, a woman pregnant for the third time (GIII)

---

**Gynaec/o**, **gyn/o**, gynaecology, woman
From a Greek word **gyne**, meaning woman. Here gynaec/o refers to a woman or the female reproductive system.

**gynaec**-ic, 1. pertaining to the female reproductive system 2. pertaining to a woman or to women

**gynaec/o**-gen-ic, pertaining to woman-forming (feminizing)

**gynaec/o**-graphy, technique of making a recording or X-ray picture of a woman's reproductive system

**gynaec**-oid, resembling a woman

**gynaec/o**-log-ical, 1. pertaining to gynaecology 2. pertaining to the study of women (anatomy, diseases and treatment of the female reproductive system)

**gynaec/o**-log-ist, a specialist who studies gynaecology (the anatomy, diseases and treatment of the female reproductive system)

**gynaec/o**-logy, the study of women, it refers to the study of anatomy, diseases and treatment of the female reproductive system

**gynaec/o**-man-ia, condition of mania towards women, it refers to an exaggerated sexual excitement of the male Syn. satyriasis

**gynaec/o**-mast-ia, condition of women's breasts, it refers to excessive development of the breasts in males

**gynaec/o**-mast-y, condition of women's breasts, it refers to excessive development of the breasts seen in males

**gynae**-plasty, surgical repair or reconstruction of the female reproductive system

**gyn**-andr-ia, condition of a male with a woman's characteristics, a male hermaphrodite

**gyn**-andr-ism, 1. hermaphroditism 2. condition of a male with a woman's characteristics, a male hermaphrodite 3. false female pseudohermaphroditism, a condition in which only the external genitalia of a female look like those of the male

**gyn**-andr/o-blast-oma, an (ovarian) tumour of immature cells or embryonic cells associated with masculinization

**gyn**-andr/o-morph, individual having the form of a male and a female, *i.e.* having male and female characteristics

**gyn**-andr/o-morph-ism, condition of having male and female characteristics

**gyne**-phob-ia, condition of irrational fear or dislike of women

**gyn/o**-genesis, early formation or development of a fertilized egg containing only the woman's (maternal) chromosomes

**gyn/o**-path-ic, pertaining to diseases peculiar to women, it refers to diseases of the female reproductive system

**gyn/o**-pathy, diseases peculiar to women, it refers to diseases of the female reproductive system

**gyn/o**-plast-ic, pertaining to surgical repair or reconstruction of the female reproductive system

**gyn/o**-plast-ics, the medical speciality of surgical repair or reconstruction of the female reproductive system

**gyn/o**-plasty, surgical repair or reconstruction of the female reproductive system

---

**Hyster/o**, uterus

From a Greek word **hystera**, meaning womb. Here hyster/o means the uterus, the hollow muscular organ into which the ovum is received from a Fallopian tube and where it is retained during development. The fetus is expelled from the uterus through the vagina during the second stage of labour.

**hyster**-alg-ia, condition of pain in the uterus

**hyster**-atres-ia, condition of without an opening of the uterus, an imperforate uterus

**hyster**-aux-esis, condition of increase (in size) of the uterus

**hyster**-ectomy, removal of the uterus

**hyster**-elc-osis, abnormal condition of ulceration of the uterus

**hyster**-eurynter, device (inflatable bag) used to dilate the os uteri (vaginal opening into the neck of the uterus)

**hyster**-itis, inflammation of the uterus

**hyster/o**-cele, a protrusion or hernia of the uterus Syn. metrocele

**hyster/o**-cervic/o-tomy, incision into the cervix and uterus (lower segment)

**hyster/o**-cleisis, surgical closure of the os uteri (vaginal opening into the neck of the uterus). From a Greek word *kleisis* meaning closure

**hyster/o**-colp-ectomy, surgical removal of the vagina and uterus

**hyster/o**-cyesis, a uterine pregnancy

**hyster/o**-cyst-ic, pertaining to or belonging to the urinary bladder and uterus

**hyster/o**-cyst/o-pex-ia, condition of surgical fixation of the urinary bladder and uterus (to the abdominal wall), an operation for the relief of a prolapse

**hyster/o**-cyst/o-pexy, surgical fixation of the urinary bladder and uterus (to the abdominal wall), an operation for the relief of a prolapse

**hyster/o**-dynam/o-meter, an instrument used to measure the power and frequency of uterine contractions

**hyster/o**-dyn-ia, condition of pain in the uterus

**hyster/o**-eurysis, process of dilating the os uteri (the vaginal opening into the neck of the uterus)

**hyster/o**-gram, a recording or X-ray picture of the uterus

**hyster/o**-graphy, technique of making a recording or X-ray picture of the uterus

**hyster/o**-lith, a stone or calculus in the uterus

**hyster/o**-lith-iasis, abnormal condition of stones or calculi in the uterus

**hyster/o**-lox-ia, condition of oblique displacement or flexion of the uterus. From a Greek word *loxos* meaning crosswise

**hyster/o**-lysis, surgical separation (of adhesions) in the uterus

**hyster/o**-malac-ia, condition of softening of the uterus

**hyster/o**-meter, an instrument used to measure the uterus (the depth of its cavity) Syn. uterometer

**hyster/o**-my-oma, a tumour of smooth muscle formed in the uterus

**hyster/o**-myom-ectomy, removal of a myoma (tumour of smooth muscle) from the uterus

**hyster/o**-my/o-tomy, incision into the muscle of the uterus (to remove a tumour)

**hyster/o**-oophor-ectomy, removal of the ovaries and uterus

**hyster/o**-pathy, disease of the uterus

**hyster/o**-pexy, surgical fixation of a displaced or prolapsed uterus

**hyster/o**-ptosis, a displaced or prolapsed uterus

**hyster/o**-rrhaphy, 1. stitching or suturing of the uterus 2. hysteropexy

**hyster/o**-rrhexis, rupture of the uterus Syn. metrorrhexis

**hyster/o**-rrhoea, excessive flow or discharge from the uterus

**hyster/o**-salping-ectomy, removal of the uterine tubes and uterus

**hyster/o**-salping/o-graphy, technique of making a recording or X-ray picture of the uterine tubes and uterus

**hyster/o**-salping-oophor-ectomy, removal of the ovaries, uterine tubes and uterus

**hyster/o**-salping/o-stomy, formation of an opening between a uterine tube and uterus or the name of the opening so created

**hyster/o**-salpinx, a uterine tube

**hyster/o**-scope, an instrument (endoscope) used to view or examine the uterus (and uterine cervix)

**hyster/o**-scopy, technique of viewing or examining the uterus

**hyster/o**-spasm, sudden contraction of the smooth muscle of the uterus

**hyster/o**-tomy, incision into the uterus

**hyster/o**-trachel-ectas-ia, condition of dilation of the neck of the uterus (uterine cervix) and cavity of the uterus

**hyster/o**-trachel-ectomy, removal of the neck of the uterus (uterine cervix)

**hyster/o**-trachel/o-plasty, surgical repair or reconstruction of the neck of the uterus (the uterine cervix)

**hyster/o**-trachel/o-rrhaphy, stitching or suturing the neck of the uterus (the uterine cervix)

**hyster/o**-trachel/o-tomy, incision into the neck of the uterus (uterine cervix)

**hyster/o**-tub/o-graphy, technique of making a recording or X-ray picture of the uterine tubes and uterus Syn. hysterosalpingography

pan-**hyster/o**-ectomy, removal of all the uterus

pan-**hyster/o**-salping-ectomy, removal of all the uterine tubes and uterus

ventr/o-**hyster/o**-pexy, surgical fixation of a displaced or prolapsed uterus to the abdominal wall

---

**Lact/i/o**, milk

From a Latin word **lactis**, meaning milk. Here lact/i/o means milk, the secretion produced by the mammary gland during lactation.

hyper-**lact**-ation, action of secreting above normal amounts of milk, for an extended period

**lact**-agogue, an agent stimulating or promoting milk (production)

**lact**-album-in, a chemical of the albumin class found in milk

**lact**-ase, an enzyme that acts on lactose (milk sugar)

**lact**-ate, to secrete milk

**lact**-ation, 1. the action of secreting milk 2. the period following childbirth when milk is secreted

**lact**-ic, pertaining to milk

**lact/i**-fer-ous, pertaining to carrying milk

**lact/i**-form, having the form of or resembling milk

**lact/i**-fuge, 1. an agent that suppresses milk secretion 2. suppressing or retarding milk secretion

**lact/i**-gen-ous, pertaining to forming milk

**lact/i**-ger-ous, pertaining to carrying milk. From a Latin word *gerere* meaning to carry

**lact/i**-phag-ous, pertaining to consuming milk

**lact/i**-vor-ous, living by consuming a diet of milk. From a Latin word *vorare* meaning to devour

**lact/o**-cele, a swelling or protrusion of milk, it refers to a milk-filled cyst in a mammary gland caused by obstruction of a duct Syn. galactocele

**lact/o**-crit, a device used to separate milk, it is used to measure fat content

**lact/o**-gen, an agent that stimulates or causes milk secretion

**lact/o**-gen-ic, pertaining to forming milk or originating in milk

**lact/o**-globul-in, a protein found in milk

**lact/o**-meter, an instrument used to measure milk (specific gravity)

**lact/o**-rrhoea, excessive flow of milk (can be spontaneous and/or persistent) Syn. galactorrhoea

**lact**-ose, a sugar found in milk, a disaccharide

**lact/os**-ur-ia, condition of lactose in the urine

**lact/o**-troph-in, a hormone that nourishes milk (stimulates and maintains milk secretion) Syn. prolactin

**lact/o**-trop-in, a hormone that stimulates and maintains milk secretion Syn. prolactin

pro-**lact**-in, a hormone that acts before milk *i.e.* on the breast to stimulate lactation

super-**lact**-ation, action of secreting above normal amounts of milk, for an extended period

---

**Lochi/o**, lochia

From a Greek word **lochos** meaning childbirth. Here lochi/o means lochia, the normal discharge from the uterus in the first weeks following childbirth or abortion. The lochia consists of blood, mucus, fibrin, necrotic tissue and leucocytes. First, it consists entirely of blood and then becomes paler, diminishes in quantity and finally ceases.

**lochi**-al, pertaining to lochia

**lochi/o**-colpos, a vagina containing lochia, it refers to distension of the vagina caused by failure to discharge lochia

**lochi/o**-metra, a uterus containing lochia, distension caused by retention of the lochia

**lochi/o**-metr-itis, inflammation of the uterus with lochia Syn. puerperal metritis

**lochi/o**-rrhag-ia, condition of bursting forth or copious discharge of lochia

**lochi/o**-rrhoea, excessive flow (discharge) of lochia

**lochi/o**-schesis, condition of retention of lochia. From a Greek word *schesis* meaning holding fast

**lochi/o**-stasis, 1. stopping or cessation of movement of lochia 2. retention of lochia

---

**Mamill/i/o**, nipple

From a Latin word **mamilla** meaning nipple or teat. Here mamill/o means nipple, a pigmented, conical projection on the areola of the breast into which the lactiferous ducts open. See the combining form thel/e also meaning nipple.

**mamilla**, 1. a nipple or teat 2. a nipple-like structure

**mamill-ary**, pertaining to a nipple or nipple-like structure

**mamill-ate**, having nipples or nipple-like structures

**mamill-ation**, a nipple-like structure

**mamill/i-form**, having the form or shape of a nipple

**mamill/i-plasty**, surgical repair or reconstruction of a nipple

**mamill-itis**, inflammation of a nipple

**mamill-oid**, resembling a nipple

**mamill-ose**, having many nipples or nipple-like structures

---

**Mamm/i/o**, breast, mammary gland

From a Latin word **mamma**, meaning breast. Here mamm/o means the mammary gland or breast that secretes milk during lactation following birth.

**mamma(e)**, the mammary gland(s) or breast(s)

**mammal**, an animal belonging to the class Mammalia that suckles its young with milk from mammary glands

**mamm**-alg-ia, condition of pain in a mammary gland

**mamm-ary**, pertaining to the mammary glands

**mamm-ate**, having mammary glands

**mamm-ectomy**, removal of a mammary gland Syn. mastectomy

**mamm/i-form**, having the form of or shaped like a mammary gland

**mamm/i-lingus**, licking or sucking the mammary gland

**mamm-itis**, inflammation of the mammary gland

**mamm/o-gen**, 1. an agent that stimulates the mammary gland 2. prolactin

**mamm/o-gram**, a recording or X-ray picture of a mammary gland

**mamm/o-graphy**, technique of making a recording or X-ray picture of the mammary glands

**mamm/o-plas-ia**, condition of growth or development of the mammary glands or breast tissue, it refers to an increase in the mass of cells of breast tissue

**mamm/o-plasty**, surgical repair or reconstruction of the breast

**mamm-ose**, pertaining to having (large) mammary glands or nipples

**mamm/o-therm/o-graphy**, technique of recording heat from the mammary glands

**mamm/o-tomy**, incision into a mammary gland Syn. mastotomy

**mamm/o-troph-ic**, pertaining to nourishing or stimulating the mammary glands

**mamm/o-trop-ic**, 1. pertaining to affinity for the mammary glands 2. pertaining to affecting the mammary glands

sub-**mamm-ary**, pertaining to beneath a mammary gland

---

**Mast/o**, breast

From a Greek word **mastos**, meaning breast. Here mast/o means the mammary gland or breast that secretes milk during lactation following birth.

macro-**mast-ia**, condition of abnormally large breasts

**mast-aden-oma**, a tumour of the breast

**mast-alg-ia**, condition of pain in the breast

**mast-a-trophy**, poor nourishment (wasting away) or without development of the breast

259

**mast**-ectomy, removal of the breast

**mast**-helc-osis, abnormal condition of ulceration of the breast

**mast**-itis, inflammation of a breast

**mast/o**-graphy, technique of making a recording or X-ray picture of the breast

**mast**-oid, resembling the breast

**mast**-onc-us, a tumour or swelling of the breast

**mast/o**-pathy, disease of the breast

**mast/o**-pexy, surgical fixation of the breasts, an operation to fix pendulous breasts in a new comfortable position

**mast/o**-plasty, surgical repair or reconstruction of the breast

**mast/o**-ptosis, falling or displacement of the breasts, it refers to pendulous breasts

**mast/o**-rrhag-ia, condition of bursting forth of blood (haemorrhage) from the breast

**mast/o**-scirrh-us, a hard breast or hard tumour of the breast

**mast**-osis, abnormal condition of the breasts (enlargement)

**mast/o**-stomy, formation of an opening into the breast (for drainage) or the name of the opening so created

**mast/o**-tomy, incision into a breast

para-**mast**-itis, inflammation of tissues beside a mammary gland

---

**Men/o**, menses, menstruation
From a Latin word **mensis**, meaning month. Here, men/o means the menstrual flow or menses, the monthly bleeding from the womb. The bleeding arises from the disintegration of the endometrium.

a-**men/o**-rrhoea, without menstrual flow *e.g.* ceasing of menstruation in pregnancy

crypto-**men/o**-rrhoea, hidden flow or hidden discharge of the menses, it refers to menstruation with retention caused by narrowing of the genital canal

dys-**men/o**-rrhoea, difficult or painful menstrual flow

epi-**men/o**-rrhag-ia, condition of additional bursting forth of blood or excessive menstrual flow at abnormally frequent intervals

epi-**men/o**-rrhoea, excessive flow or discharge of the menses at abnormally frequent intervals

hypo-**men/o**-rrhoea, 1. below normal (amount of) menstrual flow 2. below normal (duration) of menstrual flow

**men**-arche, the beginning of menstrual flow (menstruation)

**men/o**-lipsis, without menstrual flow, it refers to temporary cessation of menstruation. From a Greek word *leipien* meaning to fail

**men/o**-metr/o-rrhag-ia, condition of bursting forth of blood (haemorrhage) from the uterus at and between menstrual periods

**men/o**-paus-al, pertaining to the menopause

**men/o**-pause, the stopping of menstrual flow (menstruation)

**men/o**-rrhag-ia, condition of bursting forth of blood or excessive menstrual flow

**men/o**-rrh-alg-ia, condition of pain during menstrual flow Syn. dysmenorrhoea

**men/o**-rrhoea, flow or discharge of the menses (normal menstruation)

**men/o**-rrhoe-al, pertaining to menorrhoea

**men/o**-schesis, retention, suppression of the menses. From a Greek word *schesis* meaning a holding fast

**men/o**-stas-ia, 1. condition of stopping or cessation of menstrual flow Syn. amenorrhoea 2. condition of cessation of menstruation at the menopause

**men/o**-stasis, the stopping or cessation of menstrual flow Syn. amenorrhoea

**men/o**-staxis, excessive dripping of the menses, it refers to a prolonged menstrual period

**menses**, the monthly flow of blood from the lining of the uterus

**menstru**-al, pertaining to menstruation. From a Latin word *menstruare* meaning monthly

**mens**tru-ate, to have a monthly menstrual flow or menstruation. From a Latin word *menstruare* meaning monthly

**mens**tru-ation, action of producing a monthly menstrual flow. From a Latin word *menstruare* meaning monthly

oligo-**men/o**-rrhoea, reduced frequency of menstrual flow (menstruation)

para-**men**-ia, condition of wrong menses, it refers to menstrual disorder or irregularity

pre-**men**-arch-al, pertaining before the establishment of menstruation

pre-**mens**tru-al, pertaining to before menstruation. From a Latin word *menstruare* meaning monthly

---

**Metr/o**, uterus

From a Greek word **metra**, meaning womb. Here metr/o means the uterus, the hollow muscular organ into which the ovum is received from a Fallopian tube and where it is retained during development. The fetus is expelled from the uterus through the vagina during the second stage of labour.

hydro-**metr/o**-colp-us, a vagina and uterus containing a watery fluid

meso-**metr**-ium, the middle uterus, it refers to the area of the broad ligament outside the uterus below the mesovarium

**metr**-alg-ia, condition of pain in the uterus Syn. metrodynia

**metr**-a-ton-ia, condition of without (muscular) tone of the uterus

**metr**-atres-ia, condition of without an opening of the uterus, an imperforate uterus

**metr**-a-troph-ia, condition of lack of nourishment (wasting away) of the uterus

**metr**-ectas-ia, condition of dilation of the uterus (in non-gravid uterus)

**metr**-ec-top-ia, condition of an out of place uterus (uterine displacement)

**metr**-elc-osis, condition of ulceration of the uterus

**metr**-eurynter, device (inflatable bag) used to dilate the uterus (cervical canal)

**metr**-eurysis, process of dilating the cervix uteri (cervical canal) with a metreurynter

**metr**-itic, pertaining to having metritis

**metr**-itis, inflammation of the uterus

**metr/o**-campsis, abnormal condition of bending of the uterus. From a Greek word *kampsis* meaning a curving

**metr/o**-carcin-oma, a malignant tumour of the uterus

**metr/o**-cele, a protrusion or hernia of the uterus

**metr/o**-colp/o-cele, a protrusion or hernia of the uterus into the vagina

**metr/o**-cyst-osis, abnormal condition of cysts in the uterus

**metr/o**-dynam/o-meter, an instrument used to measure the force or power of uterine contractions

**metr/o**-dyn-ia, condition of pain in the uterus Syn. metralgia

**metr/o**-endo-metr-itis, inflammation of the endometrium and uterus

**metr/o**-fibr-oma, a fibrous tumour of the uterus (a uterine fibroma)

**metr/o**-graphy, technique of making a recording or X-ray picture of the uterus

**metr/o**-leuco-rrhoea, excessive white discharge from the uterus

**metr/o**-leuko-rrhoea, excessive white discharge from the uterus

**metr/o**-lox-ia, condition of oblique displacement of the uterus. From a Greek word *loxos* meaning oblique

**metr/o**-malac-ia, condition of softening of the uterus

**metr/o**-paralysis, paralysis of the uterus

**metr/o**-path-ia, condition of disease of the uterus

**metr/o**-path-ic, pertaining to disease of the uterus

**metr/o**-pathy, disease of the uterus

**metr/o**-periton-itis, inflammation of the peritoneum around the uterus

**metr/o**-phleb-itis, inflammation of veins of the uterus

**metr/o**-phyma, a tumour of the uterus

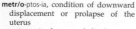 

**metr/o**-ptos-ia, condition of downward displacement or prolapse of the uterus

**metr/o**-ptosis, downward displacement or prolapse of the uterus

**metr/o**-rrhag-ia, condition of bursting forth of blood from the uterus, it refers to irregular inter menstrual bleeding

**metr/o**-rrhexis, rupture of the uterus

**metr/o**-rrhoea, excessive flow or discharge from the uterus

**metr/o**-salping-itis, inflammation of the uterine tubes and uterus

**metr/o**-salping/o-graphy, technique of making a recording or X-ray picture of the uterine tubes and uterus

**metr/o**-salpinx, a uterine tube or oviduct

**metr/o**-staxis, persistent dripping or bleeding from the uterus

**metr/o**-sten-osis, abnormal condition of narrowing of the uterus

**metr/o**-tome, an instrument used to cut the uterus

**metr/o**-tomy, incision into the uterus

para-**metr**-ic, pertaining to near or beside the uterus

---

**Nat/i/o**, birth

From a Latin word **natalis**, meaning birth. Here nat/o means birth or a new birth.

ante-**nat**-al, pertaining to before birth

**nat**-al, pertaining to birth

**nat**-al-ity, state of births, the birth rate

**nat/i**-mortal-ity, state of dead births, the proportion of stillbirths compared to live births

neo-**nat**-al, pertaining to a new birth (the first 28 days of life)

neo-**nate**, a new birth or newborn infant

neo-**nat/o**-logy, the study of new births or the newborn

neo-**nat**-us, a new birth or newborn infant

peri-**nat**-al, pertaining to around (the time) of birth

peri-**nat/o**-logy, branch of medicine that studies the fetus and infant around (the time) of birth

post-**nat**-al, pertaining to following birth

pre-**nat**-al, pertaining to before birth

---

**Nymph/o**, nymphae, the labia minora

From a Greek word **nymphe** meaning maiden. Here, nymph/o means the nymphae or labia minora, small lip-like skin folds within the labia majora bounding the vaginal opening.

**nymph**-a, labium minus. Singular of nymphae

**nymph**-ae, labia minora. Plural of nympha

**nymph**-ectomy, removal of the nymphae (labia minora)

**nymph**-itis, inflammation of the nymphae (labia minora)

**nymph/o**-man-ia, condition of mania associated with the nymphae (an exaggerated sexual desire in women)

**nymph**-onc-us, a tumour or swelling of the nymphae (labia minora)

**nymph/o**-tomy, incision into the nymphae or into the clitoris

---

**Obstetr-**, midwifery, obstetrics

From a Latin word **obstetricare** meaning to assist in delivery. Here, obstetr- means midwifery or obstetrics. Obstetrics and gynaecology are usually studied together as a medical speciality.

**obstetr**-ic, 1. pertaining to obstetrics 2. belonging to midwifery

**obstetr**-ical, 1. pertaining to obstetrics 2. belonging to midwifery

**obstetr**-ician, a medical specialist who practises obstetrics

**obstetr**-ics, the branch of medicine dealing with pregnancy, labour and the period following birth (the puerperium)

**obstetr**-ist, a medical specialist who practises obstetrics, an obstetrician

---

**Omphal/o**, navel, umbilicus, umbilical cord

From a Greek word **omphalos** meaning navel. Here omphal/o means the navel or umbilicus, a small, depressed scar on the anterior abdominal wall remaining from the separation of the umbilical cord. The umbilical cord connects the fetus to the placenta; it contains two arteries and one vein supported by embryonic connective tissue (Wharton's jelly)

**omphal**-ectomy, removal of the umbilicus (navel)

**omphal**-elc-osis, abnormal condition of ulceration of the umbilicus (navel)

**omphal**-ic, pertaining to the umbilicus (navel)

**omphal**-itis, inflammation of the umbilicus (navel)

**omphal**-cele, a protrusion or hernia (of intestine) through the umbilicus (navel)

**omphal/o**-enter-ic, pertaining to the intestine and umbilicus (navel)

**omphal/o**-genesis, formation of the umbilicus (navel)

**omphal**-oma, a tumour of the umbilicus (navel)

**omphal/o**-mesenter-ic, pertaining to the mesentery and umbilicus (navel)

**omphal**-onc-us, a tumour of the umbilicus (navel)

**omphal/o**-phleb-itis, inflammation of umbilical veins

**omphal/o**-rrhag-ia, condition of bursting forth of blood (haemorrhage) from the umbilicus (navel)

**omphal/o**-rrhexis, rupture of the umbilicus (navel)

**omphal/o**-rrhoea, excessive flow or discharge of (lymph) from the umbilicus (navel)

**omphalos**, the navel or umbilicus

**omphal/o**-tome, an instrument used to cut the umbilical cord

**omphal/o**-tomy, incision into the umbilical cord

**omphal**-us, the navel or umbilicus

---

**Oo-**, egg
From a Greek word **oon** meaning egg. Here, oo- means an ovum or egg cell. The human egg cell or ovum contains twenty-three chromosomes incorporating the maternal genes.

**oo**-blast, a germ cell or embryonic cell that produces eggs

**oo**-cyte, an egg cell or ovum

**oo**-genesis, the formation of eggs

**oo**-genet-ic, 1. pertaining to the formation of eggs 2. pertaining to oogenesis

**oo**-kinesis, movement of an egg, it refers to the movements of the nuclear material and spindle within an egg cell during its maturation and fertilization

**oo**-lemma, the sheath of the egg, it refers to the transparent layer called the zona pellucida surrounding an oocyte

---

**Oophor/o**, ovary
From a Greek word **oophoron**, meaning ovary. Here oophor/o means the ovary, the female reproductive organ or gonad that produces eggs. This organ is also a main source of the female sex-hormones oestrogen and progesterone. These steroid hormones control development of the female reproductive system and the formation of secondary sexual characteristics.

ep-**oophor**-on, a vestigial structure beside the ovary (between the ovary and uterine tube), the remains of the mesonephros (the rudimentary excretory organ of the embryo)

**oophor**-alg-ia, condition of pain in an ovary

**oophor**-ectomy, removal of an ovary

**oophor**-itis, inflammation of an ovary Syn. ovaritis

**oophor/o**-cyst-ectomy, removal of an ovarian bladder (an ovarian cyst)

**oophor/o**-cyst-osis, abnormal condition of cysts (bladders) in the ovary

**oophor/o**-gen-ous, pertaining to forming or originating in an ovary

**oophor/o**-hyster-ectomy, removal of the uterus and ovaries

**oophor**-oma, a tumour of an ovary

**oophor/o**-path-ia, condition of disease of the ovaries

**oophor/o**-pathy, disease of the ovaries

**oophor/o**-pexy, fixation of an ovary (by surgery to the abdominal wall)

**oophor/o**-plasty, surgical repair or reconstruction of an ovary

**oophor/o**-rrhag-ia, condition of bursting forth of blood (haemorrhage) from an ovary, at the site of ovulation

**oophor/o**-rrhaphy, stitching or suturing of an ovary, it refers to fixing a prolapsed ovary into position

**oophor/o**-salping-ectomy, removal of a uterine tube and its ovary

**oophor/o**-salping-itis, inflammation of a uterine tube and its ovary

**oophor/o**-stomy, formation of an opening into the ovary or the name of the opening so created

**oophor/o**-tomy, incision into an ovary

---

**Ovari/o**, ovary

From a New Latin word **ovarium**, meaning ovary, derived from **ova**, meaning egg. Here ovari/o means the ovary, the female reproductive organ or gonad that produces eggs. This organ is also a main source of the female sex-hormones oestrogen and progesterone. These steroid hormones control development of the female reproductive system and the formation of secondary sexual characteristics.

mes-**ovari**-um, the middle ovary, it refers to an area of broad ligament below the Fallopian tube that holds the ovary in position

**ovari**-an, pertaining to or belonging to an ovary

**ovari**-ectomy, removal of an ovary Syn. oophorectomy

**ovari/o**-cele, a protrusion or hernia of an ovary

**ovari/o**-centesis, puncture of an ovary

**ovari/o**-cyesis, a pregnancy developing in an ovary (an ectopic pregnancy)

**ovari/o**-gen-ic, pertaining to forming or originating in an ovary

**ovari/o**-hyster-ectomy, removal of the uterus and ovaries

**ovari/o**-lyt-ic, pertaining to breakdown of an ovary or breakdown of ovarian tissue

**ovari**-onc-us, a tumour of an ovary

**ovari/o**-pathy, disease of the ovaries

**ovari/o**-priv-al, pertaining to caused by lack of ovaries. From a Latin word *privare* meaning to deprive

**ovari/o**-rrhexis, rupture of an ovary

**ovari/o**-salping-ectomy, removal of a uterine tube and ovary

**ovari/o**-stomy, formation of an opening into an ovary (to drain the contents of a cyst) or the name of the opening so created Syn. oophorostomy

**ovari/o**-tomy, incision into an ovary

**ovari/o**-tub-al, pertaining to a uterine tube and ovary

**ovar**-itis, inflammation of an ovary Syn. oophoritis

par-**ovari**-an, 1. pertaining to beside an ovary 2. a vestigial structure beside the ovary called an epoophoron

---

**-para**, to bear, bring forth
viable offspring

From a Latin word **parere**, meaning to bear or bring forth. Here, -para refers to a woman and her previous viable pregnancies. For example Para I means a woman who has already had one pregnancy that resulted in a viable child.

multi-**para**, a woman who has had more than two viable pregnancies

multi-**par**-ity, state or condition of being a multipara

multi-**par**-ous, pertaining to a woman who has had more than two viable pregnancies

nulli-**para**, a woman who has never borne a viable child

nulli-**par**-ity, state or condition of being a nullipara

nulli-**par**-ous, pertaining to a woman who has never borne a viable child

primi-**para**, 1. a woman who has had one pregnancy that resulted in a viable child 2. Para I

primi-**par**-ity, state or condition of being a primipara

primi-**par**-ous, pertaining to a a woman who has had one pregnancy that resulted in a viable child quadri-**para**, 1. a woman who has had four pregnancies that resulted in viable offspring 2. Para IV

quinti-**para**, 1. a woman who has had five pregnancies that resulted in viable offspring 2. Para V

secundi-**para**, 1. a woman who has had two pregnancies that resulted in viable offspring 2. Para II

secundi-**par**-ity, state or condition of being a secundipara

secundi-**par**-ous, pertaining to a woman who has had two pregnancies that resulted in viable offspring

terti-**para**, 1. a woman who has had three pregnancies that resulted in viable offspring 2. Para III

uni-**para**, 1. pertaining to a a woman who has had one pregnancy that resulted in a viable child 2. Para I

uni-**par**-ous, 1. pertaining to a a woman who has had one pregnancy that resulted in a viable child 2. pertaining to producing one offspring at a time

vivi-**par**-ous, pertaining to bearing live young that develop within the female

---

**Part-, parturi/o,** childbirth, labour, parturition
From the Latin words **partus** meaning a bringing forth and **parturire** meaning to have the pains of labour. Here the words part- and parturi/o mean childbirth or labour.

ante-**part**-al, pertaining to occurring before childbirth

ante-**part**-um, occurring before childbirth

intra-**part**-um, occurring within or during childbirth

parturi-**ent**, 1. in the process of giving birth 2. pertaining to parturition 3. a woman in the process of giving birth or in labour

parturi-**o**-meter, an instrument used to measure the force of uterine contractions during labour

parturi-**tion**, the process of giving birth

part-us, labour or childbirth

post-**part**-um, pertaining to the period immediately after childbirth

pre-**part**-al, pertaining to before the onset of labour

---

**Perine/o,** perineum
From a Greek word **perineos** meaning perineum. Here perine/o means the perineum or perineal body, the area between the external genitalia and the rectum; it consists of the muscles of the pelvic floor and connective tissue covered with skin.

perine-**al**, pertaining to the perineum

perine/o-**cele**, a protrusion or hernia of the perineum (it forms between the vagina and rectum in females)

perine/o-**meter**, an instrument used to measure the perineum, it refers to measuring the strength of contraction of muscles in the pelvic floor

perine/o-**plasty**, surgical repair or reconstruction of the perineum

perine/o-**rrhaphy**, stitching or suturing of the perineum

perine/o-**stomy**, formation of an opening into the perineum or the name of the opening so created (a perineal urethrostomy)

perine/o-**synthesis**, process of making a perineum, it refers to repair of a ruptured or lacerated perineum

perine/o-**tomy**, incision into the perineum

perine/o-**vagin**-al, pertaining to the vagina and perineum

perine/o-**vagin**/o-rect-al, pertaining to the rectum, vagina and perineum

perine/o-**vulv**-ar, pertaining to the vulva and perineum

perine-**um**, the perineum or perineal body

---

**Placent/o,** placenta
From a Latin word **plakoenta**, meaning a flat cake. Here placent/o means the placenta, the temporary, hormone-secreting vascular structure that facilitates the exchange of materials between the fetal and maternal blood. The placenta is expelled from the uterus along with the fetal membranes during

the third stage of labour as the after-birth.

**extra-placent**-al, pertaining to outside or independent of the placenta

**placent**-al, pertaining to or belonging to the placenta

**placent**-ation, process of forming the placenta

**placent**-itis, inflammation of the placenta

**placent/o**-graphy, a technique of making a recording or X-ray picture of the placenta

**placent**-oid, resembling the placenta

**placent**-oma, a tumour formed from or originating in the placenta

**placent/o**-pathy, disease of the placenta

trans-**placent**-al, pertaining to through or across the placenta

---

**Pub/i/o**, pubis, pubic region
From a Latin word **pubes** meaning private parts. Here, pubi/o means the pubic bone or *os pubis* forming the centre bone of the front of the pelvis. The right and left pubic bones meet in the median plane to form the pubic symphysis. Pub/o is also used to mean the pubic region covering the pubic bones.

**pub**es, the hairs covering the pubic bones, pubic hair

**pub**-ic, 1. pertaining to the pubic region 2. pertaining to pubes 3. pertaining to the os pubis

**pubi/o**-plasty, surgical repair or reconstruction of the pubic region

**pubi/o**-tomy, incision into the os pubis, to facilitate delivery

**pub/o**-coccyg-eal, pertaining to the coccyx and the os pubis

**pub/o**-femor-al, pertaining to the femur and os pubis

**pub/o**-prostat-ic, pertaining to the prostate gland and os pubis

**pub/o**-vesic-al, pertaining to the bladder and os pubis

---

**Pudend-**, pudendum, vulva
From a Latin word **pudens** meaning modest. Here pudend- means the

pudendum, the external genitalia especially of the female, comprising the mons pubis, labia majora and minora, the clitoris, the vaginal orifice, the vestibule, the hymen and the greater vestibular glands (Bartholin's glands).

**pudend**-agra, pain in the pudendum or vulva

**pudend**-al, pertaining to the pudendum or vulva

---

**Puerper-**, puerperium
From a Latin word **puerperus** meaning relating to childbirth. Here, puerper means the puerperium, the period of about 6–8 weeks following childbirth when the reproductive organs return to their normal condition (involution).

**puerper**-a, a woman who has just given birth to a child

**puerper**-al, pertaining to the puerperium

**puerper**-al-ism, condition of disease resulting from childbirth

**puerper**-ium, period immediately following childbirth when the reproductive organs return to normal (involution)

---

**Salping/o**, Fallopian tube, oviduct, uterine tube
From a Greek word **salpingos**, meaning trumpet tube. Here salping/o means the trumpet-shaped oviduct known as a Fallopian tube or uterine tube. The uterine tube collects eggs ovulated from the ovary and passes them to the uterus. While in the uterine tube eggs may be fertilized by sperm that have managed to traverse the cervix and uterus.

endo-**salping**-itis, inflammation within the uterine tube, it refers to inflammation of its mucous lining

endo-**salping**-oma, a tumour of the lining of a uterine tube, an adenomyoma

pachy-**salping**-itis, inflammation of a uterine tube with thickening

pachy-**salping/o**-ovar-itis, inflammation of an ovary and uterine tube with thickening of the uterine tube

**salping**-ectomy, removal of a uterine tube

**salping**-ian, pertaining to a uterine tube

**salping**-ic, pertaining to a uterine tube

**salping**-itic, pertaining to having salpingitis

**salping**-itis, inflammation of a uterine tube

**salping/o**-cele, a protrusion or hernia of a uterine tube

**salping/o**-cyesis, a pregnancy developing in a uterine tube, an ectopic pregnancy

**salping/o**-gram, a recording or X-ray picture of a uterine tube (made following injection of a dye)

**salping/o**-graphy, technique of making a recording or X-ray picture of a uterine tube (following injection of a dye)

**salping/o**-lith-iasis, abnormal condition of stones or calculi (calcareous deposits) in a uterine tube

**salping/o**-lysis, separation of a uterine tube, it refers to separation of adhesions within a uterine tube by surgery

**salping/o**-oophor-ectomy, removal of an ovary and its uterine tube

**salping/o**-oophor-itis, inflammation of an ovary and its uterine tube

**salping/o**-oophor/o-cele, a protrusion or hernia of an ovary and uterine tube

**salping/o**-ovari-ectomy, removal of an ovary and its uterine tube

**salping/o**-ovari/o-tomy, incision into an ovary and its uterine tube Syn. salpingo-oophorectomy

**salping/o**-ovar-itis, inflammation of an ovary and its uterine tube

**salping/o**-periton-itis, inflammation of the peritoneum associated with a uterine tube

**salping/o**-pexy, surgical fixation of a uterine tube

**salping/o**-plasty, surgical repair or reconstruction of a uterine tube

**salping/o**-rrhaphy, stitching or suturing of a uterine tube

**salping/o**-stomy, formation of an opening into a uterine tube or the name of the opening so created

**salping/o**-tomy, incision into a uterine tube

---

**Terat/o**, monster-like, monstrosity

From a Greek word **teras** meaning monster. Here, terat/o means a monster, a malformed embryo or fetus produced by defective growth processes in the early stages of development.

**terat**-ic, pertaining to a monster or monster-like

**terat**-ism, 1. condition of having formed a monster 2. the occurrence of a monster-like abnormality

**terat/o**-gen, an agent that forms monster-like defects (malformations) in an embryo or fetus

**terat/o**-genesis, formation of monster-like defects (malformations) in an embryo or fetus

**terat/o**-genet-ic, pertaining to teratogenesis

**terat/o**-gen-ic, 1. pertaining to the formation of monster-like defects (malformations) in the embryo or fetus 2. pertaining to the capability of an agent to form monster-like defects (malformations) in the embryo or fetus

**terat/o**-gen-ic-ity, quality or ability to form monster-like defects (malformations) in an embryo or fetus

**terat/o**-gen-ous, pertaining to forming a monster, it refers to forming a monster-like structure from elements of the embryo or fetus

**terat**-oid, resembling a monster

**terat/o**-log-ic, 1. pertaining to teratology 2. pertaining to study of monster-like malformations in an embryo or fetus

**terat/o**-log-ical, 1. pertaining to teratology 2. pertaining to study of monster-like malformations in an embryo or fetus

**terat/o**-log-ist, a specialist who studies teratology

**terat/o**-logy, the study of monsters, it refers to the study of monster-like malformations in an embryo or fetus

**terat**-oma, a monster-like tumour of embryonic origin composed of different tissues in the wrong positions. Teratomas are often malignant and are found most commonly in the ovaries and testes.

**terat**-osis, abnormal condition of a monster-like abnormality

---

**Thel/e/o**, nipple

From a Greek word **thele** meaning a nipple or teat. Here thel/e means nipple, a pigmented, conical projection on the areola of the breast into which the lactiferous ducts open. See the combining form mamill/o also meaning nipple

poly-**thel**-ia, condition of many nipples or supernumerary nipples

**thel**-alg-ia, condition of pain in a nipple

**thel**-arche, beginning of nipples, it refers to the development of the breasts at puberty

**thele**, a nipple

**thele**-ectomy, removal of a nipple

**thele**-plasty, surgical repair or reconstruction of a nipple

**thel**-erethism, condition of erection of a nipple. From a Greek word *erethisma* meaning a stirring

**thel**-itis, inflammation of a nipple

**thel**-ium, a nipple

**thel**-onc-us, a tumour or growth on a nipple

**thel**-rrhag-ia, condition of bursting forth of blood (haemorrhage) from a nipple

---

**Toc/o, toko**, childbirth, labour

From a Greek word **tokos**, meaning birth or labour. Here toc/o means labour or childbirth. There are three stages: 1. From onset, until full dilation of the cervical os 2. Full dilation until the baby is expelled 3. Expulsion of the placenta and fetal membranes, and control of bleeding.

brady-**toc**-ia, condition of slow birth or slow labour

dys-**toc**-ia, condition of difficult or painful birth

eu-**toc**-ia, condition of good (normal) birth

oxy-**toc**-in, an agent that produces a quick birth, it refers to a hormone secreted by the posterior pituitary gland (or synthetic preparation) that stimulates uterine contractions

**toc/o**-dyna-graph, 1. an instrument that records the force or power of labour (uterine contractions) 2. a recording obtained by a tocodynamometer

**toc/o**-dynam/o-meter, an instrument that measures the force or power of labour, it refers to measuring the force of uterine contractions Syn. tocometer

**toc/o**-erg/o-metry, technique of measuring the work of labour, it refers to measuring the force of uterine contractions

**toc/o**-graph, an instrument that records labour, *i.e.* the force and frequency of uterine contractions

**toc/o**-graphy, technique of recording labour, *i.e.* the force and frequency of uterine contractions

**toc/o**-logy, the study of labour or childbirth

**toc/o**-lyt-ic, an agent that relaxes uterine muscle

**toc/o**-meter, an instrument used to measure the force or power of labour, it refers to measuring the force of uterine contractions Syn. tocodynamometer

**toc/o**-phob-ia, condition of irrational fear of labour or childbirth

**toc**-us, childbirth

**tok/o**-dynam/o-meter, an instrument that measures the force or power of labour, it refers to measuring the force of uterine contractions Syn. tocometer, tocodynamometer

---

**Tub/o**, Fallopian tube, oviduct, tube, uterine tube

From a Latin word **tubus** meaning tube. Here tub/o means the Fallopian tube or uterine tube. The uterine tube collects eggs ovulated from the ovary and passes them to the uterus. While in the uterine tube eggs may be fertilized by sperm that have managed to traverse the cervix and uterus.

**tub/o**-abdomin-al, pertaining to the abdomen and uterine tube

**tub/o**-ligament-ous, pertaining to the broad ligament (of the uterus) and uterine tube

**tub/o**-ovari-an, pertaining to an ovary and its uterine tube

**tub/o**-ovari/o-tomy, incision into an ovary and uterine tube (for removal)

**tub/o**-ovar-itis, inflammation of an ovary and uterine tube Syn. salpingo-oophoritis

**tub/o**-peritone-al, pertaining to the peritoneum and uterine tube

**tub/o**-plasty, surgical repair or reconstruction of a uterine tube

**tub/o**-torsion, twisting of a uterine tube

**tub/o**-uter-ine, pertaining to or belonging to the uterus and uterine tubes

**tub/o**-vagin-al, pertaining to the vagina and uterine tubes

---

**Uter/o**, uterus

From a Latin word **uterus**, meaning womb. Here uter/o means the uterus, the hollow muscular organ into which the ovum is received from a Fallopian tube and where it is retained during development. The fetus is expelled from the uterus through the vagina during the second stage of labour.

retro-**uter**-ine, pertaining to behind the uterus

**uter**-alg-ia, condition of pain in the uterus

**uter**-ectomy, removal of the uterus

**uter**-ine, pertaining to the uterus

**uter**-itis, inflammation of the uterus

**uter/o**-abdomin-al, pertaining to the abdomen and uterus

**uter/o**-cele, a protrusion or hernia of the uterus

**uter/o**-cervic-al, pertaining to the cervix uteri and the uterus

**uter/o**-col-ic, pertaining to the colon and uterus, it refers to the colon adjacent to the uterus

**uter/o**-gestat-ion, process of development of a fetus in the uterus (a normal pregnancy). From a Greek word *gestare* meaning to bear

**uter/o**-graphy, technique of making a recording or X-ray picture of the uterus

**uter/o**-intestin-al, pertaining to the intestine and uterus

**uter/o**-lith, a stone or calculus in the uterus

**uter/o**-meter, an instrument used to measure the uterus (the depth of its cavity) Syn. hysterometer

**uter/o**-metry, technique of measuring the uterus (its size)

**uter/o**-ovari-an, pertaining to or characteristic of the ovaries and uterus

**uter/o**-pariet-al, pertaining to the walls of the abdomen and uterus. From a Greek word *paries* meaning wall

**uter/o**-pelv-ic, pertaining to the pelvis and uterus

**uter/o**-pex-ia, condition of surgical fixation of the uterus (into the abdominal wall or vaginal peritoneum)

**uter/o**-pexy, surgical fixation of the uterus (into the abdominal wall or vaginal peritoneum)

**uter/o**-placent-al, pertaining to the placenta and uterus

**uter/o**-plasty, surgical repair or reconstruction of the uterus

**uter/o**-rect-al, pertaining to the rectum and uterus

**uter/o**-sacr-al, pertaining to or belonging to the sacrum and uterus

**uter/o**-salping/o-graphy, technique of making a recording or X-ray picture of the uterine tubes and uterus

**uter/o**-scler-osis, abnormal condition of hardening of the uterus

**uter/o**-scope, an instrument used to view or examine the uterus

**uter/o**-tome, an instrument used to cut the uterus

**uter/o**-tomy, incision of the uterus

**uter/o**-ton-ic, 1. pertaining to (an increased) tone of the (smooth muscle) of the uterus 2. an agent that restores tone to the uterus

**uter/o**-tractor, an instrument used to grasp and pull the uterus (during surgical removal of the uterus)

**uter/o**-tub-al, pertaining to the uterine tubes and uterus

**uter/o**-tub/o-graphy, technique of making a recording or X-ray picture of the uterine tubes and uterus Syn. utero-salpingography

**uter/o**-vagin-al, pertaining to the vagina and uterus

**uter/o**-ventr-al, pertaining to the abdomen and uterus

**uter/o**-vesic-al, pertaining to the bladder and uterus

---

**Vagin/o**, vagina

From a Latin word **vagina**, meaning sheath. Here vagin/o means the vagina, the musculo-membranous passage extending from the cervix uteri to the vulva. The vagina acts as the receptacle for the penis during coitus, and provides an elastic passageway through which the baby passes during childbirth.

pachy-**vagin**-itis, inflammation of the vagina with thickening of its walls

para-**vagin**-itis, inflammation of tissue beside the vagina

supra-**vagin**-al, pertaining to above the vagina

**vagin**-al, pertaining to the vagina

**vagin**-ectomy, removal of the vagina

**vagin**-ismus, spasm of the vagina, it refers to a sudden contraction of muscles of the vagina

**vagin**-itis, inflammation of the vagina

**vagin/o**-abdomin-al, pertaining to the abdomen and vagina

**vagin/o**-cele, a protrusion or hernia of the vagina

**vagin/o**-dyn-ia, condition of pain in the vagina

**vagin/o**-fixation, surgical fixation of the vagina e.g. to the wall of the abdomen

**vagin/o**-gen-ic, 1. pertaining to forming the vagina 2. pertaining to originating in the vagina

**vagin/o**-labi-al, pertaining to the labia and vagina

**vagin/o**-myc-osis, abnormal condition of fungi in the vagina

**vagin/o**-pathy, disease of the vagina

**vagin/o**-perine-al, pertaining to the perineum and vagina

**vagin/o**-perine/o-rrhaphy, stitching or suturing of the perineum and vagina

**vagin/o**-perine/o-tomy, incision into the perineum and vagina

**vagin/o**-peritone-al, pertaining to the peritoneum and vagina

**vagin/o**-pexy, surgical fixation of the vagina e.g. to the wall of the abdomen Syn. vaginofixation

**vagin/o**-plasty, surgical repair or reconstruction of the vagina

**vagin/o**-scope, an instrument used to view or examine the vagina

**vagin/o**-scopy, technique of viewing or examining the vagina

**vagin/o**-osis, abnormal condition of the vagina (bacterial infection)

**vagin/o**-tome, an instrument used to cut the vagina

**vagin/o**-tomy, incision into the vagina

**vagin/o**-vesic-al, pertaining to the bladder and vagina

**vagin/o**-vulv-ar, pertaining to the vulva and vagina

---

**Vulv/o**, vulva

From a Latin word **vulva**, meaning womb. Here vulv/o means the vulva, pudendum femina or external genitalia The vulva comprises the mons pubis, labia majora and minora, the clitoris, the vaginal orifice, the vestibule, the hymen and the greater vestibular glands (Bartholin's glands).

**vulv**-al, pertaining to the vulva

**vulv**-ar, pertaining to the vulva

**vulv**-ectomy, removal of the vulva

**vulv**-ismus, spasm of the vulva

**vulv**-itis, inflammation of the vulva

**vulv/o**-crur-al, pertaining to the crura (of the clitoris) and vulva. From a Latin word *crus* meaning a leg or leg-like part

**vulv/o**-pathy, disease of the vulva

**vulv/o**-uter-ine, pertaining to the uterus and vulva

**vulv/o**-vagin-al, pertaining to the vagina and vulva

**vulv/o**-vagin-itis, inflammation of the vagina and vulva

**vulv/o**-vagin/o-plasty, surgical repair or reconstruction of the vagina and vulva

**Zygot-**, a fertilized egg, a zygote
From a Greek word **zygon** meaning yolk. Here zygot- means a zygote, a fertilized egg.

di-**zygot**-ic, pertaining to (formed from) two zygotes or two fertilized eggs

mono-**zygot**-ic, pertaining to (formed from) a single zygote or a single fertilized egg, as in identical twins

pre-**zygot**-ic, pertaining to before the zygote forms or before fertilization is complete

**zygot**-ic, pertaining to a zygote or fertilized egg

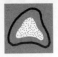

# Section 17
# The endocrine system

The endocrine system consists of:

- one pituitary gland
- two ovaries in the female
- one thyroid gland
- two testes in the male
- four parathyroid glands
- one pineal gland
- two adrenal (suprarenal) glands
- one thymus gland
- the Islets of Langerhan's in the pancreas.

The endocrine system is a diverse group of glands that secrete hormones directly into the bloodstream. Once released, a hormone circulates in the blood to all tissues and organs but only certain parts, called target tissues or target organs, respond. Each hormone exerts a specific regulatory effect on the activity of its target tissue and by doing so controls the metabolism, growth or development of cells.

The maintenance of a constant internal environment of the body (homeostasis), is regulated partly by the autonomic nervous system and partly by the endocrine system. The autonomic nervous system is concerned with rapid responses while the endocrine hormones are mainly involved in slower responses.

The concentration of hormones in the blood is precisely regulated: too much or too little of a hormone disrupts homeostasis. Normal control is achieved mainly by the brain and endocrine glands operating negative feedback mechanisms that prevent too much or too little hormone accumulating in the blood stream. Endocrine disorders brought about by changes in the output of hormones produce symptoms that range from minor to severely disabling. If untreated, some endocrine disorders may result in loss of homeostatic control and death.

Figure 26 shows combining forms of roots associated with the endocrine system.

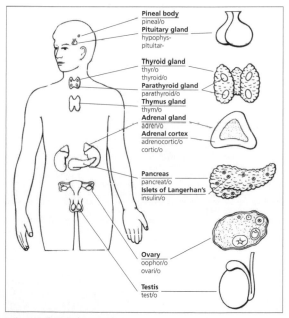

**Pineal body**
pineal/o
**Pituitary gland**
hypophys-
pituitar-

**Thyroid gland**
thyr/o
thyroid/o
**Parathyroid gland**
parathyroid/o
**Thymus gland**
thym/o
**Adrenal gland**
adren/o
**Adrenal cortex**
adrenocortic/o
cortic/o

**Pancreas**
pancreat/o
**Islets of Langerhan's**
insulin/o

**Ovary**
oophor/o
ovari/o

**Testis**
test/o

Figure 26  The endocrine system

## Roots and combining forms, meanings

**Adrenal-, adren/o**, adrenal gland
From the Latin words **ad** meaning near and **renes** meaning kidneys. Here adren/o means the adrenal gland, a small triangle-shaped gland that lies above each kidney. The inner part of the gland, called the medulla, secretes adrenalin and the outer part called the cortex, secretes steroid hormones.

**adren**-al, 1. the adrenal gland 2. pertaining to the adrenal gland

**adrenal**-ectom-ize, action of removing the adrenal glands

**adrenal**-ectomy, removal of an adrenal gland

**adrenal**-ine, a chemical (hormone) produced by the adrenal gland Syn. epinephrine

**adrenal**-in-ur-ia, condition of adrenaline (epinephrine) in the urine

**adrenal**-ism, condition of the adrenal, it refers to ill health caused by dysfunction of the adrenal glands

**adrenal**-itis, inflammation of the adrenal glands

**adren**-erg-ic, 1. pertaining to being stimulated by adrenaline. From a Greek word *ergon* meaning work 2. pertaining to nerve fibres that liberate adrenaline (epinephrine) or noradrenaline (norepinephrine) at a synapse when an impulse occurs. Most sympathetic nerves release noradrenaline

**adren**-itis, inflammation of the adrenal glands Syn. adrenalitis

**adren/o**-ceptor, a molecular site on an effector structure innervated by a sympathetic nerve fibre. There are two main types, alpha receptors that respond to noradrenalin (norepinephrine), and beta receptors that respond to adrenaline (epinephrine)

**adren/o**-genit-al, pertaining to the genitalia (reproductive organs) and adrenal glands

**adren/o**-gram, a recording or X-ray picture of the adrenal glands

**adren/o**-graphy, technique of making a recording or X-ray picture of the adrenal glands

**adren/o**-leuco-dys-trophy, poor nourishment of the adrenal glands (adrenal atrophy) with abnormal white matter in the cerebrum, it refers to a recessive inherited disorder linked to the X chromosome in males

**adren/o**-lyt-ic, 1. pertaining to breaking down (inhibiting) the action of adrenergic nerve fibres 2. pertaining to breaking down (inhibiting) the reaction to adrenaline (epinephrine)

**adren/o**-medull/o-blast-oma, a tumour of immature cells originating in the medulla (inner layer) of the adrenal gland

**adren/o**-megaly, enlargement of the adrenal gland

**adren/o**-mimet-ic, an agent that mimics or has action similar to adrenaline (epinephrine)

**adren/o**-pathy, disease of the adrenal glands

**adren/o**-receptor, a molecular site on an effector structure innervated by a sympathetic nerve fibre. There are two main types, alpha receptors respond to noradrenalin (norepinephrine), and beta receptors that respond to adrenaline (epinephrine)

**adren/o**-stat-ic, pertaining to stopping or inhibiting the adrenal gland (its activity)

**adren/o**-tox-in, an agent poisonous to the adrenal glands

**adren/o**-troph-ic, pertaining to nourishing or stimulating the adrenal glands

hyper-**adrenal**-ism, condition of above normal secretion of the adrenal gland

---

**Adrenocortic/o**, adrenal cortex
From the Latin words **ad** meaning near, **renes** meaning kidneys and **cortic/o** meaning bark or outer part. Here adrenocortic/o means the adrenal cortex, the outer layer of the adrenal gland that secretes steroid hormones.

See the combining form cortic/o also meaning adrenal cortex.

**adrenocortic**-al, pertaining to the adrenal cortex

**adrenocortic/o**-hyper-plas-ia, condition of above normal growth of cells of the adrenal cortex

**adrenocortic/o**-mimet-ic, an agent that mimics or has action similar to hormones of the adrenal cortex

**adrenocortic/o**-troph-ic, pertaining to nourishing or stimulating the adrenal cortex

**adrenocortic/o**-troph-in, an agent (hormone) secreted by the anterior pituitary gland that nourishes or stimulates the adrenal cortex Syn. corticotropin

**adrenocortic/o**-trop-in, an agent (hormone) secreted by the anterior pituitary gland that nourishes or stimulates the adrenal cortex Syn. corticotropin

hyper-**adrenocortic**-ism, condition of above normal secretion of the adrenal cortex

---

**Aldosteron-**, aldosterone

A chemical name. Aldosterone is an adrenocortical steroid hormone that acts on the distal renal tubules to regulate electrolyte metabolism; because of this action it is called a mineralocorticoid. Aldosterone increases the excretion of potassium and conserves sodium and chloride ions.

**aldosteron**-ism, condition due to above normal secretion of aldosterone

**aldosteron**-ur-ia, condition of excess aldosterone in the urine

hyper-**aldosteron**-ism, condition due to above normal secretion of aldosterone

hypo-**aldosteron**-ism, condition due to below normal secretion of aldosterone

pseudo-hypo-**aldosteron**-ism, a false hypo-aldosteronism, a congenital condition due to lack of a response of the distal renal tubules to aldosterone

---

**Andr/o**, male, masculine

From a Greek word **aner** meaning man. Here andr/o means male or masculine.

**andr/o**-blast-oma, 1. a (benign) tumour of immature male cells, it refers to a virilizing ovarian tumour in women that contains cells that mimic those of the testis by secreting testosterone 2. an arrhenoblastoma 3. a rare (benign) tumour of immature cells or embryonic cells of the testis seen in males

**andr/o**-gen, an agent that produces male or masculine characteristics *e.g.* testosterone

**andr/o**-gen-ic, pertaining to producing male or masculine characteristics

**andr/o**-gen-ous, pertaining to producing male or masculine characteristics

**andr/o**-gloss-ia, condition of having a male tongue (masculine sound to a woman's voice)

**andr/o**-gyne, male with secondary sexual organs like a woman (male pseudo-hermaphrodite)

**andr/o**-gyn-ism, female with male characteristics (female hermaphrodite)

**andr/o**-gyn-oid, a male resembling a female (male hermaphrodite)

**andr/o**-gyn-ous, pertaining to male and female (of doubtful sex, hermaphroditic)

**andr**-oid, resembling a male

**andr/o**-logy, the study of the male (particularly the anatomy, diseases of and treatment of the male reproductive system)

**andr/o**-pathy, disease of the male, it refers to any disease found only in a male

**andr/o**-phob-ia, condition of irrational fear or dislike of men

**andr/o**-sterone, a steroid hormone that produces male or masculine characteristics (a breakdown product of testosterone found in urine)

**Corti/c/o**, adrenal cortex

Form a Latin word **cortex** meaning bark or outer layer. Here, cortic/o means the adrenal cortex, the outer layer of the adrenal gland. The cortex is composed of three layers of cells, the zona glomerulosa on the outside, followed by the zona fasciculata and the zona reticularis on the inside. The cortex secretes a variety of steroid hormones, grouped into three main types: androgens (male sex hormones), glucocorticoids (controlling metabolism of glucose, fats and protein) and mineralocorticoids (regulating fluid and electrolytes).

See the combining form adrenocortic/o also meaning adrenal cortex.

**cortic**-oid, 1. resembling (an action) similar to that of a hormone of the adrenal cortex 2. a steroid hormone of the adrenal cortex

**cortic/o**-steroid, a steroid produced by the adrenal cortex

**cortic/o**-sterone, a mineralocorticoid produced by the adrenal cortex with some glucocorticoid activity

**cortic/o**-troph-ic, 1. pertaining to nourishing or stimulating the adrenal cortex 2. any agent (hormone) that nourishes or stimulates the adrenal cortex

**cortic/o**-troph-in, an agent (hormone) secreted by the anterior pituitary gland that nourishes or stimulates the adrenal cortex Syn. corticotropin

**cortic/o**-trop-in, an agent (hormone) secreted by the anterior pituitary gland that nourishes or stimulates the adrenal cortex Syn. corticotrophin

**corti**-sol, a glucocorticoid (hydrocortisone) produced by the adrenal cortex

**corti**-sone, a glucocorticoid from the adrenal cortex with some mineralocorticoid actions (inactive in man until converted to cortisol). Synthetically prepared cortisones are used as anti-inflammatory agents and for replacement of adrenocortical hormones

**Gluc/o**, glucose, sugar

From a Greek word **glykys** meaning sweet. Here, gluc/o means glucose, the physiologically-active, six-carbon, hexose sugar that circulates in the blood.

**gluc**-agon, a hormone secreted by cells of the Islets of Langerhan's, it acts to raise blood glucose concentration

**gluc**-agon-oma, a tumour of the cells that produce the pancreatic hormone glucagon that raises blood glucose

**gluc/o**-cortic-oid, a steroid hormone produced by the adrenal cortex that regulates carbohydrate metabolism

**gluc/o**-genesis, the formation or synthesis of glucose

**gluc/o**-gen-ic, pertaining to forming glucose

**gluc/o**-meter, an instrument used to measure glucose, used for home blood glucose monitoring HBGM

**gluc/o**-neo-genesis, the formation of new glucose from non-carbohydrate sources

**gluc/o**-regulat-ion, the action of regulating or controlling glucose metabolism

**glucos**-ur-ia, condition of glucose in the urine Syn. glycosuria

**Glyc/o**, glucose, sugar

From a Greek word **glykys** meaning sweet. Here, glyc/o means glucose, the physiologically-active, six-carbon, hexose sugar that circulates in the blood.

**glyc**-aem-ia, condition of glucose in the blood

**glyc/o**-genesis, the formation of glycogen from glucose

**glyc/o**-lysis, breakdown of glucose, it refers to a series of reactions in which glucose is broken down to pyruvate or lactate

**glyc/o**-lyt-ic, 1. pertaining to glycolysis 2. pertaining to breakdown of glucose, it refers to a series of reactions in which glucose is broken down to pyruvate or lactate

**glyc/o**-neo-genesis, the formation of new sugar, from non-carbohydrates

**glyc/o**-pen-ia, condition of a deficiency of sugar

**glyc/o**-phil-ia, condition of loving sugar, it refers to a condition in which a small intake of glucose results in hyperglycaemia

**glyc/o**-rrhoea, excessive flow or discharge of sugar *e.g.* glycosuria

**glyc/o**-stat-ic, pertaining to a constant glucose level (a controlled level)

**glyc/o**-trop-ic, 1. pertaining to having affinity for glucose 2. pertaining to stimulating glucose, it refers to any action causing hyperglycaemia

**glyc/o**-ur-esis, abnormal condition of glucose in the urine

**glycos**-ur-ia, condition of glucose in the urine

hyper-**glyc**-aem-ia, condition of above normal levels of glucose in the blood

hypo-**glyc**-aem-ia, condition of below normal levels of glucose in the blood

**Glycogen/o**, glycogen
From the Greek words **glykys** meaning sweet and **genein** meaning to produce. Here glycogen/o means glycogen, a storage polysaccharide composed of many glucose units. Glycogen is formed in the liver and muscle cells and is stored as granules; it can be broken down to glucose and released into the blood when required.

**glycogen**-ase, an enzyme necessary for the breakdown of glycogen into glucose

**glycogen**-e-tic, pertaining to glycogenesis

**glycogen/o**-lysis, breakdown of glycogen yielding glucose

**glycogen/o**-lyt-ic, 1. pertaining to glycogenolysis 2. pertaining to the breakdown of glycogen

**glycogen**-osis, abnormal condition of glycogen, it refers to glycogen storage disease

**Hypophys-, hypophyse/o, hypophysis**, pituitary gland
From the Greek words **hypo**- meaning below and **-physis** meaning growth. Here, hypophys- means the pituitary gland or hypophysis cerebri, a growth below the brain. The pituitary gland consists of an anterior glandular section called the adenohypophysis and a posterior neural part called the neurohypophysis.
See the root **pituitar**- also meaning pituitary gland.

**hypophys**-eal, pertaining to or belonging to the hypophysis

**hypophys**-ectom-ize, action of removing the hypophysis

**hypophys**-ectomy, removal of the hypophysis

**hypophyse/o**-port-al, pertaining to the portal system of the hypophysis

**hypophyse/o**-priv-ic, pertaining to loss of function of the hypophysis (deficient secretion)

**hypophysis**, the growth below (the brain), *i.e.* the pituitary gland

**hypophys**-itis, inflammation of the hypophysis

pre-**hypophysis**, front hypophysis, it refers to the anterior lobe of the pituitary gland

**Insul-, Insulin/o**, insulin, Islets of Langerhan's
From a Latin word **insula** meaning island. Here, insulin/o means the Islets of Langerhan's, small patches of endocrine tissue in the pancreas. The ß-cells of the islets secrete the hormone insulin directly into the blood so insulin/o is also used to mean insulin.

hyper-**insulin**-ism, process of secreting above normal levels of insulin

hypo-**insulin**-ism, process of secreting below normal levels of insulin

**insul**-ar, pertaining to the Islets of Langerhan's

**insulin**-aem-ia, condition of (excess) insulin in the blood

**insulin**-itis, inflammation of the Islets of Langerhan's

**insulin**-lip/o-dys-trophy, poor nourishment with loss of fat due to treatment with insulin

**insulin/o**-genesis, the formation of insulin (from the Islets of Langerhan's)

**insulin/o**-gen-ic, pertaining to originating in the Islets of Langerhan's

**insulin**-oma, a tumour of the Islets of Langerhan's

**insul**-itis, inflammation of the Islets of Langerhan's

insul/o-path-ic, pertaining to disease caused by abnormality of secretion of the Islets of Langerhan's

**insul/o**-pen-ic, pertaining to reduction in insulin (in the circulation)

pro-**insulin**, before insulin, it refers to a precursor of insulin

---

**Ket/o, keton-**, ketone, ketone bodies

From a German word **keton**. Here, ket/o means a ketone, an organic chemical containing a carbonyl (keto) group. Small quantities of ketones form from normal fatty acid metabolism. Abnormally high concentrations of ketones or ketone bodies appear in uncontrolled diabetes mellitus.

**ket/o**-acid-osis, condition of acidosis (low pH of body fluids) caused by an accumulation of ketone bodies

**ket/o**-acid-ur-ia, condition of keto-acids in the urine

**ket/o**-genesis, the formation of ketone bodies

**ket/o**-genet-ic, 1. pertaining to ketogenesis 2. pertaining to the formation of ketone bodies

**ket/o**-gen-ic, pertaining to the formation of ketone bodies

**ket/o**-lysis, the breakdown or splitting of ketone bodies

**ket/o**-lyt-ic, pertaining to the breakdown or splitting of ketone bodies

**keton**-aem-ia, condition of ketone bodies (acetone) in the blood

**keton**-aem-ic, pertaining to ketone bodies (acetone) in the blood

**keton**-ic, pertaining to or belonging to ketones or ketone bodies

**keton**-ization, process or action of forming into ketones or ketone bodies

**keton**-ur-ia, condition of ketone bodies in the urine

**ket**-ose, a sugar containing a keto (carbonyl) group

**ket**-osis, abnormal condition of ketone bodies (excessive amounts in tissues)

**ket/o**-steroid, a steroid containing ketone (carbonyl) groups

---

**Oestr/a/o**, oestrogen

From a Greek word **oistros** meaning mad desire. Here oestr/o means oestrus or oestrogen. Oestrus is a period of intense sexual excitement in female mammals other than humans associated with fluctuations in levels of sex-hormones. In humans the sex-hormone oestrogen regulates the growth of the female reproductive system, the menstrual cycle and the development of secondary sexual characteristics.

**oestr/a**-diol, a potent human oestrogen

**oestr**-in-iz-ation, action or process of producing changes in the vagina that are characteristic of oestrus

**oestr**-iol, a weak human oestrogen, a metabolite of oestradiol found in urine

**oestr/o**-gen, a hormone that stimulates oestrus, in humans oestrogens regulate the growth of the female reproductive system, the menstrual cycle and the development of secondary sexual characteristics e.g. oestradiol

**oestr/o**-gen-ic, 1. having an action similar to oestrogen 2. pertaining to forming oestrus

**oestr/o**-gen-ous, 1. having an action similar to oestrogen 2. pertaining to forming oestrus

**oestr**-one, an oestrogen found in human urine and the placenta during pregnancy, similar to oestradiol

**oestr**-ous, pertaining to oestrus

**oestr**-us, a period of intense sexual excitement in female mammals other than humans pro-**oestr/o**-gen, before oestrogen, it refers to a precursor of oestrogen

## Oophor/o, ovary

From a Greek word **oophoron**, meaning ovary. Here oophor/o means the ovary, the female reproductive organ or gonad that produces eggs. This organ is also a main source of the female sex-hormones oestrogen and progesterone. These steroid hormones control development of the female reproductive system and the formation of secondary sexual characteristics.

## Ovari/o, ovary

From a New Latin word **ovarium**, meaning ovary, derived from **ova**, meaning egg. Here ovari/o means the ovary, the egg-bearing gland.

Words associated with the anatomy and pathology of the ovaries are listed in Section 16 The female reproductive system.

## Pancre/a/t/o, pancreas

From the Greek word **pankreas**, **pan** meaning all and **kreas** meaning flesh. Here pancreat/o means the pancreas, a large gland situated below and behind the stomach approximately 18 cm long. The exocrine part of the gland secretes pancreatic juice that plays a major role in the digestion of fats, proteins and carbohydrates. The pancreas also contains the Islets of Langerhan's, patches of endocrine tissue that secrete the hormones insulin and glugagon.

**pancreat**-ectomy, removal of the pancreas

**pancreat**-ic, pertaining to or belonging to the pancreas

**pancreat**-in, mixture of enzymes from the pancreas

**pancreat**-itis, inflammation of the pancreas

**pancreat/o**-duoden-ectomy, removal of the duodenum and (head of) the pancreas

**pancreat/o**-gen-ous, pertaining to forming or arising in the pancreas

**pancreat/o**-graphy, technique of making a recording or X-ray picture of the pancreas

**pancreat/o**-lith-ectomy, removal of a stone from the pancreas

**pancreat/o**-lith-iasis, presence of stones or calculi in the pancreas, they may be in the duct system or parenchyma of the pancreas

**pancreat/o**-lith/o-tomy, incision into the pancreas to remove a stone

**pancreat/o**-lysis, breakdown or disintegration of the pancreas

**pancreat/o**-lyt-ic, pertaining to the breakdown or disintegration of the pancreas

**pancreat/o**-megaly, enlargement of the pancreas

**pancreat/o**-tomy, incision into the pancreas

**pancreat/o**-trop-ic, pertaining to having an affinity for the pancreas

**pancrea**-troph-ic, pertaining to nourishing or having an influence on the pancreas

**pancreo**-priv-ic, pertaining to lacking a pancreas

**pancreo**-zym-in, hormone secreted by the duodenum that stimulates the flow of pancreatic juice Syn. cholecystokinin

## Parathyr/o, parathyroid/o, parathyroid gland

From a Greek word **thyreoidos**, meaning the thyroid gland and **para**-meaning beside. Here parathyroid/o means the parathyroid glands that lie beside the thyroid. There are four parathyroid glands lying near the posterior surface of the thyroid gland. The parathyroids secrete parathyroid hormone (PTH) that regulates serum calcium levels.

hyper-**parathyroid**-ism, process of secreting above normal levels of parathyroid hormone

hypo-**parathyroid**-ism, process of secreting below normal levels of parathyroid hormone

**parathyroid**-al, pertaining to or belonging to a parathyroid gland

**parathyroid**-ectom-ize, action of removing the parathyroid glands

**parathyroid**-ectomy, removal of the parathyroid glands

**parathyroid**-oma, a tumour derived from a parathyroid gland

**parathyr/o**-pathy, disease of the parathyroid glands

**parathyr/o**-troph-ic, pertaining to nourishing or stimulating the growth of the parathyroid glands

**parathyr/o**-trop-ic, pertaining to having an affinity for or stimulating the parathyroid glands

---

**Pineal/o**, **pine/o**, pineal gland, pineal body

From a Latin word **pineus** meaning a pine cone. Here pineal/o refers to the pineal body or pineal gland, a small reddish-grey conical structure on the dorsal surface of the mid-brain. The pineal body secretes a hormone melatonin that coordinates circadian and diurnal rhythms such as sleep and inhibits the secretion of luteinizing hormone. The secretion of melatonin is linked to the amount of light entering the eye.

**pine**-al, 1. pertaining to the pineal body 2. pertaining to resembling the shape of a pine cone

**pineal**-ectomy, removal of the pineal body

**pineal**-ism, condition due to abnormal secretion of the pineal body

**pineal/o**-blast-oma, an invasive tumour of immature cells or embryonic cells of the pineal body

**pineal/o**-cyte, a cell of the pineal body

**pineal**-oma, a tumour of the pineal body composed of large epithelial cells

**pineal/o**-pathy, disease of the pineal body

**pine/o**-cyt-oma, a tumour of mature pineal cells

---

**Pitui-**, **pituitar-**, pituitary gland

From a Latin word **pituita**, meaning slime or phlegm. Here, pituitar- means

the pituitary gland, a small gland that grows from the base of the brain on a stalk. The pituitary gland is commonly called the 'master' gland of the endocrine system because it releases tropic hormones that regulate other endocrine glands. The pituitary is also called the hypophysis cerebri, it consists of an anterior glandular section called the adenohypophysis and a posterior neural part called the neurohypophysis.

See the combining form hypophyse/o also meaning the pituitary gland.

hyper-**pituitar**-ism, process of secreting above normal levels of a pituitary hormone

hypo-**pituitar**-ism, process of secreting below normal levels of a pituitary hormone

pan-hypo-**pituitar**-ism, process of secreting below normal levels of all pituitary hormones, due to absence of a pituitary gland or a damaged pituitary gland

**pitui**-cyte, a cell of the pituitary gland, found in the neurohypophysis

**pituitar**-ism, a condition of dysfunction of the pituitary gland

---

**Proge/st/er/o**, progesterone

From the Greek word **pro-** meaning before and Latin **-gestare** meaning to carry used together they mean before pregnancy. Here, progester/o means progesterone, an ovarian hormone secreted by the corpus luteum following ovulation. Progesterone prepares the endometrium to receive a fertilized egg and bring about implantation.

**progest**-ation-al, 1. pertaining to having an action like progesterone 2. pertaining to the phase of the menstrual cycle when the corpus luteum is secreting progesterone before the onset of menstruation

**proge**-sterone, the main steroid hormone produced by the corpus luteum in the ovary (also produced in the placenta and adrenal gland), it prepares the endometrium to receive a fertilized egg and bring about implantation

**progest**-in, a crude extract of the corpus luteum containing progesterone

**progest/o**-gen, an agent that produces progesterone-like actions

---

**Test/o**, testicle, testis

From a Latin word **testiculus** meaning testicle, or testis. Here, test/o means the testicle or testis. These male reproductive organs are present in pairs, and their function is to produce spermatozoa and the male sex-hormones called androgens. Androgens stimulate the formation of the male sexual characteristics.

Note: words associated with the anatomy and pathology of the testes can be found in Section 15 The male reproductive system.

**test/o**-sterone, a steroid hormone produced by the testis (the principal androgenic hormone)

---

**Thym/o**, thymus gland

From a Greek word **thymos**, meaning soul or emotion. Here thym/o means the thymus gland, a structure that lies behind the breast above the aorta and extends upward as far as the thymus gland. The thymus controls the development of the immune system in early life reaching its greatest size towards puberty.

The maturation of the thymus and T-lymphocytes is stimulated by thymosin, an endocrine hormone secreted by the epithelial cells that form the framework of the thymus gland.

Note: words associated with the anatomy and pathology of the thymus can be found in Section 6 The lymphatic system and immunology.

**thym**-in, an agent (hormone) produced by the thymus gland that stimulates differentiation of precursor lymphocytes into thymocytes Syn. thymopoietin

**thym/o**-poiet-in, an agent (hormone) that forms the thymus, it refers to a ladle

hormone that stimulates differentiation of precursor lymphocytes into thymocytes

**thymos**-in, an agent (hormone) secreted by the thymus gland that promotes the maturation of T-cells

---

**Thyr/o**, thyroid gland

From a Greek word **thyreoidos**, meaning resembling a shield. Thyr/o means the shield-shaped thyroid gland that lies above the trachea. The thyroid gland secretes the hormones tri-iodothyronine, $T_3$ and thyroxine, $T_4$, that control the metabolic rate of all cells.

anti-**thyroid**, 1. acting against the thyroid 2. an agent that acts against the thyroid, particularly against the synthesis of thyroid hormones

hyper-**thyroid**-ism, process of secreting above normal levels of thyroid hormone

hypo-**thyroid**-ism, process of secreting below normal levels of thyroid hormone

para-**thyroid**, beside or near the thyroid, it refers to the parathyroid glands near the posterior surface of the thyroid

peri-**thyroid**-itis, inflammation around the thyroid gland, it refers to inflammation of the thyroid capsule

**thyr/o**-aden-itis, inflammation of the thyroid gland

**thyr/o**-a-plas-ia, condition of lack of development of the thyroid gland (cells) with resulting deficient secretion

**thyr/o**-arytenoid, pertaining to the arytenoid cartilage (the jug-shaped laryngeal cartilage) and the thyroid gland. From a Greek word *arytainoeides* meaning shaped like a ladle

**thyr/o**-calciton-in, a hormone produced by the thyroid gland that regulates calcium metabolism, it reduces serum calcium and phosphate levels by its action on the kidneys and bone Syn. calcitonin

**thyr/o**-cardi-ac, pertaining to the heart and thyroid gland

**thyr/o**-card-itis, inflammation of the heart due to the thyroid (hyperthyroidism)

**thyr/o**-cele, a swelling or protrusion of the thyroid gland (a tumour)

**thyr/o**-chondr/o-tomy, incision into the cartilage of the thyroid gland

**thyr/o**-cric/o-tomy, incision into the cricothyroid membrane (of the larynx)

**thyr/o**-epiglott-ic, pertaining to the epiglottis and thyroid gland

**thyr/o**-gen-ic, 1. pertaining to originating in the thyroid gland 2. pertaining to derived from thyroid gland

**thyr/o**-gen-ous, 1. pertaining to originating in the thyroid gland 2. pertaining to derived from thyroid gland

**thyr/o**-globul-in, a thyroid protein stored in thyroid follicles from which thyroxine and triiodothyronine form

**thyr/o**-gloss-al, pertaining to the tongue and thyroid gland

**thyr/o**-hy-al, pertaining to or belonging to the hyoid bone (of the larynx) and thyroid gland

**thyr/o**-hyoid, pertaining to or belonging to the hyoid bone (of the larynx) and thyroid gland or thyroid cartilage

**thyroid**-ectom-ize, action of removing the thyroid gland

**thyroid**-ectomy, removal of the thyroid gland

**thyroid**-itis, inflammation of the thyroid gland

**thyroid/o**-tomy, incision into the thyroid gland

**thyr/o**-laryng-eal, pertaining to the larynx and thyroid gland

**thyr/o**-lingu-al, pertaining to the tongue and thyroid gland

**thyr/o**-megaly, enlargement of the thyroid gland Syn. goitre

**thyr/o**-mimet-ic, an agent that mimics or has action similar to thyroid hormones

**thyr/o**-parathyroid-ectomy, removal of the parathyroid glands and thyroid

**thyr/o**-priv-al, 1. pertaining to loss of function of the thyroid gland 2. pertaining to effect or symptoms resulting from loss of thyroid function

**thyr/o**-priv-ic, 1. pertaining to loss of function of the thyroid gland 2. pertaining to the effect or symptoms resulting from loss of thyroid function

**thyr/o**-ptosis, falling or downward displacement of the thyroid gland

**thyr/o**-therapy, treatment using preparations of the thyroid gland

**thyr/o**-tome, an instrument used to cut the thyroid gland

**thyr/o**-tomy, incision of the thyroid gland or thyroid cartilage

**thyr/o**-tox-ic, 1. pertaining to poisoning by the thyroid gland (due to excessive secretion of thyroid hormones 2. pertaining to having thyrotoxicosis

**thyr/o**-toxic-osis, condition of poisoning by the thyroid, due to overstimulation of the thyroid gland and excessive secretion of thyroid hormones $T_3$ and $T_4$ Syn. Graves' disease, hyperthyroidism

**thyr/o**-troph-ic, pertaining to nourishing or stimulating the thyroid gland

**thyr/o**-troph-in, an agent (hormone produced by the anterior pituitary gland) that stimulates the thyroid gland Syn. thyrotropin

**thyr/o**-trop-ic, pertaining to affinity for or stimulating the thyroid gland

**thyr/o**-trop-in, an agent (hormone produced by the anterior pituitary gland) that stimulates the thyroid gland

# Section 18
# Radiology and nuclear medicine

Radiology is the study of the diagnosis of disease by the use of radiant energy (radiation). In the past this meant the use of X-rays to make an image of the internal components of the body. Today many other forms of radiation are used to aid both diagnosis and treatment of disease. Developments in physics and technology are bringing rapid changes to this branch of medicine.

---

**Roots and combining forms,** meanings

**Cinemat/o, cine/o,** motion, movement
From a Greek word **kinein,** meaning movement. Here cinemat/o means a motion picture on film, video or other recording device.

**cine-**angi/o-cardi/o-graphy, technique of making a moving X-ray recording or film of the heart and (blood) vessels (the pictures are made from fluoro-scopic images)

**cine-**angi/o-graphy, technique of making a moving X-ray recording or film of (blood) vessels (the pictures are made from fluoroscopic images)

**cinemat/o-**radi/o-graphy, technique of making a moving X-ray recording or film of body structures (the pictures are made from fluoroscopic images) Syn. cineradiography

**cine-**oesophag/o-gram, a moving X-ray recording or film of the oesophagus

**cine-**radi/o-graph, a moving X-ray recording or film

**cine-**radi/o-graphy, technique of making a moving X-ray recording or film of body structures (the pictures are made from fluoroscopic images)

**cine**-radi/o-logy, the study of X-ray techniques applied to making moving images

---

**Ech/o**, echo, ultrasound echo

From a Greek word **echo** meaning sound. Here, ech/o means an ultrasound echo, the reflection of ultrasound by an obstacle. When pulses of high-frequency sound waves between 1 and 10 megahertz are directed at the body, internal organs and masses reflect the sound to a different extent. They are said to have different echo textures. These internal echoes are detected and converted into an image. The size and shape of easily recognized organs can be investigated using this technique, and it is widely used for examining a fetus *in utero*.

See the combining form son/o meaning sound or ultrasound.

**echo**-cardi/o-gram, a picture or recording of the heart made using ultrasound echoes

**echo**-cardi/o-graphy, technique of making a picture or recording of the heart (movement) using ultrasound echoes

**echo**-encephal/o-gram, a picture or recording of the brain made using ultrasound echoes

**echo**-encephal/o-graphy, technique of making a picture or recording of the brain using ultrasound echoes

**echo**-gen-ic, pertaining to forming or generating echoes

**echo**-gram, a picture or recording made using ultrasound echoes

**echo**-graphy, technique of making a picture or recording using ultra-sound echoes

**echo**-phon/o-cardi/o-graphy, technique of making a picture or recording of the heart using ultrasound echoes and phonocardiography (a technique of recording sounds from the heart)

**echo**-ranging, using ultrasound echoes to determine position of body structures

**Fluor/o**, fluorescent, luminous

From a Latin word **fluere** meaning to flow. Here fluor/o means emitting light, fluorescent or luminous. The movement of internal parts of the body can be observed using the technique known as fluoroscopy. In this procedure X-rays pass through the body onto a phosphor screen (a fluorescent screen, from which light flows). As the X-rays strike the screen, the phosphor emits light, producing an image which is viewed as it is generated. Fluoroscopy is useful for observing movement of the oesophagus, stomach and heart and a recording can be made of the light image from the screen.

**fluor/o**-scope, an instrument used to view or examine the motion of body structures by means of X-rays projected onto a fluorescent screen, the fluoroscope is used for direct viewing of an X-ray image

**fluor/o**-scop-ical, pertaining to fluoroscopy

**fluor/o**-scopy, technique of viewing or examining internal structures of the body with a fluoroscope

tele-**fluor/o**-scopy, technique of viewing a fluoroscopic image at a distant location, by television

---

**Radi/o**, radiation, radioactivity, X-rays

From a Latin word **radius**, meaning a ray. Here radi/o means radiation, radioactivity or X-rays, the invisible rays produced by an X-ray machine. Radio- is also used as a prefix before the name of a chemical element to indicate a radioactive isotope; for example, radio-iodine refers to any radioactive isotope of the element iodine.

auto-**radi/o**-graph, a recording of 'oneself' using radiation, it refers to a radiograph produced by radiation emitted from a specimen that directly exposes a photographic plate Syn. radioautograph

auto-**radi/o**-graphy, technique of making an autoradiograph micro-**radi/o**-graphy, technique of making a recording or X-ray picture the small detail of which can be examined microscopically or enlarged to show more detail

**radi**-ation, 1. action of emitting electromagnetic waves or particles charged or uncharged with electricity 2. in medicine the use of radioactive substances to diagnose and treat disease.

**radi/o**-act-ive, having the property of radioactivity

**radi/o**-activ-ity, property of certain chemicals (nuclides) or emitting electromagnetic waves or particles charged or uncharged with electricity

**radi/o**-auto-graph, a recording of 'oneself' using radiation, it refers to a radiograph produced by radiation emitted from a specimen that directly exposes a photographic plate Syn. autoradiograph

**radi/o**-auto-graphy, technique of making a radioautograph Syn. autoradiography

**radi/o**-bio-log-ical, 1. pertaining to radiobiology 2. pertaining to the effects of radiation on living tissue

**radi/o**-bio-logy, the study of the effects of radiation on living tissue

**radi/o**-bismuth, radioactive bismuth, example $^{206}$Bi

**radi/o**-caesium, radioactive caesium, examples $^{132}$Cs, $^{137}$Cs

**radi/o**-calcium, radioactive calcium, examples $^{45}$Ca, $^{47}$Ca

**radi/o**-carbon, radioactive carbon, examples $^{14}$C, $^{11}$C

**radi/o**-cardi/o-graphy, technique of recording radiation from the chambers of the heart, from an isotope injected intravenously

**radi/o**-chemic-al, 1. pertaining to radiochemistry 2. a radioactive chemical

**radi/o**-chemistry, the science dealing with the chemistry of radioactive materials (preparation, purification and properties)

**radi/o**-chromium, radioactive chromium, example $^{51}$Cr

**radi/o**-cinemat/o-graph, an instrument that records moving images produced by an X-ray machine

**radi/o**-cobalt, radioactive cobalt, examples $^{57}$Co, $^{58}$Co, $^{60}$Co

**radi/o**-copper, radioactive copper, examples $^{64}$Cu, $^{67}$Cu

**radi/o**-cyst-itis, inflammation of the bladder caused by radiation

**radi/o**-dens-ity, state or property of impeding the passage of radiant energy or X-rays

**radi/o**-dermat-itis, inflammation of the skin caused by radiation

**radi/o**-diagnosis, the diagnosis of disease using X-rays or radiographs

**radi**-odont-ics, the science of dental radiology

**radi**-odont-ist, a specialist who studies and practises dental radiology

**radi/o**-element, an element that exhibits radioactivity

**radi/o**-epiderm-itis, inflammation of the epidermis caused by radiation

**radi/o**-fluorine, radioactive fluorine, example $^{18}$F

**radi/o**-gallium, radioactive gallium, example $^{67}$Ga

**radi/o**-gold, radioactive gold, example $^{198}$Au

**radi/o**-gram, a picture or recording made using X-rays, the term radiograph is preferred

**radi/o**-graph, a picture or recording made using X-rays

**radi/o**-graph-er, one who makes an X-ray, a technician not medically qualified

**radi/o**-graphy, technique of making a recording or X-ray picture

**radi/o**-immun-ity, state or property of being immune to radiation, it refers to a diminished sensitivity to radiation

**radi/o**-immun/o-sorbent (test), a radioimmunoassay test (RIST) that measures total serum immunoglobulin E (IgE)

**radi/o**-immun/o-assay, technique of using radioactive (radiolabelled) substances in antigen-antibody reactions to identify and measure hormones, drugs and proteins in the blood

**radi/o**-immun/o-diffusion, the diffusion of radioactive (radiolabelled) antibodies or antigens in a gel or other substance

**radi/o**-iodine, radioactive iodine, examples $^{123}I$, $^{125}I$, $^{127}I$, $^{131}I$, $^{132}I$

**radi/o**-iron, radioactive iron, examples $^{55}Fe$, $^{59}Fe$

**radi/o**-isotope, an unstable chemical element whose atoms decay emitting alpha, beta or gamma radiation, those used in medicine are artificially produced by the nuclear industry and are known as radionuclides

**radi/o**-ligand, a radioisotope-labelled substance such as an antigen

**radi/o**-log-ical, 1. pertaining to radiology 2. pertaining to the study of radiation or radioactive substances

**radi/o**-log-ist, a specialist who studies radiology, medically qualified

**radi/o**-logy, 1. the study of radiation 2. the study of radioactive substances in relation to the diagnosis and treatment of disease

**radi/o**-lucent, permitting X-rays to pass through. From a Latin word *lucere* meaning to shine Syn. roentgeno-lucent. Structures that are radio-lucent appear dark on exposed X-ray film

**radi/o**-mimet-ic, pertaining to mimicking or having a similar effect to radiation, the term is applied to the action of some cytotoxic drugs

**radi/o**-mut-ation, a change to the nature of a cell brought about by exposure to radiation. From a Latin word *mutare* meaning to change

**radi/o**-necr-osis, abnormal condition of death of tissue due to radiation

**radi/o**-neur-itis, inflammation of nerves or nervous tissue caused by radiation

**radi/o**-nuclide, a radioisotope, isotopes are forms of elements that have the same atomic number but different mass numbers, radioisotopes are unstable and exhibit the property of spontaneous nuclear disintegration with the emission of radiation

**radi**-opac-ity, state or property of impeding the passage of radiant energy or X-rays

**radi/o**-opaque, property of impeding the passage of radiant energy or X-rays, structures that are radio-opaque appear light on exposed X-ray film

**radi/o**-path/o-logy, the study of disease caused by radiation

**radi/o**-pelvi-metry, technique of measuring the pelvis using X-rays or radiography

**radi/o**-pharmaceut-ical, 1. a radioactive pharmaceutical (drug) used for diagnosis or therapy 2. pertaining to radioactive pharmaceuticals (drugs)

**radi/o**-phob-ia, condition of irrational fear of radiation or X-rays

**radi/o**-resistance, state or property of relative resistance of living tissue to damage by radiation

**radi/o**-scopy, technique of viewing or examining internal structures of the body with a fluoroscope Syn. fluoroscopy

**radi/o**-sensitive, state or property of being sensitive to radiation or X-rays

**radi/o**-sensitiv-ity, state or property of being radiosensitive

**radi/o**-therap-ist, a specialist who treats (disease) using radiation or X-rays, medically qualified

**radi/o**-therapy, treatment using radiation or X-rays

**radi/o**-tox-aem-ia, condition of poisoning of the blood due to the effects of radiation

**radi/o**-tracer, a radioactive isotope administered to the body that can be traced or detected by a Geiger-Muller tube or gamma camera

**radi/o**-transparent, permitting X-rays to pass through Syn. radiolucent. Structures that are radiotransparent appear dark on exposed X-ray film

**radi/o**-trop-ic, pertaining to responding to radiation or X-rays

**radi**-um, a radioactive element Symbol Ra, it emits alpha, beta and gamma radiation

tele-**radi/o**-graphy, technique of making a recording or X-ray picture from a distance, so the rays are parallel Syn. teleroentgenography

xero-**radi**/o-graphy, technique of making a dry X-ray, a process producing a non-transparent print that uses a selenium plate exposed to X-rays

**Roentgen/o,** Roentgen rays, X-rays
From the name of Wilhelm K. **Roentgen,** a German physicist who discovered X-rays. Here, Roentgen/o means roentgen rays or X-rays.

**roentgen,** international unit of dose of X-rays or gamma rays Symbol **R**

**roentgen**-kym/o-gram, a roentgenogram (X-ray picture or film) made by roentgenokymography

**roentgen**-kym/o-graphy, technique of making a recording of the movements of body organs on X-ray film

**roentgen/o**-cardi/o-gram, an roentgenogram (X-ray picture) of the heart

**roentgen/o**-cinemat/o-graphy, technique of making a recording of a moving X-ray picture

**roentgen/o**-gram, an X-ray picture or radiograph

**roentgen/o**-graph, an X-ray picture or radiograph

**roentgen/o**-graph-ic, 1. pertaining to roentgenography 2. pertaining to making an X-ray picture or roentgenograph

**roentgen/o**-graphy, technique of making a roentgenogram (radiograph)

**roentgen/o**-log-ist, a specialist who studies roentgenology, medically qualified

**roentgen/o**-logy, the study roentgen rays (X-rays), a branch of radiology dealing with diagnostic and therapeutic uses of X-rays

**roentgen/o**-lucent, permitting roentgen rays (X-rays) to pass through. From a Latin word *lucere* meaning to shine Syn. radiolucent Structures that are roentgenolucent appear dark on exposed X-ray film

**roentgen/o**-meter, an instrument used for measuring roentgen rays (intensity of X-rays)

**roentgen/o**-metry, 1. technique of measuring roentgen rays (intensity) 2. technique of measuring structures outlined on a roentgenograph (radiograph)

**roentgen/o**-scope, an instrument used to view or examine a moving image produced by roentgen rays (X-rays) on a screen Syn. fluoroscope

**roentgen/o**-scopy, technique of viewing or examining a moving image produced by roentgen rays (X-rays) on a screen Syn. fluoroscopy

tele-**roentgen/o**-graphy, technique of making a roentgenograph (radiograph) from a distance, so the rays are parallel Syn. teleradiography

**Scint/i, scintill/a/o,** spark, emitting light
From a Latin word **scintillatio,** meaning a sparkling. Here, scint/i means a scintillation, the emission of light from a scintillator. Scintigraphy is the technique of producing a scintiscan or radioisotope scan. A radioisotope with an affinity for a particular organ or tissue is injected into the body and the distribution of the radioactivity is followed using an instrument called a scintillation counter (scintiscanner). This device contains a scintillator, a substance that emits light when in contact with ionizing radiation. There is a flash of light for each ionizing event and the number of flashes (or counts) is related to the radioactivity present in the area being scanned. Scintillation counters can be moved over the outer surface of the body to locate radioisotopes within particular organs and build an image (scintigram/scintiscan) of their distribution. The gamma camera is a scintillation counter.

**scint/i**-gram, a picture or recording of sparks, it refers to a recording of the distribution of radioactivity within the body Syn. scintiscan

**scint/i**-graphy, technique of making a scintigram or radioisotope scan

**scintilla**-scope, a device for viewing scintillations on a fluorescent screen

**scintill**-ation, 1. action or process of emitting sparks, it refers to rays or particles from a radioactive isotope colliding with a scintillator 2. a particle emitted when a radioactive element disintegrates

**scintilla**-tor, an agent that has the property of emitting sparks or light when in contact with ionizing radiation

**scintill/o**-graphy, technique of making a scintigram or radioisotope scan Syn. scintigraphy, scintiscanning

**scint/i**-scan, a recording of sparks or light, due to gamma rays from a radioactive isotope colliding with a scintillator, it shows the concentration of a radioactive isotope in a particular tissue or organ

**scint/i**-scanning, technique of making a scintiscan

---

**Son/o**, sound, ultrasound
From a Latin word **sonus**, meaning sound. Here, son/o refers to the use of ultrasound, that is sound waves having a frequency of more than 20 000 Hz, the limit of human hearing. When pulses of high-frequency sound waves between 1 and 10 megahertz are directed at the body, internal organs and masses reflect the sound to a different extent. They are said to have different echo textures. These internal echoes are detected and converted into an image. The size and shape of easily recognized organs can be investigated using this technique, and it is widely used for examining a fetus *in utero*.

See the combining form **ech/o** meaning ultrasound echo.

**son/o**-cardi/o-metry, technique of measuring the heart (size of) using ultrasound

**son/o**-graph, a picture or recording produced using ultrasound

**son/o**-graph-ic, 1. pertaining to sonography 2. pertaining to making a recording or image of part of the body using ultrasound

**son/o**-graphy, technique of using ultrasound to make a recording or image

of part of the body Syn. ultrasonography

**ultra-son**-ic, pertaining to beyond sound, it refers to sound waves having a frequency of more than 20 000 Hz, the limit of human hearing

**ultra-son**-ics, the science of studying ultrasound or ultrasonic sound waves

**ultra-son/o**-cardi/o-graphy, technique of making a picture or recording of the heart using ultrasound Syn. echocardiography

**ultra-son/o**-gram, a picture or recording produced using ultrasound

**ultra-son/o**-graph-ic, 1. pertaining to ultrasonography 2. pertaining to making a recording or picture using ultrasound

**ultra-son/o**-graphy, technique of making a recording or picture using ultrasound

---

**tele-**, far away, operating at a distance
From a Greek word **tele** meaning far off. Here tele- means operating at a distance.

**tele**-fluor/o-scopy, technique of viewing a fluoroscopic image at a distant location, by television

**tele**-radi/o-graphy, technique of making an X-ray picture from a distance, approximately 2 m away to make the rays parallel

**tele**-roentgen/o-graphy, technique of making a recording or X-ray picture from a distance, approximately 2 m away to make the rays parallel

**tele**-roentgen/o-therapy, treatment by radiation at a distance from the body, using a radiotherapy machine that produces roentgen rays (X-rays)

**tele**-therapy, treatment by radiation at a distance from the body, using a radiotherapy machine

---

**Therm/o**, heat
From a Greek word **therme** meaning heat. Here therm/o means heat.

**therm**-al, pertaining to heat or of the nature of heat

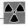

**therm**-ic, pertaining to heat or of the nature of heat

**therm/o**-genesis, the formation of heat

**therm/o**-gen-ic, pertaining to the formation of heat

**therm/o**-gram, 1. a picture or recording of infrared heat in the body 2. a picture or recording obtained by thermography 3. a recording of a patient's temperature variations

**therm/o**-graph, 1. an instrument used to record temperature of infrared heat in the body 2. a recording instrument used for thermography 3. a recording of temperature variations Syn. thermogram

**therm/o**-graphy, technique of making a recording or picture of the distribution of infrared heat in the body

**therm/o**-metry, the technique of measuring temperatures

**therm/o**-placent/o-graphy, technique of recording the position of the placenta using thermography

---

**Tom/o**, section, slice

From a Greek word **tomos**, meaning a slice or section. Here, tom/o means

an X-ray of a slice through the body. Computed tomography also called computerized axial tomography or CAT scanning is a technique of making detailed cross-sectional images of the body using X-rays.

poly-**tom/o**-gram, a recording or X-ray picture produced by polytomography

poly-**tom/o**-graphy, technique of making a recording or X-ray picture of many slices or sections through the body at predetermined planes

**tom/o**-gram, a recording or X-ray picture of a slice or section through the body

**tom/o**-graph, an instrument used to make a recording or X-ray picture of a slice or section through the body, it produces a cross-sectional image

**tom/o**-graph-ic, 1. pertaining to tomography 2. pertaining to producing a recording or X-ray picture of a slice or section through the body

**tom/o**-graphy, technique of making a recording or X-ray picture of a slice or section through the body

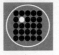

# Section 19
# Oncology

Oncology is the branch of medicine that deals with the study and treatment of malignant tumours commonly called cancers. A tumour is a mass or swelling forming from dividing cells that appear to be out of control. Benign tumours remain localized and do not threaten life but malignant tumours spread and may lead to death. Tumours spread when they release cells into the blood and lymph; the tumour cells multiply in new sites forming secondary growths or **metastases** (from Greek *meta* + *histanai*, *meta* meaning changed in form, *histanai* to place/set, *i.e.* a growth changed in form and position).

As tumours grow they consume nutrients, depriving normal cells of essential metabolic components. A clinical feature called **cachexia** is seen in advanced stages of disease (from Greek *kakos* meaning bad and *hexis* meaning state). The body appears to suffer from malnutrition and becomes thin and 'wastes' away.

In this section we list terms that relate to common types of tumour.

## Cancer classification

Cancers are classified in two ways:

- by the type of tissue in which the cancer originates (histological type)
- by the the location or primary site where the cancer first developed

## Histological types of cancer

There are hundreds of different types of cancer grouped into six main categories:

## Carcinoma

A carcinoma is a malignant cancer of epithelial origin. Epithelial tissue consists of epithelial membranes and epithelial glands that form the internal and external linings of the body. Carcinomas are divided into two major subtypes: adenocarcinoma, which develop from glands, and squamous cell carcinoma, which develop from squamous epithelium. Carcinomas often affect glands or organs with epithelial membranes capable of secretion. such as the breast, prostate gland, bronchus or colon. Examples of carcinomas are:

**Basal cell carcinoma of the skin**
**Adenocarcinoma of the breast**

## Sarcoma

A sarcoma is a malignant cancer that originates in connective tissue such as cartilage, bone or adipose tissue, and in muscle tissue. A sarcoma usually forms a painful mass in a bone or other tissue and resembles the tissue from which it originates. There are many types of sarcoma named after the tissue in which they originate. For example:

**Chondr/o-sarcoma**
a sarcoma originating in cartilage
**Oste/o-sarcoma**
a sarcoma originating in bone
**Angi/o-sarcoma**
a sarcoma originating in blood vessels
**Leiomy/o-sarcoma**
a sarcoma originating in smooth muscle
**Myx/o-sarcoma**
a sarcoma originating in primitive embryonic connective tissue

## Myeloma

A myeloma is a cancer that originates in the plasma cells of bone marrow. The cancerous cells produce many of the proteins found in blood. For example, in multiple myeloma plasma cells derived from ß lymphocytes produce an abnormal amount of immuno-globulin.

## Leukaemia

Leukaemia is a cancer of the blood-forming cells in the bone marrow. The disease affects the immature cells that produce leucocytes, hence the term leuk-aem-ia, meaning condition of white blood or too many white cells.

Leucocytes normally protect us from disease but the leukaemic white cells lose their ability to protect us against infectious organisms leaving the patient prone to infection. Leukaemia can also affect the immature cells that produce erythrocytes. resulting in the symptoms and signs of anaemia and interference with blood clotting.

There are many types of leukaemia:

**Granulocytic leukaemia**
a malignancy of the granulocytic series of leucocytes

**Lymphocytic leukaemia**
a malignancy of the lymphocytic series of blood cells

**Polycythaemia vera**
a malignancy of many blood cells with red cells predominating

## Lymphoma

Lymphoma develops in the nodes and organs of the lymphatic system. A lymphoma is a solid cancer that arises in an organ such as the spleen, tonsil, thymus gland or in a lymph node. Extra-nodal lymphomas are also found in other organs such as the stomach or brain. Lymphomas are classified into two sub-types:

**Hodgkin's lymphoma**
(Hodgkin's disease)
**Non-Hodgkin's lymphoma**

## Mixed tumours

In mixed tumours the cells may be of different origins and be classified in different categories:

**Carcinosarcoma**
a malignant tumour composed of cells originating in epithelial and connective tissue

**Adenosquamous carcinoma**
a malignant tumour composed of cells that originate in squamous epithelia and glandular tissue

## Diagnosis of malignant tumours

Precise classification of malignant tumours is essential for determining their likely growth characteristics. Once a tumour has been classified, appropriate treatment can be planned and the patient can be given a prognosis, which is a forecast of the probable course of his/her disease.

Attempts to develop an international language for describing the extent of malignant disease have been made.

One of these is in widespread use and is known as the **TNM** system:

**T** – tumour
categorizes the primary tumour and its size

**N** – nodes
defines the number of lymph nodes that have been invaded

**M** – metastases
indicates the presence or absence of metastases.

The extent of malignant disease defined by these categories is termed **staging**. Staging defines the size of tumour, its growth and progression at any one point.

Many different staging systems are in use for different cancers. It is not possible to study them here, but a basic system is outlined below:

**T**

| | |
|---|---|
| $T_0$ | no primary tumour |
| $T_1$ | primary tumour limited to site of origin |
| $T_{2-4}$ | progressive increase in size of primary tumour |
| $T_x$ | primary tumour cannot be assessed |
| $T_{is}$ | primary tumour in situ |

**N**

| | |
|---|---|
| $N_0$ | no evidence of spread to nodes |
| $N_1$ | spread to nodes in immediate area |
| $N_{2-4}$ | increasing number of lymph nodes invaded |
| $N_x$ | lymph nodes cannot be assessed |

**M**

| | |
|---|---|
| $M_0$ | no evidence of metastases |
| $M_{1-3}$ | ascending degrees of metastases |

Using the above system, a cancer could be at stage $T_2 N_1 M_0$.

This would indicate that the primary tumour is large and has spread to deeper structures ($T_2$). It has spread to one lymph node draining the area ($N_1$) and there is no evidence of a distant metastasis ($M_0$).

Staging is not an exact description of a tumour's progress but it is a useful way to estimate the course of the disease when planning treatment.

**Roots and combining forms**, meanings

**Aden/o**, gland, glandular tissue
From a Greek word **aden** meaning gland. Here aden/o means gland but the following set of words refers mainly to adenoma, a tumour formed from glandular tissue.

Other words containing aden/o can be found in Section 6 The lymphatic system.

**aden/o**-acanth-oma, a tumour containing squamous cells and glandular tissue (the squamous cells may show differentiation into cells like those of the prickle-cell layer of the epidermis)

**aden/o**-amel/o-blast-oma, a tumour of immature cells or embryonic cells that form the dental tissue that gives rise to tooth enamel with glandular elements

**aden/o**-angi/o-sarc-oma, a malignant tumour of connective tissue and endothelial tissue of (blood) vessels with glandular elements

**aden/o**-blast, an immature cell or embryonic cell that forms glandular tissue

**aden/o**-carcin-oma, a malignant epithelial tumour derived from glandular tissue

**aden/o**-cele, a swelling or tumour containing adenomatous tissue

**aden/o**-chondr-oma, a tumour containing cartilage and glandular elements

**aden/o**-cyst-oma, a tumour of glandular epithelium in the form of a cyst or swelling

**aden/o**-epitheli-oma, a tumour containing epithelial and glandular elements

**aden/o**-gen-ous, pertaining to or originating in glandular tissue

**aden**-oid, 1. resembling a gland 2. resembling lymphoid tissue

**aden/o**-lei/o-my/o-fibr-oma, 1. a tumour of smooth muscle fibres and glandular

tissue 2. a leiomyofibroma with glandular elements

**aden/o**-lip-oma, a tumour with fatty and glandular elements

**aden/o**-lip-omat-osis, abnormal condition of having multiple adenolipomas

**aden/o**-lymph-oma, a tumour containing lymphatic and glandular elements

**aden**-oma, a tumour derived from a glandular epithelium

**aden**-omat-a, plural of adenoma

**aden**-omat-oid, resembling an adenoma

**aden**-omat-osis, abnormal condition of the presence of multiple adenomas (adenomata)

**aden**-omat-ous, 1. pertaining to or of the nature of an adenoma 2. pertaining to growth or hyperplasia of gland tissue

**aden/o**-my/o-fibr-oma, a tumour of fibrous connective tissue with muscular and glandular elements

**aden/o**-my-oma, a tumour of muscle and glandular tissue, found in the uterus

**aden/o**-my-omat-osis, abnormal condition of the presence of multiple adenomyomas

**aden/o**-my/o-sarc-oma, a tumour of connective tissue, (striated) muscle and glandular tissue

**aden/o**-myx-oma, a tumour containing mucoid tissue and glandular tissue

**aden**-onc-us, a tumour or swelling of a gland

**aden/o**-pathy, disease of a gland, especially lymph nodes

**aden/o**-sarc-oma, a tumour of connective tissue and glandular tissue

**aden/o**-sarco-rhabd/o-my-oma, a tumour in which there are elements of striated muscle, connective tissue and glandular tissue

---

**Blast/o**, embryonic cell, immature cell, undifferentiated cell
From a Greek word **blastos** meaning bud or germ. Here blast/o means an immature stage in cell development, an undifferentiated cell or a stem cell that is forming something. Here, we are relating blast/o to tumours that form from immature, undifferentiated cells.

293

Other words containing blast/o can be found in Section 1 Cells, tissues, organs and systems.

**blast/o**-cyte, an immature cell or undifferentiated embryonic cell

**blast/o**-cyt-oma, a tumour consisting of blastocytes

**blast**-oma, a tumour of immature cells or undifferentiated embryonic cells

**blastomat**-a, plural of blastoma

**blastomat**-oid, resembling a blastoma

**blastomat**-osis, abnormal condition of the presence of multiple blastomas (blastomata)

**blastomat**-ous, pertaining to or of the nature of a blastoma

---

**Cancer/i/o, cancr/i,** cancer

From a Latin word **cancer**, meaning crab. Here carcin/o means cancer a general term used for any malignant tumour.

**cancer**-aem-ia, condition of cancer cells in the blood

**cancer/i**-gen-ic, pertaining to forming cancer

**cancer/o**-cid-al, pertaining to killing a cancer or cancer cells

**cancer/o**-phob-ia, condition of irrational fear of developing cancer

**cancer/o**-phob-ic, 1. pertaining to having an irrational fear of developing cancer 2. pertaining to having cancerophobia

**cancer**-ous, pertaining to cancer or of the nature of cancer

**cancr/i**-form, having the form of cancer

**cancr**-oid, 1. resembling cancer 2. an epithelioma or skin cancer showing a mild degree of malignancy

---

**Carcin/o, carcinomat-,** carcinoma

From a Greek word **karkinos**, meaning crab. Here carcin/o and carcinomat- mean carcinoma, a malignant tumour or cancer arising from epithelial tissue.

**carcin**-ectomy, removal of a carcinoma

**carcin/o**-embryon-ic, pertaining to the embryo and carcinoma

**carcin/o**-gen, an agent that causes carcinomas (cancer)

**carcin/o**-gen-ic, pertaining to formation of a carcinoma (cancer)

**carcin/o**-genic-ity, state or tendency to form carcinomas (cancer)

**carcin**-oid, 1. resembling a carcinoma 2. a tumour derived from argentaffin cells, an argentaffinoma

**carcin/o**-lysis, destruction or disintegration of a carcinoma

**carcin**-oma, a malignant tumour of epithelial cells

**carcin**-omat-oid, resembling a carcinoma

**carcin**-omat-osis, abnormal condition of multiple carcinomas, it refers to the spread of a cancer throughout the body

**carcin**-omat-ous, pertaining to or of the nature of a carcinoma

**carcin/o**-phob-ia, condition of irrational fear of cancer

**carcin/o**-sarc-oma, a malignant tumour of connective tissue (sarcoma) and epithelial tissue (carcinoma)

**carcin**-osis, abnormal condition of carcinomas Syn. carcinomatosis

**carcin/o**-stat-ic, pertaining to stopping the growth of a carcinoma

pro-**carcin/o**-gen, before a carcinogen, it refers to an agent that enters the body and only becomes carcinogenic after being altered by metabolic processes

---

**Leukaem/o,** leukaemia

From the Greek words **leukos**, meaning white and **-aem-** meaning blood. Here, leukaem/o means leukaemia, a malignant cancer of the haemopoietic tissue that forms white blood cells.

**leukaem**-ia, condition of white blood, it refers to a malignant cancer of haemopoietic tissue showing an abnormal increase in the number of leucocytes in the circulation Syn. leukocythaemia

**leukaem**-ic, pertaining to leukaemia

**leukaem/o**-gen, an agent that produces or causes leukaemia

**leukaem/o**-genesis, formation of leukaemia

**leukaem/o**-gen-ic, pertaining to forming or causing leukaemia

**leukaem**-oid, resembling leukaemia, it refers to the clinical picture of this condition

pre-**leukaem**-ia, condition before leukaemia, it refers to a bone marrow disorder before the onset of acute myelogenous leukaemia

pre-**leukaem**-ic, 1. pertaining to before the onset of leukaemia 2. pertaining to having a bone marrow disorder before the onset of acute myelogenous leukaemia

---

**Lymph/o**, lymph

**Lymphomat-**, **lymphoma**, a tumour forming from lymph tissue

From a Greek word **lympha**, meaning water. Here, lymph/o means the fluid lymph or lymphatic tissue. The words listed below are mainly associated with tumours (lymphomas) of the lymphatic system.

Other words containing lymph/o can be found in Section 5 on The blood and and Section 6 on The lymphatic system and immunology.

**lymph**-aden-oma, tumour of a lymph node Syn. lymphoma

**lymph**-aden-omat-osis, abnormal condition of tumours of the lymph nodes or presence of multiple lymphomas

**lymph**-aden-oid, resembling a lymph node

**lymph**-aden/o-path-ic, pertaining to disease of lymph nodes

**lymph**-aden/o-pathy, disease of lymph nodes

**lymph**-aden-osis, abnormal condition or disease of lymph nodes, it refers to hypertrophy of lymph tissue

**lymph**-angi/o-endotheli-oma, a malignant tumour originating in the endothelial cells lining lymphatic vessels

**lymph**-angi/o-fibr-oma, a tumour composed of fibrous tissue and lymph vessels (benign)

**lymph**-angi-oma, a tumour similar to an angioma but filled with lymph, it contains lymph spaces and channels

**lymph**-angi/o-my-oma, a tumour of smooth muscle and lymph vessels or lymphatic elements

**lymph**-angi/o-my-omat-osis, abnormal condition of multiple lymph-angiomyomas, often present in the lung and mediastinum as nodules or diffuse

**lymph**-angi/o-sarc-oma, a malignant tumour of lymph vessels

**lymph/o**-blast, an immature cell or embryonic cell that forms into a mature lymphocyte

**lymph/o**-blast-oma, a malignant tumour that arises from lymphoblasts

**lymph/o**-cyt-ic, pertaining to lymphocytes

**lymph/o**-cyt-oma, a malignant tumour composed of lymphocytes Syn. lymphocytic lymphoma

**lymph/o**-epitheli-oma, a malignant tumour (carcinoma) arising from the epithelium covering lymph tissue (found in the nasopharynx)

**lymph/o**-granul-oma, 1. a granular tumour of lymphatic tissue 2. Hodgkin's disease

**lymph/o**-granul-omat-osis, 1. abnormal condition of having multiple lymphogranulomas 2. Hodgkin's disease

**lymph**-oid, resembling lymph

**lymph/o**-ect-omy, removal of lymphatic tissue

**lymph**-oma, a tumour forming from lymph tissue

**lymph**-omata, lymphomas, plural of lymphoma

**lymph**-omat-oid, resembling a lymphoma

**lymph**-omat-osis, abnormal condition of or formation of multiple lymphomas

**lymph**-omat-ous, pertaining to or having characteristics of a lymphoma

**lymph/o**-myel-oma, a tumour of bone marrow that contains many cells resembling lymphocytes

**lymph/o**-myx-oma, a tumour of mucoid tissue and lymph, it refers to a soft, benign growth of lymphoid tissue

**lymph/o**-nod-us, a lymph node

295

**lymph/o**-path-ia, condition of disease of lymph vessels or nodes

**lymph/o**-pathy, disease of the lymph vessels or nodes

**lymph/o**-proliferative, pertaining to the proliferation (increase) of lymphoid tissue

**lymph/o**-sarc-oma, a malignant tumour of lymphoid tissue

---

**Melan/o**, melanin
**Melanomat-**, melanoma, a tumour of darkly pigmented melanin-containing cells

From a Greek word **melas** meaning black. Here, melan/o means melanin, the black pigment found in hair, skin and the choroid of the eye. Tumours containing melanin (melanomas) develop from the melanocytes that produce pigmentation of the skin and other structures.

**melan**-ism, condition of excessive pigmentation of the skin or other tissues

**melan/o**-blast, an immature cell or embryonic cell that develops into a melanocyte

**melan/o**-blast-oma, a tumour formed from melanoblasts

**melan/o**-blast-osis, abnormal condition of melanoblasts, it refers to a tumour composed of melanoblasts

**melan/o**-carcin-oma, a carcinoma containing melanin

**melan/o**-cyte, a pigment cell, a cell containing melanin

**melan/o**-cyt-oma, a tumour composed of melanocytes

**melan/o**-epatheli-oma, a tumour of epithelial tissue in which melanin is produced

**melan/o**-gen, an agent (a colourless chromogen) found in the body that can be converted into melanin

**melan/o**-genesis, the formation of melanin

**melan**-oid, resembling melanin

**melan**-oma, a tumour of darkly pigmented melanin-containing cells

*e.g.* malignant melanoma in the skin

**melan/o**-malignancy, a malignant tumour of cells containing melanin

**melan**-omat-osis, abnormal condition of having multiple (malignant) melanomas

**melan/o**-path-ia, disease condition accompanied by pigmentation or darkening of the skin or other tissue

**melan/o**-pathy, disease accompanied by pigmentation or darkening of the skin or other tissue

**melan/o**-phore, a pigment cell containing melanin

**melan/o**-sarc-oma, a malignant fleshy tumour containing melanin

**melan/o**-sarc-omat-osis, abnormal condition of having multiple malignant melanosarcomas

**melan**-osis, abnormal condition of pigment deposition in the skin or other tissues

**melan/o**-tic, 1. pertaining to melanosis 2. pertaining to affected by melanosis

**melan/o**-troph, a cell that nourishes melanin, it refers to a cell in the pituitary gland that produces MSH, melanocyte-stimulating hormone

**melan/o**-trop-ic, pertaining to having an affinity for melanin

**melan**-ur-ia, condition of melanin or dark pigment in the urine

---

**Myel/o**, bone marrow, bone marrow cell, myelocyte
**Myelomat-**, a myeloma, a tumour of myeloid tissue (bone marrow cells)

From a Greek word **myelos**, meaning marrow. Here myel/o means the bone marrow, a substance that fills the medullary cavities of cancellous bone. Bone marrow contains haemopoietic tissue that produces blood cells. Myel/o also refers to myelocytes, precursor cells of the polymorphonuclear series of granulocytes found in the bone marrow.

Words containing myel/o are also listed in Section 5 on The blood and Section 8 on The nervous system.

**myel/o**-blast, 1. an immature cell of the marrow 2. the earliest precursor cell of the granular series of leucocyte

**myel/o**-blast-oma, a tumour composed of myeloblasts, seen in myelocytic leukaemia

**myel/o**-cyte, 1. marrow cell 2. a precursor cell of the polymorphonuclear series of granulocytes

**myel/o**-cyt-haem-ia, condition of the blood containing myelocytes as in myeloid leukaemia

**myel/o**-cyt-ic, pertaining to or of the nature of myelocytes

**myel/o**-cyt-oma, a tumour of myelocytes Syn. myeloma

**myel/o**-cyt-osis, abnormal condition of myelocytes in the blood

**myel/o**-genet-ic, pertaining to originating or forming in bone marrow

**myel/o**-gen-ous, pertaining to originating or forming in bone marrow

**myel**-oid, 1. resembling bone marrow 2. derived from bone marrow 3. pertaining to bone marrow 4. resembling myelocytes but not originating in bone marrow

**myel**-oid-osis, abnormal condition (hyperplasia) of myeloid tissue

**myel/o**-lip-oma, a tumour of fatty tissue and myeloid cells, it refers to a benign tumour of the adrenal gland

**myel**-oma, a tumour of myeloid tissue (bone marrow cells), multiple myeloma is a malignant tumour of plasma cells that are derived from β-lymphocytes

**myel**-omat-oid, resembling a myeloma

**myel**-omat-osis, abnormal condition of having multiple myelomas Syn. multiple myeloma

**myel**-omat-ous, pertaining to myelomas

**myelo**-path-ic, pertaining to disease of the bone marrow

**myel/o**-pathy, disease of the bone marrow

**myel/o**-proliferative, proliferation or increase in one or more of the cellular components of bone marrow

**myel/o**-sarc-oma, a malignant tumour of connective tissue (sarcoma) composed of myeloid tissue (bone marrow cells)

**myel**-osis, abnormal condition of (increase) in bone marrow tissue producing myelocytic leukaemia

**myel/o**-suppressive, 1. action of suppression or inhibition of bone marrow activity 2. an agent that has such an action

**myel/o**-therapy, treatment with bone marrow preparations

---

**Myx/o**, mucus, mucoid tissue

**Myxomat-**, amyxoma, a tumour of embryonic connective tissue

From a Greek word **myxa** meaning mucus. Here myx/o means mucus, or mucoid tissue. Mucoid tissue is a loose, gelatinous mass of connective tissue cells resembling mesenchyme, the embryonic connective tissue.

**myx**-aden-itis, inflammation of a mucous gland

**myx**-aden-oma, a tumour derived from a glandular epithelium with mucous elements or the structure of a mucous gland

**myx/o**-blast-oma, a tumour of immature cells or embryonic cells that form mucoid tissue

**myx/o**-chondr-oma, a tumour containing cartilage and mucoid tissue elements

**myx/o**-chondr/o-fibr/o-sarc-oma, a malignant tumour of connective tissue containing fibrous, cartilaginous and mucoid elements

**myx/o**-chondr/o-sarc-oma, a malignant tumour of connective tissue containing cartilaginous and mucoid elements

**myx/o**-cyst-oma, a tumour in the form of a cyst containing mucoid tissue

**myx/o**-endotheli-oma, a tumour of the endothelium (of blood vessels) with myxomatous elements

**myx/o**-fibr-oma, a tumour of fibrous connective tissue containing mucoid tissue

**myx/o**-gli-oma, a tumour of neuroglial cells with myxomatous degeneration

297

**myx**-oid, resembling mucus

**myx/o**-lip-oma, a tumour of fatty and myxomatous tissue

**myx**-oma, a tumour of mucoid tissue, it resembles mesenchyme, the embryonic fibrous connective tissue

**myx**-omat-a, plural of myxoma

**myx**-omat-osis, 1. abnormal condition of the presence of myxomata (multiple myxomas) 2. myxomatous degeneration 3. a viral disease of rabbits

**myx**-omat-ous, pertaining to or of the nature of a myxoma

**myx/o**-sarc-oma, a malignant tumour of connective tissue with myxomatous elements

**myx/o**-sarc-omat-ous, pertaining to or of the nature of a myxosarcoma

pseudo-**myx**-oma, a false myxoma, it refers to a mass of mucus from epithelial cells resembling a myxoma

---

**Onc/o**, tumour

From a Greek word **ogkos**, meaning bulk. Here onc/o means a tumour.

**onc/o**-cyte, a tumour cell, it refers to an abnormal epithelial cell that may undergo neoplastic change

**onc/o**-cyt-ic, pertaining to an oncocyte

**onc/o**-dna-virus, a tumour or cancer, forming virus that contains DNA

**onc/o**-fet-al, pertaining to tumour, associated substances present in fetal tissue

**onc/o**-gene, a gene that has the potential to form malignant changes in cells

**onc/o**-genesis, pertaining to formation of a tumour

**onc/o**-gen-ic, pertaining to forming tumours

**onc/o**-gen-ous, 1. pertaining to originating in a tumour 2. pertaining to forming from a tumour

**onc/o**-log-ist, a medical specialist who studies and treats tumours

**onc/o**-logy, the study of tumours

**onc/o**-lys-ate, an agent that lyses or destroys tumour cells

**onc/o**-lysis, destruction or disintegration of a tumour

**onc/o**-lyt-ic, pertaining to destruction or disintegration of a tumour

**onc/o**-rna-virus, a tumour or cancer forming virus that contains RNA

**onc**-osis, abnormal condition of tumours

**onc/o**-therapy, the treatment of tumours

**onc/o**-tic, pertaining to or resulting from a tumour

**onc/o**-tomy, incision into a tumour

**onc/o**-trop-ic, pertaining to an affinity for tumours

**onc/o**-virus, a virus (infectious particle) that causes tumours or cancer

---

**-plas/t-**, forming cells or tissue, capable of changing shape or being moulded

From a Greek word **plassein** meaning to mould. Here -plast means the formation of new cells or tissues as in the development of a benign or malignant tumour.

ana-**plas**-ia, condition of reversion or going back of a specialized tissue to less differentiated type

ana-**plast**-ic, 1. reversion or going back of a specialized tissue to less differentiated type 2. pertaining to anaplasia

anti-neo-**plast**-ic, 1. pertaining to acting against neoplasms (new growths of malignant cells) 2. an agent that acts against neoplasms

anti-**plast**-ic, 1. pertaining to against growth or healing 2. an agent that suppresses the formation of cells particularly blood cells

a-**plas**-ia, condition of lack of formation of cells or tissue

a-**plast**-ic, 1. pertaining to lack of formation of cells or tissue 2. pertaining to aplasia 3. unable to form new tissue

cata-**plas**-ia, condition in which cells or tissues revert or atrophy to an earlier stage of development

dys-**plas**-ia, condition of poor growth of cells and tissues, it refers to abnormalities of size, shape and organization of cells

heter/o-meta-**plas**-ia, condition of replacement of normal tissue by different tissue that is not natural to the position in which it is produced heter/o-**plas**-ia, 1. condition in which normal cells are in the wrong or different position 2. condition of replacement of normal tissue by different tissue that is not natural to the position in which it is produced

heter/o-**plast**-ic, pertaining to heteroplasia

home/o-**plas**-ia, condition of formation of new cells or tissue similar to the normal tissue of the part

home/o-**plast**-ic, pertaining to homeoplasia

hyper-**plas**-ia, condition of above normal number of normal cells in a tissue or organ

hyper-**plast**-ic, pertaining to hyperplasia

meta-**plas**-ia, condition of change of form of adult cells in a tissue into another type abnormal to that tissue

neo-**plas**-ia, condition of forming a neoplasm, an abnormal new growth of cells

neo-**plas**m, a new growth, it refers to a new growth of cells or tissue forming a tumour. Neoplasms can be benign or malignant

neo-**plast**-ic, 1. pertaining to a neoplasm or neoplasia 2. pertaining to abnormal formation of new cells or tissues giving rise to a tumour

para-neo-**plast**-ic, pertaining to changes beyond a neoplasm, it refers to changes in tissues at sites away from a tumour or its metastases

**plast**-ic, 1. pertaining to forming tissue 2. capable of being moulded

poly-**plast**-ic, 1. pertaining to many changes in form of cells and tissues 2. pertaining to composed of many different structural elements

retro-**plas**-ia, condition of backward development or degeneration of cells to a more primitive type

---

**Polyp-**, polyp

From the Greek words **polys** meaning many and **pous** meaning foot. Here polyp- means a polyp, a tumour with a stalk arising from a mucous membrane or body surface.

polyp-ectomy, removal of a polyp

polyp-oid, resembling a polyp

polyp-osis, abnormal condition of having many polyps e.g. familial polyposis in which numerous polyps grow in the colon

polyp-ous, polyp-like

polyp-us, a polyp

pseudo-**polyp**, false polyp, it refers to a hypertrophied tag of mucous membrane possibly a result of inflammation

---

**Sarc/o**, connective tissue, flesh

**Sarcomat-**, sarcoma, a malignant tumour of connective tissue

From a Greek word **sarkoma**, meaning a fleshy growth. Here sarc/o means flesh or connective tissue. Malignant tumours of the connective tissues (sarcomas) can form from bone, cartilage, blood, lymph and muscle.

sarc/o-aden-oma, a mixed tumour with glandular and sarcomatous tissue

sarc/o-blast, an immature cell or embryonic cell that forms a muscle cell

sarc/o-carcin-oma, a mixed tumour with elements of a carcinoma and sarcoma

sarc/o-cele, a fleshy swelling, protrusion or tumour (of the testicles)

sarc/o-en-chondr-oma, a sarcoma within which there are elements of cartilage

sarc/o-gen-ic, pertaining to forming flesh

sarc/o-gen-ous, pertaining to forming flesh

sarc/o-hydro-cele, a fleshy swelling, protrusion or tumour (of a testicle) with a hydrocele, a swelling containing water or fluid

sarc-oid, 1. resembling flesh 2. sarcoidosis 3. an obsolete term for a sarcoma-like tumour

sarc-oid-osis, abnormal condition of sarcoma-like tumours, it refers to a granulomatous disease of unknown origin forming tubercles of non-necrotizing epithelioid tissue, especially in the lungs with resulting fibrosis

**sarc/o**-lysis, breakdown or disintegration of flesh

**sarc/o**-lyt-ic, 1. pertaining to sarcolysis 2. pertaining to breakdown or disintegration of flesh

**sarc**-oma, a malignant tumour of connective tissue

**sarcoma**-gen-ic, pertaining to the development of a sarcoma

**sarcomat**-a, sarcomas, plural of sarcoma

**sarcomat**-oid, resembling a sarcoma

**sarcomat**-osis, abnormal condition of having sarcomas at many sites

**sarcomat**-ous, pertaining to or of the nature of a sarcoma

**sarc**-omphal/o-cele, a fleshy tumour of the umbilicus

**sarc/o**-plast-ic, pertaining to forming flesh (muscle tissue)

**sarc/o**-poiet-ic, pertaining to forming flesh (muscle tissue)

**sarc**-osis, abnormal condition of fleshy growths

**sarc**-ost-osis, abnormal condition of bone element formation in flesh (muscle tissue)

**sarc**-ous, pertaining to flesh (muscle tissue)

# Section 20
## Anatomical position

This section lists the components of medical words that indicate the position of organs within the body and their relationship to each other. Many of these terms are used by doctors and other health care workers to indicate the position of injuries, pain or surgical procedures.

The anatomical position of the body (Figure 27) is a reference system that all medical staff and anatomical texts use when describing the location of parts of the body. We always refer positions and directions in a patient as if he/she were standing upright with arms at

the sides and palms of the hands facing forward, head erect and eyes looking forward.

With the body in the anatomical position we can draw an imaginary line down the middle of the body (Figure 27). This is called the **midline** or **median line** and it bisects the body into right and left sides. *Note that right and left refer to the sides of the patient in the anatomical position, not those of the observer.*

## Directions

We can now see how the imaginary midline can be used to indicate directions when a body is in the anatomical position. Parts that lie nearer to the median line of the body than another are described as **medial** to that part. Any part that lies further away is said to be **lateral** to the first part (Figure 28). Other directions are also shown with the body in this position.

## Locating anatomical parts

### External anatomy
With the body in the anatomical position a number of combining forms of word roots are used for the external anatomy. The two reference boxes on page 303 list combining forms of word roots associated with the external anatomy.

### Locative prefixes
There are many prefixes that can tell us about the location of anatomical parts;

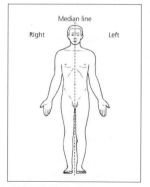

Figure 27 The anatomical position

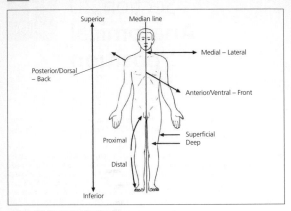

Figure 28  Anatomical directions

**Table 5**
**Examples of the use of directional terms**

| Direction | Meaning | Example |
|---|---|---|
| **Superior** | towards the head, upper | The eyes are **superior** to the mouth. |
| **Inferior** | away from the head, lower | The mouth is **inferior** to the nose. |
| **Anterior** (ventral) | front, towards the front | The sternum is **anterior** to the vertebral column. |
| **Posterior** (dorsal) | back, towards the back | The ear is **posterior** to the eye. |
| **Proximal** | pertaining to near the point of attachment or point of origin | The ankle is **proximal** to the toes. |
| **Distal** | pertaining to further from the point of attachment or origin | The wrist is **distal** to the elbow. |
| **Superficial** | pertaining to near the surface of the body | The ribs are **superficial** to the lungs. |
| **Deep** | away from the surface of the body | The lungs are **deep** to the ribs. |
| **Ventral** (anterior) | front, towards the front | The thymus gland is **ventral** to the aorta. |
| **Dorsal** (posterior) | back, towards the back | The lungs are **dorsal** to the sternum. |
| **Medial** | pertaining to towards the median line (or midline) | The nose is **medial** to the eye. |
| **Lateral** | pertaining to away from the median line (or midline) | The ear is **lateral** to the eye |

**Quick Reference**

Combining forms relating to external anatomy:

| | |
|---|---|
| **Axill/o** | armpit |
| **Blephar/o** | eyelid |
| **Brachi/o** | arm |
| **Bucc/o** | buccal cavity, cheek |
| **Cephal/o** | head |
| **Cervic/o** | neck |
| **Crur/o** | leg |
| **Digit/o** | finger or toe |
| **Faci/o** | face |
| **Femor/o** | femur, thigh |
| **Hallux** | great toe |
| **Ili/o** | flank (the side between ribs and ilium) |
| **Mamm/o** | breast, mammary gland |
| **Mast/o** | breast, mammary gland |
| **Nas/o** | nose |
| **Ocul/o** | eye |
| **Omphal/o** | umbilicus |
| **Ophthalm/o** | eye |
| **Orbit/o** | eye-socket |
| **Or/o** | mouth |
| **Ot/o** | ear |
| **Palm/o** | palm |
| **Palpebr/o** | eyelid |
| **Patell/o** | patella, knee cap |
| **Ped/o** | foot |
| **Phalang/o** | phalanx, finger, toe |
| **Pollex** | thumb |
| **Pub/o** | pubic region |
| **Rhin/o** | nose |
| **Stomat/o** | mouth |
| **Thorac/o** | thorax |
| **Umbilic-** | umbilicus |
| **Vol/o** | palm |

**Quick Reference**

Common words and combining forms relating external anatomy:

| | |
|---|---|
| Arm | **brachi/o** |
| Armpit | **axill/o** |
| Breast | **mamm/o, mast/o** |
| Buccal cavity | **bucc/o** |
| Cheek | **bucc/o** |
| Ear | **ot/o** |
| Eye | **ocul/o, ophthalm/o** |
| Eyelid | **blephar/o, palpebr/o** |
| Eye-socket | **orbit/o** |
| Face | **faci/o** |
| Femur | **femor/o** |
| Finger | **digit/o, phalang/o** |
| Flank | **ili/o** |
| Foot | **ped/o** |
| Great toe | **hallux** |
| Head | **cephal/o** |
| Knee cap | **patell/o** |
| leg | **crur/o** |
| mammary gland | **mamm/o, mast/o** |
| mouth | **or/o, stomat/o** |
| neck | **cervic/o** |
| nose | **nas/o, rhin/o** |
| palm | **palm/o, vol/o** |
| patella | **patell/o** |
| phalanx | **phalang/o** |
| pubic region | **pub/o** |
| side of the body | **ili/o** |
| thigh | **femor/o** |
| thumb | **pollex** |
| toe | **digit/o, phalang/o** |
| umbilicus | **omphal/o, umbilic-** |

| Prefix | Root | Suffix | Meaning |
|---|---|---|---|
| **epi-** | -gastr- | -ic | pertaining to upon or above the stomach |
| **endo-** | -gastr- | -ic | pertaining to within the stomach |
| **hypo-** | -gastr- | -ic | pertaining to below the stomach |

they act as prepositions when placed in front of word roots. A single word root can be modified by prefixes to form different medical words for example using the root **gastr-** meaning stomach:

The next two reference boxes list prefixes that can be used to indicate a position or direction of a part in relation to the anatomical position:

**Quick Reference**
Locative prefixes and their meanings:

| Locative prefix | Meaning | Example word |
|---|---|---|
| ab- | away or separate | **ab**duct |
| ad- | towards or near | **ad**nerval |
| af- | towards or near | **af**ferent |
| ag- | towards or near | **ag**gregation |
| ante- | before or in front | **ante**brachium |
| antero- | anterior or in front | **antero**lateral |
| anti- | against or opposite | **anti**clinal |
| ap- | towards or near | **ap**position |
| apo- | away or separate | **apo**crine |
| as- | towards or near | **as**sociation |
| at- | towards or near | **at**traction |
| circum- | around | **circum**oral |
| contra- | against or opposed | **contra**lateral |
| dextro- | right | **dextro**cardia |
| dia- | through or across | **dia**condylar |
| dis- | apart or separate | **dis**location |
| dors- | dorsal or back | **dors**ad |
| dorsi- | dorsal or back | **dorsi**flexion |
| dorso- | dorsal or back | **dorso**ventral |
| e- | out or away | **e**visceration |
| ec- | out or away | **ec**centric |
| ect- | outside | **ect**osteal |
| ef- | out or away | **ef**ferent |
| em- | in | **em**pyema |
| en- | in | **en**ophthalmos |
| endo- | in or inside | **endo**cardium |
| ento- | inside | **ento**retina |
| ep- | above or upon | **ep**axial |
| epi- | above or upon | **epi**gastric |
| ex- | out or away | **ex**crescence |
| exo- | out or outside | **exo**cardial |
| extra- | outside | **extra**cellular |
| hyp- | below or under | **hyp**arterial |
| hypo- | below or under | **hypo**glossal |
| hyper- | above | **hyper**phoria |
| in- | in | **in**version |
| infra- | beneath or under | **infra**tracheal |
| inter- | between | **inter**costal |
| intra- | inside | **intra**cellular |
| juxta- | adjoining | **juxta**glomerular |
| laevo- | left | **laevo**cardia |
| later- | side | **later**al |
| latero- | side | **latero**flexion |
| medi- | middle | **medi**al |
| meso- | middle | **meso**tympanum |
| meta- | next or after | **meta**carpal |
| opistho- | behind or backwards | **opisth**otic |
| para- | beside or near | **para**rectal |
| per- | through | **per**cutaneous |
| peri- | around | **peri**anal |
| post- | after or behind | **post**ganglionic |
| pre- | before or in front | **pre**vesical |
| pro- | before or in front | **pro**cephalic |

| Locative prefix | Meaning | Example word |
|---|---|---|
| re- | back | **re**curvation |
| retro- | behind or backwards | **retro**cervical |
| sub- | below or under | **sub**cutaneous |
| super- | above | **super**lateral |
| supra- | above | **supra**hepatic |
| sym- | together or with | **sym**podia |
| syn- | together or with | **syn**dactyly |
| trans- | through or across | **trans**urethral |
| ultra- | beyond | **ultra**ligation |
| ventr- | ventral or in front | **ventr**al |
| ventro- | ventral or in front | **ventro**lateral |

**Quick Reference**
Common words relating to locative prefixes

| Common word | Locative prefix |
|---|---|
| Above | ep-, epi-, hyper-, super-, supra-, |
| Across | dia, trans- |
| Adjoining | juxta- |
| After | meta-, post- |
| Against | anti, contra- |
| Anterior | antero- |
| Apart | dis- |
| Around | circum-, peri- |
| Away | ab-, apo-, e-, ec-, ef-, ex |
| Back | dors-, dorsi-, dorso-, re-, retro- |
| Backward | opistho-, retro |
| Before | ante-, pre-, pro- |
| Behind | opistho-, post-, retro- |
| Below | hyp-, hypo-, infra-, sub- |
| Beneath | hyp-, hypo-, infra-, sub- |
| Beside | para- |
| Between | inter- |
| Beyond | ultra- |
| Front | antero-, pro-, ventr-, ventro- |
| In | em-, en-, endo-, ento-, in-, intra- |

| | |
|---|---|
| In front | ante-, antero-, pre-, pro-, ventr-, ventro- |
| Inside | em-, en-, endo-, ento-, intra- |
| Left | laevo- |
| Middle | medi-, meso- |
| Near | ad-, af-, ag-, ap-, as, at-, para- |
| Next | meta- |
| Opposed | anti-, contra- |
| Opposite | anti-, contra- |
| Out | e-, ec-, ect-, ef-, ex-, exo-, extra- |
| Outside | ect-, ef-, exo-, extra- |
| Right | dextro- |
| Separate | ab-, apo-, dis- |
| Side | later-, latero- |
| Through | dia-, per-, trans- |
| To | ad-, af-, ag-, ap-, as, at- |
| Together | sym-, syn- |
| Towards | ad-, af-, ag-, ap-, as, at- |
| Under | hyp-, hypo-, infra-, sub- |
| Upon | ep-, epi- |
| Ventral | ventr-, ventro- |
| With | sym-, syn- |

# Section 21
# Microbiology

Microbiology is the study of organisms too small to be seen with the naked eye. Many microorganisms, including bacteria, fungi, protozoa and viruses, are pathogenic and are responsible for the spread of infectious disease. Swabs, fluids and tissues taken from patients suspected of having an infection are sent to the microbiology laboratories for analysis. The microbiology laboratory is often part of the pathology department in a large hospital. This section examines common words associated with microorganisms.

Microbiology is divided into the following specialities:

- **Bacteri**ology
  the study of bacteria
- **Myc**ology
  the study of fungi
- **Vir**ology
  the study of viruses
- **Protozoo**logy
  the study of protozoa

## Bacteriology

Bacteria are small single-celled organisms that can only be seen with an optical microscope. There are thousands of different types classified according to their shape, group arrangement, colony characteristics, structure, and chemical characteristics. The combining form bacteri/o is used to mean bacteria (from the Greek *bakterion* meaning staff).

## Classification of bacteria using the Gram staining reaction

For more than a century bacteria have been classified using the **Gram**-staining reaction named after Christian Gram who devised it in 1884. His method is

| Quick Reference | | |
|---|---|---|
| Combining forms relating to microbiology: | | |
| | | Page |
| **Bacill/i** | bacilli, | |
| | bacillus | 309 |
| **Bacteri/o** | bacterium, | |
| | bacteria | 310 |
| **Cocc/o** | cocci, coccus | 310 |
| **Fung/i** | fungus | 311 |
| **Micro-** | small | 311 |
| **Myc/o** | fungus | 311 |
| **Protozo/a** | protozoon, | |
| | protozoa | 312 |
| **Spirill/i** | spirilla, | |
| | spirillum | 312 |
| **Staphyl/o** | staphylococcus | 312 |
| **Staphylococc/i** | staphylococcus | 312 |
| **Strept/o** | streptococcus | 312 |
| **Streptococc/i** | streptococcus | 312 |
| **Vir/o** | virus, virion | 313 |

| Quick Reference | | |
|---|---|---|
| Common words and combining forms relating to microbiology: | | |
| | | Page |
| Bacteria | **bacteri/o** | 310 |
| Bacterium | **bacteri/o** | 310 |
| Bacilli | **bacill/i** | 309 |
| Bacillus | **bacill/o** | 309 |
| Cocci | **cocc/o** | 310 |
| Coccus | **cocc/o** | 310 |
| Fungus | **fung/i,** | |
| | **myc/o** | 311 |
| Protozoa | **protozo/o** | 312 |
| Protozoon | **protozo/o** | 312 |
| Small | **micro-** | 311 |
| Spirilla | **spirill/i** | 312 |
| Spirillum | **spirill/i** | 312 |
| Staphylococcus | **staphyl/o,** | |
| | **staphylococc/i** | 312 |
| Streptococcus | **strept/o,** | |
| | **streptococc/i** | 312 |
| Virion | **vir/o** | 313 |
| Virus | **vir/o** | 313 |

based upon the ability of bacteria to retain the purple crystal violet–iodine complex when stained and treated with organic solvents:

**Gram-positive bacteria** (Gram +ve) retain the stain and appear purple
**Gram-negative bacteria** (Gram −ve) cannot retain the purple dye complex and need to be stained with a red dye before they can be seen with an optical microscope

## Classification by shape and grouping

Individual bacteria have one of three basic shapes, they are either spherical, cylindrical or spiral. Spherical cells are called **cocci** (singular – **coccus**), cylindrical cells **bacilli** (singular – **bacillus**) and helical or spiral cells **spirilla** (singular – **spirillum**).

### 1 The coccus (plural – cocci)

The word coccus comes from a Greek word *kokkos* meaning berry. They are usually round but can be ovoid or flattened on one side when adhering to another cell. Cocci can grow in several different arrangements or groups depending on the plane of cell division, and whether the new cells remain together. Each arrangement is typical of a species and contributes to an organism's classification. When a coccus divides in one plane and the two new cells remain together, the arrangement is called a **diplococcus**.

When cocci divide repeatedly in one plane and remain together to form a twisted row of cells they are called **streptococci** (*strepto-* from a Greek word meaning twisted, singular -streptococcus). Others divide in three planes and remain together in irregular, grape-like patterns: these are called **staphylococci** (*staphylo-* from a Greek word meaning grapes, singular – staphylococcus). See Figure 29A–D for examples of cocci.

Some cocci are of great medical importance. For example:

**Gram +ve**
*Streptococcus pneumoniae* – causes pneumonia and meningitis
*Staphylococcus aureus* – causes serious infection in hospitals (MRSA-methicillin resistant *Staphylococcus aureus*)
**Gram −ve**
*Neisseria gonorrhoeae* – causes gonorrhoea
*Neisseria meningitidis* – causes meningitis
(*Neisseria* are sometimes seen in pairs and are grouped as diplococci)

### 2 The bacillus (plural – bacilli)

These are rod-shaped bacteria (*bacillus* is a Latin word meaning a stick or rod). They are also classified using the Gram-staining procedure (see Figure 29E). There are large differences in the length and width of bacilli, and their ends can be square, rounded or tapered.

Some bacilli are of medical importance. For example:

**Gram +ve**
*Bacillus anthracis* – causes anthrax. Produces highly resistant spores that are difficult to destroy except at high temperatures
*Clostridium tetani* – found in soil. Causes tetanus

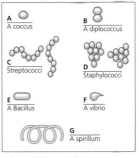

A — A coccus
B — A diplococcus
C — Streptococci
D — Staphylococci
E — A Bacillus
F — A vibrio
G — A spirillum

Figure 29 Shapes and group arrangements of bacteria

**Gram −ve**

*Escherichia coli* – found in the human gut. Certain strains are pathogenic

*Salmonella typhi* – causes typhoid

Gram −ve bacilli that appear curved in shape (like a comma) are called vibrios (see Figure 29F). Example:

*Vibrio cholerae* – causes cholera, a water-borne infection

### 3 The Spirillum (plural – spirilla)

The spirilla (from a Greek word *speira* meaning coil) are spiral or helical-shaped bacteria that look like tiny corkscrews (see Figure 29G). Those that belong to the genus *Spirillum* consist of Gram-ve, non-flexous (non-flexible) spiral-shaped filaments. Another group distinguished by their flexibility belong to the genus *Spirochaeta*. (Note: the use of this group is becoming obsolete and most of the bacteria assigned to it have been transferred to other genera.) Examples:

*Spirillum minus* – causes rat-bite fever in man

*Treponema pallidum* – a spirochaete (*Am. spirochete*) that belongs to the Order Spirochaetales and causes syphilis.

It should be noted that the cells of a given species are rarely arranged in exactly the same pattern. It is the predominant arrangement that is important when studying bacteria.

Some terms denoting shape, for example bacillus, may be used as generic names, as in *Bacillus anthracis*.

### Culture and sensitivity testing

Infected swabs, fluids and tissues are sent to microbiology laboratories for culture and sensitivity testing. To culture an organism, it is placed at an optimum temperature in a special culture medium (broth or agar jelly) that contains all the nutrients required for growth. In ideal conditions the microorganism multiplies rapidly, producing a huge clone of identical cells. Samples from the culture are then exposed to a range of different antibiotics. If an organism is sensitive to a particular antibiotic, it will be destroyed or its growth inhibited. Antibiotics that are found to destroy the cultured organisms are administered to the patient to try to rid them of the infection.

## Mycology

Fungi are non-green plants that act as decomposers in the environment, breaking down the dead bodies of plants and animals. The group includes the familiar mushrooms and toadstools, and microscopic moulds and yeasts. Certain types of moulds and yeasts are pathogenic and infect the body causing disease. When they infect the skin they are called **dermatophytes** (*demat/o* meaning skin, *-phyte* plant). A common condition is Athlete's foot caused by several species of fungi, e.g. *Trichophyton rubrum*, which infects skin between the toes. In warm, moist conditions, the fungi grow and digest the skin causing it to itch and split. The fungal spores that generate the infection are usually picked up on changing room floors, so the condition is common among sports enthusiasts. Athlete's foot is easily treated and harmless, unlike some fungal infections found in tropical climates.

When round, red patches of skin infected with fungi begin to heal they often take on a ring-like appearance. Because of this the infection became inaccurately known as 'ringworm'. The medical name for Athlete's foot is **Tinea pedis** or ringworm of the foot (*Tinea* is a Latin word meaning gnawing worm, and *-pedis* means the foot). Other super-ficial fungal infections of the skin are named in a similar way: **Tinea capitis** (ringworm of the head); **Tinea corporis** (ringworm of the body).

Fungal infections are life-threatening in patients whose immune system is compromised. For example, *Candida*

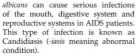

*albicans* can cause serious infections of the mouth, digestive system and reproductive systems in AIDS patients. This type of infection is known as Candidiasis (*-iasis* meaning abnormal condition).

Fungi are named according to the binomial system with a generic and specific name, as in *Candida albicans*.

## Virology

A virus (virion) is an extremely small infectious particle that does not show the usual characteristics of life; for example, it does not move, respire, feed or respond to stimuli.

Viruses do reproduce but only within a specific host cell. (Note: a host is an organism that harbours a parasite.) When a virus comes into contact with a host cell, it inserts its genes. Once inside the viral genes alter the metabolism of the host cell and instruct it to make new viruses. The host cell fills with copies of the original virus and may burst, releasing the new infectious particles into the surrounding environment.

Viruses have characteristic shapes, different chemical structures and different methods of replication. They can only be seen with an electron microscope that produces a large magnification and has the ability to resolve their fine detail. Characteristics of viruses and the conditions they cause are incorporated into their names.

Examples: the words have been split to show their meaning.

Onco-rna-**virus** – a type of virus that causes cancer (onc/o) and contains ribonucleic acid (-rna-)

Papo-va-**virus** – a type of virus that causes vacuoles (va) inside host cells and the formation of papillomas (papo -papilloma)

Pico-rna-**virus** – a type of virus that is very small (pico-) and contains ribonucleic acid (-rna-)

Retro-**virus** – a type of virus that carries the enzyme reverse transcriptase that catalyses the conversion of RNA back into DNA (retro-back)

Rhino-**virus** – a type of virus that infects the nose (rhin/o- nose)

Entero-**virus** – a type of virus that infects the intestines

Bacterio-phage – a type of virus that uses a bacterium as a host, destroying it in the process

## Protozoology

This is a branch of medicine concerned with single-celled animals called protozoa. Some of these organisms are pathogenic and responsible for serious disease. Infection with protozoa is generally referred to as a protozoiasis. Examples:

*Plasmodium falciparum* (a type of sporozoan) – causes malaria

*Trypanosoma gambiense* (a type of flagellate) – causes African sleeping sickness

*Entamoeba histolytica* (a type of amoeba) – causes amoebic dysentery

---

**Roots and combining forms**, meanings

**Bacill/i/o**, bacillus, bacilli
From a Latin word **bacillus** meaning a small rod or staff. Here bacill/o means bacilli, rod-shaped spore-forming bacteria belonging to the genus Bacillus (Family Bacillaceae).

**bacill**-aem-ia, condition of bacilli in the blood

**bacill**-ary, 1. pertaining to bacilli 2. pertaining to being rod-like

**bacilli**, 1. rod-shaped, spore-forming microorganisms of the genus Bacillus (Family Bacillaceae) 2. the plural of bacillus

**bacill/i**-cid-al, pertaining to killing or destroying bacilli

**bacill/i**-cide, an agent that kills or destroys bacilli

**bacill/i**-form, having the form or shape of a bacillus

**bacill**-in, an agent (antibiotic) produced by *Bacillus subtilis*

**bacill**-osis, abnormal condition or disease caused by infection with bacilli

**bacill**-ur-ia, condition of bacilli in the urine

**bacill**-us, 1. a rod-shaped, spore-forming microorganism of the genus Bacillus (Family Bacillaceae) 2. the singular of bacilli

---

**Bacter/i/o**, bacteria, bacterium
From a Greek word **bakterion** meaning small staff. Here bacteri/o means bacteria, single-celled prokaryotic microorganisms responsible for many types of infection.

anti-**bacteri**-al, 1. pertaining to acting against or destroying bacteria 2. an agent that destroys bacteria

**bacter**-aem-ia, condition of bacteria in the blood Syn. bacteriaemia

**bacter**-aem-ic, 1. pertaining to having bacteraemia 2. pertaining to having bacteria in the blood

**bacter**ia, the plural of bacterium, single-celled prokaryotic microorganisms

**bacteri**-aem-ia, condition of bacteria in the blood Syn. bacteraemia

**bacteri**-al, pertaining to bacteria

**bacteri**-cid-al, pertaining to killing bacteria

**bacteri**-cide, any agent that kills bacteria

**bacteri**-cid-in, an agent that kills bacteria, it refers to a bactericidal antibody

**bacteri/o**-cid-al, pertaining to killing bacteria

**bacteri/o**-gen-ic, 1. pertaining to originating in bacteria 2. pertaining to forming bacteria

**bacteri/o**-log-ical, pertaining to bacteriology

**bacteri/o**-log-ist, a specialist who studies bacteria

**bacteri/o**-logy, the study of bacteria

**bacteri/o**-lys-in, an agent that lyses or splits bacteria, it refers to a bactericidal antibody

**bacteri/o**-lysis, lysis or breakdown of bacterial cells

**bacteri/o**-lyt-ic, 1. pertaining to bacteriolysis 2. pertaining to lysis or breakdown of bacterial cells

**bacteri/o**-pexy, the fixation of bacteria, by phagocytic histiocytes

**bacteri/o**-phage, a virus that lyses or splits bacteria

**bacteri**-opson-in, an agent that acts on bacteria, it refers to an antibody or complement proteins that render bacteria more susceptible to phagocytosis. From a Greek word *opsonein* meaning to provide with food

**bacteri/o**-stat, any agent that stops or inhibits the growth of bacteria

**bacteri/o**-stat-ic, 1. pertaining to stopping or inhibiting the growth of bacteria 2. an agent that stops or inhibits the growth of bacteria

**bacteri/o**-tox-aem-ia, condition of bacterial poisons or toxins in the blood

**bacteri**-um, 1. a single-celled prokaryotic microorganism 2. the singular of bacteria

**bacteri**-ur-ia, condition of bacteria in the urine

---

**Cocc/i/o**, cocci, coccus
From a Greek word **kokkos** meaning berry. Here cocc/o means a coccus, a spherical bacterium less than 1μ in diameter.

**cocc**-al, pertaining to or originating in cocci

**cocc**i, the plural of coccus, spherical bacteria less than 1μ in diameter

**cocc/i**-gen-ic, pertaining to produced by cocci

**cocc/o**-bacillus, a short bacillus resembling a coccus, intermediate between a bacillus and coccus

**cocc/o**-bacteria, a general name for spherical bacteria, cocci of any kind

**cocc/o**-gen-ous, pertaining to forming cocci

**cocc**-oid, 1. resembling a coccus 2. spherical or berry-like

**cocc**-us, 1. a spherical bacterium less than 1μ in diameter 2. the singular of cocci

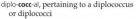

diplo-**cocc**-al, pertaining to a diplococcus or diplococci

diplo-**cocc**-aem-ia, condition of diplococci in the blood

diplo-**cocc**-oid, resembling a diplococcus

diplo-**cocc**-us, a spherical coccus that occurs in pairs as a result of incomplete cell division in one plane

---

**Fung/i/os**, fungus

From a Greek word **fungus** meaning mushroom. Here fung/i means a fungus or fungal infection.

anti-**fung**-al, 1. pertaining to acting against fungi 2. an agent that acts against fungi or against a fungal infection

**fung**-al, pertaining to or caused by a fungus

**fung**-ate, 1. having fungus-like growths 2. to grow rapidly like a fungus, sometimes used to describe the growth of fungus-like tumours

**fungi**-cid-al, pertaining to killing fungi

**fungi**-cide, an agent that kills fungi

**fungi**-form, having the form of a fungus

**fungi**-stasis, the stopping of the growth of fungi

**fungi**-stat-ic, pertaining to stopping the growth of fungi

**fungi**-tox-ic, pertaining to poisonous to fungi

**fung**-oid, resembling a fungus

**fungos**-ity, 1. condition of resembling a fungus 2. a fungus-like growth

**fung**-ous, pertaining to fungi or a fungus-like growth

---

**Micro-**, small

From a Greek word **mikros** meaning small. Here micro- is used with words associated with microbiology. Other words associated with cells and microscopy are listed in Section 1 Cells, tissues, organs and systems.

**micro**-be, a general term for a microorganism especially one causing disease. From the Greek words *mikros* meaning small and *bios* meaning life

**micro**be-cide, an agent that destroys microbes

**microb**-ial, 1. pertaining to to a microbe or microorganism 2. having the characteristics of a microbe or microorganism

**microb**-ic, pertaining to or caused by microbes or microorganisms

**micro**-bio-log-ical, pertaining to the study of microbiology

**micro**-bio-log-ist, a specialist who studies microbiology or microorganisms

**micro**-bio-logy, the study of small life, it refers to the study of microorganisms

**micro**-bio-phot/o-meter, an instrument that measures light passing through microbes, it detects turbidity in a bacterial culture medium

**micro**-fauna, small (microscopic) animals of a region

**micro**-flora, small (microscopic) plants of a region

**micro**-organism, a small organism, any plant or animal of microscopic size, a protozoon, fungus, alga, bacterium or virus

**micro**-path/o-log-ical, pertaining to micropathology

**micro**-path/o-logy, 1. the study of small pathological changes 2. the study of diseases due to microorganisms

**micro**-zoon, a small (microscopic) animal

---

**Myc/o, mycot-**, fungus

From a Greek word **mykes** meaning fungus. Here myc/o means a fungus or fungi.

anti-**mycot**-ic, 1. an agent that acts against fungi or against a fungal infection 2. pertaining to acting against fungi

**myc/o**-log-ist, a specialist who studies fungi

**myc/o**-logy, the study of fungi

**myc/o**-myring-itis, inflammation of the tympanic membrane (ear drum) caused by fungi

**myc**-osis, abnormal condition or disease caused by fungi

**mycot**-ic, pertaining to caused by fungi

**myc/o**-toxic-osis, 1. condition of poisoning by eating fungi 2. condition of poisoning with a fungal toxin

**myc/o**-tox-in, a poisonous agent produced by a fungus

---

**Protozo/a, protozo/o,** protozoon, protozoa

From the Greek words **protos** meaning first and **zoon** meaning animal. Here protozo/a means a protozoon, a single-celled animal; some types of protozoa can infect humans and are of great medical importance *e.g.* malaria.

**protozoa**, 1. single-celled animals belonging to the Subkingdom Protozoa 2. the plural of protozoon

**protozo/a**-cide, an agent that kills or destroys protozoa

**protozo**-al, 1. pertaining to protozoa 2. pertaining to caused by protozoa

**protozo**-an, 1. pertaining to protozoa 2. pertaining to caused by protozoa

**protozo**-iasis, abnormal condition or disease caused by protozoa

**protozo/o**-logy, the study of protozoa

**protozoon**, 1. single-celled animal belonging to the Subkingdom Protozoa 2. the singular of protozoa

**protozo/o**-phage, a cell that 'eats' protozoa, meaning a cell that destroys protozoa by phagocytosis

---

**Spirill/i,** spirillum, spirilla

From a Greek word **speira** meaning coil. Here, spirill/i means Spirillum, a genus of corkscrew-shaped, non-flexous, Gram-negative bacteria. Some spirilla are potential pathogens causing disease in man.

**spirilla**, the plural of spirillum, a corkscrew-shaped, non-flexous, Gram-negative bacterium belonging to the genus Spirillum

**spirill**-aem-ia, condition of spirilla in the blood

**spirill/i**-cid-al, pertaining to killing or destroying spirilla

**spirill/i**-cide, an agent that kills or destroys spirilla

**spirill**-osis, abnormal condition or disease caused by spirilla

**spirill**-um, 1. corkscrew-shaped, non-flexous, Gram-negative bacterium belonging to the genus Spirillum 2. the singular of spirilla

---

**Staphyl/o,** staphylococc/i, staphylococcus, staphylococci

From the Greek words **staphyle** meaning bunch of grapes and **kokkos** meaning berry. Here, staphyl/o and staphylococc/i refer to staphylococci, Gram-positive bacteria growing in grape-like clusters that belong to the genus Staphylococcus. Staphylococci are potential pathogens causing serious disease.

**staphylococc**-aem-ia, condition of staphylococci in the blood

**staphylococc**-al, pertaining to or caused by staphylococci

**staphylococci**, 1. clusters of berry-like bacteria belonging to the genus Staphylococcus 2. the plural of staphylococcus

**staphylococc**-ic, pertaining to or caused by staphylococci

**staphylococc/i**-cide, an agent that kills or destroys staphylococci

**staphylococc**-us, 1. a berry-like bacterium that joins with others to form grape-like clusters belonging to the genus Staphylococcus 2. the singular of staphylococci

**staphyl/o**-derma, presence of staphylococci in the skin

**staphyl/o**-dermat-itis, inflammation of the skin caused by staphylococcal infection

**staphyl/o**-lys-in, an agent produced by staphylococci that lyses or breaks down blood cells

---

**Strept/o,** streptococc/i, streptococcus, streptococci

From the Greek words **streptos** meaning curved and **kokkos** meaning berry. Here, strept/o and streptococc/i refer to Streptococcus, a genus of Gram-positive bacteria growing in curved chains of varying length. Streptococci are potential pathogens causing serious disease.

**streptococc**-aem-ia, condition of streptococci in the blood

**streptococc**-al, pertaining to or caused by streptococci

**streptococci**, 1. curved chains of berry-like bacteria belonging to the genus Streptococcus 2. the plural of streptococcus

**streptococc**-ic, pertaining to or caused by streptococci

**streptococc/i**-cide, an agent that kills or destroys streptococci

**streptococc/i**-osis, abnormal condition or disease caused by streptococci

**streptococc**-us, 1. a berry-like bacterium belonging to the genus Streptococcus that joins with others to form curved chains 2. the singular of streptococcus

**strept/o**-derma, presence of streptococci in the skin

**strept/o**-dermat-itis, inflammation of the skin caused by streptococcal infection

**strept/o**-dorn-ase, an enzyme produced by streptococci that catalyses the depolymerization of deoxyribose nucleic acid (DNA). Used with streptokinase as desloughing agents to liquefy clots and pus

**strept/o**-kin-ase, an enzyme produced by streptococci that breaks down fibrin, used as a thrombolytic agent

**strept/o**-lys-in, an agent produced by streptococci that lyses or breaks down blood cells

**strept/o**-septic-aem-ia, condition of septicaemia (blood poisoning) caused by streptococci

---

**Vir/i/o/u**, virion, virus

From a Greek word **virus**, meaning poison. Here vir/o means a virus, a minute infectious particle that replicates only within a living host cell. Each particle consists of viral genes (DNA or RNA) enclosed in a protein coat.

anti-retro-**vir**-al, 1. pertaining to acting against retroviruses such as HIV 2. an agent that acts against retroviruses

anti-**vir**-al, 1. pertaining to acting against viruses or a viral infection 2. an agent that acts against viruses or a viral infection

**vir**-aem-ia, condition of having viruses in the blood

**vir**-al, 1. pertaining to a virus 2. caused by a virus

**vir/i**-cide, agent that kills viruses

**vir/i**-on, a complete mature viral particle or virus

**vir/o**-log-ical, 1. pertaining to virology 2. pertaining to the study of viruses and viral diseases

**vir/o**-lact-ia, condition of secretion viruses in milk

**vir/o**-log-ist, a specialist who studies virology

**vir/o**-logy, the study of viruses and viral diseases

**vir/u**-cid-al, pertaining to destroying viruses

**vir/u**-cide, an agent that destroys viruses

**vir**-ur-ia, condition of viruses in the urine

# Section 22
# Pharmacology

Pharmacology is the science that deals with the study of drugs. By drugs we mean medicinal substances that can be used to treat, prevent or diagnose disease and illness. Research into the properties and potential use of substances showing physiological activity has enabled the pharmaceutical industry to market new and more effective drugs. This section lists the main words associated with pharmacy and a list of the main drug classifications.

---

**Roots and combining forms**, meanings

## Pharmac/o

From a Greek word **pharmakon** meaning drug. Here pharmac/o means a drug or pharmaceutical.

**pharmac**-ist, a specialist who dispenses drugs, a pharmaceutical chemist

---

**Quick Reference**
Drug classification relating to body systems and infections:

**pharmac/o**-dynam-ics, the study of the action of drugs, that is what the drug does to the body

**pharmac/o**-gnosy, the study of crude drugs of vegetable and animal origin. From a Greek word *gnosis* meaning knowledge of

**pharmac/o**-kine-tics, the study of movement of drugs, the study of how drugs are absorbed, metabolized and excreted, *i.e.* what the body does to the drug and how it moves through the body

**pharmac/o**-log-ist, 1. a specialist who studies drugs 2. a specialist who studies pharmacology

**pharmac/o**-logy, the scientific study of drugs (their chemistry, actions and uses)

**pharmac/o**-psych-osis, abnormal condition of a psychosis induced by drugs

**pharmac**-y, 1. the study of the process of preparing and dispensing medicinal drugs 2. a place where drugs are compounded or dispensed

There are several individual specialisms related to pharmacology including:

**Therapeutics** – the branch of medicine that deals with the treatment of disease. Treatment can be **palliative** *i.e.* alleviates symptoms, or **curative**. In common usage, therapeutics refers mainly to the use of drugs to treat disease.

**Chemotherapy** – the treatment of disease using chemical agents, a main type of treatment for cancer.

**Toxicology** – the study of poisons and other toxic substances and their effect on the body.

## Naming drugs

Drugs are known by several different names.

### The brand, trade or proprietory name

Following extensive research and development, pharmaceutical companies assign brand names to their products for marketing purposes. Each drug and its name is the exclusive property of the company with patent rights to its manufacture. The patent will expire after a fixed time (usually seventeen years) allowing time for development costs to be recouped. When the patent has expired the drug may be manufactured by other companies under different brand names or under the drug's generic name.

### The generic name

Each drug has an official non-proprietory or generic name. This name is assigned to it in its early stage of development and often a description of its chemical composition or class. A generic drug may be manufactured by any number of companies under different brand names once the patent has expired.

A recent EEC directive requires the use of a Recommended International Non-propriety Name (rINN) for medicinal substances. Many British Approved Names (BANs) have been changed or modified to comply with the rINN directive.

### The chemical name

This name indicates a drug formula and is used by a manufacturer or pharmacist when making up a formulation.

Authoritative information about the use, structure, manufacture, and the dosage of medicinal drugs is documented in large reference texts known as a *pharmacopoeia*.

In pharmacology certain suffixes are used to denote types of substance:

| Suffix | Meaning | Examples |
|---|---|---|
| -ase | indicates an enzyme | amyl**ase**/ sucr**ase** |
| -gen | a precursor or agent that produces | trypsino**gen** |
| -ic | denotes a type of medicinal drug | mucolyt**ic** |
| -in | non-specific suffix denoting chemical agent | tristerl**in** |
| -ine | substance derived from ammonia | am**ine**/ alan**ine** |
| -ite | end product | metabol**ite** |
| -ose | a type of sugar | gluc**ose**/ malt**ose** |

## Drug classification

Drugs can be classified by their therapeutic use or action. There follows a list of general drug classifications used to treat infections and disorders associated with the body systems listed in this book.

Note: the suffixes -al, -ant, -ent -ic, and -ive are all used to mean *pertaining to* but they can all be used in pharmacology to indicate a type of drug.

## Drug classifications associated with body systems

### The digestive system

**ant-acid,** a drug used to neutralize stomach acid, used as a treatment for dyspepsia or heartburn

**anti-diarrhoe-al,** a drug that acts against diarrhoea

**anti-spasmod-ic,** a drug that acts against an intestinal spasm (reduces symptoms of)

**$H_2$-receptor antagonist,** a drug that prevents the secretion of acid by the gastric mucosa and promotes the healing of ulcers

**laxative,** an agent that promotes evacuation of the bowels

## The respiratory system

**anti-histam-ine**, a drug that acts against the effects of histamine, a chemical released during allergic reactions such as asthma

**anti-tuss-ive**, a drug that acts against coughs

**bronch/o-dilat-or**, a drug that dilates bronchi

**cortic/o-steroid**, a drug used to reduce inflammation. Here they are used for prophylaxis in the treatment of asthma by reducing inflammation in the bronchial mucosa (lining).

**decongestant**, a drug used to reduce the feeling of congestion in the nose

**muc/o-lyt-ic**, a drug that breaks up mucus

## The cardiovascular system and blood

**alpha-blocker**, a drug that blocks alpha-adrenoceptors causing vasodilation, used as a long-acting antihypertensive to reduce blood pressure

**angiotensin-converting enzyme inhibitor (ACE inhibitor)**, a drug that inhibits the conversion of angiotensin I to angiotensin II, used for treatment of heart failure and high BP (hypertension)

**anti-a-rrhyth-ic**, a drug that acts against arrhythmias (an arrhythmia is an abnormal heart beat that is one without a rhythm)

**anti-coagul-ant**, a drug that acts against coagulation (clotting of blood), it prevents the formation of blood clots

**anti-fibrin/o-lyt-ic**, a drug that acts against the break down of clots, it is used to promote clotting in severe haemorrhage

**anti-hypertens-ive**, a drug that acts against hypertension, it reduces high blood pressure

**anti-platelet**, a drug that acts against platelet aggregation in arteries and thereby inhibits clot formation

**beta-adrenoceptor blocking drug (beta-blocker)**, a drug that blocks the beta-adrenoceptors in the heart, peripheral vessels, bronchi, pancreas and liver. They reduce BP and heart rate and are used in management of angina and hypertension

**diuret-ic**, a drug used to promote the excretion of urine thereby relieving the oedema of heart failure

**fibrin/o-lyt-ic**, a drug that breaks down fibrin, it is used to break down fibrin found in blood clots or thrombi

**haem/o-stat-ic**, a drug that brings about haemostasis (the clotting of blood)

**inotrop-ic**, a drug used to increase the force of contraction of heart muscle (a positive inotropic)

**scleros-ant (local)**, a chemical irritant that hardens blood vessels, used to treat haemorrhoids

**sympath/o-mimet-ic**, a drug that mimics the action of the sympathetic nervous system raising blood pressure

**vas/o-dilator anti-hypertens-ive**, a drug that dilates blood vessels, thereby reducing high blood pressure *i.e.* reducing hypertension

## The immune system

Drugs in this section are used mainly to suppress the cells that bring about the rejection of transplanted organs in their recipients or to treat autoimmune diseases. (*auto-* meaning self), autoimmunity is an abnormal response of the immune system to the body's own tissues.

**cortic/o-steroid**, a steroid drug used to suppress the immune system and prevent organ transplant rejection, they are also used to reduce inflammation

**cyt/o-tox-ic**, a drug that is toxic or poisonous to cells and kills them

**immun/o-suppress-ant**, a drug that suppresses the immune system and immune response, they are used to suppress the cells that bring about the rejection of transplanted organs

**interferon**, an immune system regulator used to treat patients with multiple sclerosis *e.g.* interferon beta 1b

**monoclonal antibody**, rituximab is a type of monoclonal antibody that can destroy β-lymphocytes

## The urinary system

**alpha-blocker**, a drug that blocks alpha-adrenoceptors, it is used to relax smooth muscle producing an increased flow rate of urine in benign prostatic hyperplasia

**anti-diuretic hormone**, a hormone that acts on the kidney stimulating reabsorption of water thereby reducing the formation of urine

**anti-muscarin-ic**, a drug used to treat urinary frequency by increasing bladder capacity (antimuscarinic means acting against cholinergic effects similar to those produced by the action of muscarine, an alkaloid found in poisonous fungi)

**diuret-ic**, a drug used to promote the excretion of urine

**uricos-ur-ic**, a drug used to increase the excretion of uric acid in urine thereby relieving the symptoms of gout

**xanthine-oxidase inhibitor**, a drug used for the palliative treatment of gout, it reduces the formation of uric acid from purines

## The nervous system

**an-alges-ic**, a drug used to relieve pain, opioid analgesics are used to relieve moderate to severe pain particularly of visceral origin (opioid refers to a synthetic narcotic resembling but not derived from opium)

**anti-depress-ant**, a drug that acts against depression, it prevents or relieves depression

**anti-emet-ic**, a drug that acts against or prevents vomiting (emesis)

**anti-epilept-ic**, a drug that acts against epilepsy

**anti-man-ic**, a drug used to control acute attacks of mania and prevent their reoccurrence

**anxi/o-lyt-ic**, a drug that breaks down anxiety, *i.e.* relieves the symptoms of anxiety

**anti-psychot-ic**, a drug that acts against a psychosis or relieves the symptoms of a psychosis such as schizophrenia

**CNS stimul-ant**, a drug that has limited use for treating narcolepsy, a recurrent, uncontrollable desire to sleep

**hypnot-ic**, a drug that induces sleep

## The eye

**an-aesthet-ic (local)**, a drug used to reduce sensation in the eye

**anti-infect-ive preparation (topical)**, antibacterial, antifungal or antiviral applied directly to the eye

**cortic/o-steroid (topical)**, an anti-inflammatory steroid drug applied directly to the eye

**cycl/o-pleg-ic**, a drug used to paralyse the ciliary body of the eye for examination of the eye

**eye lotion**, a solution for irrigation of the eye

**mydriat-ic**, a drug used to dilate the pupil or cause mydriasis for examination of the eye

**miot-ic**, a drug used to treat glaucoma, a side effect being that the pupil is reduced in diameter

## The ear

**anti-infect-ive preparation (topical)**, an antibacterial or antifungal applied directly to the external ear for treatment of otitis externa

**astring-ent (topical)**, a drug used to treat inflammation and dry up secretion of fluid

## The skin

**anti-perspir-ant**, a drug used against sweating, used for the treatment of excessive sweating (hyperhidrosis)

**anti-prurit-ic**, a drug that acts against pruritus, it reduces itching

**cortic/o-steroid (topical)**, an anti-inflammatory steroid applied directly to the skin to reduce inflammation in non-infective conditions such as eczema

**desloughing agent**, an agent that removes dead tissue from a wound

**emollient**, an agent that softens or soothes the skin

**kerat/o-lyt-ic**, a drug that breaks down the epidermis, it is used to remove warts, overgrowths of the epidermis caused by viral infection

**retinoid (oral)**, a drug used for the treatment of severe psoriasis that is resistant to other forms of treatment

**vehicle**, an inert substance added to drugs that gives a suitable consistency for transfer into the body, vehicles do not possess therapeutic properties

---

### The nose and mouth

**anti-histamine (oral)**, a drug that reduces the symptoms of histamine, used for treatment of nasal allergy

**nasal decongest-ant (topical)**, a drug applied directly to the nose as drops or spray to relieve congestion

**nasal decongest-ant (systemic)**, a drug used for symptomatic relief in chronic nasal obstruction given by mouth or injection

---

### The musculoskeletal system

**anti-cholinesterase**, a drug that acts against cholinesterase, used to enhance neuromuscular transmission in voluntary and involuntary muscle in the condition myasthenia gravis

**cortic/o-steroid**, an anti-inflammatory steroid used to treat inflammation in rheumatic disease. Intra-articular injection of local corticosteroids can relieve pain and inflammation in a joint

**disease modifying anti-rheumat-ic**, a drug that acts against rheumatism, it relieves the signs and symptoms of rheumatism. These drugs are sometimes known as DMARDs *i.e.* disease-modifying antirheumatic drugs

**muscle relax-ant**, a drug that blocks the neuromuscular junction and produces relaxation of muscles, they are widely used in anaesthesia

**non-steroidal anti-inflammatory drug (NSAID)**, a non-steroid drug that has analgesic and anti-inflammatory effects. NSAIDs are used to treat painful inflammatory conditions such as rheumatic disease, aspirin is a familiar example

**rubefaci-ent**, a topical antirheumatic agent that produces a counter irritant effect on the skin and relieves the pain from muscles, tendons and joints

**uricos-ur-ic**, a drug that promotes the excretion of uric acid in the urine thereby relieving the symptoms of gout

---

### The reproductive system and obstetrics

**andro-gen**, a male sex-hormone *e.g.* testosterone, used for hormone replacement therapy in castrated males or those with hypogonadal conditions

**anti-androgen**, an agent that acts against androgens, used in the treatment of sexual deviation and hypersexuality in males

**anti-oestrogen**, a drug that acts against oestrogen

**contracept-ive**, an agent or drug used to prevent conception *i.e.* the fertilization of an egg by a sperm. Family planning pills contain sex hormones that inhibit the release of eggs from the ovary thereby preventing a pregnancy

**gonad/o-troph-in**, a drug used to stimulate the gonads (reproductive organs)

**myometrial relax-ant**, a beta$_2$ agonist that relaxes the smooth muscle of the uterus and thereby prevents premature delivery Syn. beta$_2$-sympathomimetic, beta$_2$ adrenoceptor stimulant

**oestro-gen**, a female sex-hormone used in hormone replacement therapy and in oral contraceptive pills

**oxy-toc-ic**, a drug used to induce labour, resulting in a quick birth

**prostagland-in**, a drug used to induce abortion, augment labour and to minimize blood loss from the placental site

**progesto-gen**, a female sex-hormone used in the treatment of endometriosis, hormone replacement therapy and oral contraception

**sex hormone**, a steroid used for hormone replacement therapy (HRT) for example, menopausal symptoms are relieved by small doses of the female sex hormone oestrogen. The male sex hormones called androgens are used for replacement therapy in castrated males

### The endocrine system
This section deals with examples of drug classifications associated with the endocrine system other than those that act on the reproductive system.

**anti-diabet-ic**, a drug that acts against diabetes, it is used for treatment of non-insulin dependent diabetes mellitus and acts by stimulating insulin secretion by the pancreas

**anti-thyroid**, a drug that acts against the thyroid, especially against the synthesis of thyroid hormones

**cortic/o-steroid**, a steroid produced by the adrenal cortex or a synthetic equivalent used for replacement therapy when secretion by the adrenal glands is insufficient

**human growth hormone**, a growth hormone of human origin (somatotrophin) has been used to stimulate growth in patients of short stature. This has been replaced by somatotropin, a biosynthetic human growth hormone that has a similar effect

**anabolic steroid**, a protein-building drug with androgenic activity, little used in medicine but abused by body builders and some athletes

**insulin**, a hormone that lowers blood glucose in patients with diabetes mellitus. Many different forms of

insulin *e.g.* short, intermediate and long-acting are available for injection

**thyroid hormone**, a hormone used to treat hypothyroidism, it acts to increase metabolic rate

### Oncology
Drugs used in oncology aim to prevent the replication of cancer cells and destroy them by interfering with their metabolism. The process of using drugs in this way to destroy tumours is called chemotherapy.

**alkylating drug**, a drug that damages DNA (the genetic material of the cell) and interferes with the replication of cancer cells

**anti-metabolite**, a drug that acts against a metabolite, it refers to a drug that combines with an end-product or inhibits formation of an end-product such as a vital cell enzyme

**cyt/o-tox-ic**, a drug that is toxic or poisonous to cells and kills them, cytotoxics are used to destroy cancer cells as in chemotherapy

**anti-neo-plast-ic**, a drug that acts against a neoplasm (a new growth of cancer cells and kills them)

**vinca alkaloid**, a drug originally derived from the plant species *Vinca* that has the ability to directly interrupt the process of cell division.

### Infections and Infestations

**acari-cide**, a drug that acts against or destroys mites belonging to the order Acarina (mites and ticks)

**amoebi-cide**, a drug that kills amoebae (amoebae are single-celled animals belonging to the Subkingdom Protozoa some are pathogenic *e.g.* *Entamoeba histolytica*, which causes amoebic dysentery)

**ant-helmint-ic**, a drug that acts against or destroys worm infections such as roundworms, tapeworms, threadworms etc.

**anti-amoeb-ic**, a drug that acts against or destroys amoebae (amoebae are single-celled animals belonging to the Subkingdom Protozoa some are pathogenic *e.g. Entamoeba histolytica*, which causes amoebic dysentery)

**anti-bacteri-al**, a drug that acts against or destroys bacteria

**anti-bilharzi-al**, a drug that acts against or destroys Bilharzia or Schistosoma, a trematode worm (fluke) infestation that causes schistosomiasis *e.g. S. haematobium*, a fluke that lives in the genito-urinary veins of humans

**anti-biot-ic**, a drug that acts against life, it is used to destroy bacteria and fungi

**anti-fung-al**, a drug that acts against or destroys fungi Syn. antimycotic

**anti-giardi-al**, a drug that acts against or destroys species of flagellate protozoa belonging to the genus Giardia that are parasitic in the intestine of man, *e.g. G. lamblia*

**anti-leprot-ic**, a drug that acts against or destroys leprosy, a disease caused by infection with the bacillus *Mycobacterium leprae*

**anti-malari-al**, a drug that acts against or destroys malarial parasites

**anti-microb-ial**, a drug that acts against or destroys microbes

**anti-mycot-ic**, a drug that acts against or destroys fungi Syn. antifungal

**anti-parasit-ic**, any agent that acts against or destroys parasites

**anti-protozo-al**, a drug that acts against or destroys protozoa (single-celled animals belonging to the Subkingdom Protozoa some are pathogenic, *e.g. Entamoeba histolytica* that causes amoebic dysentery)

**anti-pseudomon-al**, a drug that acts against or destroys infections caused by the Gram-negative bacillus *Pseudomonas aeruginosa*

**anti-retrovir-al**, a drug that acts against or destroys retroviruses *e.g.* HIV

**anti-schistosom-al**, a drug that acts against or destroys Bilharzia or Schistosoma, a trematode worm (fluke) infestation that causes schistosomiasis *e.g. S. haematobium*, a fluke that lives in the genito-urinary veins of humans

**anti-sept-ic**, a substance that acts against sepsis, it can be applied to the skin surface to destroy or inhibit the growth of microorganisms

**anti-tuberculous drug**, a drug that acts against or destroys tuberculosis, a disease caused by infection with bacilli belonging to the genus Mycobacterium *e.g. M. tuberculosis* in which the lung is a principal seat of infection

**anti-vir-al**, a drug that acts against or destroys viruses

**ascari-cide**, a drug that kills species of parasitic, nematode roundworms belonging to the genus Ascaris *e.g. A. lumbricoides* found in the human intestine

**filari-cide**, a drug that kills microfilariae (prelarval stages) and adult filarial worms, these are species of parasitic nematode worms that live in subcutaneous tissues and lymphatics *e.g. Wuchereria bancrofti* and *Loa loa*

**leishmania-cide**, a drug that kills protozoa causing leishmaniasis, an infection with *Leishmania* species transmitted to man by bites from sand flies

**schistosomi-cide**, a drug that kills schistosomes. Schistosomiasis or bilharziasis is caused by a trematode worm (fluke) infestation *e.g. S. haematobium*, a fluke that lives in the genito-urinary veins of humans

**taeni-cide**, a drug that kills species of parasitic tapeworms belonging to the genus Taenia *e.g. T. solium* found in the human intestine, a result of eating inadequately cooked pork

**trichomona-cide**, a drug that acts against or destroys species of flagellate protozoa belonging to the genus Trichomonas that are parasitic in man, *e.g. T. vaginalis* found in the vagina and male genital tract

**trypano-cide**, a drug that kills trypanosomes, species of parasitic protozoa of the genus Trympanosoma *e.g. T. gambiense* that causes African sleeping sickness

**vir/u-cide**, an agent that destroys viruses

# Abbreviations

The abbreviations listed here have been extracted from recent health care publications and the medical records of patients. Students should be aware that while certain abbreviations are standard, others are not and their meaning may vary from one health care setting to another. Abbreviations with several meanings should be carefully interpreted to avoid confusion.

| | |
|---|---|
| A | anaemia (Am. anemia) |
| AAA | abdominal aortic aneurysm/acute anxiety attack |
| AAAAA | aphasia, agnosia, agraphia, alexia and apraxia |
| A & E | accident and emergency |
| AAFB | acid alcohol fast bacilli |
| AAH | atypical adenomatous hyperplasia |
| AB1 | one abortion |
| Ab, ab | abortion/antibody |
| ABC | airway, breathing, circulation |
| Abdo | abdomen |
| ABE | acute bacterial endocarditis |
| ABG | arterial blood gases |
| abor | abortion |
| ABX | antibiotics |
| AC | air conduction |
| ac | ante cibum (before meals/food) |
| ACBS | aortocoronary bypass surgery |
| Accom | accommodation of eye |
| ACE | angiotensin converting enzyme |
| ACh | acetylcholine |
| ACS | acute confused state |
| ACT | alpha$_1$-antichymotrypsin |
| ACTH | adrenocorticotrophic hormone |
| ACU | acute care unit |
| AD or ad | Alzheimer's disease/auris dextra (right ear) |
| ADA | adenosine deaminase |
| ADC | AIDS dementia complex |
| ADD | attention deficit disorder |
| ADH | antidiuretic hormone |
| ADL | aids to daily living |
| ADR | adverse drug reaction |
| ADU | acute duodenal ulcer |
| AED | anti-epileptic drug |
| AEM | ambulatory electrocardiogram monitoring |
| AF | amniotic fluid/atrial fibrillation |
| AFB | acid-fast bacilli |
| AFP | alphafeto protein |

| | |
|---|---|
| A/G | albumin/globulin ratio |
| Ag | antigen |
| AGA | appropriate for gestational age |
| AGL | acute granulocytic leukaemia (Am. leukemia) |
| AGN | acute glomerulonephritis |
| AI | aortic incompetence/aortic insufficiency/artificial insemination |
| AID | artificial insemination by donor |
| AIDS | acquired immunodeficiency syndrome |
| AIH | artificial insemination by husband |
| A/K | above knee (amputation) |
| ALD | alcoholic liver disease |
| ALG | anti-lymphocyte immunoglobulin |
| ALL | acute lymphocytic leukaemia (Am. leukemia) |
| ALS | amyotrophic lateral sclerosis |
| ALs | activities of living |
| ALT | alanine aminotransferase/alanine transaminase |
| amb | ambulant/ambulatory |
| AMI | acute myocardial infarction |
| AML | acute myeloid leukaemia (Am. leukemia) |
| ANC | absolute neutrophil count |
| ANF | antinuclear factor |
| ANS | autonomic nervous system |
| ANT or ant | anterior |
| antib | antibiotic |
| A & O | alert and orientated |
| AOB | alcohol on breath |
| AP | antepartum/anteroposterior/appendicectomy/auscultation and percussion |
| APB | atrial premature beat |
| APH | antepartum haemorrhage (Am. hemorrhage) |
| APPY | appendicectomy |
| APSAC | acylated plasminogen streptokinase activator complex (anistreplase) |
| APTT | activated partial thromboplastin time |
| A-R | apical-radial (pulse) |
| ARC | aids related complex |
| ARD | acute respiratory disease |
| ARDS | adult respiratory distress syndrome |
| ARF | acute renal failure |
| AS | alimentary system/aortic stenosis/auris sinistra (left ear) |
| A-S | Adams-Stokes attack |
| 5-ASA | 5-aminosalicylic acid |
| ASC | altered state of consciousness |
| ASCVD | arteriosclerotic cardiovascular disease |
| ASD | atrial septal defect |
| ASHD | arteriosclerotic heart disease |
| ASO | antistreptolysin O |
| ASOM | acute suppurative otitis media |
| AST | aspartate transaminase |
| Astigm | astigmatism of eye |
| ASX | asymptomatic |

| | |
|---|---|
| ATG | anti-thymocyte immunoglobulin |
| ATN | acute tubular necrosis |
| ATP | adenosine triphosphate |
| ATS | anti tetanus serum |
| aud | audiology |
| aur dextr | to the right ear |
| AV | arteriovenous/atrioventricular bundle/atrioventricular node/aortic valve |
| AVM | arteriovenous malformation |
| AVP | vasopressin |
| AVR | aortic valve replacement |
| A & W | alive and well |
| AXR | abdominal X-ray |
| AZT | azidothymidine |
| | |
| Ba | barium |
| BaE | barium enema |
| BAL | blood alcohol level |
| BBA | born before arrival |
| BBB | blood–brain barrier/bundle branch block |
| BBBB | bilateral bundle branch block |
| BBT | basal body temperature |
| BBx | breast biopsy |
| BC | birth control/bone conduction |
| BCC | basal cell carcinoma |
| BCG | bacille-Calmette-Guérin |
| BD or b.d. | bis diurnal (twice a day) |
| BDA | British Diabetic Association |
| BE | bacterial endocarditis/barium enema |
| BI | bone injury |
| BID | brought in dead |
| bid | bis in die (twice daily) |
| B/KA | below knee (amputation) |
| BM | bowel movement |
| BMI | body mass index |
| BMR | basal metabolic rate |
| BM (T) | bone marrow (trephine) |
| BMT | bone marrow transplant |
| BNF | British National Formulary |
| BNO | bowels not open |
| BOO | bladder outlet obstruction |
| BOR | bowels open regularly |
| BP | blood pressure/British Pharmacopoeia/bypass |
| BPD | bronchopulmonary dysplasia |
| BPH | benign prostatic hyperplasia |
| BPM | beats per minute |
| BRO | bronchoscopy |
| BS | blood sugar/bowel sounds/breath sounds |
| BSA | body surface area |
| BSE | bovine spongiform encephalopathy/breast self-examination |
| BSO | bilateral salpingo-oophorectomy |
| BSS | blood sugar series |

| | |
|---|---|
| BT | bedtime/bone tumour/brain tumour/breast tumour |
| BTS | blood transfusion service |
| BUN | blood urea nitrogen |
| BW | body weight |
| BX, Bx or bx | biopsy |
| | |
| C | Celsius |
| c | with |
| C 1–7 | cervical vertebra |
| CA, Ca or ca | cancer/carcinoma/cardiac arrest/coronary artery |
| CABG | coronary artery bypass grafting |
| CACX | cancer of the cervix |
| CAD | coronary artery disease |
| CAG | closed angle glaucoma |
| CAH | chronic active hepatitis/congenital adrenal hyperplasia |
| CAL | computer assisted learning |
| CAPD | continuous ambulatory peritoneal dialysis |
| CAT | computer assisted tomography/computerized axial tomography |
| CAVH | continuous arteriovenous haemofiltration (Am. hemofiltration) |
| CAVHD | continuous arteriovenous haemodialysis (Am. hemodialysis) |
| CBC | complete blood count |
| CBE | clinical breast examination |
| CBF | cerebral blood flow |
| CCCC | closed-chest cardiac compression |
| CCF | chronic cardiac failure/congestive cardiac failure |
| CCIE | counter current immunoelectrophoresis |
| CCU | coronary care unit |
| CD | Crohn's disease/cluster designation |
| CDH | congenital dislocation of the hip joint |
| CDI | colour Doppler imaging |
| CEA | carcino embryonic antigen |
| CF | cancer free/cardiac failure/cystic fibrosis |
| CFT | complement fixation test |
| CFTR | cystic fibrosis transmembrane regulator |
| CGL | chronic granulocytic leukaemia |
| CGN | chronic glomerulonephritis |
| CH | cholesterol |
| CHD | coronary heart disease |
| CHF | congestive heart failure |
| CHI | creatinine height index |
| CHOP | cyclophosphamide, hydroxydaunorubicin, Oncovin and prednisolone |
| CHR | chronic |
| CI | cardiac index/cerebral infarction/confidence interval |
| CIBD | chronic inflammatory bowel disease/disorder |
| CIN | cervical intraepithelial neoplasia |
| CJD | Creutzfeldt–Jakob disease |
| CK | creatine kinase |
| CL | clubbing |
| CLD | chronic liver disease/chronic lung disease |

| | |
|---|---|
| CLL | chronic lymphocytic leukaemia (Am. leukemia) |
| CMF | cyclophosphamide, methotrexate, 5-fluorouracil |
| CML | chronic myeloid leukaemia (Am. leukemia) |
| CMV | cytomegalovirus |
| CN | cranial nerve |
| CNS | central nervous system |
| CO | carbon monoxide/cardiac output/complains of |
| COAD | chronic obstructive airways disease |
| COD | cause of death |
| COLD | chronic obstructive lung disease |
| COPD | chronic obstructive pulmonary disease |
| COP | colloid osmotic pressure |
| C & P | cystoscopy and pyelogram |
| CP | cor pulmonale/cerebral palsy |
| CPA | cardiopulmonary arrest |
| CPAP | continuous positive airways pressure |
| CPK | creatinine phosphokinase |
| CPN | community psychiatric nurse |
| CPPV | continuous positive pressure ventilation |
| CPR | cardiopulmonary resuscitation |
| CrCl | creatine clearance |
| CRD | chronic renal disease |
| CRF | chronic renal failure |
| CRH | corticotrophin-releasing hormone |
| C+S | culture and sensitivity (test) |
| C-sect, or c/sect | Caesarean section (Am. Cesarean) |
| CSF | cerebrospinal fluid |
| CSH | chronic subdural haematoma (Am. hematoma) |
| CSM | cerebrospinal meningitis |
| CSOM | chronic suppurative otitis media |
| CSR | Cheyne–Stokes respiration/correct sedimentation rate |
| CSU | catheter specimen of urine |
| CT | cerebral tumour/clotting time/computerized tomography/continue treatment/coronary thrombosis |
| CUG | cystourethrogram |
| CV | cardiovascular/cerebrovascular |
| CVA | cerebrovascular accident (stroke)/costovertebral angle |
| CVD | cardiovascular disease |
| CVP | central venous pressure |
| CVS | cardiovascular system/chorionic villus sampling |
| CVVH | continuous venovenous haemofiltration (Am. hemofiltration) |
| CVVHD | continuous venovenous haemodialysis (Am. hemodialysis) |
| Cx | cervical/cervix |
| CXR | chest X-ray |
| Cy | cyanosis |
| cyclic AMP | cyclic adenosine monophosphate |
| Cysto | cystoscopy |
| | |
| D | diagnosis |
| db | decibel |
| DBP | diastolic blood pressure |
| D & C | dilatation and curettage |

| | |
|---|---|
| DC or d/c | decrease/direct current/discharge/discontinue |
| DCCT | diabetes control and complications trial |
| DD | differential diagnosis |
| DDA | Dangerous Drugs Act |
| DDAVP | desmopressin (synthetic vasopressin) |
| ddC/DDC | dideooxycytidine/zalcitabine |
| ddI/DDI | didanosine/dideoxyinosine |
| DDx | differential diagnosis |
| D & E | dilatation and evacuation |
| Derm, derm | dermatology |
| DES | diethylstilbestrol |
| DH | delayed hypersensitivity/drug history |
| DIC | disseminated intravascular coagulation |
| DIDMOAD | diabetes insipidus, diabetes mellitus, optic atrophy and deafness |
| Diff | differential blood count (of cell types) |
| DIMS | disorders of initiating and maintaining sleep |
| DIOS | distal intestinal obstruction syndrome |
| DIP | distal interphalangeal |
| DJK | degenerative joint disease |
| DKA | diabetics ketoacidosis |
| DLE | discoid lupus erythematosus/disseminated lupus erythematosus |
| DM | diabetes mellitus/diastolic murmur |
| DMD | Duchenne muscular dystrophy |
| dmft | decayed missing and filled teeth (deciduous) |
| DMFT | decayed missing and filled teeth (permanent) |
| D/N | day/night (frequency of urine) |
| DNA | deoxyribose nucleic acid/did not attend |
| DOA | dead on arrival |
| DOB | date of birth |
| DOD | date of death |
| DOE | dyspnoea on exertion (Am. dyspnea) |
| DOES | disorders of excessive somnolence |
| DRE | digital rectal examination |
| DS | Down's syndrome |
| D/S | dextrose and saline |
| DSA | digital subtraction angiography |
| DTP | diphtheria, tetanus and pertussis (vaccine) |
| DTR | deep tendon reflex |
| DTs | delerium tremens |
| DU | duodenal ulcer |
| DUB | dysfunctional uterine bleeding |
| D & V | diarrhoea and vomiting |
| DVT | deep venous thrombosis |
| Dx | diagnosis |
| DXT | deep X-ray therapy |
| DXRT | deep X-ray radiotherapy |
| | |
| EBM | expressed breast milk |
| EBV | Epstein–Barr virus |
| ECF | extracellular fluid |

| | |
|---|---|
| ECFV | extracellular fluid volume |
| ECG | electrocardiogram |
| ECHO | echocardiogram |
| ECSL | extra corporeal shockwave lithotripsy |
| ECT | electroconvulsive therapy |
| EDC | expected date of confinement |
| EDD | expected date of delivery |
| EDV | end-diastolic volume |
| EEG | electroencephalography/gram |
| EENT | eyes, ears, nose and throat |
| EFM | electronic fetal monitoring |
| ELBW | extremely low birth weight |
| ELISA | enzyme-linked immunosorbent assay |
| Em | emmetropia (good vision) |
| EMD | electromechanical dissociation |
| EMG | electromyogram/electromyography |
| EMI | elderly mentally infirm/etoposide-methotrexate-ifosfamide |
| EMU | early morning urine |
| EN | erythema nodosum |
| ENG | electronystagmogram |
| ENT | ear, nose and throat |
| EOG | electrooculogram |
| EOM | extraocular movement |
| EP | ectopic pregnancy |
| EPSP | excitatory postsynaptic potential |
| ERCP | endoscopic retrograde cholangiopancreatography |
| ERG | electroretinogram |
| ERT | estrogen replacement therapy (Am.) |
| ERV | expiratory reserve volume |
| ESM | ejection systolic murmur |
| ESN | educationally subnormal |
| ESP | end-systolic pressure |
| ESR | erythrocyte sedimentation rate |
| ESRD | end-stage renal disease |
| ESRF | end-stage renal failure |
| ESV | end-systolic volume |
| ESWL | extracorporeal shock wave lithotripsy |
| ET | embryo transfer/endotracheal/endotracheal tube |
| ET CPAP | endotracheal continuous positive airways pressure |
| ETF | Eustachian tube function |
| ETT | endotracheal tube/exercise tolerance test |
| EUA | examination under anaesthesia (Am. anesthesia) |
| EX | examination |
| EXP | expansion |
| Ez | eczema |
| | |
| F | Fahrenheit |
| FA | folic acid |
| FAS | fetal alcohol syndrome |
| FB | fasting blood sugar/finger breadth/foreign body |
| FBC | full blood count |
| FBE | full blood examination |

| | |
|---|---|
| FBS | fasting blood sugar |
| FDIU | fetal death *in utero* (Am. fetal) |
| FET | forced expiratory technique |
| FEV | forced expiratory volume |
| FEV$_1$ | forced expiratory volume in 1 sec |
| FFA | free fatty acids |
| FFP | fresh frozen plasma |
| FH | family history |
| FLP | fasting lipid profile |
| FMH | family medical history |
| FNAB | fine needle aspiration biopsy |
| FOB | faecal occult blood (Am. fecal) |
| FOBT | faecal occult blood testing (Am. fecal) |
| FP | false positive |
| FRC | functional reserve capacity/functional residual capacity |
| FROM | full range of movement |
| FSH | follicle stimulating hormone |
| FSHRH | follicle stimulating hormone releasing hormone |
| FT | full term |
| FT$_4$ | free thyroxine |
| FTI | free thyroxine index |
| FTND | full term, normal delivery |
| FUO | fever of unknown origin |
| FVC | forced vital capacity |
| FX, Fx or fx | fracture |
| | |
| g | gauge |
| GI and GII | gravida I and gravida II (first and second pregnancy) |
| GA | general anaesthesia (Am. anesthesia)/general appearance |
| GABA | gamma-aminobutyric acid |
| GB | gall bladder/Guillain-Barré (syndrome) |
| GC | gonococci |
| GCSF | granulocyte colony stimulating factor |
| GE | gastroenterology |
| GF | glomerular filtration/gluten-free |
| GFR | glomerular filtration rate |
| GGTP | gamma glutamyl transpeptidase |
| gGT ($\gamma$GT) | gamma glutamyl transferase |
| GH | growth hormone |
| GHIH | growth hormone inhibiting hormone |
| GHQ | general health questionnaire |
| GHRH | growth hormone releasing hormone |
| GHRIH | growth hormone release-inhibiting hormone |
| GI | gastrointestinal |
| GIFT | gamete intrafallopian transfer |
| ging | gingiva (gum) |
| GIS | gastrointestinal system |
| GIT | gastrointestinal tract |
| GKI | glucose/potassium/insulin |
| GM | grand mal seizure |
| GN | glomerulonephritis |
| GNDC | Gram-negative diplococci |

| | |
|---|---|
| GnRH | gonadotrophin releasing hormone |
| GP | general practitioner |
| GR1 | gravida one (pregnant for the first time) |
| grav | gravid (pregnant) |
| GS | general surgery/genital system |
| G&S/XM | group and save/cross match |
| GTN | glyceryl trinitrate |
| gtt | guttae (drops) |
| GTT | glucose tolerance test |
| GU | gastric ulcer/genitourinary/gonococcal urethritis |
| GUS | genitourinary system |
| GVHD | graft versus host disease |
| Gyn | gynaecology (Am. gynecology) |
| | |
| H | hypodermic |
| HAD | hospital anxiety and depression scale |
| HAV | hepatitis A virus |
| HB | heart block |
| Hb | haemoglobin (Am. hemoglobin) |
| HBAg | hepatitis B antigen |
| HBGM | home blood glucose monitoring |
| HBO | hyperbaric oxygenation |
| HBP | high blood pressure |
| HBsAg | Hepatitis B surface antigen |
| HBV | Hepatitis B virus |
| HC | head circumference |
| HCG(hCG) | human chorionic gonadotrophin |
| H/ct or/h.ct | haematocrit (Am. hematocrit) |
| HCV | Hepatitis C virus |
| HCVD | hypertensive cardiovascular disease |
| HD | haemodialysis (Am. hemodialysis)/Hodgkin's disease/ Huntington's disease |
| HDLs | high density lipoproteins |
| HDN | haemolytic disease of newborn (Am. hemolytic) |
| HDV | hepatitis delta virus |
| HEENT | head, eyes, ears, nose and throat |
| HF | heart failure |
| HGH or hGH | human growth hormone |
| HGP | human genome project |
| HHNK | hyperglycaemic (Am. hyperglycemic) hyperosmolar nonketonic |
| HHV | human herpes virus |
| Hib | *Haemophilus influenzae* type b |
| Hist. | histology (lab) |
| HIV | human immunodeficiency virus |
| HIVD | herniated intervertebral disc |
| H & L | heart and lungs |
| HLA | human leucocyte antigen (Am. leukocyte) |
| HMG(hMG) | human menopausal gonadotrophin |
| HOCM | hypertrophic obstructive cardiomyopathy |
| HO | house officer |
| H & P | history and physical |

| | |
|---|---|
| HPC | history of present condition |
| HPEN | home parenteral and enteral nutrition |
| hpf | high power field |
| HPI | history of present illness |
| HR | heart rate |
| HRM | human resource management |
| HRT | hormone replacement therapy |
| HSA | human serum albumin |
| HSV | *Herpes simplex* virus |
| 5-HT | 5-hydroxytryptamine |
| HT | hypertension |
| HTLV | human T-cell leukaemia-lymphoma virus (Am. leukemia) |
| HTN | hypertension |
| HTVD | hypertensive vascular disease |
| HUS | haemolytic uraemic syndrome (Am. hemolytic uremic syndrome) |
| HVD | hypertensive vascular disease |
| Hx | history |
| | |
| IABP | intra-aortic balloon pump |
| IBC | iron binding capacity |
| IBD | inflammatory bowel disease |
| IBS | irritable bowel syndrome |
| IC | intercostal/intracerebral/intracranial |
| ICA | islet cell antibody |
| ICF | intracellular fluid |
| ICH | intracerebral haemorrhage (Am. hemorrhage) |
| ICM | intracostal margin |
| ICP | intracranial pressure |
| ICS | intercostal space |
| ICSH | interstitial cell stimulating hormone |
| ICU | intensive care unit |
| ID or id | identity/intradermal |
| I & D | incision and drainage |
| IDDM | insulin-dependent diabetes mellitus |
| IDL | intermediate-density lipoprotein |
| IFN | interferon |
| Ig | immunoglobulin (*e.g.* IgA, IgG) |
| IGT | impaired glucose tolerance |
| IHD | ischaemic heart disease (Am. ischemic) |
| IHR | intrinsic heart rate |
| i.m. | intramuscular |
| IM | infectious mononucleosis/intramuscular |
| IMHP | intramuscular high potency |
| IMI | inferior myocardial infarction |
| IMP | impression |
| IMV | intermittent mandatory ventilation |
| IN | internist (Am.) |
| inf | inferior |
| inf.MI | inferior myocardial infarction |
| INR | international normalized ratio |
| int | between/inter |

| | |
|---|---|
| I & O | intake and output |
| IOFB | intra-ocular foreign body |
| IOL | intraocular lens |
| IOP | intraocular pressure |
| *in utero* | within uterus |
| i.p. | intraperitoneal |
| IPA | immunosuppressive acid protein |
| IPD | idiopathic Parkinson's disease |
| IPF | idiopathic pulmonary fibrosis |
| IPPA | inspection, palpation, percussion, auscultation |
| IPPB | intermittent positive pressure breathing |
| IPPV | intermittent positive pressure ventilation |
| IQ | intelligence quotient |
| IRDS | idiopathic respiratory distress syndrome |
| IRV | inspiratory reserve volume |
| ISQ | idem status quo (*i.e.* unchanged) |
| IT | intrathecal |
| ITCP | idiopathic thrombocytopenia purpura |
| ITP | idiopathic thrombocytopenic purpura |
| ITT | insulin tolerance test |
| ITU | intensive therapy unit |
| IU | international units |
| IUC | idiopathic ulcerative colitis |
| IUCD | intra-uterine contraceptive device |
| IUD | intra-uterine death/intra-uterine device |
| IUFB | intra-uterine foreign body |
| IUGR | intra-uterine growth retardation |
| IV or i.v. | intravenous |
| IVC | inferior vena cava/intravenous cholecystogram |
| IVD | intervertebral disc |
| IVF | *in vitro* fertilization/*in vivo* fertilization |
| IVH | intraventricular haemorrhage (Am. hemorrhage) |
| IVHP | intravenous high potency |
| IVI | intravenous infusion |
| IVP | intravenous pyelogram/intravenous pyelography |
| IVSD | interventricular septal defect |
| IVT | intravenous transfusion |
| IVU | intravenous urography |
| | |
| J | jaundice |
| JVD | jugular venous distension |
| JVP | jugular vein pressure/jugular venous pressure |
| | |
| KA | ketoacidosis |
| KCCT | kaolin–cephalin clotting time |
| KCO | transfer factor for carbon monoxide |
| KJ | knee jerk |
| KLS | kidney, liver, spleen |
| KO | keep open |
| KS | Karposi's sarcoma |
| KUB | kidney, ureters and bladder |
| KVO | keep vein open |

| | |
|---|---|
| L | lymphadenopathy |
| (L) | left/lower |
| L 1–5 | lumbar vertebrae |
| L & A | light and accommodation |
| LA | left arm/left atrium/local anaesthetic (Am. anesthetic) |
| La | labial (lips) |
| LAD | left axis deviation |
| LaG | labia and gingiva (lips and gums) |
| LAS | lymphadenopathy syndrome |
| LAT or lat. | lateral |
| LBBB | left bundle branch block |
| LBM | lean body mass |
| LBW | low birth weight |
| LCCS | low cervical caesarean section (Am. cesarean) |
| LD | lethal dose/loading dose |
| LDH | lactic dehydrogenase |
| LDL | low density lipoprotein |
| LE | lupus erythematosus |
| LFT | liver function test |
| LGA | large for gestational age |
| LH | luteinizing hormone |
| LH-RH | luteinizing hormone-releasing hormone |
| LIF | left iliac fossa |
| LIH | left inguinal hernia |
| LKKS | liver, kidney, kidney, spleen |
| LL | left leg/left lower/lower lobe |
| LLETZ | large loop excision of the transformation zone |
| LLL | left lower lid (eye)/left lower lobe (lung) |
| LLQ | left lower quadrant |
| LMP | last menstrual period |
| LMN | lower motor neuron |
| LN | lymph node |
| LNMP | last normal menstrual period |
| LOC | level of consciousness |
| LOM | limitation of movement |
| LP | lumbar puncture |
| LPA | left pulmonary artery |
| LPN | licensed practical nurse (Am.) |
| LRI | lower respiratory infection |
| LS | left side/liver and spleen/lumbosacral/lymphosarcoma |
| LSB | long stay bed (geriatric) |
| LSCS | lower section caesarean section |
| LSD | lysergic acid diethylamide |
| LSK | liver, spleen, kidneys |
| LSM | late systolic murmur |
| LTC | long term care |
| LTOT | long term oxygen therapy |
| L & U | lower and upper |
| LUL | left upper lobe |
| LUQ | left upper quadrant |
| LV | left ventricle |
| LVDP | left ventricular diastolic pressure |

| | |
|---|---|
| LVE | left ventricular enlargement |
| LVEDP | left ventricular end-diastolic pressure |
| LVEDV | left ventricular end-diastolic volume |
| LVET | left ventricular ejection time |
| LVF | left ventricular failure |
| LVH | left ventricular hypertrophy |
| LVP | left ventricular pressure |
| L & W | living and well |
| Lymphos | lymphocytes |
| | |
| M | male/married/murmur |
| MAb | monoclonal antibody |
| MABP | mean arterial blood pressure |
| MAC | mid-arm circumference/*Mycobacterium avium* complex |
| MAMC | mid-arm muscle circumference |
| mane | in the morning |
| MAOI | mono-amine oxidase inhibitor |
| MAP | mean arterial pressure/muscle action potential |
| MCH | mean corpuscular (red cell) haemoglobin (Am. hemoglobin) |
| MCHC | mean corpuscular haemoglobin concentration (Am. hemoglobin) |
| MCL | mid clavicular line |
| MCP | metacarpophalangeal |
| MCV | mean corpuscular (cell) volume |
| MD | maintenance dose/mitral disease/muscular dystrophy |
| MDI | metered dose inhaler |
| MDM | mid diastolic murmur |
| MDRTB | multidrug resistant tuberculosis |
| ME | myalgic encephalopathy |
| med | medial |
| MEN | multiple endocrine neoplasia |
| meQ | milli-equivalent |
| mEq/l | milli-equivalent per litre |
| Metas | metastasis |
| MF | mycoses fungoides/myocardial fibrosis |
| MFT | muscle function test |
| MG | myasthenia gravis |
| MGN | membranous glomerulonephritis |
| MH | medical history/menstrual history |
| MHC | major histocompatability complex |
| MHz | megahertz (megacycles per second) |
| MI | mitral incompetence/mitral insufficiency/myocardial infarction |
| MIBG | meta-iodo benzyl guanidine |
| MIC | minimum inhibitory concentration |
| MID | multi-infarct dementia |
| ML | middle lobe/midline |
| MLT | medical laboratory technician/technologist |
| mm³ | cubic millimetre |
| mmHg | millimetres of mercury |
| MMM | Mitozantrone, Methotrexate, Mitomycin C |
| mmol | millimole |

| | |
|---|---|
| MNJ | myoneural junction |
| MODY | maturity onset diabetes of the young |
| MOFS | multiple organ failure syndrome |
| MOPP | **m**ustine, **O**ncovin (vincristine), **p**rocarbazine, **p**rednisolone |
| MPJ | metacarpophalangeal joint |
| MPQ | McGill Pain Questionnaire |
| MR | mitral regurgitation |
| MRC | Medical Research Council |
| MRDM | malnutrition-related diabetes mellitus |
| MRI | magnetic resonance imaging |
| mRNA | messenger ribonucleic acid |
| MRSA | methicillin resistant *Staphylococcus aureus* |
| MS | mitral stenosis/multiple sclerosis/muscle shortening/ muscle strength/musculoskeletal/musculoskeletal system |
| MSAFP | maternal serum alphafetoprotein |
| MSE | mental state examination |
| MSH | melanocyte-stimulating hormone |
| MSL | midsternal line |
| MSOF | multisystem organ failure |
| MSSU | midstream specimen of urine |
| MSU | midstream urine |
| MTA | mid-thigh amputation |
| MTP | metatarsophalangeal |
| MV | mitral valve |
| MVP | mitral valve prolapse |
| MVR | minute volume of respiration/mitral valve replacement |
| My, my | myopia |
| | |
| N | normal |
| NAD | nothing abnormal discovered/no acute distress/normal axis deviation |
| NAG | narrow angle glaucoma |
| NANB | non A, non B viruses |
| NAP | neutrophil alkaline phosphatase |
| NAS, nas | nasal/no added salt |
| NBM | nil (nothing) by mouth |
| NCVs | nerve conduction velocities |
| NEC | necrotizing enterocolitis |
| NFTD | normal full term delivery |
| NG | nasogastric |
| NGU | non-gonococcal urethritis |
| NHL | non-Hodgkin's lymphoma |
| NHS | National Health Service |
| NIDDM | non insulin-dependent diabetes mellitus |
| NIH | National Institutes of Health (USA) |
| NK | natural killer (cells) |
| NMR | nuclear magnetic resonance |
| NO | nitric oxide |
| #NOF | fractured neck of femur |
| NP | nasopharynx |
| NPN | non protein nitrogen |

| NPO, npo | non per os/nothing by mouth |
| NPV | non-positive predictive value |
| NREM | non rapid eye movement (sleep) |
| NRS | numerical rating scale |
| NS | nephrotic syndrome/nervous system/no specimen |
| NSAIDs | non-steroidal anti-inflammatory drugs |
| NSFTD | normal spontaneous full-term delivery |
| NSR | normal sinus rhythm |
| NST | non shivering thermogenesis |
| NSU | nonspecific urethritis |
| NT | nasotracheal/nasotracheal tube |
| N & T | nose and throat |
| NTP | normal temperature and pressure |
| N & V | nausea and vomiting |
| NVD | nausea, vomiting and diarrhoea |
| | |
| O | oedema (Am. edema) |
| O & A | observation and assessment |
| OA | on admission/osteoarthritis |
| OAD | obstructive airway disease |
| OAG | open angle glaucoma |
| OB | occult blood |
| Ob-Gyn | obstetrics and gynaecology (Am. gynecology) |
| Obst-Gyn | obstetrics and gynaecology (Am. gynecology) |
| OC | oral cholecystogram/oral contraceptive |
| OCP | oral contraceptive pill |
| OD | oculus dexter (right eye), oculo dextro (in the right eye)/overdose |
| od | every day |
| Odont | odontology |
| ODQ | on direct questioning |
| OE | on examination/otitis externa |
| OGD | oesophago-gastro-duodenoscopy |
| OGTT | oral glucose tolerance test |
| OH | occupational history |
| OHS | open heart surgery |
| OM | olim mane (once daily in the morning)/otitis media |
| OOB | out of bed |
| OPA | outpatient appointment |
| OPD | outpatient department |
| Ophth | ophthalmology |
| OPT | orthopantomogram |
| OR | operating room |
| ORT | operating room technician |
| Ortho | orthopaedics (Am. orthopedics) |
| Orthop | orthopnoea (Am. orthopnea) |
| OS | oculus sinister (left eye), oculo sinistro (in left eye) |
| Os | mouth |
| osteo | osteomyelitis |
| OT | occupational therapy/old tuberculin/oxytocin |
| OTC | over the counter (remedies) |
| oto | otology |

| | |
|---|---|
| OU | oculus unitas (both eyes together)/oculus uterque (for each eye)/oculus utro (in each eye) |
| P | pressure |
| PA | pernicious anaemia (Am. anemia)/posteroanterior/pulmonary artery |
| P & A | percussion and auscultation |
| PABA | para-aminobenzoic acid |
| PACG | primary angle closure glaucoma |
| PADP | pulmonary artery diastolic pressure |
| PAH | pulmonary artery hypertension |
| PAP | primary atypical pneumonia |
| Pap | Papanicolaou smear test |
| PAS | $p$-aminosalycilic acid |
| PAT | paroxysmal atrial tachycardia |
| PAWP | pulmonary artery wedge pressure |
| PBC | primary biliary cirrhosis |
| PBI | protein bound iodine |
| pc | post cibum (after meals/food) |
| PCA | patient controlled analgesia |
| PCAS | patient controlled analgesia system |
| PCN | penicillin |
| PCNL | percutaneous nephrolithotomy |
| $pCO_2$ | partial pressure carbon dioxide |
| PCP | *Pneumocystis carinii* pneumonia |
| PCR | polymerase chain reaction |
| PCT | prothrombin clotting time |
| PCV | packed cell volume |
| PCWP | pulmonary capillary wedge pressure |
| PD | Parkinson's disease/peritoneal dialysis |
| PDA | patent ductus arteriosus |
| PE | physical examination/pleural effusion/pulmonary embolism |
| PEC | pneumoencephalogram |
| PED | paediatrics (Am. pediatrics) |
| PEEP | positive end expiratory pressure |
| PEF | peak expiratory flow |
| PEFR | peak expiratory flow rate |
| PEG | percutaneous endoscopic gastrostomy/pneumoencephalogram |
| PEJ | percutaneous endoscopic jejunostomy |
| PEM | protein–energy malnutrition |
| PERLAC | pupils equal, react to light, accommodation consensual |
| PERRLA | pupils equal, round, react to light, accommodation consensual |
| PET | positron emission tomography/pre-eclamptic toxaemia (Am. toxemia) |
| PF | peak flow |
| PFT | peak flow rate |
| PFTs | pulmonary function tests |
| PG | prostaglandin |
| PGL | persistent generalized lymphadenopathy |
| PH | past history/patient history/prostatic hypertrophy/pulmonary hypertension |

| | |
|---|---|
| pH | hydrogen ion concentration |
| PID | pelvic inflammatory disease/prolapsed intervertebral disc |
| PIH | prolactin inhibiting hormone |
| PIN | prostatic intra-epithelial neoplasia |
| PIP | proximal interphalangeal |
| PIVD | protruded intervertebral disc |
| PKU | phenylketonuria |
| PLCO | prostate, lung, colon and ovary |
| PM | post mortem |
| PMB | post menopausal bleeding |
| PMH | past medical history |
| PMI | past medical history/point of maximum impulse |
| PML | progressive multifocal leucoencephalopathy (Am. leukoencephalopathy) |
| PMN | polymorphonuclear leucocytes (Am. leukocyte) |
| PMS | premenstrual syndrome |
| PMT | premenstrual tension |
| PMV | prolapsed mitral valve |
| PN | percussion note/peripheral nerve/peripheral neuropathy |
| PND | paroxysmal nocturnal dyspnoea (Am. dyspnea)/post nasal drip |
| PNS | peripheral nervous system |
| PO or po | per os/by mouth |
| pO$_2$ | partial pressure oxygen |
| POAG | primary open angle glaucoma |
| POLY | polymorphonuclear leucocytes (Am. leukocytes) |
| POP | plaster of Paris |
| pos | position |
| post | posterior |
| PPAM | pneumatic post-amputation mobility |
| PPD | packs per day/purified protein derivative (of tuberculin) |
| PPE | personal protective equipment |
| PPH | postpartum haemorrhage (Am. hemorrhage) |
| PPS | plasma protein solution |
| PPT | partial prothrombin time |
| PPV | positive-pressure ventilation/positive predictive value |
| p.r. or PR | per rectum/plantar reflex |
| PRH | prolactin releasing hormone |
| PRL | prolactin |
| PRN or p.r.n. | pro re nata (as required) |
| PROG | progesterone |
| PROM | premature rupture of membranes |
| PRV | polycythaemia rubra vera (Am. polycythemia) |
| pros | prostate |
| prox | proximal |
| PS | pulmonary stenosis/pyloric stenosis |
| PSA | prostate specific antigen |
| PSAD | prostate specific antigen density |
| PSCT | pain and symptom control team |
| PSD | personal and social development |
| PSG | presystolic gallop |

| | |
|---|---|
| PSVT | paroxysmal supraventricular tachycardia |
| pt or PT | patient/physical therapy/prothrombin time/physical therapist (Am.) |
| PTA | prior to admission |
| PTC | percutaneous transhepatic cholangiogram/graphy |
| PTCA | percutaneous transluminal coronary angioplasty |
| PTD | permanent and total disability |
| PTH | parathormone/parathyroid hormone |
| PTR | prothrombin ratio |
| PTT | partial thromboplastin time |
| PTX | pneumothorax |
| PU | peptic ulcer/per urethra |
| PUO | pyrexia of unknown origin |
| PUVA | psoralen + ultraviolet light A |
| PV | per vagina |
| P & V | pyloroplasty and vagotomy |
| PVC | premature ventricular contraction |
| PVD | peripheral vascular disease |
| PVP | pulmonary venous pressure |
| PVT | paroxysmal ventricular tachycardia |
| PX | physical examination |
| Px | past history/prognosis |
| | |
| QDS or qds | quater diurnale summensum (four times a day) |
| qid | quater in die (four times a day) |
| | |
| (R) | right |
| RA | rheumatoid arthritis/right auricle/atrium |
| Ra | radium |
| RAD | radiation absorbed dose/right axis deviation |
| rad | radical |
| RAS | reticular activating system |
| RAST | radio-allergosorbent test |
| RBBB | right bundle branch block |
| RBC | red blood cell/red blood (cell) count |
| RBS | random blood sugar |
| RCC | red cell concentrate/red cell count |
| RCT | randomized controlled trial |
| RDA | recommended dietary allowance |
| rDNA | recombinant deoxyribose nucleic acid |
| RDS | respiratory distress syndrome |
| RE | rectal examination |
| REM | rapid eye movement (in sleep) |
| RES | reticulo endothelial system |
| RF | renal failure/rheumatoid factor/rheumatic fever |
| RFLA | rheumatoid factor like activity |
| RFT | respiratory function tests |
| Rh | Rhesus |
| RHD | rheumatic heart disease |
| RHL | right hepatic lobe |
| RIA | radioimmunoassay |
| RIF | right iliac fossa |

| | |
|---|---|
| RK | radial keratotomy/right kidney |
| RL | right leg/right lung |
| RLC | residual lung capacity |
| RLD | related living donor |
| RLE | right lower extremity |
| RLL | right lower lobe |
| RLQ | right lower quadrant |
| RM | radical mastectomy |
| RN | registered nurse |
| RNA | ribose nucleic acid |
| R/O | rule out |
| ROM | range of movement (exercises) |
| ROS | review of symptoms |
| RP | radial pulse |
| RPE | retinal pigment epithelial (cells, layer) |
| RQ | respiratory quotient |
| RR | recovery room/respiratory rate |
| RR & E | round, regular and equal |
| RRR | regular rate and rhythm |
| RS | respiratory system/Reye's syndrome |
| RSI | repetitive strain injury |
| RSV | respiratory syncytial virus |
| RT | radiologic technologist (Am.)/radiotherapy |
| RTA | renal tubular acidosis/road traffic accident |
| RUL | right upper lobe |
| RUQ | right upper quadrant |
| RV | residual volume/right ventricle |
| RVF | right ventricular failure |
| RVH | right ventricular hypertrophy |
| | |
| s | without |
| S1 | first heart sound |
| S2 | second heart sound |
| SA | sarcoma/sinoatrial (node)/sinus arrhythmia/Stokes–Adams (attacks) |
| SACD | subacute combined degeneration |
| SAD | seasonal affective disorder |
| SAH | subarachnoid haemorrhage (Am. hemorrhage) |
| SB | seen by |
| SBE | subacute bacterial endocarditis |
| SBO | small bowel obstruction |
| SBP | systolic blood pressure |
| s.c. | subclavian/subcutaneous |
| SCA | sickle-cell anaemia |
| SCC | squamous cell carcinoma |
| SCD | sequential pneumatic compression device/sudden cardiac death |
| SCID | severe combined immunodeficiency syndrome |
| SDH | subdural haematoma (Am. hematoma) |
| SDS | same day surgery |
| SED | skin erythema dose |
| SEM | systolic ejection murmur |

| | |
|---|---|
| SG | skin graft/specific gravity |
| SGA | small for gestational age |
| SGOT | serum glutamic oxaloacetic transaminase now serum aspartate transferase |
| SGPT | serum glutamic pyruvic transaminase |
| SF | synovial fluid |
| SH | social history |
| SIADH | syndrome of inappropriate antidiuretic hormone |
| SIDS | sudden infant death syndrome |
| SIG | sigmoidoscope/sigmoidoscopy |
| SIMV | synchronized intermittent mandatory ventilation |
| s.l. | sublingual |
| SLE | systemic lupus erythematosus |
| SLS | social and life skills |
| SMD | senile macular degeneration |
| SNS | somatic nervous system |
| SOA | swelling of ankles |
| SOB | short of breath/stools for occult blood |
| SOBOE | short of breath on exertion |
| SOS | swelling of sacrum |
| SP | systolic pressure |
| SPF | sun protection factor |
| SPP | suprapubic prostatectomy |
| SR | sedimentation rate/sinus rhythm |
| SS S/S | saline solution/signs and symptoms |
| ST | sinus tachycardia/skin test |
| STD | sexually transmitted disease/skin test dose |
| STS | serological tests for syphilis |
| STU | skin test unit |
| Subcu | subcutaneous |
| subling | sublingual/under the tongue |
| sup | superior |
| SV | stroke volume |
| SVC | superior vena cava |
| SVI | stroke volume index |
| SVR | systemic venous resistance |
| SVT | supraventricular tachycardia |
| SWS | slow wave sleep |
| Sx | symptoms |
| syph. | syphilis |
| | |
| T | temperature/tumour |
| t | terminal |
| T 1–12 | thoracic vertebrae |
| $T_3$ $T_4$ | triiodothyronine, tetraiodothyronine (thyroid hormones) |
| T & A | tonsils and adenoids or tonsillectomy/adenoidectomy |
| T.A. | toxin–antitoxin |
| TAH | total abdominal hysterectomy |
| TAS | transabdominal sonography |
| Tb or TB | tuberculosis (tubercle bacillus) |
| TBA | to be arranged |
| TBG | thyroid binding globulin |

| | |
|---|---|
| TBI | total body irradiation |
| TBW | total body water/total body weight |
| T & C | type and cross match |
| TCP | thrombocytopenia |
| TD | thymus dependent cells |
| TDM | therapeutic drug monitoring |
| TDS | ter diurnale summensum (three times a day) |
| TED | thromboembolic deterrent (stockings) |
| TENS | transcutaneous electrical nerve stimulation |
| TH | thyroid hormone (thyroxine) |
| THR | total hip replacement |
| TI | thymus independent cells |
| TIA | transient ischaemic attack (Am. ischemic) |
| TIBC | total iron-binding capacity |
| t.i.d. | ter in die (three times daily) |
| TIP | terminal interphalangeal |
| TIPS | transjugular intrahepatic portosystemic shunting |
| TJ | triceps jerk |
| TKVO | to keep vein open |
| TLC | tender loving care/total lung capacity |
| TLD | thoracic lymph duct |
| TM | tympanic membrane |
| TMJ | temporomandibular joint |
| TMR | transmyocardial revascularization |
| TNF | tumour necrosis factor |
| TNM | tumour, node, metastases (a system of pathological staging of tumours) |
| TOP | termination of pregnancy |
| tPA | recombinant tissue-type plasminogen activator |
| TPHI | *Treponema pallidum* haemagglutination inhibition (Am. hemagglutination) |
| TPI | *Treponema pallidum* immobilization |
| TPN | total parenteral nutrition |
| TPR | temperature, pulse, respiration |
| TRH | thyrotrophin-releasing hormone |
| TRUS | transrectal ultrasound |
| TSA | tumour specific antigen |
| TSF | triceps skin fold thickness |
| TSH | thyroid stimulating hormone |
| TSS | toxic shock syndrome |
| TT | tetanus toxoid/thrombin clotting time |
| TTA | transtracheal aspiration |
| TTO | to take out (to home) |
| TUIP | transurethral incision of the prostate |
| TUR | transurethral resection (of prostate) |
| TURB | transurethral resection of bladder |
| TURP | transurethral resection of the prostate |
| TURT | transurethral resection of tumour |
| TV | tidal volume |
| TVS | transvaginal sonography |
| Tx | therapy/transfusion/treatment |
| T & X | type and cross match |

| U | unit |
|---|---|
| UA | uric acid/urinalysis |
| UAC | umbilical artery catheter |
| UC | ulcerative colitis |
| UDO | undetermined origin |
| U & E | urea and electrolytes |
| UG | urogenital |
| UGH | uveitis + glaucoma + hyphaema syndrome (Am. hyphema) |
| UGI | upper gastrointestinal |
| UIBC | unsaturated iron-binding capacity |
| ung | ointment (unguentum) |
| URI | upper respiratory (tract) infection |
| URT | upper respiratory tract |
| URTI | upper respiratory tract infection |
| US | ultrasonography/ultrasound/urinary system |
| USS | ultrasound scan |
| UTI | urinary tract infection |
| UVA | ultraviolet light A |
| UVB | ultraviolet light B |
| UVC | ultraviolet light C |
| UTI | urinary tract infection |

| VA | visual acuity |
|---|---|
| VAC | **V**incristine, **A**driamycin, **C**yclophosphamide |
| VAS | visual analogue scale |
| VC | vital capacity/vulvovaginal candidiasis |
| VD | venereal disease |
| VDRL | venereal disease research laboratory (test) |
| VE | vaginal examination |
| VF | ventricular fibrillation/visual field |
| VHD | valvular heart disease |
| VLBW | very low birth weight |
| VLDL | very low density lipoprotein |
| VMA | vanillyl-mandelic acid |
| VP | venous pressure |
| VPC | ventricular premature contraction |
| VRS | verbal rating scale |
| VS | vital signs |
| VSD | ventricular septal defect |
| VT | ventricular tachycardia |
| VUR | vesicouretic reflux |
| VWF | von Willebrand factor |
| VV | varicose veins/vulva and vagina |

| WBC | white blood (cell) count/white blood cell |
|---|---|
| WCC | white cell count |
| WNL | within normal limits |
| WPW | Wolff–Parkinson–White (syndrome) |
| WR | Wasserman reaction (test for syphilis) |

| X-match | cross-match |
|---|---|
| XOP | exophoria |

| | |
|---|---|
| XOT | exotropia |
| XR | X-ray |
| XRT | X-ray therapy |
| | |
| ZE | Zollinger–Ellison (syndrome) |
| ZN | Ziel–Nielsen Stain |

## Symbols

| | |
|---|---|
| ♂ | male |
| ♀ | female |
| * | birth |
| α | alpha |
| β | beta |
| γ | gamma |
| Δ | delta/diagnosis |
| ΔΔ | differential diagnosis |
| # | fracture |
| † | dead |

# Glossary

The glossary contains a list of prefixes, suffixes and combining forms used in common medical terms. The meaning of each word component is given with an example of its use in a medical term.

Use the list to decipher the meaning of unfamiliar words. Note that a dash is added to indicate whether the component usually precedes or follows the other elements of a compound word; for example, ante- precedes a word root as in **ante**natal while -stomy follows the root as in colo**stomy**. Some components are composed of a root with a suffix; for example -**plegia** contains the root **pleg**- meaning paralysis with the suffix **-ia** meaning condition of.

The vowels of combining forms are used or dropped by the application of 'rules' described in the introduction of this book. Some roots are listed with more than one combining vowel, for example, **ren**/i/o. Both vowels may be used in combination with the root as in **ren**ipelvic and **ren**ography.

|  | Meaning | Medical term |
|---|---|---|
| a- | without, not (n is added before words beginning with a vowel) | a**phasia** |
| -a | noun ending/a name | burs**a** |
| ab- | away from | **ab**duct |
| abdomin/o | abdomen | **abdomino**pelvic |
| -able | capable of/having ability to | palp**able** |
| -ac | pertaining to/to/toward/near/person affected by something | ac**cretion** |
| acanth/o | spiny | **acanth**osis |
| acarin/o | mites of the order Acarina | **acarin**osis |
| acar/i/o | mites of the order Acarina | **acar**icide |
| acetabul/o | acetabulum | **acetabulo**plasty |
| acet/o | vinegar | *Acetobacter* |
| aceton- | ketones/acetone | **aceton**aemia |
| achill/o | Achilles tendon | **achillo**tomy |
| acid/o | acid | **acido**phil |
| acin/i | sac-like dilation | **acin**us |
| acne/o | acne/point/peak | **acne**genic |
| acou- | hear/hearing | **acou**metric |
| -acousia | condition of hearing | dys**acousia** |
| acoust/o | hear/hearing/sound | **acoust**ic |
| acro- | extremities, point | **acro**megaly |
| acromi/o | acromion (point of the shoulder) | **acromio**clavicular |
| act- | do, drive, act | **act**ion |
| actin/o | rays *e.g.* of sun/ultra violet radiation | **actino**therapy |
| acu- | hear/hearing/severe/sudden | **acu**te |
| -acusia | condition/sense of hearing | dys**acusia** |

| | | |
|---|---|---|
| ad- | to/toward/in the direction of the midline/near | **ad**duct |
| adamant/o | dental enamel | **adamant**ine |
| aden/o | gland | **aden**oid |
| adenoid/o | adenoids | **adenoid**ectomy |
| adip/o | adipose tissue/fat | **adip**osity |
| adnex/o | bound to/conjoined | **adnex**a |
| adrenal/o | adrenal gland | **adrenal**ectomy |
| adren/o | adrenal gland | **adren**ogenital |
| adrenocortic/o | adrenal cortex | **adrenocortic**al |
| -aem- | blood (Am. -em-) | an**aem**ia |
| -aemia | condition of blood (Am. -emia) | leuk**aemia** |
| aer/o | air/gas | **aero**phagia |
| aesthe/s/i/o | sensation/sensitivity (Am. esthe/s/i/o) | an**aesthesio**logy |
| aeti/o | causation (of disease) (Am. eti/o) | **aeti**ology |
| af- | to/towards/near | **af**ferent |
| ag- | to/towards/near | **ag**glutinate |
| agglutin/o | sticking/clumping together | **agglutin**ation |
| -ago | abnormal condition/disease | lumb**ago** |
| -agogic | pertaining to inducing/ stimulating | dacry**agogic** |
| -agogue | inducing/promoting | lact**agogue** |
| agora- | market place, open space | **agora**phobia |
| -agra | seizure/sudden pain | pod**agra** |
| -aise | comfort/ease | mal**aise** |
| -al[1] | pertaining to | bronchi**al** |
| -al[2] | used in pharmacology to mean a drug or drug action | antifung**al** |
| albin/o | white | **albin**ism |
| alb/i/o | white | **alb**us |
| album- | white | **album**in |
| albumin/o | albumin/albumen | **albumin**uria |
| aldosteron- | aldosterone | **aldosteron**ism |
| -algesia | condition of pain | an**algesia** |
| alges/i/o | sense of pain | **alges**iometer |
| -algia | pain | neur**algia** |
| alg/e/i/o | pain | **alg**aesthesia |
| aliment/o | to nourish | **aliment**ary |
| all/o | other/different from normal | **all**ogenic |
| alve/o | trough/channel/cavity | **alve**us |
| alveol/o | alveoli (of lungs) | **alveol**itis |
| ambi- | both/on both sides | **ambi**lateral |
| ambly/o | dull/dim | **ambly**opia |
| ameb/o (Am.) | ameba, a type of protozoan | **ameb**iasis (Am.) |
| amel/o | dental enamel | **amel**oblast |
| -amine | nitrogen containing compound | catechol**amine** |
| amni/o | amnion/fetal membrane | **amnio**centesis |
| amnion/o | amnion/fetal membrane | **amnion**ic |
| amoeb/o | amoeba a type of protozoan (Am. ameb/o) | **amoeb**iasis |
| amph/i | both/doubly/on both sides | **amphi**gonadism |

| | | |
|---|---|---|
| amyl/o | starch | **amyl**oid |
| an- | without/not | **an**encephalic |
| -an | pertaining to/characteristic of | ovari**an** |
| ana- | backward/apart/up/again | **ana**plastic |
| ancyl/o | crooked/stiffening/fusing/bent | **ancylo**stomiasis |
| andr/o | male/masculine | **andr**ology |
| -ane | a saturated, open-chain hydrocarbon | meth**ane** |
| aneurysm/o | aneurysm | **aneurysmo**plasty |
| angi/o | vessel | **angio**plasty |
| an-iso- | unequal/dissimilar | **aniso**coria |
| ankyl/o | crooked/stiffening/fusing/bent | **ankylo**sis |
| an/o | anus | **an**orectal |
| -ant | having the characteristic of/an agent that . . . | stimul**ant** |
| ante- | before in time or place/in front of/forward | **ante**natal |
| anter/o | front/in front of/anterior to | **antero**lateral |
| anthrac/o | coal dust | **anthrac**osis |
| anthrop/o | man/human | **anthropo**metry |
| anti- | against | **anti**fungal |
| antr/o | antrum/maxillary sinus | **antro**tomy |
| anxi/o | anxiety | **anxio**lytic |
| aort/o | aorta | **aorto**rrhaphy |
| ap- | to/towards/near/separated from | **ap**position |
| -aph- | touch | hyper**aph**ia |
| -apheresis | removal | leuk**apheresis** |
| aphth/o | ulcer | **aphth**ous |
| apic/o | apex | **apic**al |
| ap/o | away from/detached/derived from/separate | **apo**physis |
| aponeur/o | aponeurosis (flat tendon) | **aponeuro**rrhaphy |
| append/ic/o | appendix | **appendic**ectomy |
| aqu/a/e/o | water | **aque**ous |
| -ar | pertaining to | lob**ar** |
| arachn/o | spider | **arachn**ophobia |
| arc/o | arch/bow-shaped | **arc**us |
| -arch/e- | beginning | men**arch** |
| arrhen/o | male/masculine | **arrheno**blastoma |
| arter/i/o | artery | **arterio**sclerosis |
| arteriol/o | arteriole | **arteriolo**necrosis |
| arthr/o | joint | **arthro**desis |
| articul/o | joint | **articul**ate |
| -ary | pertaining to/connected with | pulmon**ary** |
| as- | to/towards/near | **as**sociation |
| -ase | an enzyme | amyl**ase** |
| -asia | state or condition | euthan**asia** |
| -asis | state or condition | elephanti**asis** |
| -asthenia | condition of weakness | my**asthenia** |
| asthen/o | weakness | **astheno**coria |
| astr/o | star-shaped/star | **astro**cyte |

| | | |
|---|---|---|
| at- | to/towards/near | **at**tenuation |
| -ate | in a state/acted upon/possessing/chemical from a specific source | stimul**ate** |
| atel/o | imperfect/incomplete | **atel**ocardia |
| ather/o | porridge-like plaque lining a blood vessel | **ather**osclerosis |
| -ation | action/condition | ejacul**ation** |
| -atresia | condition of occlusion/closure/absence of opening | anal **atresia** |
| atret/o | closure of a normal opening/imperforation | **atret**ometria |
| atri/o | atrium | **atri**oventricular |
| audi/o | hearing/sense of hearing | **audi**ometry |
| audit/o | hearing/sense of hearing | **audit**ory |
| -aural | pertaining to the ear | mon**aural** |
| auricul/o | auricle/pinna | **auricul**oplasty |
| aur/i/o | ear/hearing | **aur**iscope |
| auto- | self | **auto**lysis |
| aux/i | increase | **aux**ilytic |
| -auxis | increase | onych**auxis** |
| aux/o | increase | **auxo**cardia |
| -ax | noun ending/a name | thor**ax** |
| axill/o | armpit | **axill**ary |
| ax/i/o | axis | **axi**petal |
| axon/o | axis/axon of neuron | **axon**al |
| azot/o | urea/nitrogen | **azot**aemia |
| | | |
| ba- | go/walk/stand | hypno**ba**tia |
| bacill/o | bacillus/a rod-shaped bacterium | **bacill**uria |
| bacter/i/o | bacterium/bacteria | **bacter**iophage |
| balan/o | glans penis | **balan**itis |
| ballist/o | throw/movement | **ballist**ocardiograph |
| bar/o | weight/pressure | **baro**trauma |
| bartholin/o | Bartholin's glands/greater vestibular glands of the vagina | **bartholin**itis |
| basi- | base/basic/alkaline | **basi**chromatin |
| bas/o | base/basic/alkaline | **baso**phil |
| bathy- | deep | **bathy**pnoea |
| bi- | two/twice/double | **bi**pedal |
| bil/i | bile | **bil**iary |
| bin- | two each/double | **bin**ocular |
| bio- | life/living | **bio**logy |
| -blast | germ cell/immature cell/embryonic cell/developing stage | osteo**blast** |
| blast/o | germ cell/immature cell/embryonic cell/developing stage | retino**blast**oma |
| blenn/o | mucus | **blenn**oid |
| blephar/o | eyelid | **blephar**optosis |
| bol/o | ball | **bol**us |
| brachi/o | arm | **brachi**al |
| brachy- | short | **brachy**gnathia |

| | | |
|---|---|---|
| brady- | slow | **brady**cardia |
| brev/i | short | **brevi**flexor |
| bromidr/o | stench/smell of sweat | **bromidr**osis |
| bronch/i/o | bronchus/bronchial tube/ windpipe | **broncho**scopy |
| bronchiol/o | bronchiole | **bronchiol**itis |
| bront/o | thunder | **bronto**phobia |
| bucca- | cheek | **bucca**l |
| bucc/o | cheek | **bucco**pharyngeal |
| bulb/o | bulb/medulla oblongata | **bulb**ar |
| burs/o | bursa (fluid-filled sac) | **burs**itis |
| byssin/o | cotton dust | **byssin**osis |
| | | |
| cac/o | bad/ill/abnormal | **caco**cholia |
| caec/o | caecum (Am. cecum) | **caeco**cele |
| calcane/o | calcaneus/heel bone | **calcaneo**plantar |
| calc/i/o | calcium/lime/heel | **calci**penia |
| calcin/o | calcium | **calcin**osis |
| calcul/o | stone/little stone | **calcul**us |
| calic- | calyx (Am. calix)/a cup-shaped organ or cavity | **calic**ectasis |
| calor/i | heat | **calori**metry |
| calyc- | calyx (Am. calix)/a cup-shaped organ or cavity | **calyc**ulus |
| cancer/o | cancer (general term) | **cancero**phobia |
| canth/o | canthus (corner of the eye) | **cantho**plasty |
| capill/o | hair/blood capillary | **capill**ary |
| capit/o | head | **capit**ate |
| -capnia | condition of carbon dioxide | hyper**capnia** |
| caps- | container | **caps**itis |
| capsul/o | capsule | **capsul**ar |
| carb/o | carbon/bicarbonate | **carbo**hydrate |
| carcin/o | cancerous/malignant tumour of epithelial tissue | **carcin**oma |
| carcinomat- | carcinoma | **carcinomat**ous |
| -cardia | condition of heart | tachy**cardia** |
| cardi/o | heart | **cardi**ologist |
| cari/o | rot/decay (of teeth) | **cario**genesis |
| carp/o | carpal/wrist bones | **carpo**ptosis |
| cary/o | nucleus | eu**cary**otic |
| cat/a | down/negative/against | **cata**bolic |
| caud/o | tail/towards the tail/lower part of body | **caud**al |
| caus- | burn/corrosive | **caus**tic |
| caut- | burn | **caut**ery |
| cav- | hollow | **cav**ity |
| cec/o (Am.) | cecum | **ceco**cele |
| -cele | swelling/protrusion/hernia | vesico**cele** |
| celi/o | hollow/abdomen | **celio**scope |
| cell- | cell | **cell**ular |
| cellul- | cell | a**cellul**ar |
| cel/o (Am.) | hollow/abdomen/celom | **celo**schisis (Am.) |

| | | |
|---|---|---|
| cement/o | cementum of a tooth | **cemento**clasia |
| cen/o | new/empty/common | **cen**osis |
| -centesis | surgical puncture to remove fluid | amnio**centesis** |
| centi- | hundred/one hundredth | **centi**grade |
| centr/i/o | centre/central location | **centri**lobular |
| cephal/o | head | hydro**cephal**ic |
| cerat/o | horny/epidermis/cornea (Syn. kerat/o) | **cerato**cricoid |
| cerebell/o | cerebellum | **cerebell**ar |
| cerebr/i/o | cerebrum/brain | **cerebr**oma |
| cer/o | wax | **cer**oma |
| cerumin/o | cerumen/ear wax | **cerumin**ous |
| cervic/o | cervix | **cervic**al |
| -chalasis | slackening/loosening | blepharo**chalasis** |
| chancr- | chancre, a destructive sore | **chancr**oid |
| cheil/o | lip | **cheil**oplasty |
| cheir/o | hand | **cheir**omegaly |
| chem/i/c/o | chemical | **chemo**receptor |
| -chezia | condition of defaecation especially of foreign substances | uro**chezia** |
| chil/o | lip | **chil**oplasty |
| chir/o | hand | **chir**opody |
| chlor/o | green/chlorine | **chlor**oma |
| cholangi/o | bile vessel/bile duct | **cholangi**ogram |
| cholecyst/o | gall bladder | **cholecysto**lithiasis |
| choledoch/o | common bile duct | **choledocho**lithiasis |
| chol/e/o | bile | **chol**uria |
| cholester/o | cholesterol | **cholester**osis |
| chondr/o | cartilage | **chondro**sarcoma |
| chord/o | string/cord | **chord**otomy |
| chore/o | chorea/dance/jerky movement | **chore**a |
| chori/o | chorion/outer fetal membrane | **chorio**allantois |
| choroid/o | choroid layer of eye | **choroid**itis |
| chromat/o | colour | **chromat**opsia |
| -chromia | condition of haemoglobin/colour | hypo**chromia** |
| chrom/o | colour | **chromo**cystoscopy |
| chron/o | time | **chron**ic |
| chrys/o | gold | **chryso**derma |
| chyl/e/o | chyle, lymphatic fluid formed by lacteals in the intestine, a product of digestion | **chylo**thorax |
| chym/o | chyme, creamy material produced by digestion of food/juice | **chymo**poiesis |
| -cidal | pertaining to killing | bacterio**cidal** |
| -cide | agent that kills/killing | acari**cide** |
| cili/o | cilia/ciliary body of eye/eyelash | **cili**ectomy |
| cinemat/o | movement/motion (picture) | **cinemat**ography |
| cine/o | movement/motion | **cine**angiography |
| cinesi/o | movement/motion | **cinesi**ology |
| circum- | around | **circum**cision |
| cirrh/o | yellow | **cirrh**osis |

| | | |
|---|---|---|
| cirs/o | varicose vein/varix | **cirs**ectomy |
| cis- | on the near side/this side | **cis** position |
| -cis- | cut/kill | ex**cis**ion |
| cistern/o | cistern/enclosed space (sub arachnoid space) | **cistern**ography |
| -clasia | condition of breaking | osteo**clasia** |
| -clasis | breaking | osteo**clasis** |
| -clast | a cell that breaks/an instrument that breaks | osteo**clast** |
| claustr/o | barrier/enclosed | **claustr**ophobia |
| clavic/o | clavicle | **clavic**otomy |
| clavicul/o | clavicle | **clavicul**ar |
| -cle | small | vesi**cle** |
| cleid/o | clavicle | **cleid**otomy |
| clin/o | bend/incline | **clin**odactyly |
| clitor/i/o | clitoris | **clitor**ism |
| clon/o | clone of cells | mono**clon**al |
| -clonus | violent action | myo**clonus** |
| -clysis | infusion/injection/irrigation | veno**clysis** |
| co- | with/together | **co**factor |
| coccid/i | type of parasitic protozoa of the Order Coccidia | **coccid**iosis |
| cocc/i/o | coccus, a berry-shaped bacterium | **cocc**ogenous |
| -coccus | a berry-shaped bacterium | strepto**coccus** |
| coccyg/o | coccyx | **coccyg**eal |
| cochle/o | cochlea | **cochle**ovestibular |
| -coel(e) | hollow/abdomen | blasto**coel(e)** |
| coel/o | hollow/abdomen/coelom (Am. cel/o) | **coel**om |
| col- | with/together | **col**lateral |
| collagen/o | collagen | **collagen**ase |
| col/o | colon | **col**ostomy |
| colon/o | colon | **colon**ic |
| colp/o | vagina | **colp**ohysterectomy |
| com- | with/together | **com**mensal |
| con- | with/together | **con**centric |
| condyl/o | condyle | **condyl**ar |
| coni/o | dust | **coni**osis |
| conjunctiv/o | conjunctiva | **conjunctiv**itis |
| contra- | against/opposed/opposite | **contra**ception |
| -conus | cone-like protrusion | kerato**conus** |
| copr/o | faeces | **copr**olith |
| cor- | with/together | **cor**rosive |
| cord/o | a cord | **cord**otomy |
| cor/e/o | pupil | **core**omorphosis |
| -coria | condition of the pupils | aniso**coria** |
| corne/o | cornea/horny (consisting of keratin) | **corne**oblepharon |
| coron/ar- | crown-like projection/encircling/coronary vessels of heart | **coron**ary |
| corpor/o | body | **corpor**al |

| | | |
|---|---|---|
| -cortex- | outer part/bark | adrenal **cortex** |
| cortic/o | adrenal cortex/cortex/outer region | **cortic**otrophic |
| cost/o | rib | inter**cost**al |
| cox/o | hip/hip joint | **cox**ofemoral |
| cranl/o | cranium/skull | **cranl**otomy |
| cren/o | crenated | **cren**ocytosis |
| -crescent | grow/crescent | epithelial **crescent** |
| -crine | secrete | exo**crine** |
| crin/o | secrete | endo**crin**ology |
| -crit | separate/device for measuring cells | haemato**crit** |
| crur/o | leg | **crur**al |
| cry/o | relating to cold | **cry**ostat |
| crypt/o | hidden | **crypt**orchism |
| cubit/o | elbow | **cubit**us |
| culd/o | cul-de sac/Douglas pouch/recto-uterine pouch | **culd**oscope |
| -cule | small | animal**cule** |
| cult/o | cultivate | **cult**ure |
| cune/i | wedge (shape) | **cune**iform |
| cutane/o | skin | **cutane**ous |
| cut/i | skin | **cut**icle |
| cyan/o | blue | **cyan**osis |
| cycl/o | ciliary body/circle | **cycl**otomy |
| cyes/i/o | pregnancy | **cyes**iology |
| -cyesis | pregnancy | pseudo**cyesis** |
| cylindr/o | cylinder | **cylindr**oid |
| cyll/o | deformity | thoraco**cyll**osis |
| cyn/o | dog | **cyn**ophobla |
| cyrt/o | curved/abnormal curvature | **cyrt**ometer |
| cyst/i/o | bladder | **cyst**ostomy |
| -cyte | cell | melano**cyte** |
| cyt/o | cell | **cyt**ology |
| -cytosis | condition of cells, usually an abnormal increase | thrombo**cytosis** |
| dacry/o | tear/lacrimal apparatus | **dacry**olith |
| dacryocyst/o | lacrimal sac | **dacryocyst**otomy |
| dactyl/o | digits/fingers or toes | **dactyl**omegaly |
| de- | down/away from/loss of/reversing | **de**calcification |
| deca- | ten | **deca**gram |
| deci- | one tenth | **deci**litre |
| demi- | half | **demi**facet |
| dendr/i/o | tree/tree-like (dendrite of a neuron) | **dendr**itic |
| dentin/o | dentine of tooth | **dentin**ogenesis |
| dent/i/o | tooth | **dent**ist |
| derm/a/o | skin | **derm**abrasion |
| dermat/o | skin | **dermat**ology |
| descemet/o | Descemet's membrane (of cornea) | **descemet**ocele |

| | | |
|---|---|---|
| -desis | fixation/to bind together by surgery/sticking together | arthro**desis** |
| desm/o | band/ligament | **desmo**pathy |
| deuter/o | second | **deuter**anopia |
| dextro- | right | **dextro**cardia |
| di- | two/twice/double | **di**coria |
| dia- | through/apart/across/between | **dia**physis |
| -dialysis | separate | haemo**dialysis** |
| diaphor/o | sweating (excessive) | **diaphor**esis |
| diaphragmat/o | diaphragm | **diaphragmat**algia |
| diastol- | diastole | **diastol**ic |
| didym- | twins | epi**didym**is |
| digit/o | finger/toe | **digito**plantar |
| dipl/o- | double | **dipl**opia |
| dips/o | thirst | poly**dips**ia |
| dis- | apart/reversal/separation/duplication/free from | **dis**location |
| disc/o | intervertebral disc | **disco**graphy |
| disk/o (Am.) | intervertebral disc | **disk**ectomy |
| dist/o | far from point of origin | **dist**al |
| diverticul/o | diverticulum | **diverticul**itis |
| doch/o | duct/to receive | chole**doch**itis |
| dolich/o | long | **dolicho**cranial |
| dolor/i/o | pain (dol-unit of pain) | **doloro**genic |
| -dorsal | pertaining to the back (of the body) | ventro**dorsal** |
| dors/i/o | dorsal/the back (of the body) | **dorso**ventral |
| -drome | a course/conduction/flowing | syn**drome** |
| drom/o | a course/conduction/flowing | **dromo**tropic |
| -duct- | tube to lead material to or away from a structure | ovi**duct** |
| duoden/o | duodenum | **duoden**ostomy |
| dur/o | dura mater/hard | epi**dural** |
| dynam/o | force/power (of movement) | **dynam**ic |
| -dynia | condition of pain | pleuro**dynia** |
| dys- | difficult/disordered/painful/bad | **dys**phasia |
| | | |
| e- | away from/out from/outside/without | **e**masculation |
| -e | noun ending/a name | trigon**e** |
| -eal | pertaining to | oesophag**eal** |
| ec- | away from/out from/outside/without | **ec**cyesis |
| ech/o | reflected sound/echo/ultrasound echo | **echo**lalia |
| ect- | out/outside/outer part | **ect**ethmoid |
| ecto- | out/outside/outer part | **ecto**derm |
| ectopia- | condition of displacement | **ectopia** lentis |
| ectop/o | displaced away from normal position | **ectop**ic |

| | | |
|---|---|---|
| -ectasia | condition of dilation or stretching | pneumon**ectasia** |
| -ectasis | dilation, stretching | bronchi**ectasis** |
| -ectomy | removal, excision | appendic**ectomy** |
| ectro- | congenital absence/miscarriage | **ectro**dactylia |
| edema- (Am.) | swelling due to fluid | **edema**tous (Am.) |
| ef- | out/away from | **ef**ferent |
| eikon/o | icon | **eikon**ometer |
| elae/o | oil | **elae**opathia |
| elast/o | elastic/elastic tissue/elastin | **elast**osis |
| electro- | electrical | **electro**cardiograph |
| ellipto- | shaped like an ellipse | **ellipto**cytosis |
| em- | in | **em**pathy |
| -ema (Am.) | swelling/distension | myx**edema** |
| embol/o | embolus/plug/blockage | **embol**ism |
| embry/o | embryo | **embry**ogenesis |
| -emesis | vomiting | haemat**emesis** |
| emet/o | vomiting | **emet**ic |
| -emia (Am.) | condition of blood | an**emia** (Am.) |
| emmetr/o | in due measure/normally proportioned | **emmetr**opia |
| -emphraxis | blocking/stopping up | salping**emphraxis** |
| en- | within/in | **en**sheathed |
| encephal/o | brain | **encephal**itis |
| endo- | within/inside/inner | **endo**scope |
| endocardi/o | endocardium | **endocardi**tis |
| endocrin/o | endocrine (gland) | **endocrin**ologist |
| endometri/o | endometrium of uterus (lining) | **endometri**osis |
| endotheli/o | endothelium | **endotheli**al |
| enter/o | intestine | **enter**itis |
| -ent | person/agent | dilu**ent** |
| ento- | within/inside | **ento**cranial |
| eosin/o | red/dawn coloured/like eosin, a red acid dye | **eosin**ophil |
| ep- | above/upon/on | **ep**arterial |
| epi- | above/upon/on/in addition | **epi**dermis |
| epiderm/o | epidermis | **epiderm**al |
| epididym/o | epididymis | **epididym**ovasectomy |
| epiglott/o | epiglottis | **epiglott**itis |
| epilept/i/o | epilepsy | **epilept**iform |
| epipl/o | omentum | **epipl**oplasty |
| episi/o | pudendum/vulva | **episi**otomy |
| epitheli/o | epithelium | **epitheli**al |
| -er | one who/a person/an agent | radiograph**er** |
| erg/o/n/o | work | **ergo**nometer |
| -erysis | drag/draw/suck out | phaco**erysis** |
| erythr/o | red | **erythr**ocyte |
| -esis | abnormal state/condition | ur**esis** |
| es/o | within/inwards | **eso**deviation |
| esophag/o (Am.) | esophagus/gullet | **esophag**ostomy (Am.) |
| esthesi/o (Am.) | sensation | an**esthesi**ology (Am.) |
| estr/o (Am.) | estrogen/female/estrus | **estro**genic (Am.) |

| | | |
|---|---|---|
| ethm/o | ethmoid bone | **ethm**oidonasal |
| ethmoid/o | ethmoid bone | **ethmoido**palatal |
| eti/o (Am.) | causation (of disease) | **eti**ology (Am.) |
| eu- | good/normal/easy | **eu**tocia |
| eury- | wide/broad | **eury**cephalic |
| ex- | out/away from/outside | **ex**ophthalmos |
| exo- | out/away from/outside | **exo**gastric |
| -externa | external | otitis **externa** |
| extr/a/o | outside of/beyond/outward | **extra**hepatic |
| | | |
| faci/a/o | face | **facio**maxillary |
| faec/o | faeces | **faec**olith |
| falc/i | falx/sickle-shaped structure | **falci**form |
| fasicul/o | fascicle | **fasicul**ar |
| fasci/o | fascia/fibrous tissue *e.g.* covering muscles | **fascio**tomy |
| febr/o | fever | **febr**ile |
| fec/o (Am.) | feces/waste | **fec**al (Am.) |
| femor/o | femur/thigh | **femor**al |
| -ferent | carrying/to carry/to bear | e**fferent** |
| fer/o | to carry/to bear | urini**ferous** |
| ferr/o | iron | **ferro**protein |
| fet/i/o (Am.) | fetus | **fet**ometry (Am.) |
| fibrill/o | muscular twitching | **fibrill**ation |
| fibrin/o | fibrinogen | **fibrin**olytic |
| fimbri/o | fringe | **fimbri**ate |
| fibr/o | fibre | **fibr**osis |
| fibul/o | fibula | **fibulo**calcaneal |
| fil/o | thread | **filo**pressure |
| fissur- | split/cleft | **fissur**al |
| fistul/o | tube/pipe | **fistul**a |
| flagell/o | flagellum/whip | **flagell**osis |
| flav/o | yellow | **flavo**protein |
| -flect | bend | re**flect** |
| -flex- | bend | **flex**ion |
| fluor/o | fluorescent/luminous/flow | **fluoro**scopy |
| foet/o | foetus (Am. fet/o) | **foet**al |
| follicul/o | small sac/follicle | **follicul**itis |
| fore- | before/in front of | **fore**brain |
| -form | having form/structure of | epilepti**form** |
| foss/o | depression | **foss**a |
| fove/o | pit | **fove**a |
| fraen/o | fraenum or fraenulum/restraining structure *e.g.* fraenulum of the lip | **fraen**al |
| fren/o (Am.) | frenum or frenulum/restraining structure *e.g.* frenulum of the lip | **freno**plasty (Am.) |
| front/o | front/forehead | **fronto**temporal |
| -fuge | agent that suppresses/gets rid of | lacti**fuge** |
| fund/o | bottom/base (of an organ) | **fund**us |
| fung/i | fungus | **fungi**cide |
| furc/o | branching | bi**furc**ation |

| galact/o | milk | **galacto**poiesis |
| gamet/o | gametes/sperm or eggs | **gameto**genesis |
| gangli/o | ganglion/swelling/plexus | **gangli**form |
| ganglion- | ganglion/swelling/plexus | **ganglion**ectomy |
| gastr/o | stomach | **gastro**pathy |
| -gen | agent that produces/precursor | pepsino**gen** |
| -genesis | capable of causing/pertaining to formation | spermato**genesis** |
| -genic | pertaining to formation/originating in | oestro**genic** |
| genicul/o | knee | **genicul**ar |
| geni/o | chin | **genio**glossal |
| genit/o | genitals/reproductive organs/produced by birth | **genit**al |
| gen/o | cause/produce/originate | **geno**phobia |
| -genous | arising from/produced by/producing | andro**genous** |
| ger/i/o | old age/the aged | **ger**iatric |
| geront/o | old age/the aged | **geront**ology |
| gingiv/o | gum | **gingiv**itis |
| gli/a/o | glue-like (pertains to neuroglial supporting cells of CNS) | **gli**oma |
| glisson- | Glisson's capsule (around the liver) | **glisson**itis |
| -globin | protein | myo**globin** |
| -globulin | protein | immuno**globulin** |
| -globus | globe/like a small ball | kerato**globus** |
| glomerul/o | glomerulus of kidney | **glomerul**itis |
| gloss/o | tongue | **gloss**ectomy |
| glott- | glottis (vocal apparatus and its opening) | **glott**al |
| gluc/o | glucose/sugar/sweet | **gluco**neogenesis |
| glyc/o | glucose/sugar/sweet | **glyco**protein |
| glycogen/o | glycogen, a polysaccharide | **glycogen**osis |
| glycos- | sugar (obsolete variant of glucose) | **glycos**uria |
| gnath/o | jaw | **gnatho**plasty |
| -gnomy | science or means of judging | patho**gnomy** |
| -gnos- | to know/known or knowledge/judgment | **gnos**ia |
| -gnosia | condition of knowing/receiving/recognizing | hyper**gnosia** |
| -gnosis | to know/known or knowledge/judgment | pro**gnosis** |
| gonad/o | gonads (ovaries or testes) | **gonad**otrophin |
| gonecyst/o | seminal vesicle | **gonecyst**olith |
| gon/e/o | seed/semen/sperm/knee | **gono**coccus |
| goni/o | angle/corner | **goni**oscopy |
| gony/o | knee | **gony**oncus |
| -grade | to go | retro**grade** |
| -gram | X-ray/tracing/recording/one thousandth of a kilogram (g) | mammo**gram** |
| granul/o | granule/granular | **granul**oma |

| | | |
|---|---|---|
| -graph | usually recording instrument/ a recording/X-ray/mathematical curve representing data | electrocardio**graph** |
| -graphy | technique of recording/making an X-ray | electrocardio**graphy** |
| -gravida | pregnancy/pregnant woman | primi**gravida** |
| gravid/o | pregnancy | **gravid**ocardiac |
| gyn- | woman | **gyn**andrism |
| gynaec/o | gynaecology/female reproductive system/woman | **gynaec**ology |
| gynec/o (Am.) | gynecology/female reproductive system/woman | **gynec**ological (Am.) |
| gyn/o | gynaecology/female reproductive system/woman | **gyn**opathy |
| -gyric | pertaining to circular motion | oculo**gyric** |
| haemangi/o | blood vessel | **haemangi**oma |
| haem/a/o | blood (Am. hem/a) | **haem**odynamometer |
| haemat/o | blood (Am. hemat/o) | **haemat**ology |
| haemoglobin/o | haemoglobin | **haemoglobin**uria |
| halit/o | breath | **halit**osis |
| hallux | great toe | **hallux** rigidus |
| hal/o | salts | **hal**ogen |
| hapl/o | single/simple | **hapl**opia |
| hapt/o | touch | **hapt**ometer |
| hecto- | one hundred | **hecto**gram |
| helc/o | ulcer | **helc**osis |
| heli/o | sun | **heli**osis |
| helic/o | helix/spiral form | **helic**oid |
| helmint/h/o | worms | ant**helmint**hic |
| hem/a/o (Am.) | blood | **hem**ocytoblast (Am.) |
| hemat/o (Am.) | blood | **hemat**ology (Am.) |
| hemi- | half/on one side | **hemi**plegia |
| hepatic/o | hepatic bile duct | **hepatic**ostomy |
| hepat/o | liver | **hepat**ocyte |
| hept/a | seven | **hept**achromic |
| herni/o | hernia | **herni**orrhaphy |
| heter/o | other/another/different | **heter**osexual |
| hex- | six/hold/being | **hex**ose |
| hidraden/o | sweat gland | **hidraden**itis |
| hidr/o | sweat/perspiration | **hidr**osis |
| histi/o | histiocyte, a type of macrophage | **histi**ocytosis |
| hist/o | tissue | **hist**ology |
| hol/o | entire/whole | **hol**ocrine |
| homeo- | the same/resembling/ unchanging/constant | **homeo**stasis |
| homo- | the same/resembling | **homo**zygous |
| humer/o | humerus | **humer**oradial |
| hyal/o | glass-like | **hyal**oid |
| hydatid/i/o | hydatid cyst | **hydatid**osis |
| hydr/a/o | water | **hydr**onephrosis |
| hygr/o | moisture | **hygr**oblepharic |

| | | |
|---|---|---|
| hymen/o | hymen | **hymeno**tomy |
| hy/o | hyoid bone | **hyo**mandibular |
| hyp- | below/below normal/under | **hyp**hidrosis |
| hyper- | above/above normal/excessive/over | **hyper**chromia |
| hypn/o | sleep | **hypn**otic |
| hypo- | below normal/under | **hypo**thyroidism |
| hypophys- | hypophysis/pituitary gland | **hypophys**ectomy |
| hyster/o | uterus | **hyster**ectomy |
| | | |
| -ia | condition of/abnormal condition/disease | poly**uria** |
| -ial | pertaining to | bronch**ial** |
| -ian | belonging to/characteristic of | salping**ian** |
| -iasis | abnormal condition/process or condition resulting from/disease | lith**iasis** |
| -iatrics | medical speciality | paed**iatrics** |
| iatr/o | medical treatment by a doctor | **iatr**ogenic |
| -iatry | treatment by a doctor/speciality (of doctor) | psych**iatry** |
| -ible | capable of/able | flex**ible** |
| -ic[1] | pertaining to | gastr**ic** |
| -ic[2] | used in pharmacology to mean a drug or drug action | diuret**ic** |
| -ical | pertaining to | cytolog**ical** |
| ichthy/o | dry/scaly/fish like | **ichthy**osis |
| -ician | person associated with/specialist | techn**ician** |
| -ics | art or science of | genet**ics** |
| -ictal | pertaining to seizure/sudden attack | pre**ictal** |
| icter/o | jaundice | **icter**ogenic |
| -ide | binary chemical compound | glycos**ide** |
| idi/o | self/one's own/peculiar to an organism | **idi**opathic |
| -igo | attack/abnormal condition | vert**igo** |
| il- | in/none | **il**legitimate |
| -ile | capable of/able | contract**ile** |
| ile/o | ileum | **ile**ocolitis |
| ili/o | ilium/flank | **ili**ofemoral |
| im- | in/within/none/not | **im**potence |
| immun/o | immune/immunity | **immun**ology |
| in- | in/none/not | **in**cision |
| -in | used as suffix for various chemicals | glycer**in** |
| incud/o | anvil/incus (the anvil-shaped ear ossicle) | **incudo**malleal |
| -ine | pertaining to/a suffix for chemicals derived or thought to be derived from ammonia | am**ine** |
| infer/o | inferior/below/beneath | **infer**olateral |
| infra- | below/beneath/inferior to | **infra**mammary |

| | | |
|---|---|---|
| lumb/o | loin/lower back | **lumbo**costal |
| lump- | lump/swelling | **lump**ectomy |
| lute/o | yellow/corpus luteum of ovary | **luteo**trophic |
| lymph/a/t/o | lymph | **lymph**oma |
| lymphaden/o | lymph node (lymph gland) | **lymphaden**itis |
| lymphangi/o | lymph vessel | **lymphangio**graphy |
| lymphocyt/o | lymphocyte | **lymphocyto**sis |
| lymphomat/o | lymphoma | **lymphomat**osis |
| lyo- | water soluble/solvent/dissolve | **lyo**phil |
| -lys/o | break down/disintegration/dissolving | **lys**in |
| -lysis | break down/disintegration/dissolving | auto**lysis** |
| -lytic | pertaining to break down/disintegration | haemo**lytic** |
| | | |
| macro- | large | **macro**phage |
| macul/o | spot/blotch | **maculo**papular |
| mal- | bad/diseased or impaired | **mal**nutrition |
| -malacia | condition of softening | myo**malacia** |
| malac/o | softening | **malac**ic |
| malign- | bad/harmful | **malign**ant |
| malle/o | hammer/malleus (the hammer-shaped ear ossicle) | **malle**otomy |
| mamill/i/o | nipple | **mamilli**plasty |
| mamm/a/o | breast/mammary gland | **mammo**graphy |
| mammill/i/o | nipple | **mammill**itis |
| mandibul/o | mandible (lower jaw bone) | **mandibulo**plasty |
| mani- | mental disorder/madness | **mani**ac |
| -mania | condition of mental disorder/psychosis | hyper**mania** |
| man/o | pressure | **mano**metry |
| manus- | hand | **manus** extensa |
| mast/o | breast/mammary gland | **mast**algia |
| mastoid/o | nipple-shaped/mastoid process/mastoid air cells | **mastoid**ectomy |
| maxill/o | maxilla (upper jaw bone) | **maxillo**facial |
| meat/o | meatus/opening/external orifice *e.g.* of the urethra | **meato**tomy |
| medi/o | middle/midline | **medi**al |
| -media | middle | otitis **media** |
| medull/o | inner part/medulla | adrenal **medulla** |
| mega- | abnormally large | **mega**colon |
| megal/o | abnormally large | **megalo**glossia |
| -megaly | enlargement | acro**megaly** |
| melan/o | melanin/dark pigment | **melan**oma |
| melanomat- | melanoma | **melanomat**osis |
| melit/o | sugar/honey | **melit**uria |
| mel/o | limb/cheek | **mel**agra |
| melon/o | cheek | **melono**plasty |
| mening/i/o | membranes (of CNS) | **mening**itis |
| menisc/o | meniscus/crescent-shaped | **menisco**cyte |

| men/o | menses/menstruation/monthly flow | **men**orrhagia |
| ment/o | chin/mind | **mento**plasty |
| mes/o | middle/intermediate | **meso**derm |
| meta- | change in form, position or order/after/next/between | **meta**plasia |
| metacarp/o | metacarpus | **meta**carpal |
| metatars/o | metatarsal | **metatars**algia |
| -meter | measuring instrument/a measure | audio**meter** |
| metr/a/i/o | uterus/womb | endo**metr**iosis |
| -metrist | person who measures | audio**metrist** |
| -metry | process of measuring | audio**metry** |
| micro- | small/one millionth | **micro**glia |
| mid- | middle | **mid**brain |
| -mileusis | to carve | kerato**mileusis** |
| milli- | one thousandth | **milli**litre |
| -mimesis | simulation/imitation | patho**mimesis** |
| -mimetic | simulation of a specific effect | sympatho**mimetic** |
| -mimia | condition of expressing through gestures | macro**mimia** |
| mi/o | make smaller/less | **mi**opia |
| mito- | thread-like/mitosis | **mito**tic |
| mono- | one/single | **mono**somy |
| monocyt/o | monocyte | **monocyt**openia |
| -morph | shape/form | ecto**morph** |
| morph/o | shape/form | **morph**ogenesis |
| mort/o | death | **mort**al |
| -motor- | moving/action/set in motion | oculo**motor** |
| muc/o | mucus | **muc**ous |
| multi- | many | **multi**gravida |
| muscul/o | muscle | **musculo**cutaneous |
| my- | (from myein) to close/squint | **my**opic |
| mycet/o | fungus | **mycet**oid |
| myc/o | fungus | broncho**myc**osis |
| myelin/o | myelin/myelin sheath | **myelin**ated |
| myel/o | bone marrow/spinal cord | **myel**oma |
| myelomat/o | myeloma | **myelomat**osis |
| my/o | muscle | **my**oglobin |
| myocardi/o | myocardium (heart muscle) | **myocardi**opathy |
| myomat/o | myoma | **myomat**osis |
| myop- | short sighted | **myop**ia |
| myos/o | muscle | **myos**itis |
| myring/o | eardrum/tympanic membrane | **myring**otome |
| myx/o | mucus/mucoid tissue (embryonic connective tissue) | **myx**adenitis |
| myxomat- | myxoma | **myxomat**osis |
| nano- | one billionth ($10^{-9}$) | **nano**metre |
| narc/o | stupor/numbness | **narc**otic |
| nas/o | nose | **naso**pharyngitis |
| nasopharyng/o | nasopharynx | **nasopharyngo**scope |

| | | |
|---|---|---|
| -natal | pertaining to birth | ante**natal** |
| nat/o | birth | neo**nat**ology |
| natr/i | sodium | **natr**iuresis |
| necr/o | death/dead tissue | **necr**osis |
| neo- | new/recent | **neo**plasia |
| nephr/o | kidney | **nephr**itis |
| neur/o | nerve (rarely tendon) | **neur**ology |
| neuron/o | neuron | **neuron**al |
| neutr/o | neutral | **neutr**ophil |
| noc/i | harm | **noc**iceptor |
| noct/i | night/darkness | **noct**uria |
| nod/o | knot/swelling | **nod**ule |
| nom/o | distribute/law/custom | **nom**otopic |
| non- | without/no | **non** compos mentis |
| normo- | normal | **normo**cytosis |
| nos/o | disease | **nos**ology |
| not/o | back | **not**ochord |
| nucle/o | nucleus | **nucle**oprotein |
| nulli- | none | **nulli**para |
| nyctal/o | night/darkness | **nyctal**opia |
| nyct/o | night/darkness | **nyct**algia |
| nymph/o | labia minora/nymphae | **nymph**omania |
| -nyxis | perforation/pricking/puncture | kerato**nyxis** |
| | | |
| obstetr- | midwifery/obstetrics | **obstetr**ician |
| occipit/o | occiput, posterior region of the skull | **occipit**ocervical |
| occlus/o | shut/close up | **occlus**ion |
| octa/i/o- | eight | **octi**gravida |
| ocul/o | eye | bin**ocul**ar |
| odont/o | tooth/teeth | orth**odont**ics |
| -oedema | swelling due to fluid (Am. edema) | myx**oedema** |
| oes/o | within (Am. es/o) | **oes**ogastritis |
| oesophag/o | oesophagus/gullet (Am. esophago) | **oesophag**ostomy |
| oestr/o | oestrogen (a female sex-hormone)/oestrus (Am. estr/o) | **oestr**ogenic |
| -oid | resembling | lip**oid** |
| -ola | small | arteri**ola** |
| -ole | small | arteri**ole** |
| olecran/o | elbow/olecranon (bony projection of ulna) | **olecran**arthropathy |
| ole/o | oil | **ole**ogranuloma |
| olfact/o | sense of smell/smell | **olfact**ory |
| olig/o | deficiency/few/little | **olig**uria |
| -olisthesis | slipping | spondylol**isthesis** |
| -oma | tumour/swelling | sarc**oma** |
| oment/o | omentum (peritoneal fold of stomach) | **oment**oplasty |
| om/o | shoulder | **om**oclavicular |
| omphal/o | navel/umbilical cord/umbilicus | **omphal**ogenesis |

| | | |
|---|---|---|
| onc/o | tumour/mass | oncology |
| -one | hormone | progesterone |
| onych/o | nail | onychodystrophy |
| oo- | egg | oocyte |
| oophor/o | ovary | oophorectomy |
| -op- | seeing/looking at | presbyopia |
| ophthalm/o | eye | ophthalmoscope |
| -ophthalmos | eye | exophthalmos |
| -opia | condition of vision/defective vision | amblyopia |
| opistho- | backward/behind | opisthognathism |
| -opsia | condition of vision/defective vision | hemiachromatopsia |
| -opsy | to view/process of viewing | biopsy |
| optic/o | vision/eye/optic nerve | optical |
| opt/o | vision/eye | optometry |
| orbit/o | the orbit (the bony cavity of the eye) | orbitonasal |
| -or | person or agent | donor |
| orchid/o | testicle/testis | orchidopathy |
| orch/i/o | testicle/testis | orchioplasty |
| -orexia | condition of appetite | anorexia |
| organ/o | organ | organogenesis |
| or/o | mouth | oral |
| orth/o- | correct/normal/straight | orthoptics |
| -ory | pertaining to | sensory |
| os- | bone/a mouth/an orifice | os uteri |
| osche/o | scrotum | oscheoplasty |
| -ose | carbohydrate/sugar/starch/full of/pertaining to/having form of | glucose |
| -osis | abnormal condition/disease of/abnormal increase | leucocytosis |
| osm/o | odour/smell/osmosis | osmodysphoria |
| osphresi/o | odour/olfaction/smell | osphresiology |
| osse/o | bone | osseous |
| oss/i | bone | ossicle |
| ossicul/o | ear ossicles/ear bones | ossiculectomy |
| ost/e/o | bone | osteoarthritis |
| ot/o | ear | otology |
| oul/o | scar/gum | oulectomy |
| -ous | pertaining to | uriniferous |
| ovari/o | ovary | ovariotomy |
| ov/i/o | egg/ovum | oviduct |
| -oxia | condition of oxygen | hypoxia |
| ox/i/o | oxygen | oximetry |
| oxy- | oxygen/sharp/quick | oxytocic |
| | | |
| pachy- | thick | pachydermia |
| paed/o | child (Am. ped/o) | paediatric |
| palae/o | old/primitive (Am. pale/o) | palaeocortex |
| palat/o | palate | palatoplasty |
| pale/o (Am.) | old/primitive | paleocortex (Am.) |

| | | |
|---|---|---|
| palm/o | palm | **palm**ar |
| palpebr/o | eyelid | **palpebr**itis |
| pan- | all | **pan**carditis |
| pancreatic/o | pancreatic duct | **pancreatico**enterostomy |
| pancreat/o | pancreas | **pancreato**lysis |
| pannicul/o | fatty layer *e.g.* of abdomen | **pannicul**itis |
| pant/o | all/entire | **pant**atrophy |
| papill/i/o | nipple-like/optic disc/optic papilla | **papillo**retinitis |
| para- | beside/near/beyond/accessory to/wrong | **para**nephric |
| -para(re) | to bear/bring forth offspring/ a woman who has borne viable young | primi**para** |
| parasympath/o | parasympathetic nervous system | **parasympatho**mimetic |
| parathyr/o | parathyroid gland | **parathyro**trophic |
| parathyroid/o | parathyroid gland | **parathyroid**ectomy |
| -paresis | slight paralysis | juvenile **paresis** |
| parotid/o | parotid gland | **parot**itis |
| -parous | pertaining to production of live young | nulli**parous** |
| -partum | birth/labour | post **partum** |
| parturi- | childbirth/labour/parturition | **parturi**ent |
| patell/o | patella/knee cap | **patello**femoral |
| -pathia | condition of disease | psycho**pathia** |
| -pathic | pertaining to disease | idio**pathic** |
| path/o | disease | **patho**logist |
| -pathy | disease/emotion | gastro**pathy** |
| -pause | stopping | meno**pause** |
| pect- | chest/breast/thorax | **pect**us |
| pector/o | chest/breast/thorax | **pector**al |
| pedicul/o | lice | **pedicul**osis |
| ped/i/o | foot/child | **ped**iatrics (Am.) |
| pelli- | skin/hide | **pelli**cle |
| pelv/i/o | pelvis | **pelv**imeter |
| -penia | condition of deficiency or lack of | erythro**penia** |
| pen/o | penis | **pen**itis |
| peps- | digestion/pepsin | **peps**inogen |
| -pepsia | condition of digestion | brady**pepsia** |
| pepsin/o | digestion/pepsin | **pepsin**ogen |
| pept- | digestion/pepsin | **pept**ic |
| per- | through/completely/excessive | **per**cutaneous |
| peri- | around | **peri**corneal |
| pericardi/o | pericardium | **pericard**itis |
| perine/o | perineum | **perineo**rrhaphy |
| periton/e/o | peritoneum | **periton**itis |
| petr/o | stone/rock | osteo**petr**osis |
| -pexis | surgical fixation/fix in place/ storage | glyco**pexis** |
| -pexy | surgical fixation/fix in place/ storage | arthro**pexy** |
| phac/o | lens | **phaco**scopy |

| phae/o | dusky/dark (Am. phe/o) | **phae**ochromocyte |
| -phagia | condition of eating/swallowing | poly**phagia** |
| phag/o | eating/consuming/phagocyte | **phago**cyte |
| -phagy | eating or swallowing | copro**phagy** |
| phak/o | lens | **phak**itis |
| phalang/o | phalanx/finger/toe | **phalang**eal |
| phall/o | penis | **phall**ic |
| phaner/o | visible/manifesting | **phaner**ogenic |
| pharm/ac/o | drug/medicine | **pharm**acology |
| pharyng/o | pharynx | **pharyng**itis |
| -phasia | condition of speaking/speech | dys**phasia** |
| phas/i/o | speech | a**phas**iology |
| phe/o | dusky/dark | **pheo**chromocyte (Am.) |
| -phil | love/affinity for/cell type with affinity for | neutro**phil** |
| -philia | condition of love/affinity for | haemo**philia** |
| -phily | condition of love/affinity for | necro**phily** |
| phleb/o | vein | **phleb**ectomy |
| -phobia | condition of irrational fear/aversion | hydro**phobia** |
| -phonia | condition of having voice | a**phonia** |
| phon/o | speech/sound/voice | **phono**cardiograph |
| -phony | sound/type of speech | tracheo**phony** |
| -phore | a carrier | chromato**phore** |
| -phoresis | movement in a specified way/bearing/carrying/driving ions | electro**phoresis** |
| -phoria | condition of mental state/feeling/bearing/deviation of the eyes/heterophoria | eu**phoria** |
| phor/o | mental state/bearing/carrier (*e.g.* of disease) | **phor**ology |
| phosph/o | phosphate/phosphorus/phosphoric acid | **phospho**lipid |
| phot/o | light | **photo**sensitive |
| phrenic/o | diaphragm/mind/phrenic nerve | **phrenic**ectomy |
| phren/i/o | diaphragm/mind/phrenic nerve | **phreno**gastric |
| -phthisis | wasting away | neuro**phthisis** |
| -phylaxis | protection | pro**phylaxis** |
| -phyma | tumour/boil/swelling | rhino**phyma** |
| phys/i/o | nature/physical things/physiology | **physio**therapy |
| -physis | growth | hypo**physis** |
| -phyt/e/o | plant/fungus | dermato**phyte** |
| pico- | small/a quantity multiplied by $10^{-12}$ | **pico**gram |
| pil/o | hair | **pilo**sebaceous |
| pineal/o | pineal body/pineal gland | **pineal**ocyte |
| pituitar- | pituitary gland | hypo**pituitar**ism |
| placent/o | placenta | **placent**ography |
| -plakia | condition of broad/flat (patch) | leuko**plakia** |
| -plania | condition of wandering *e.g.* a cell moving position | leucocyto**plania** |

| | | |
|---|---|---|
| plan/o | flat | **plano**cellular |
| plant/i | sole of foot | **plant**ar |
| -plasia | condition of growth due to formation of cells | hyper**plasia** |
| -plasm | formative substance/growth | cyto**plasm** |
| plasma- | plasma cell/fluid of blood | **plasma**therapy |
| plasm/o | anything moulded, shaped or formed/formative substance/ growth/plasma | |
| | | **plasmo**cyte |
| plast- | forming cells or tissues/plastic | a**plast**ic |
| -plastic | pertaining to formation of cells or tissues | |
| | | neo**plastic** |
| -plasty | surgical repair/reconstruction | kerato**plasty** |
| platy- | flat | **platy**onychia |
| -plegia | condition of paralysis/stroke | para**plegia** |
| pleo- | more | **pleo**cytosis |
| plethysm/o | volume | **plethysmo**graph |
| pleur/o | pleural membranes/rib/side | **pleuro**dynia |
| plex/o | network of nerves, blood or lymph vessels | |
| | | **plex**us |
| -plex-ia | condition from a stroke or serious occurrence | |
| | | apo**plexia** |
| -plexy | strike/paralyse | apo**plexy** |
| -ploid(y) | chromosome sets in a cell | di**ploid** |
| pluri- | several/more | **pluri**glandular |
| -pnea (Am.) | breathing | a**pnea** (Am.) |
| pne/o | breath/breathing | **pne**oscope |
| pneum/a/o | gas/air/lung/breathing | **pneumo**thorax |
| pneumat/o | gas/air/lung/breathing | **pneumato**metry |
| pneumon/o | lung | **pneumon**ectomy |
| -pnoea | breathing (Am. pnea) | dys**pnoea** |
| pod/o | foot | **pod**iatry |
| pogon/o | beard | **pogon**iasis |
| -poiesis | formation | erythro**poiesis** |
| poikil/o | varied/irregular | **poikilo**cyte |
| polio- | grey matter (of CNS)/ poliomyelitis | |
| | | **polio**myelitis |
| pollex | thumb | **pollex** flexus |
| poly- | many/too much | **poly**uria |
| polyp/o | polyp/small growth | **polyp**ectomy |
| pont/o | pons (part of metencephalon of brain) | |
| | | **ponto**cerebellar |
| por/o | passage/pore | osteo**porosis** |
| port/o | portal vein | **porto**graphy |
| post- | after/behind | **post**-ganglionic |
| poster/o | back of body/behind/posterior to | |
| | | **postero**superior |
| posth/o | prepuce/foreskin | balano**posthitis** |
| -prandial | pertaining to a meal | post**prandial** |
| -praxia | condition of purposeful movement or conduct | |
| | | a**praxia** |
| pre- | before/in front of | **pre**tracheal |

| | | |
|---|---|---|
| preputi/o | prepuce/foreskin | **prepu**tiotomy |
| presby/o | old man/old age | **presby**opia |
| primi- | first | **primi**gravida |
| priv-ia | condition of loss or deprivation | calci**privia** |
| pro- | before/favouring/in front of | **pro**drome |
| proct/o | rectum/anus | **proct**algia |
| progest/o | progesterone | **progest**ogen |
| prosop/o | face | **prosop**oplegia |
| prostat/o | prostate gland | **prostat**ism |
| prosth/o | adding (replacement part) | **prosth**odontics |
| proto- | first | **proto**diastole |
| protoz/o | protozoa | **protoz**oiasis |
| proxim/o | near | **proxim**al |
| prurit/o | itching | **prurit**ic |
| pseud/o | false | **pseud**oplegia |
| psych/o | mind | **psych**osis |
| psychr/o | cold | **psychr**algia |
| -ptosis | falling/displacement/prolapse | blepharo**ptosis** |
| -ptotic | pertaining to falling/displacement/prolapse/affected with a ptosis | nephro**ptotic** |
| ptyal/o | saliva | **ptyal**ography |
| -ptysis | spitting/coughing up | pyo**ptysis** |
| pub/o | pubis/pubic region | **pub**ovesical |
| pudend- | pudendum/vulva | **pudend**al |
| puerper/o | puerperium/time of childbirth | **puerper**al |
| pulm/o | lung | **pulm**o-aortic |
| pulmon/o | lung | **pulmon**ary |
| pupill/o | pupil | **pupill**ometry |
| purul/o | pus-filled | **purul**oid |
| pustul/o | infected pimple/pustule | **pustul**osis |
| pyel/o | pelvis/trough of kidney | **pyel**olithotomy |
| pykn/o | compact/thick/frequent | **pykn**osis |
| pyle/o | portal (vein) | **pyle**phlebitis |
| pylor/o | pylorus | **pylor**ic |
| py/o | pus | **py**ogenic |
| pyret/o | heat/fire/burning/fever | **pyret**ic |
| pyr/o | heat/fire/burning/fever | **pyr**ogen |
| quadr/i/u- | four | **quadr**iplegia |
| quinque- | five | **quinque**cuspid |
| quint- | five | **quint**an |
| rachi/o | backbone/spine/vertebral column | **rachi**opathy |
| radic/o | nerve root | **radic**otomy |
| radicul/o | spinal nerve root | **radicul**itis |
| radi/o | radioactivity/radiation/X-ray/radius | **radi**otherapy |
| re- | back/contrary/again | **re**position |
| rect/o | rectum | **recto**sigmoid |
| ren/i/o | kidney | **ren**ography |

| | | |
|---|---|---|
| reticul/o | net-like/reticulum | **reticulo**cytosis |
| reticuloendotheli/o | reticuloendothelial system | **reticuloendothelium** |
| retin/o | retina | **retino**blastoma |
| retro- | backwards/behind | **retro**verted |
| rhabd/o | rod/rod-shaped | **rhabd**oid |
| rhabdomy/o | striated muscle | **rhabdomy**oma |
| rhe/o | electric current/flow of fluid | **rhe**ology |
| rheumat/o | rheumatism | **rheumat**ism |
| rhin/o | nose | **rhino**plasty |
| rhiz/o | root/spinal nerve root | **rhizo**tomy |
| rhod/o | red | **rhod**opsin |
| rhytid/o | wrinkle | **rhytido**plasty |
| roentgen/o | X-ray/Roentgen rays | **roentgeno**graphy |
| rostr/i | superior/a rostrum/beak | **rostr**al |
| -rrhage | bursting forth/excessive flow | haemo**rrhage** |
| -rrhagia | condition of bursting forth/ excessive flow | oto**rrhagia** |
| -rrhaphy | suture/suturing/stitching | teno**rrhaphy** |
| -rrhea (Am.) | excessive discharge/flow | rhino**rrhea** (Am.) |
| -rrhexis | breaking/rupturing | ovario**rrhexis** |
| -rrhoea | excessive discharge/flow (Am. -rrhea) | rhino**rrhoea** |
| (r)rhythm/o | rhythm | ar**rhythm**ia |
| rubr- | red | **rub**or |
| rug/o | wrinkle/fold/ridge | **rug**a |
| | | |
| sacchar/o | sugar/sweet | **saccharo**lytic |
| saccul/o | saccule of inner ear | **saccul**ar |
| sacr/o | sacrum | **sacro**coccygeal |
| salping/o | Eustachian (auditory) tube/ Fallopian tube | **salpingo**stomy |
| sanguin/o | blood/bloody | **sanguin**olent |
| sapr/o | decay/decayed matter | **sapro**dontia |
| sarc/o | flesh/connective tissue | **sarc**oid |
| -sarcoma | malignant (fleshy) tumour of connective tissue | Kaposi's **sarcoma** |
| sarcomat- | sarcoma (malignant fleshy tumour of connective tissue) | **sarcomat**osis |
| scapul/o | scapula | **scapulo**clavicular |
| scat/o | faeces/faecal matter | **scato**logy |
| -schisis | cleaving/splitting/parting | palato**schisis** |
| schist/o | cleaving/splitting/parting | **schisto**cephalus |
| schistosom/o | parasitic worm of Genus Schistosoma | **schistosom**iasis |
| schiz/o | split/cleft/divided | **schizo**trichia |
| scint/i | scintillation/spark/flash of light | **scinti**scan |
| scirrh/o | hard | **scirrh**us |
| scler/o | hard/sclera (the white of the eye) | **sclero**tome |
| -sclerosis | abnormal condition of hardening | arterio**sclerosis** |
| scoli/o | crooked/twisted/lateral curvature of the spine | **scoli**osis |
| -scope | instrument to view/examine | endo**scope** |

| | | |
|---|---|---|
| -scopic | pertaining to examining/viewing | microscopic |
| -scopist | specialist who examines or uses a viewing instrument | endoscopist |
| -scopy | visual examination/examination | endoscopy |
| scot/o | darkness/scotoma | scotopia |
| scotom/o | blind spot/scotoma | scotomagraph |
| scrot/o | scrotum | scrotocele |
| seb/o | sebum/sebaceous gland | sebolith |
| -sect(ion) | cut | Caesarean section |
| secund/- | second | secundigravida |
| semi- | half/partly | semicomatose |
| semin/i | semen | seminoma |
| sen/i | old | senile |
| sens/o | sense | sensomotor |
| sensor/i | sense/sensation | sensorium |
| -sepsis | infection | asepsis |
| septi- | seven | septipara |
| septic/o | sepsis/infection/putrefaction | septicaemia |
| sept/o | septum e.g. nasal septum | septotomy |
| sequestr- | sequestrum, a portion of dead bone | sequestrectomy |
| ser/o | serum | seropositive |
| sex/i | six | sexidigital |
| sialaden/o | salivary glands | sialadenitis |
| sial/o | saliva/salivary gland or duct | sialography |
| sider/o | iron | sideropenia |
| sigmoid/o | sigmoid colon | sigmoidoscopy |
| silic/o | glass/silica | silicosis |
| sinistr/o | left/left side | sinistrocardia |
| sin/o | sinus | sinoatrial |
| sinus- | sinus | sinus venosus |
| sinus/o | sinus | sinusitis |
| -sis | abnormal condition/action/state of | centesis |
| -sitia | condition of appetite for food | eusitia |
| sit/o | food | sitophobia |
| somatic/o | body | somaticosplanchnic |
| somat/o | body | somatotrophic |
| somn/i/o | sleep | somnial |
| son/o | sound/ultrasound | ultrasonography |
| -spadia(s) | condition of drawing out/cleft or rent of the male urethra | hypospadia |
| span/o | scanty or scarce | spanomenorrhoea |
| -spasm | involuntary contraction of muscle | blepharospasm |
| spasm/o | spasm/involuntary muscle contraction | spasmodyspnoea |
| spermat/o | sperm | spermatogenesis |
| sperm/i/o | sperm | spermicidal |
| sphen/o | sphenoid bone/wedge shaped | sphenomandibular |
| spher/o | sphere-shaped/round | spherophakia |

| | | |
|---|---|---|
| sphincter/o | sphincter/ring-like muscle | **sphincter**oplasty |
| sphygm/o | pulse | **sphygmo**manometer |
| -sphyx- | pulsing | a**sphyx**ia |
| spirill/i | spiral-shaped bacteria of Genus Spirillum | **Spirillum** minus |
| spir/o | to breathe | **spir**ometry |
| spirochaet/o | spirochaete (a spiral-shaped bacterium) | **spirochaet**e |
| spirochet/o (Am.) | spirochaete (a spiral-shaped bacterium) | **spiroch**ete (Am.) |
| splanchnic/o | splanchnic nerve | **splanchnic**ectomy |
| splanchn/i/o | viscera/splanchnic nerve | **splanchnic** |
| splen/o | spleen | **splen**ectomy |
| spondyl/o | vertebra | **spondyl**itis |
| spongi/o | sponge | **spongi**form |
| spor/o | spore | **sporo**mycosis |
| squam/o | scale/scale-like | **squam**ous |
| -stalsis | contraction | peri**stalsis** |
| stapedi/o | stirrup/stapes (the stirrup-shaped ear ossicle) | **stapedio**tenotomy |
| staphyl/o | staphylococcus/a grape-like cluster/the uvula | **staphylo**coccal |
| staphylococc/o | staphylococcus | **staphylococc**aemia |
| -stasis | stopping/controlling/cessation of movement | haemo**stasis** |
| -stat | agent/device that prevents change, regulates or stops something | cryo**stat** |
| -static | pertaining to stopping/controlling/standing or without motion | haemo**static** |
| -staxis | dripping/a dropping *e.g.* of blood | epi**staxis** |
| stear/i/o | fat | **stear**iform |
| steat/o | fat | **steat**oma |
| sten/o | narrow/constricted | **steno**coriasis |
| -stenosis | abnormal condition of narrowing | urethro**stenosis** |
| sterc/o | faeces | **sterc**olith |
| ster/e/o | solid/three dimensional | **stereo**scopic |
| stern/o | sternum | **sterno**costal |
| steth/o | chest/breast | **stetho**scope |
| -sthenia | condition of strength/full power | mya**sthenia** |
| sthen/o | strength/full power | a**sthen**ic |
| stomat/o | mouth | **stomat**itis |
| stom/o | mouth/mouth-like opening | **stom**al |
| -stomy | to form a new opening or outlet/ a communication/an opening | colo**stomy** |
| strabism/o | squint/strabismus | **strabism**ic |
| strab/o | squint/strabismus | **strab**otomy |
| strat/i | layer | **strat**iform |
| -ept/o | streptococcus/a twisted chain | **strepto**coccal |

| | | |
|---|---|---|
| streptococc/o | streptococcus | **strepto**coccaemia |
| striat/o | mark/stripe | **striat**ed |
| styl/o | stake/styloid process (of temporal bone) | **stylo**mastoid |
| sub- | beneath/under | **sub**cutaneous |
| sud/or/i | sweat/perspiration | **sud**oresis |
| super/o | superior/above/excess | **supero**lateral |
| supra- | superior/above/excess | **supra**hepatic |
| sy- | with/together | **sy**stole |
| sym- | with/together | **sym**melia |
| sympath/o | sympathetic nervous system/ sympathetic nerves | **sympath**olytic |
| symphysi/o | symphysis (fibro-cartilaginous joint) *e.g.* symphysis pubis | **symphysio**tomy |
| syn- | together/in association/with | **syn**chronous |
| synapt- | synapse | **synapt**ic |
| syndesm/o | ligament/connective tissue | **syndesm**ectomy |
| syndrom/o | running together | **syndrom**ic |
| -synechia | condition of synechia/adhering together | blepharo**synechia** |
| synovi/o | synovia/synovial fluid/synovial membranes | **synovi**al |
| syphil/o | syphilis | **syphil**oma |
| syring/o | tube/cavity | **syring**omyelia |
| system/o | system | **system**ic |
| systol- | systole | **systol**ic |
| | | |
| tachy- | fast | **tachy**cardia |
| tact- | touch | **tact**ile |
| tal/o | ankle/ankle bone | **tal**ar |
| tars/o | tarsus/ankle/eyelid edge | **tars**algia |
| -taxia | condition of ordered movement | a**taxia** |
| tax/o | ordered movement/ arrangement/classification | **tax**ology |
| tectori/o | covering/roof-like | **tectori**al |
| tel- | tela or web | **tel**angiectasis |
| -tela | a web-like membrane | epi**tela** |
| tele- | far away/operating at a distance | **tele**cardiography |
| telo- | end | **telo**phase |
| tendin/o | tendon | **tendin**oplasty |
| tend/o | tendon | **tendo**tome |
| ten/o | tendon | **teno**rrhaphy |
| tenont/o | tendon | **tenont**ophyma |
| ter- | three | **ter**valent |
| terat/o | monster-like/a deformed embryo or fetus | **terat**ogenic |
| testicul/o | testicle/testis | **testicul**ar |
| test/o | testicle/testis | **test**osterone |
| tetra- | four | **tetra**ploid |
| thalam/o | thalamus (part of cerebral cortex) | **thalamo**tomy |
| than/at/o | death | **thanat**ophobia |
| thec/o | sheath | **thec**al |

| thel/e/o | nipple | **thele**plasty |
|---|---|---|
| -therapy | treatment | physio**therapy** |
| -thermia | condition of heat | hypo**thermia** |
| therm/o | heat | **therm**ography |
| -thermy | state of heat/process of heating | cystodia**thermy** |
| thio- | sulphur | **thio**cyanate |
| thoracico- | thorax | **thoracico**-abdominal |
| thorac/o | thorax | **thoraco**tomy |
| -thorax | thorax/chest | pneumo**thorax** |
| thromb/o | thrombus/clot | **thromb**osis |
| thrombocyt/o | platelet/thrombocyte | **thrombocyto**penia |
| thymic/o | thymus gland | **thymico**lymphatic |
| thym/o | thymus gland | **thym**ic |
| thyr/o | thyroid gland | **thyro**trophic |
| thyroid/o | thyroid gland | hypo**thyroid**ism |
| tibi/o | tibia | **tibio**fibular |
| -tic | pertaining to | necrotic |
| tine/o | gnawing worm/ringworm | *Tinea pedis* |
| -tion | state or condition/process | resection |
| -tocia | condition of birth/labour | eu**tocia** |
| toc/o | labour/childbirth | **toco**logy |
| -tome | cutting instrument | myringo**tome** |
| tom/o | slice/section | **tomo**graphy |
| -tomy | incision into | laparo**tomy** |
| -tonia | condition of tension/tone | a**tonia** |
| ton/o | stretching/tension/tone | **tono**meter |
| tonsill/o | tonsil | **tonsill**ectomy |
| top/o | place/particular area | **topo**logy |
| tort/i | twisted | **torti**collis |
| -toxic | pertaining to poisoning | nephro**toxic** |
| toxic/o | poison | **toxico**logy |
| tox/i/o | poison | **tox**ic |
| trabecul/o | trabecula/anchoring strand of connective tissue/trabecular meshwork of the eye | **trabecul**ectomy |
| trachel/o | neck/uterine cervix | **trachelo**plasty |
| trache/o | trachea | **tracheo**stomy |
| trans- | across/through | **trans**urethral |
| -trauma | injury/wound | baro**trauma** |
| -tresia | condition of an opening/perforation | a**tresia** |
| tri- | three | **tri**cuspid |
| trichin/o | *Trichinella spiralis* (parasitic nematode worm) | **trichin**iasis |
| trich/o | hair | **trich**osis |
| trigon/o | trigone/triangular space *e.g.* at the base of the bladder | **trigon**itis |
| -tripsy | act of crushing | litho**tripsy** |
| -triptor | instrument designed to crush or fragment *e.g.* using shock waves | litho**triptor** |
| -trite | instrument designed to crush or fragment | litho**trite** |

| | | |
|---|---|---|
| -trope | influencing/a cell influencing . . .)/influenced by | gonado**trope** |
| -trophic | pertaining to nourishment/ stimulation | adreno**trophic** |
| troph/o | nourishment/food/stimulation | **troph**oblast |
| -trophy | nourishment/development/ increase in cell size | a**trophy** |
| -tropia | condition of turning/deviation/ heterotropia/strabismus | hyper**tropia** |
| -tropic | affinity for/stimulating/ changing in response to a stimulus/turning towards | thyro**tropic** |
| -tubal | pertaining to a tube | ovario**tubal** |
| tub/o | Fallopian tube/oviduct/tube/ uterine tube | |
| turbin/o | top-shaped/turbinate bone (nasal concha) | **turbin**ectomy |
| tuss/i | cough | anti**tuss**ive |
| tympan/o | tympanic membrane/middle ear | **tympano**plasty |
| typhl/o | caecum | **typhlo**cele |
| -ula | small/little | ling**ula** |
| ulcer/o | ulcer/sore/local defect in a surface | **ulcer**ogenic |
| -ule | small | ven**ule** |
| uln/o | ulna | **uln**oradial |
| ul/o/e | scar/gingiva (gums) | **ul**oid |
| ultra- | beyond | **ultra**sonography |
| -ulum | small | coag**ulum** |
| -ulus | small | sacc**ulus** |
| -um | thing/structure/noun ending/a name | ov**um** |
| un- | ~~not/opposite of/release from~~ | **un**differentiated |
| ungu/o | nail | **ungu**al |
| uni- | one | **uni**lateral |
| uran/o | palate | **urano**rrhaphy |
| urat/o | urate/a salt of uric acid (found in calculi) | **urat**uria |
| urea- | urea | **urea**poiesis |
| ur/o | urine/urinary tract | **uro**logy |
| -uresis | excrete in urine/urinate | lith**uresis** |
| ureter/o | ureter | **uretero**stenosis |
| urethr/o | urethra | **urethro**scopy |
| -uria | condition of urine/urination | poly**uria** |
| uric/o | uric acid | **uric**aemia |
| urin/a/o | urine | **urin**ometer |
| urticar/i | nettle rash/hives | **urticar**ia |
| -us | thing/structure/noun ending/a name | bronch**us** |
| uter/o | uterus | **utero**tubal |
| utricul/o | utricle of the inner ear | **utricul**itis |
| uve/o | uvea (pigmented parts of eye) | **uve**itis |

| | | |
|---|---|---|
| uvul/o | uvula | **uvulo**ptosis |
| | | |
| vagin/o | vagina | **vagin**itis |
| vag/o | vagus nerve | **vago**tomy |
| valv/o | valve | **valvo**tomy |
| valvul/o | valve | **valvulo**tome |
| varic/o | dilated veins/varicose vein/ varix | **varico**phlebitis |
| vascul/o | vessel | **vascul**ar |
| vas/o | vessel/vas deferens | **vas**ectomy |
| vel/o | soft/veil | **velo**pharyngeal |
| venacav/o | vena cava/great vein | **venacavo**graphy |
| ven/e/i/o | vein | **vene**section |
| vener/o | sexual intercourse | **vener**eal |
| ventricul/o | ventricle of heart or brain | **ventriculo**graphy |
| ventr/i/o- | belly side of body/in front/ ventral | **ventro**dorsal |
| verm/i | worm | **vermi**cide |
| -version | turning | retro**version** |
| vertebr/o | vertebra | **vertebr**al |
| vesic/o | bladder/blister | **vesico**prostatic |
| vesicul/o | seminal vesicle | **vesicul**itis |
| vestibul/o | vestibule/vestibular apparatus/ space leading to the entrance of a canal *e.g.* in the ear | **vestibulo**tomy |
| vibri/o | comma-shaped bacterium of the Genus Vibrio | **vibrio**cidal |
| vibr/o | vibration | **vibro**cardiogram |
| vir/o/u | virus/virion | **viro**lactia |
| viscer/o | viscera/internal organs (esp. of the abdomen) | **viscero**peritoneal |
| vit/o | life | **vit**al |
| vitre/o | glass/vitreous body of eye | **vitreo**retinal |
| viv/i | life | **vivi**section |
| vol/o | palm | **vol**ar |
| vulv/o | vulva | **vulv**itis |
| | | |
| xanth/o | yellow | **xanth**oma |
| xen/o | strange/foreign | **xeno**graft |
| xer/o | dry | **xer**ophthalmia |
| xiph/i/o | xiphoid process | **xiphi**costal |
| | | |
| -y | process/condition/noun ending/a name | apoplex**y** |
| -yl- | substance | but**yl**ene |
| | | |
| zo/o | animal | **zo**oid |
| zyg/o | joined | **zygo**dactyly |
| zygomatic/o | zygomatic arch | **zygomatico**temporal |
| zygot- | fertilized egg/zygote | **zygot**ic |
| -zyme | fermentation/enzyme | lyso**zyme** |
| zym/o | fermentation/enzyme | **zym**osis |

# Appendix 1
# Units of measurement

## Units of measurement — International System of Units (SI), the metric system, and conversions

The International System of Units (SI) or Système International d'Unités is the measurement system used for scientific, medical and technical purposes in most countries. In the United Kingdom SI units have replaced those of the Imperial System, *e.g.* the kilogram is used for mass instead of the pound (in everyday situations, both mass and weight are measured in kilograms although weight, which varies with gravity, is really a measure of force).

The SI comprises seven base units with several derived units. Each unit has its own symbol and is expressed as a decimal multiple or submultiple of the base unit by using the appropriate prefix, *e.g.* millimetre is one thousandth of a metre.

### Base units

| Quantity | Base unit and symbol |
|---|---|
| length | metre (m) |
| mass | kilogram (kg) |
| time | second (s) |
| amount of substance | mole (mol) |
| electric current | ampere (A) |
| thermodynamic temperature | kelvin (°K) |
| luminous intensity | candela (cd) |

### Derived units
Derived units for measuring different quantities are reached by multiplying or dividing two or more base units.

| Quantity | Derived unit and symbol |
|---|---|
| work, energy, quantity of heat | joule (J) |
| pressure | pascal (Pa) |
| force | newton (N) |
| frequency | hertz (Hz) |
| power | watt (W) |
| electrical potential, electromotive force, potential difference | vol volt (v) |
| absorbed dose of radiation | gray (Gy) |
| radioactivity | becquerel (Bq) |
| dose equivalent | sievert (Sv) |

Version from Appendix 2, *Churchill Livingstone's Dictionary of Nursing*, pages 479–82.

## Factor, decimal multiples and submultiples of SI units

| Multiplication factor | Prefix | Symbol |
|---|---|---|
| $10^{12}$ | tera | T |
| $10^9$ | giga | G |
| $10^6$ | mega | M |
| $10^3$ | kilo | k |
| $10^2$ | hecto | h |
| $10^1$ | deca | da |
| $10^{-1}$ | deci | d |
| $10^{-2}$ | centi | c |
| $10^{-3}$ | milli | m |
| $10^{-6}$ | micro | μ |
| $10^{-9}$ | nano | n |
| $10^{-12}$ | pico | p |
| $10^{-15}$ | femto | f |
| $10^{-18}$ | atto | a |

## Rules for using units and writing large numbers and decimals

- The symbol for a unit is unaltered in the plural and should not be followed by a full stop except at the end of a sentence:
  5 cm not 5 cm. or 5 cms.
- Large numbers are written in three-digit groups (working from right to left) with spaces not commas (in some countries the comma is used to indicate a decimal point):
  fifty thousand is written as 50 000
  five hundred thousand is written as 500 000
- Numbers with four digits are written without the space, *e.g.* four thousand is written as 4000.
- The decimal sign between digits is indicated by a full stop positioned near the line, *e.g.* 50.25. If the numerical value of the decimal is less than 1, a zero should appear before the decimal sign:
  0.125 not .125
  Decimals with more than four digits are also written in three-digit groups, but this time working from left to right, *e.g.* 0.00025.
- 'Squared' and 'cubed' are expressed as numerical powers and not by abbreviation:
  square centimetre is $cm^2$ not sq. cm.

## Commonly used measurements requiring further explanation

- Temperature – although the SI base unit for temperature is the kelvin, by international convention temperature is measured in degrees Celsius (°C).
- Energy – the energy of food or individual requirements for energy are measured in kilojoules (kJ); the SI unit is the joule (J). In practice many people still use the kilocalorie (kcal), a non-SI unit, for these purposes.
- calorie = 4.2 J.
- kilocalorie (large calorie) = 4.2 kJ.
- Volume – volume is calculated by multiplying length, width and depth. Using the SI unit for length, the metre (m), means ending up with a cubic metre ($m^3$), which is a huge volume and is certainly not appropriate for most purposes. In

clinical practice the litre (L or l) is used. A litre is based on the volume of a cube measuring 10 cm × 10 cm × 10 cm. Smaller units still, *e.g.* millilitre (mL) or one thousandth of a litre, are commonly used in clinical practice.

- Time – the SI base unit for time is the second (s), but it is acceptable to use minute (min), hour (h) or day (d). In clinical practice it is preferable to use 'per 24 hours' for the excretion of substances in urine and faeces: g/24 h
- Amount of substance – the SI base unit for amount of substance is the mole (mol). The concentration of many substances is expressed in moles per litre (mol/L) or millimoles per litre (mmol/L) which replaces milliequivalents per litre (mEq/L). Some exceptions exist and include haemoglobin and plasma proteins in grams per litre (g/L); and enzyme activity in International Units (IU, U or iu).
- Pressure – the SI unit of pressure is the pascal (Pa), and the kilopascal (kPa) replaces the old non-SI unit of millimetres of mercury pressure (mmHg) for blood pressure and blood gases. However, mmHg is still widely used for measuring blood pressure. Other anomalies include cerebrospinal fluid, which is measured in millimetres of water (mmH$_2$O); and central venous pressure, which is measured in centimetres of water (cmH$_2$O).

## Measurements, equivalents and conversions (SI or metric and imperial)

### Length

| | | |
|---|---|---|
| 1 kilometre (km) | = | 1000 metres (m) |
| 1 metre (m) | = | 100 centimetres (cm) or 1000 millimetres (mm) |
| 1 centimetre (cm) | = | 10 millimetres (mm) |
| 1 millimetre (mm) | = | 1000 micrometres (µm) |
| 1 micrometre (µm) | = | 1000 nanometres (nm) |

### Conversions

| | | |
|---|---|---|
| 1 metre (m) | = | 39.370 inches (in) |
| 1 centimetre (cm) | = | 0.3937 inches (in) |
| 30.48 centimetres (cm) | = | 1 foot (ft) |
| 2.54 centimetres (cm) | = | 1 inch (in) |

### Volume

| | | |
|---|---|---|
| 1 litre (L) | = | 1000 millilitres (mL) |
| 1 millilitre (mL) | = | 1000 microlitres (µL) |

NB The millilitre (mL) and the cubic centimetre (cm$^3$) are usually treated as being the same.

### Conversions

| | | |
|---|---|---|
| 1 litre (L) | = | 1.76 pints (pt) |
| 568.25 millilitres (mL) | = | 1 pint (pt) |
| 28.4 millilitres (mL) | = | 1 fluid ounce (fl oz) |

### Weight or mass

| | | |
|---|---|---|
| 1 kilogram (kg) | = | 1000 grams (g) |
| 1 gram (g) | = | 1000 milligrams (mg) |
| 1 milligram (mg) | = | 1000 micrograms (µg) |
| 1 microgram (µg) | = | 1000 nanograms (ng) |

NB To avoid any confusion with milligram (mg) the word microgram (µg) should be written in full on prescriptions.

## Conversions

| 1 kilogram (kg) | = | 2.204 pounds (lb) |
|---|---|---|
| 1 gram (g) | = | 0.0353 ounce (oz) |
| 453.59 grams (g) | = | 1 pound (lb) |
| 28.34 grams (g) | = | 1 ounce (oz) |

## Temperature conversions

*To convert Celsius to Fahrenheit:*
multiply by 9, divide by 5, and add 32 to the result,
*e.g.* 36°C to Fahrenheit:
$36 \times 9 = 324 \div 5 = 64.8 + 32 = 96.8°F$
therefore 36°C = 96.8°F

*To convert Fahrenheit to Celsius:*
subtract 32, multiply by 5, and divide by 9,
*e.g.* 104°F to Celsius:
$104 - 32 = 72 \times 5 = 360 \div 9 = 40°C$
therefore 104°F = 40°C

## Temperature comparison

| °Celsius | °Fahrenheit | °Celsius | °Fahrenheit |
|---|---|---|---|
| 100 | 212 | 37.5 | 99.5 |
| 95 | 203 | 37 | 98.6 |
| 90 | 194 | 36.5 | 97.7 |
| 85 | 185 | 36 | 96.8 |
| 80 | 176 | 35.5 | 95.9 |
| 75 | 167 | 35 | 95 |
| 70 | 158 | 34 | 93.2 |
| 65 | 149 | 33 | 91.4 |
| 60 | 140 | 32 | 89.6 |
| 55 | 131 | 31 | 87.8 |
| 50 | 122 | 30 | 86 |
| 45 | 113 | 25 | 77 |
| 44 | 122.2 | 20 | 68 |
| 43 | 109.4 | 15 | 59 |
| 42 | 107.6 | 10 | 50 |
| 41 | 105.8 | 5 | 41 |
| 40 | 104 | 0 | 32 |
| 39.5 | 103.1 | −5 | 23 |
| 39 | 102.2 | −10 | 14 |
| 38.5 | 101.3 | NB Boiling point = 100°C = 212°F | |
| 38 | 100.4 | Freezing point = 0°C = 32°F | |

# Appendix 2
# Normal values

The values below represent an 'average' reference range, in adults, for blood, cerebrospinal fluid, urine and faeces. These ranges should be used as a guide only. Reference ranges vary between individual laboratories and readers should consult their own laboratory for those used locally. This is especially important where reference values depend upon the analytical equipment and temperatures used.

## Blood (haematology)

| Test | Reference range |
|------|-----------------|
| Activated partial thromboplastin time (APTT) | 30–40 s |
| Bleeding time (Ivy) | 2–8 min |
| Erythrocyte sedimentation rate (ESR) | |
|     Adult women | 3–15 mm/h |
|     Adult men | 1–10 mm/h |
| Fibrinogen | 1.5–4.0 g/L |
| Folate (serum) | 4–18 μg/L |
| Haemoglobin | |
|     Women | 115–165 g/L (11.5–16.5 g/dL) |
|     Men | 130–180 g/L (13–18 g/dL) |
| Haptoglobins | 0.3–2.0 g/L |
| Mean cell haemoglobin (MCH) | 27–32 pg |
| Mean cell haemoglobin concentration (MCHC) | 30–35 g/dL |
| Mean cell volume (MCV) | 78–95 fl |
| Packed cell volume (PCV or haematocrit) | |
|     Women | 0.35–0.47 (35–47%) |
|     Men | 0.4–0.54 (40–54%) |
| Platelets (thrombocytes) | $150-400 \times 10^9$/L |
| Prothrombin time | 12–16s |
| Red cells (erythrocytes) | |
|     Women | $3.8-5.3 \times 10^{12}$/L |
|     Men | $4.5-6.5 \times 10^{12}$/L |
| Reticulocytes (newly formed red cells in adults) | $25-85 \times 10^9$/L |
| White cells total (leucocytes) | $4.0-11.0 \times 10^9$/L |

Version from Appendix 3, *Churchill Livingstone's Dictionary of Nursing*, pages 483–5.

## Blood-venous plasma (biochemistry)

| Test | Reference range |
| --- | --- |
| Alanine aminotransferase (ALT) | 10–40 U/L |
| Albumin | 36–47 g/L |
| Alkaline phosphatase | 40–125 U/L |
| Amylase | 90–300 U/L |
| Aspartate aminotransferase (AST) | 10–35 U/L |
| Bicarbonate (arterial) | 22–28 mmol/L |
| Bilirubin (total) | 2–17 µmol/L |
| Caeruloplasmin | 150–600 mg/L |
| Calcium | 2.1–2.6 mmol/L |
| Chloride | 95–105 mmol/L |
| Cholesterol (total) | ideally below 5.2 mmol/L |
| HDL–Cholesterol | |
|     Women | 0.6–1.9 mmol/L |
|     Men | 0.5–1.6 mmol/L |
| $PaCO_2$ (arterial) | 4.4–6.1 kPa |
| Copper | 13–24 µmol/L |
| Cortisol (at 08.00 h) | 160–565 nmol/L |
| Creatine kinase (total) | |
|     Women | 30–150 U/L |
|     Men | 30–200 U/L |
| Creatinine | 55–150 µmol/L |
| Gamma-glutamyl-transferase (γGT) | |
|     Women | 5–35 U/L |
|     Men | 10–55 U/L |
| Globulins | 24–37 g/L |
| Glucose (venous blood, fasting) | 3.6–5.8 mmol/L |
| Glycosylated haemoglobin ($HbA_1$) | 4–6% |
| Hydrogen ion concentration (arterial) | 35–44 nmol/L |
| Iron | |
|     Women | 10–28 µmol/L |
|     Men | 14–32 µmol/L |
| Iron-binding capacity total (TIBC) | 45–70 µmol/L |
| Lactate (arterial) | 0.3–1.4 mmol/L |
| Lactate dehydrogenase (total) | 230–460 U/L |
| Lead (adults, whole blood) | <1.7 µmol/L |
| Magnesium | 0.7–1.0 mmol/L |
| Osmolality | 275–290 mmol/kg |
| $PaO_2$ (arterial) | 12–15k Pa |
| Oxygen saturation (arterial) | >97% |
| pH | 7.36–7.42 |
| Phosphate (fasting) | 0.8–1.4 mmol/L |
| Potassium (serum) | 3.6–5.0 mmol/L |
| Protein (total) | 60–80 g/L |
| Sodium | 136–145 mmol/L |
| Transferrin | 2–4 g/L |
| Triglycerides (fasting) | 0.6–1.8 mmol/L |

| Test | Reference range |
|------|-----------------|
| Urate | |
|   Women | 0.12–0.36 mmol/L |
|   Men | 0.12–0.42 mmol/L |
| Urea | 2.5–6.5 mmol/L |
| Uric acid | |
|   Women | 0.09–0.36 mmol/L |
|   Men | 0.1–0.45 mmol/L |
| Vitamin A | 0.7–3.5 μmol/L |
| Vitamin C | 23–57 μmol/L |
| Zinc | 11–22 μmol/L |

## Cerebrospinal fluid

| Test | Reference range |
|------|-----------------|
| Cells | 0–5 mm³ |
| Chloride | 120–170 mmol/L |
| Glucose | 2.5–4.0 mmol/L |
| Pressure (adult) | 50–180 mm/H$_2$O |
| Protein | 100–400 mg/L |

## Urine

| Test | Reference range |
|------|-----------------|
| Albumin/creatinine ratio | <3.5 mg albumin/mmol creatinine |
| Calcium (diet dependent) | <12 mmol/24 h (normal diet) |
| Copper | 0.2–0.6 μmol/24 h |
| Cortisol | 9–50 μmol/24 h |
| Creatinine | 9–17 mmol/24 h |
| 5-Hydroxyindole-3-acetic acid (5H1AA) | 10–45 μmol/24 h |
| Magnesium | 3.3–5.0 mmol/24 h |
| Oxalate | |
|   Women | 40–320 mmol/24 h |
|   Men | 80–490 mmol/24 h |
| pH | 4–8 |
| Phosphate | 15–50 mmol/24 h |
| Porphyrins (total) | 90–370 nmol/24 h |
| Potassium (depends on intake) | 25–100 mmol/24 h |
| Protein (total) | no more than 0.3 g/L |
| Sodium (depends on intake) | 100–200 mmol/24 h |
| Urea | 170–500 mmol/24 h |

## Faeces

| Test | Reference range |
| --- | --- |
| Fat content (daily output on normal diet) | <7 g/24 h |
| Fat (as stearic acid) | 11–18 mmol/24 h |

# Appendix 3
# Chemical symbols and formulae

| | | | |
|---|---|---|---|
| Aluminium | Al | Lithium | Li |
| Ammonia | $NH_3$ | Magnesium | Mg |
| Ammonium | $NH_4$ | Manganese | Mn |
| Barium | Ba | Mercury | Hg |
| Calcium | Ca | Molybdenum | Mo |
| Carbon | C | Nitrogen | N |
| Caesium | Cs | Nitrate | $NO_3$ |
| Carbon dioxide | $CO_2$ | Oxygen | O |
| Chlorine | Cl | Phosphate | $PO_4$ |
| Chromium | Cr | Phosphorus | P |
| Cobalt | Co | Potassium | K |
| Copper | Cu | Radium | Ra |
| Fluorine | F | Selenium | Se |
| Gold | Au | Silicon | Si |
| Helium | He | Silver | Ag |
| Hydrogen | H | Sodium | Na |
| Hydrogen carbonate | | Strontium | Sr |
| (bicarbonate) | $HCO_3$ | Sulphate | $SO_4$ |
| Hydrogen phosphate | $HPO_4$ | Sulphur | S |
| Hydroxide | OH | Technetium | Tc |
| Iodine | I | Vanadium | V |
| Iridium | Ir | Water | $H_2O$ |
| Iron | Fe | Yttrium | Y |
| Lead | Pb | Zinc | Zn |

Version from Appendix 3, *Mosby Nurse's Pocket Dictionary*, page 392.